TWO-DIMENSIONAL ECHOCARDIOGRAPHY
AND
CARDIAC DOPPLER

Second Edition

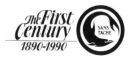

TWO-DIMENSIONAL ECHOCARDIOGRAPHY
AND
CARDIAC DOPPLER
Second Edition

EDITORS

JAY N. SCHAPIRA, M.D., F.A.C.C., F.A.C.P.

Assistant Clinical Professor of Medicine
UCLA School of Medicine
Attending Physician
Cedars-Sinai Medical Center and Century City Hospital
Los Angeles, California

JOHN G. HAROLD, M.D., F.A.C.C., F.A.C.P.

Assistant Clinical Professor of Medicine
UCLA School of Medicine
Attending Physician
Division of Cardiology
Department of Medicine
Cedars-Sinai Medical Center
Los Angeles, California

ASSOCIATE EDITOR

CLAIN BEEDER, M.A.

Executive Director
Ventura Heart Institute
HCA Los Robles Regional Medical Center
Thousand Oaks, California

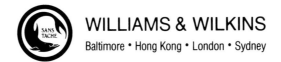

WILLIAMS & WILKINS
Baltimore • Hong Kong • London • Sydney

Editor: Jonathan W. Pine
Associate Editor: Carol Eckhart
Copy Editor: Shelley Hyatt-Blankman
Designer: Norman Och
Illustration Planner: Ray Lowman
Production Coordinator: Barbara Felton

Accurate indications, adverse reactions, and dosage schedules for drugs are provided in this book, but it is possible that they may change. The reader is urged to review the package information data of the manufacturers of the medications mentioned.

Printed in the United States of America

First Edition 1982

Library of Congress Cataloging-in-Publication Data

Two-dimensional echocardiography and cardiac Doppler / editors, Jay N.
  Schapira, John G. Harold; associate editor, Clain Beeder.—2nd
  ed.
    p.   cm.
  Rev. ed. of: Two-dimensional echocardiography. c1982.
  Includes bibliographies and index.
  ISBN 0-683-07522-5
  1. Two-dimensional echocardiography.   2. Doppler echocardiography.
I. Schapira. Jay N.   II. Harold, John G.   III. Beeder, Clain.
IV. Two-dimensional echocardiography.
  [DNLM: 1. Echocardiography—methods.   WG 141.5.E2 T9742]
RC683.5.U5T87   1989
616.1′207543—dc19
DNLM/DLC
for Library of Congress   88-39699
                                                                                   CIP

                                                        90 91 92 93 94
                                            1   2   3   4   5   6   7   8   9   10

TO THE SCHAPIRAS
Phyllis, Beth, Jamie, Gwen, Leslie, Ruth, and Roy

TO THE HAROLDS
my wife, Ellen, my mother, Ann, and to the memory of my father, John

TO THE BEEDERS
my parents, Lee and Betty

PREFACE
TO THE SECOND EDITION

In the seven years since the first edition of this book was published, there have been enormous changes in two-dimensional echocardiography. Initially, the physics of ultrasound provided equipment capable of answering questions that had yet to be asked. Today, there are a number of established clinical applications around which new technology can build. It is an exciting time, a period in which the maturity gained from experience helps in both refining existing applications and spurring the development of new ones.

New contributions continue to come from physicists, physiologists, engineers, research scientists, radiologists, veterinarians, and physicians in clinical practice. All of these disciplines share one overriding concern—the desire to make the techniques used by the clinician easier and more rewarding. Our book has the same purpose: to present practical information in the most efficient way—but without losing the subtleties that enrich the basic information.

In this endeavor, we have been aided by contributors who represent all these disciplines but who write from the point of view of the clinical echocardiographer. Our intention is always to put practical matters first without sacrificing the insights unique to each specialty.

The two-dimensional echocardiographic illustrations in this book were made by photographing a stop-frame videotape image. The subsequent photograph contains half of a single video frame of information from an interlacing dual videotape imaging system containing 0.016 second of video information. This results in an observable and unavoidable degradation in image quality, as well as loss of the dynamic information contained on the videotape. The photographs have not been retouched. When the image was not self-explanatory, labels and arrows were added or line drawings made to clarify the anatomy.

Jay N. Schapira, M.D., F.A.C.C., F.A.C.P.
John G. Harold, M.D., F.A.C.C., F.A.C.P.
Clain Beeder, M.A.

PREFACE
TO THE FIRST EDITION

Over the past 8 years, two-dimensional echocardiography has gained wide acceptance and has improved vastly in its technical capabilities. Although this growth and refinement has just begun, it was felt that the progress to this point demanded publication of a book about this rapidly expanding dynamic field.

Because there is a plethora of books on M-mode echocardiography, it was decided to have this book deal primarily with two-dimensional echocardiography and include M-mode echocardiography only when it complemented the two-dimensional echocardiographic discussion. An obligation was felt to make this endeavor of practical usefulness to physicians, to echocardiographic technicians who are learning the technique for the first time and to those who wish to refine their knowledge and skills, but who already possess the basic knowledge of two-dimensional echocardiography. In this book, therefore, the basic principles of normal two-dimensional echocardiographic anatomy, standard nomenclature and the physics of instrumentation of two-dimensional echocardiography are emphasized before the reader proceeds to discussions of pediatric and adult two-dimensional echocardiographic cardiac pathology.

The development of two-dimensional echocardiography has come from many sources—physicists, engineers, basic scientists, radiologists and pediatric and adult clinical cardiologists. Therefore, a likewise diverse group of contributors from these disciplines was enlisted to write this book. However, despite the variability of backgrounds, each contributor directed his material to the people who use this technique in a clinical manner for patient care. The editors of this book are primarily clinical cardiologists who utilize echocardiography in addition to other invasive and noninvasive modalities in the evaluation of their patients. Therefore, this book is intended to aid other clinicians who also use two-dimensional echocardiography as a part of their overall evaluation of patients. In this regard, the utility of two-dimensional echocardiography in evaluating a particular patient is emphasized, especially in terms of its diagnostic capabilities, limitations, descriptive appearance and the proper technique to obtain maximum diagnostic data.

A comment must be included about the two-dimensional echocardiographic illustrations. The pictures in this book were made by photographing a stop frame videotape image. Photographs from such video images contain half of a single frame of information from an interlacing dual videotape imaging system containing 0.016 seconds of video information, resulting in a definite degradation in stop image quality as well as the obvious loss of the dynamic information contained on the videotape. None of the photographs in this book have been retouched, and when the two-dimensional echocardiogram was not self-explanatory, labels and arrows were added to the photograph or line drawings were made to clarify the anatomy.

This book is intended to provide a basis for understanding the principles and techniques of two-dimensional echocardiography and for solving diagnostic problems with this modality in patients with heart disease. There is no doubt that future developments will require a constant updating of knowledge and skill in two-dimensional echocardiography, but we feel that this book will provide a firm foundation in two-dimensional echocardiography and prepare the individual for acquiring future knowledge and skill in this area.

Jay N. Schapira, M.D.
Yzhar Charuzi, M.D.
Robert M. Davidson, M.D.

ACKNOWLEDGMENTS

This book coalesced around the talents of a number of dedicated individuals. Special thanks are due to Rosella Hansen Shea for her invaluable assistance during the preparation of this book. We are also indebted to Debra Schlobohm and Helen Maryman.

CONTRIBUTORS

Howard N. Allen, M.D., F.A.C.C.
Attending Physician
Cedars-Sinai Medical Center
Los Angeles, CA

Clain Beeder, M.A.
Executive Director
Ventura Heart Institute
HCA Los Robles Regional Medical Center
Thousand Oaks, CA

David J. Benefiel, M.D.
Assistant Professor in Residence
Department of Anesthesiology
University of California, San Francisco
Director of Cardiovascular Anesthesia
Pacific Presbyterian Medical Center
San Francisco, CA

Robert J. Bryg, M.D., F.A.C.C., F.A.C.P.
Assistant Professor of Medicine
Wayne State University
Assistant Director
Harper Hospital
Detroit, MI
Veterans Administration Hospital
Allen Park, MI

Michael W. Bungo, M.D., F.A.C.C.
Director of Cardiovascular Research
The Johnson Space Flight Center
National Aeronautics and Space Administration
Houston, TX

Eugenio Carmo, M.D., F.C.C.P.
Cardiac Non-invasive Laboratory
Century City Hospital
Los Angeles, CA

Robert Carroll, M.D.
Cedars-Sinai Vascular Diagnostic Service
Cedars-Sinai Medical Center
Los Angeles, CA

P. Anthony N. Chandraratna, M.D., M.R.C.P.
Professor of Medicine
Director, Echocardiography and Graphics
Section of Cardiology
Department of Medicine
University of Southern California School of Medicine
Los Angeles, CA

Yzhar Charuzi, M.D., F.A.C.C.
Associate Clinical Professor of Medicine
UCLA School of Medicine
Attending Physician
Cedars-Sinai Medical Center
Los Angeles, CA

Satyabrata Chatterjee, M.D.
Section of Cardiology
Department of Medicine
University of Southern California School of Medicine
Los Angeles, CA

David Cossman, M.D.
Cedars-Sinai Vascular Diagnostic Service
Cedars-Sinai Medical Center
Los Angeles, CA

John Michael Criley, M.D., F.A.C.C.
Professor of Medicine and Radiologic Sciences
UCLA School of Medicine
Harbor General Hospital
Torrance, CA

Philip J. Currie, M.B.B.S., F.R.A.C.P.
Head
Echocardiographic Laboratory
Michigan Heart Institute
St. Joseph's Hospital
Ann Arbor, MI

Lawrence S. C. Czer, M.D., F.A.C.C.
Assistant Professor of Medicine
UCLA School of Medicine
Associate Cardiologist
Division of Surgical Cardiology
Department of Medicine
Cedars-Sinai Medical Center
Los Angeles, CA

Robert M. Davidson, M.D., F.A.C.C.
Associate Clinical Professor of Medicine
UCLA School of Medicine
Attending Physician
Cedars-Sinai Medical Center
Los Angeles, CA

Robert Decker, M.D.
Attending Physician
Cedars Sinai Medical Center
Los Angeles, CA

Mark Durell
National Cardiology Program Manager
Acuson Computed Tomography
Mountain View, CA

Inge G. Edler, M.D.
Department of Cardiology
University Hospital
Lund, Sweden

William D. Edwards, M.D., F.A.C.C.
Professor of Pathology
Mayo Medical School
Consultant
Section of Medical Pathology
Department Pathology
Mayo Clinic
Rochester, MN

Jean Ellison, R.V.T.
Cedars-Sinai Vascular Diagnostic Service
Cedars-Sinai Medical Center
Los Angeles, CA

Stephen J. Ettinger, D.V.M., F.A.C.C.
Professor of Veterinary Medicine
UCLA School of Medicine
California Animal Hospital
Los Angeles, CA

Rodney A. Foale, M.D., M.R.C.P., F.A.C.C.
Waller Department of Cardiology
Saint Mary's Hospital
London, England

Robert E. Fowles, M.D., F.A.C.C.
Salt Lake Clinic
Salt Lake City, UT

C. D. Gresser, M.D.
Associate Professor
Department of Medicine
University of Toronto
Faculty of Medicine
Director
Non-Invasive Laboratory
Toronto General Hospital
Toronto, Ontario, Canada

Donald J. Hagler, M.D., F.A.C.C.
Professor of Pediatrics
Mayo Medical School
Consultant
Divisions of Cardiovascular Diseases and Internal
  Medicine and Pediatric Cardiology
Mayo Clinic
Rochester, MN

John G. Harold, M.D., F.A.C.C., F.A.C.P.
Assistant Clinical Professor of Medicine
UCLA School of Medicine
Attending Physician
Division of Cardiology
Department of Medicine
Cedars-Sinai Medical Center
Los Angeles, CA

Hiroshi Honma, M.D.
Clinical Research Fellow
Division of Cardiology
Department of Medicine
Cedars-Sinai Medical Center
Los Angeles, CA

Mee-Nin Kan, M.D.
Division of Cardiovascular Diseases
University of Alabama School of Medicine
Birmingham, AL

James R. Katz, M.D.
Department of Cardiology
St. Vincent's Hospital
Los Angeles, CA

David H. Knight, D.V.M.
Associate Professor of Medicine
University of Pennsylvania
School of Veterinary Medicine
Department of Clinical Studies
Philadelphia, PA

Arthur J. Labovitz, M.D., F.A.C.C., F.A.C.P.
Associate Professor of Medicine
St. Louis University School of Medicine
Director
Echocardiography Laboratory
St. Louis University Medical Center
St. Louis, MO

Robert H. Lusk, D.V.M.
California Animal Hospital
Los Angeles, CA

Donald V. Mahony, M.D., F.A.C.C., F.A.C.P.
Consultant
Non Invasive Testing Procedures
Jackson, WY
Director (Retired)
Cardiac Non-Invasive Lab
St. Jude Hospital
Fullerton, CA
Associate Clinical Professor of Medicine
Irvine, CA

Joan C. Main, R.C.P.T., R.C.T.
Cardiology Product Manager
Acuson Computed Tomography
Mountain View, CA

Gerald Maurer, M.D., F.A.C.C.
Director
Cardiac Non-Invasive Laboratory
Division of Cardiology
Department of Medicine
Cedars-Sinai Medical Center
Los Angeles, CA

Samuel Meerbaum, Ph.D., F.A.C.C.
Woodland Hills, CA

Navin C. Nanda, M.D., F.A.C.C.
Professor of Medicine and Director
Heart Station
Echocardiography and Graphics Laboratory
University of Alabama School of Medicine
Birmingham, AL

Petros Nihoyannopoulos, M.D.
Waller Department of Cardiology
St. Mary's Hospital
London, England

Ryozo Omoto, M.D.
Professor of Surgery
Vice Director
Saitama Medical School Hospital
Chairman
Department of Surgery
Saitama Medical School
Saitama, Japan

Enrique Ostrzega, M.D.
Clinical Research Fellow
Division of Cardiology
Department of Medicine
Cedars-Sinai Medical Center
Los Angeles, CA

Peter C. D. Pelikan, M.D., F.A.C.C.
Assistant Professor of Medicine
UCLA School of Medicine
Harbor General Hospital
Torrance, CA

Robert A. Quaife, M.D., F.A.C.C.
Salt Lake Clinic
Salt Lake City, UT

Shahbudin H. Rahimtoola, M.B., F.R.C.P.
Professor of Medicine
Chief
Section of Cardiology
Department of Medicine
University of Southern California School of Medicine
Los Angeles, CA

Harry Rakowski, M.D., F.R.C.P.C.
Associate Professor
Department of Medicine
University of Toronto
Faculty of Medicine
Director
Non-Invasive Laboratory
Toronto General Hospital
Toronto, Ontario, Canada

Samuel Ritter, M.D., F.A.C.C.
Childrens Heart Center
Mount Sinai Medical Center
New York, NY

Michael F. Roizen, M.D.
Professor of Anesthesiology and Medicine
Chairperson
Department of Anesthesia and Critical Care
The University of Chicago
Chicago, IL

Jay N. Schapira, M.D., F.A.C.C., F.A.C.P.
Assistant Clinical Professor of Medicine
UCLA School of Medicine
Attending Physician
Cedars-Sinai Medical Center and
  Century City Hospital
Los Angeles, CA

James B. Seward, M.D., F.A.C.C.
Professor of Internal Medicine and Associate
  Professor of Pediatrics
Mayo Medical School
Consultant
Internal Medicine (Cardiovascular Diseases) and
  Pediatric Cardiology
Mayo Clinic and Mayo Foundation
Rochester, MN

Frank G. Shellock, Ph.D., F.A.C.C.
Research Scientist
Division of Cardiology
Department of Medicine
Cedars-Sinai Medical Center
Los Angeles, CA

J. Shime, M.D.
Associate Professor
Department of Medicine
University of Toronto
Faculty of Medicine
Director
Non-Invasive Laboratory
Toronto General Hospital
Toronto, Ontario, Canada

Robert J. Siegel, M.D., F.A.C.C.
Associate Professor of Medicine
University of California
Los Angeles
UCLA School of Medicine
Cedars-Sinai Medical Center
Los Angeles, CA

Jay S. Simonson, M.D.
Division of Cardiology
Department of Medicine
Cedars-Sinai Medical Center
Los Angeles, CA

H. J. C. Swan, M.D., Ph.D., F.A.C.C., M.A.C.P.
Professor of Medicine
University of California
Los Angeles
UCLA School of Medicine
Senior Cardiologist
Division of Cardiology
Department of Medicine
Cedars-Sinai Medical Center
Los Angeles, CA

A. Jamil Tajik, M.D., F.A.C.C.
Professor of Medicine
Associate Professor of Pediatrics (Cardiology)
Mayo Medical School
Director
Echocardiography Laboratory
Mayo Clinic
Rochester, MN

Tahir Tak, M.D.
Section of Cardiology
Department of Medicine
University of Southern California School of Medicine
Los Angeles, CA

Randall G. Wilson, M.D.
Division of Cardiovascular Diseases
University of Alabama School of Medicine
Birmingham, AL

CONTENTS

INTRODUCTION

H. J. C. Swan, M.D., Ph.D.

Clinical cardiology has now matured to the degree that it functions primarily on an ambulatory or outpatient basis. Hospitalization may be required only for invasive diagnostic or therapeutic procedures or life-threatening events including the acute coronary syndromes, severe heart failure, cardiac sepsis, and serious cardiac arrhythmias. The great majority of cardiac diagnoses can be effectively made in the doctor's office; one exception is definition of the detailed anatomy of the small coronary vessels. Long-term treatment plans and assessment of efficacy are also provided as an outpatient function.

Excluding arrhythmias, what are the fundamental cardiovascular parameters that provide information necessary for cardiac diagnosis? These parameters include the detailed anatomy of the heart and surrounding structures, myocardial contractile state, valvar function, coronary perfusion, and changes in these variables under a variety of imposed stresses. In combination with historic and electrocardiographic information, a knowledge of such functional characteristics allows for effective diagnosis of the majority of cardiac disorders.

Imaging of the heart and associated structures is essential to cardiac diagnosis. Available methods include angiocardiography, radionuclear scanning procedures, computerized tomography, magnetic resonance imaging, and cardiac ultrasound. Developments in echocardiography in the past decade include high resolution two-dimensional display, exercise studies of ventricular function, estimates of flow velocity by Doppler and color-coded flow directional mapping. More recently, the developments in transesophageal techniques, which may be used in the outpatient setting, provide unique imaging of the aortic root, the outflow tract of the left ventricle, the left atrium, and the mitral valve. Additionally, approximate estimates of right ventricular and pulmonary artery systolic pressure as well as cardiac output have been made on the basis of echo-Doppler data.

Importantly, technical advances in "user-friendly" ultrasound instrumentation now provide the physician-cardiologist with a powerful modality that can render him or her substantively independent of centralized imaging centers. Effectively applied, ultrasound has the potential to satisfy the great majority of diagnostic imaging requirements in cardiology. However, the cardiologist utilizing ultrasound has a responsibility to use these applications wisely and with competence. It is not enough to meet the capital costs of expensive instrumentation and hire a technician trained at an academic center. An understanding of the physical basis of cardiac ultrasound, imaging techniques, cardiac anatomy and function, data retrieval and processing, inherent limitations and errors of the methodology, and interpretation with relevance to the clinical problem are essential for effective use of this imaging modality.

Within the hospital setting the impact of modern ultrasound techniques is no less impressive. Echo-Doppler determination of valve gradients may avoid the requirement of cardiac catheterization. Intraoperative ultrasound is now required in the evaluation of surgical repair of the mitral valve. The potential of the transesophageal technique to identify the precise anatomy of aortic dissection, the aortic valve, the left ventricular outflow tract, and the proximal coronary arteries represents an enormous advance that may replace conventional aortography in many of these critically ill patients. New Doppler flow devices have been incorporated into the tip of cardiac catheters so as to determine the efficacy of revascularization procedures such as angioplasty by the measurement of coronary arterial flow before and after the procedure. In this application, circumferentially distributed ultrasound can also define the reflectance and, potentially, the composition of the wall of a coronary artery and of an atherosclerotic lesion.

Indeed, diagnostic cardiac ultrasonography has come into its own. Hence, this text has been expanded from the 10 chapters in the first edition to 33, reflecting the explosion of applications and information in this field. New authors have been added reflecting this growth. However, the fundamental purpose of this publication remains: to provide the clinical cardiologist with a handbook to a most important cardiac imaging procedure, one that he or she personally may master and control. It would behoove all cardiologists to become intimately familiar with and gain experience in the diagnostic potential of cardiac ultrasound. It is the objective and accomplishment of the present text to enhance this process.

1

Echocardiography: A Historical Perspective

Inge G. Edler, M.D.

For more than 50 million years some species of bats have used ultrasonic echo-orientation. Until recently it was a mystery how bats could move about with such assurance and seek out and catch prey in the darkest of nights. This uncertainty wasn't for lack of attempts to discover the secret of the bat's capacity for nocturnal flight. Some of the earliest theories were along the right lines, but it required the sophisticated apparatus of modern science to prove how these amazing animals used their senses to catch even the tiniest of insects. Of course, many people long ago had a ready explanation: bats must be in possession of magic powers. Undoubtedly, these "flying mice" were the devil's own creatures.

Lazzaro Spallanzani, an Italian naturalist, made the first attempt to counter the magic theory in 1793 (1). His experiments showed that bats were able to avoid all obstacles in a darkened room, just as if they could see them. He even hung threads across the room, but at no time did the bats touch them. Further experiments demonstrated that covering or removing the bats' eyes had no effect on their powers of orientation.

When the Swiss zoologist Jurine learned about this work, he added another, decisive experiment. He plugged the ears of the bats and discovered their sense of orientation was now gone. Spallanzani repeated the experiment with the same result, but at the time, nobody believed either scientist's findings.

In 1920, the British physiologist Hartridge put forth the hypothesis that bats emit ultrasonic signals and receive the echoes of these sounds. This theory was confirmed 18 years later by Griffin, an American zoologist. He was assisted by Pierce, a physicist, who constructed an apparatus to detect ultrasound. Further refinements and collab-

oration with Galambos established that closing the mouth or nose of a bat produced disorientation. In Holland, the zoologist Dijkgraaf made another observation: if the ultrasound, transmitted from the larynx, could not pass through the bat's mouth or nose or the returning ultrasound could not be received by the bat's ear, disorientation resulted.

The use of echo-location is not exclusive to bats. Other animals, including dolphins and whales, make use of the same principle, though not to the same extent or degree of perfection. Echo-location is most advanced in the insectivorous bat Microchiroptera. The frequency range of emitted signals extends to 215 kHz, which produces a wave length of 1.6 millimeters in air. These short waves are enough to produce usable echoes from small objects, such as insects. In some species, analyzing the sound shows a sharply decreased frequency toward the end of the signal. For example, the Little Brown bat, common in America, sweeps down from 100 kHz at the start of transmission to 40 kHz at the end, only milliseconds later. Every pulse may contain only about 50 sound waves in all, no two of them having the same wavelength. If such a tone could be heard by man, it would be a chirp and not a pure tone.

However, the "sound picture" mechanism is not the same in all species of bats. Horseshoe bats do not use short frequency-modulated chirps, but emit sounds with a constant frequency. These pure tones are emitted as long pulses with a duration of 90 to 110 milliseconds. Echoes from objects less than 15 to 17 meters away return while the sound is still being emitted. Do these bats have the capability to use the Doppler effect for orientation or localization? It has been observed that these bats move their body, head and ears and emit ultrasound before flying. In this way they scan their environment.

Bats are also able to distinguish between edible and inedible objects. In one experiment meal-worms were mixed with plastic disks the same size as the mealworms. This "food mixture" was tossed into the air. At first the bats rushed at both the mealworms and the plastic disks. Within a week they could distinguish the live food from the simulated food. No one knows how the bats were able to learn the difference between the two. Could this be a form of tissue characterization?

Currently we are not able to completely explain the phenomenon of ultrasonic echolocation. Perhaps further studies will illuminate mechanisms that will be useful in advancing medical ultrasound.

THE DEVELOPMENT OF ULTRASOUND

Many doctors and technicians now using echo-cardiography don't think about the hundred years of development that made this valuable diagnostic method possible. One of the cornerstones of this work was the discovery of the piezoelectric effect. In 1880 Pierre and Jacques Curie showed that mechanical stresses on suitably cut plates of different crystals produced electric charges. This phenomenon is called the direct piezoelectric effect. For thermodynamic reasons, G. Lippman predicted in 1881 that this effect would be reversible. That same year, the Curie brothers detected a reciprocal piezoelectric effect. If a suitable quartz crystal was placed in an alternating electric field, it vibrated in a characteristic fashion.

After the Titanic disaster in 1912, Richardson proposed using submarine ultrasound to detect icebergs (2). However, it was not until 1917 that Langevin produced the first practical piezoelectric ultrasound generator (3). The frequency of an alternating electric field was matched to the resonant frequency of a quartz crystal. In this manner, powerful ultrasound waves were produced and transmitted throughout the surrounding medium. The purpose of this ultrasound device was to detect submarines. However, World War I ended before any practical application occurred.

Langevin also proposed using a piezoelectric crystal, connected to a suitable apparatus, as an ultrasound detector (4). In 1928 Hehlgans performed the first quantitative measurement of ultrasound with a piezoelectric quartz crystal (5).

This new technique was developed to detect submarines and echo-sound the depths of the sea.

When Langevin performed underwater experiments using the ultrasound generator in 1917, he observed that fish swimming into the ultrasound waves died (6). This first observation of the biological effects of ultrasound inspired further research. The first systematic investigation of biological effects was reported by Wood and Loomis in 1927 (7). They performed a variety of experiments showing the disruptive and thermal effects of ultrasonic energy. Small fish, mice, and frogs died if subjected to high-intensity ultrasound. Subsequent examination revealed intra-abdominal hemorrhages and erythrocyte destruction.

In 1940 Conte and Delorenzi observed the brain and spleen were particularly sensitive to ultrasound (8). The biological effects of ultrasound were classified as heating, stirring, microrupture, macrorupture and chemical changes.

These early investigations led scientists to suggest the use of ultrasound in medical therapy. It was first supposed that the destructive effects of ultrasound could be used to treat carcinomas. However, animal experiments did not support this theory. Ultrasound was also used without therapeutic effect in otosclerosis, bronchial asthma, Ménière's disease and Parkinson's disease. In all these experiments, high intensity ultrasound was used. Many complications were reported due to the destructive effects of high intensity ultrasound. In recent years, high intensity ultrasound has found new applications: destruction of stones in the gallbladder and kidney.

In 1939, Pohlman eliminated destructive effects and preserved heating effects by using lower intensity. A thermic therapeutic effect was obtained in this manner (9). This therapy, ultrasonic irradiation, is even used today.

ULTRASOUND AS A DIAGNOSTIC TOOL

The first attempt to use ultrasound as an aid to medical diagnosis was reported in 1942 by Dussik (10). He used the transmission method, which is somewhat similar to the way that conventional radiology uses x-rays. The region to be examined (in this case the skull) was exposed on one side to a beam of parallel ultrasonic rays. Changes in attenuation in the traversed structures were used to build an oscilloscopic picture. This method was used by Dussik (11), Ballantine (12) and Huter (13). These researchers produced pictures that they supposed represented the fluid-filled ventricular system in the brain. However, Guttner et al. showed in 1952 that this method could not visualize the ventricular system because of interference from the skull (14). After further study, Ballantine et al. also concluded this method was valueless (15).

In 1946 Denier used the transmission method in an attempt to map the position of various organs. These included the heart, liver and spleen (16,17).

Keidel used a variation of the transmission method to record fluctuations in heart volume occurring during the cardiac cycle (18). Continuous ultrasound at a frequency of 60 kHz was directed through the chest at the level of the heart. The sound intensity following passage through the thorax was recorded. Keidel found that intensity fluctuated synchronously with the heart beat. He attributed this to the constantly altering relationship along the ultrasound path between blood and heart muscle on one hand and the lung tissue on the other. This technique gave no quantitative information on cardiac volume changes. Apart from the original paper describing the method, no further information was published.

Developments in two different fields during World War II had a great impact on diagnostic ultrasound. The two new techniques were sonar (sound navigation and ranging) and radar (radio detection and ranging). Sonar, developed from early ultrasound experiments, was an echo-ranging technique with a B-mode display. This gave a visual representation of the distance and bearing of a submerged object such as a submarine. The sound frequency used was between 50 and 100 kHz.

Radar detection of airplanes required the generation and reception of very short electrical pulses. By the end of the war it was possible to measure a time interval of less than one-millionth of a second. The application of this technology to ultrasound came in 1945 when Firestone developed a technique for non-destructive testing of industrial materials (19). A quartz crystal was used as a transducer, with frequencies of 0.5, 1.0, 2.25 or 5.0 mHz.

Reflected Ultrasound

For medical diagnostic purposes the reflection technique is more practical than the transmission method. The transducer (combined transmitter and receiver) is placed on the object to be examined. Very short sound impulses are emitted at relatively long intervals. At each interface between media of differing density, a fraction of the sound is reflected. This reflected sound is represented as an echo signal on an oscilloscope. This method was anticipated as being possible by Gohr and Widekind in 1940 (20). However, they did not publish any subsequent results.

In the interval between the World Wars, almost all the basic ultrasound techniques were described by Sokoloff in Leningrad (21,22). Unfortunately, his understanding of the potential for ultrasound was in advance of technology. Inspired by radar's solution of visualization problems, many scientists hoped that reflected sound could be used to visualize internal organs in the human body. Almost 2,000 independent groups in the United States and Europe began separate investigations in varying fields and with quite different purposes.

The first practical use of this method was reported in 1949 by Ludwig and Struthers (23) in detecting gallstones and foreign bodies buried in the muscles of dogs. These researchers offered the opinion that the multiple reflections obtained from soft tissue were too erratic to be of practical value. They suggested, however, that refinements in the technique might make it possible to detect tumors. This led to further investigation by Ludwig of the velocity and acoustic impedance of sound in different tissues (24).

In 1950 Wild (25) reported using the reflection method to obtain multiple reflections from a strip of resected cancerous stomach. On an A-mode echogram the echo pattern from the carcinoma differed significantly from that of normal tissue. The same result was obtained at post-mortem examination of a cerebral tumor (26). Wild et al. next focused their attention on diagnosing breast tumors (27–29).

In 1952 Wild and Reid published a series of 18 cases of breast tumors (28). They concluded that the echo pattern in breast tumor differs significantly from that of normal breast tissue. This was the first clinical application of reflected ultrasound as a diagnostic tool in medicine. Unfortunately, these results were never verified by other investigators. Still, this marked the first attempt to use ultrasound for tissue characterization. Many scientists are now studying echo signals from various structures, such as ischemic versus normal heart muscle.

That same year, Wild and Reid also described a method for two-dimensional visualization of living tissues with their original apparatus. They recorded a two-dimensional echogram by moving the sound generator (transducer) over the breast.

At the same time, attempts to produce cross-sectional ultrasonic images were being made by the radiologist Howry and the electrical engineer Bliss. Because of the poor sound transmission in air, scans were made with the transducer inserted in water. In 1952 they published an incomplete image of an extremity placed in a bathtub (30). In 1954 they also used the method to visualize breast tumors (31) and later went on to collaborate with Dr. Joseph Holmes of Denver, Colorado.

In 1954 Howry and Holmes formulated the principle of compound scanning (32,33). This required moving the transducer in two different motion patterns simultaneously. The cathode-ray oscilloscope sweep was moved simultaneously with the transducer. The combined circular and linear motion produced a compound scan in a cross-sectional plane parallel to the surface of the water. In this way artifacts were eliminated and curved or angulated tissue interfaces could be recorded.

In the following years excellent cross-sectional pictures of the extremities and liver were obtained (33,34). Because this method required placing the patient in a water tank, it proved too cumbersome for clinical use. Overall, these initial American investigations did not produce any practical technique for medical diagnostics.

European investigations were directed toward clinical problems and were not as theoretical as the American studies. For acoustical reasons it was easy to obtain echoes from the organs under investigation. Consequently, the clinical application of ultrasound to medical diagnosis started earlier in Europe than the United States. By 1954 ultrasound was used to diagnose pericardial effusion (35) and mitral valve diseases (36–42). In 1955 Leksell used echoencephalography clinically (43,44).

In 1958 Donald et al. described the hand-operated two-dimensional contact scanner (45). Donald also introduced the use of ultrasound in obstetrics and gynecology (45,46). The principle of contact scanning is now used clinically for ultrasonic imaging of the pelvis and abdomen.

An ophthalmologic two-dimensional sector scanner was developed in the United States by Baum and Greenwood in 1958 (47). Two years later, an ophthalmologic compound scanner was developed. Baum was able to detect retinal detachment, intraocular tumors and foreign bodies (48,49). The first application of ultrasound in the United States was in ophthalmology.

The Development of Ultrasound at Lund

In the early 1950s, before the introduction of open heart surgery, mitral valve disease with pure or predominant stenosis was the only type of acquired heart disease in which surgery could be performed (closed commissurotomy). In pure mitral stenosis there was no problem assessing the need for surgery. However, this was more difficult in combined mitral valve disease.

At this time left ventricular angiography had not been introduced and it was impossible to evaluate the degree of regurgitation into the left atrium. For this reason, many cases of combined mitral valve disease with predominant stenosis were excluded from surgery. On the other hand, sometimes patients with moderate or predominant regurgitation unfortunately were sent to surgery.

As the person responsible for selecting patients for heart surgery at the University Hospital in Lund, I was very unsatisfied with this situation. A method for evaluating the degree of regurgitation was needed. Perhaps, I thought, it would be possible to use a method like radar or ultrasound to measure systolic expansion of the left atrium when blood regurgitated from the left ventricle. The problem was discussed with a physicist, who referred me to a friend—Hellmuth Hertz, at the time an assistant at the Institute of Physics, University of Lund. Hertz had just studied ultrasound and believed there was about a 50 percent chance that reflected ultrasound could be used.

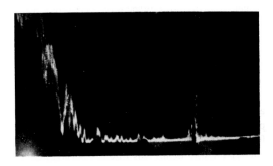

Figure 1.1. Photograph of the oscilloscope screen of the first patient investigated by ultrasound in May 1953 by Hertz and Edler. *Left:* Echoes from the anterior chest wall. *Right:* Echo signal from a structure at a distance of 8–10 cm from the anterior chest wall. This echo signal moved back and forth along the x axis of the oscilloscope screen. From Edler I: Diagnostic ultrasound; In Donald, Levi (eds): Rotterdam, Kooyker Scientific Publications, 1976, p 128.

Over a weekend we borrowed an ultrasound apparatus used at a ship wharf for non-destructive testing of materials. We applied the transducer to the precordium of a patient, directing the sound beam toward the heart. An echo signal was observed at a depth of 8–9 cm from the anterior chest wall (Fig. 1.1). The signal moved back and forth along the x-axis of the oscilloscope screen with an amplitude of about 1 cm. The relationship between these movements and the heart activity was obvious and stimulated further investigations.

In October 1953 Hertz and I were loaned an ultrasonic reflectoscope by Siemens-Reiniger Werke AG in West Germany. This machine was used in industry for non-destructive detection of flaws in materials. The first step in our investigation was to demonstrate that the blood-heart wall interface reflected ultrasound that could be detected and recorded. This was considered doubtful, since the difference in acoustic impedance between muscle and blood is small. Since the choice of sound frequency is a compromise between penetration power and resolution, Hertz selected a frequency of 2.5 megahertz (MHz).

Using transected isolated human heart preparations, we found it was possible to localize interfaces between the heart walls and the enclosed blood-filled cavities (50). Also, the thickness of the heart walls and interventricular septum could be measured. We then took a thrombus, removed from the left atrium during commissurotomy, and placed it in the left ventricle of the preparation. Multiple echoes were received from the thrombus (Fig. 1.2). Further investigations demonstrated interfaces between vessel walls and fluid (Fig. 1.3) (36). Our findings were confirmed by Effert in 1959 (42).

After the experiments on isolated heart preparations we began to investigate ultrasound using patients. The transducer was applied to the left fourth intercostal space close to the sternal margin. The sound beam was directed straight back at a right angle to the anterior chest wall. We received echo signals at a depth corresponding to the posterior part of the heart shadow, as measured on an x-ray film. We concluded that these echo signals emanated from the endocardial surface of the left ventricular posterior wall (50).

In order to study the movement patterns of echo-producing structures, a method was required to continuously record the motion seen on A-scan. A camera was placed in front of the os-

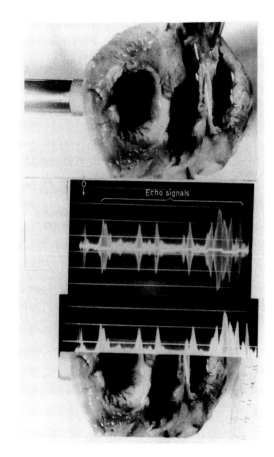

Figure 1.2. *Top,* Transected human heart with water-filled cavities, transducer applied to the left ventricular wall. *Middle,* Echogram obtained on the oscilloscope screen. *O* = outgoing sound impulse. *Bottom,* By suitably bisecting the *top panel* and the *middle panel* and placing the cut edges together, the correlation between the echo signals and heart walls is evident. From Edler I, Hertz CH: The use of ultrasonic reflectoscope for the continuous recording of movements of heart walls. *Kungl Fysiogr Sällsk i Lund Förhandl* 24:5, 1954.

cilloscope's screen and the film was advanced at a constant speed (Figs. 1.4, 1.5). Movement of echo signals along the x-axis were reproduced on the film as curves. Today this recording technique is called M-mode.

Our apparatus had a special device that permitted enlargement of a limited area of the oscillogram, allowing more detailed inspection. Intensity of the outgoing impulse and the degree of echo amplitude could be varied. This allowed adjustment of the echo signal's size. However, there

ECHOGRAM   QUARTZ - CRYSTAL

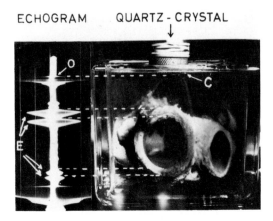

Figure 1.3. Isolated calf pulmonary artery placed in water. The transducer is placed above the artery. The echo signals correspond well to the outer and inner surfaces of the vessel. From Edler I: The diagnostic use of ultrasound in heart diseases. *Acta Med Scand Suppl* 308:32, 1955.

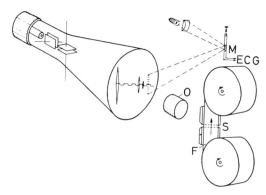

Figure 1.5. Arrangement for simultaneous recording of an M-mode echocardiogram and electrocardiogram on film. The film (*F*) passes a slot (*S*) at a constant speed. *ECG* = leads to the electrocardiograph; *M* = oscilloscope mirror of a galvanometer. This reflects light as a vertical line on the oscilloscope screen at the same level as the echo signals. Both are reproduced on the film by a lens (*O*). From Edler I, Hertz CH: The use of ultrasonic reflectoscope for the continuous recording of movements of heart walls. *Kungl Fysior Sällsk Lund Forhandl* 24:5, 1954.

was no time-gain compensation on our equipment. This made it difficult to get good quality from both the anterior and posterior part of the heart on the same recording.

The posterior left ventricular wall could be recorded in both enlarged and normal-sized hearts. Normally the left ventricular posterior wall was found at a depth of 9–11 cm from the anterior chest wall. The amplitude of systolic movement was approximately 1.0 cm. In aortic regurgitation with heart dilation, the distance to the echo from

the posterior wall was approximately 14 cm. Systolic amplitude was increased and the early diastolic movement backwards was more abrupt than normal (50). Some of the first recorded echocardiograms are shown in Figures 1.6 through 1.9.

While searching for a method to diagnose mitral regurgitation, we discovered most of the patients under investigation had mitral valve disease. We often observed fragments of a rapidly moving echo signal at a depth corresponding to 5–7 cm from the anterior chest wall. After several weeks of training it was possible to record continuous curves with the transducer placed in the third or fourth left intercostal space (Figs. 1.10, 1.11). As the movement could be correlated to both atrial and ventricular activity, we believed the echo emanated from the anterior left atrium close to the mitral annulus.

At this time mitral leaflets were believed to be situated such that it would be impossible to strike their surfaces at a 90 degree angle with the transducer on the precordium. In fact, the mitral leaflets were often referred to as "antero-medial and postero-lateral" leaflets.

Further investigation demonstrated typical echocardiograms in patients with pure mitral stenosis that were quite different from those recorded in patients with mitral regurgitation or no

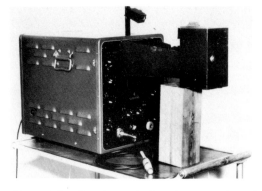

Figure 1.4. The ultrasonic flow detector adapted for echocardiography. A camera is placed in front of the oscilloscope screen, allowing continuous photographic recording of M-mode. This apparatus was used between 1953 and 1965.

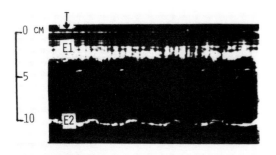

Figure 1.6. The first recorded echocardiogram: October 29, 1953. *Top*, Small scale picture. *E1* = echo from anterior chest wall; *E2* echo from the posterior wall of the *LV* at a depth of 10 cm from the transducer. *Bottom*, The posterior *LV* wall recorded at a larger scale. From Edler I: Diagnostic ultrasound. In Donald, Levi (eds): Rotterdam, Kooyker Scientific Publications 1976, p 128.

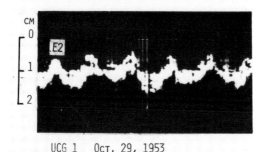

UCG 1   Oct. 29, 1953

heart disease (Figs. 1.10, 1.11) (36–39). A correlation between the speed of diastolic downstroke and the size of the ostium estimated at surgery (closed commissurotomy) was reported in 40 patients with pure mitral stenosis (40). The speed of diastolic downstroke decreased as the size of the mitral orifice decreased. After commissurotomy, the speed of diastolic downstroke increased (37,40).

In atrial flutter, the "atrial wall echo" showed rapid fluctuations corresponding to the electrocardiographic flutter waves (36,40). We showed

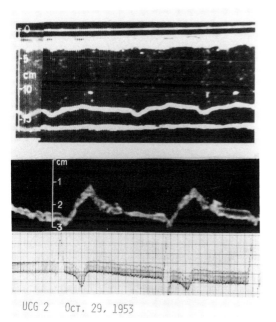

UCG 2   Oct. 29, 1953

Figure 1.7. The second echocardiogram ever recorded, from a patient with aortic regurgitation and dilatation of the heart. The echo signal from the posterior wall of the left ventricle is about 14 cm from the transducer. The amplitude of systolic movement is approximately 1.5 cm. Another echo at a depth of 16 cm may represent the posterior pericardium. From Edler I, Hertz CH: The use of ultrasonic reflectoscope for the continuous recording of movements of heart walls. *Kung Fysior Sällsk Lund Forhandl* 24:5, 1954.

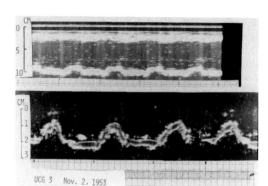

Figure 1.8. Echocardiogram from a patient demonstrating normal heart size. The posterior wall is at a depth of 9–10 cm and the amplitude of systolic motion is 0.9 cm.

echocardiograms of left atrial thrombosis and pericardial effusion in 1954 at the XXIV Scandinavian Congress for Internal Medicine in Stockholm (36) (Figs. 1.12, 1.13).

Starting in 1954, echocardiography was routinely used at Lund for the diagnosis and follow-

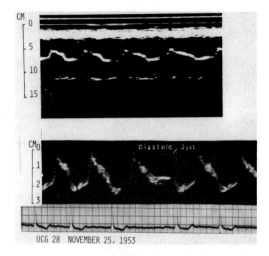

Figure 1.10. Echocardiogram from the patient in Figure 1.9, with combined mitral valve disease. This represents the first satisfactory recording of motion of the anterior mitral leaflet. At the time the recording was made, the nature of the echo-producing structure was unknown. At surgery, a moderate regurgitation was found. From Edler I: The diagnostic use of ultrasound in heart diseases. *Acta Med Scand Suppl* 308: 32, 1955.

up study of pericardial effusion (Fig. 1.14). This was the first clinical application of echocardiography (35). As our equipment had no time-gain compensation, we investigated only the anterior part of the heart in pericardial effusion. By 1955

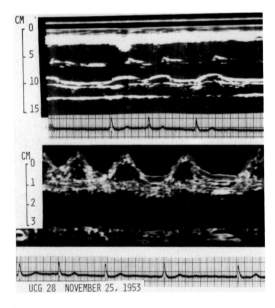

Figure 1.9. Echocardiogram from a patient with mitral valve disease. The posterior wall of the left ventricle is seen at a depth of 9–10 cm. Echoes from another structure appear at a depth of 6 cm. When the transducer was directed upward and laterally, echoes from a structure with a large amplitude of movement were recorded at a 6–8 cm depth from the transducer.

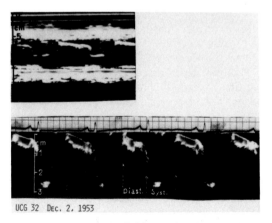

Figure 1.11. The first successful recording of an echocardiogram of the anterior mitral leaflet in a patient with pure mitral stenosis. From Edler I, Hertz CH: The use of ultrasonic reflectoscope for the continuous recording of movements of heart walls. Kungl *Fysior Sällsk Lund Forhandl* 24:5, 1954.

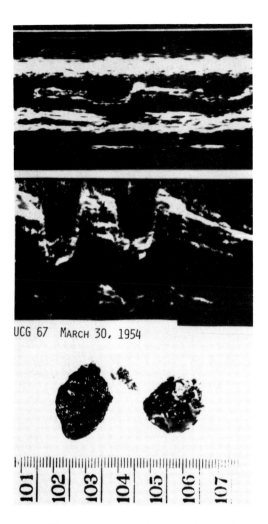

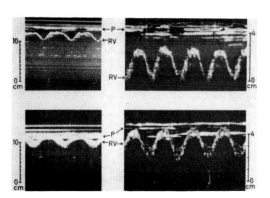

UCG 67 MARCH 30, 1954

Figure 1.12. Echocardiogram from a patient with mitral stenosis and left atrial thrombi. Multiple echoes are seen during diastole behind the anterior mitral echo. The multiple echoes are not exactly parallel to the mitral echo. At surgery, two thrombi were removed. The postoperative echocardiograms no longer showed multiple echoes. From Edler I: The diagnostic use of ultrasound in heart diseases. *Acta Med Scand Suppl* 308:32, 1955.

echocardiography was routinely used to evaluate and follow up patients with mitral stenosis after commissurotomy (Fig. 1.15).

The most fascinating episode to occur during the first 3 years of clinical use was in 1956. A patient with suspected mitral stenosis was sent to us for an echocardiogram. The left atrium was almost completely filled with echo-producing structures (Fig. 1.16). As the patient was in sinus rhythm and the echoes differed in appearance from those of an atrial thrombosis, we believed the mass was a myxoma. The diagnosis was con-

Figure 1.13. Echocardiogram from a patient with pericardial effusion. P = pericardium; RV = right ventricular wall. The *top left* and *right panels* are recorded with the patient in a sitting position, the *bottom left* and *right* in a recumbent position. The *top left* and *bottom right panels* are recorded on the large scale. It is apparent that the distance between the pericardium and anterior heart wall increases in the recumbent position. From Edler I: The diagnostic use of ultrasound in heart diseases. *Acta Med Scand Suppl* 308:32, 1955.

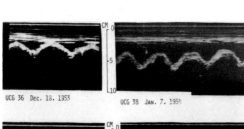

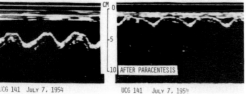

Figure 1.14. Echocardiograms from a patient with a mediastinal malignant tumor and pericardial effusion. The *top left* and *right panels* show progression of the disease over 3 weeks. The *bottom left* and *right* show the effect of paracentesis. From Edler I: Ultrasoundcardiogram in pericardial effusion: Follow up of six cases. Scientific session, Swedish Society of Internal Medicine, Lund, Sweden, June 4, 1955.

firmed at surgery; however, we did not publish this observation until 1960 (51). The first published report of left atrial myxoma diagnosed by echocardiography was done by Effert in 1959 (52).

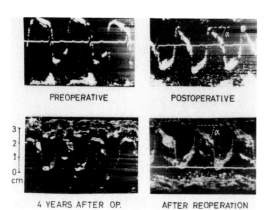

Figure 1.15. Echocardiograms showing follow-up studies of a patient with mitral stenosis. *Top left*, Presurgical echocardiogram, March 1955. *Top right*, Echo taken in April 1955, following closed commissurotomy. *Bottom left*, By July 1959, restenosis is apparent. *Bottom right*, Echocardiogram taken in October 1959, following reoperation. At both operations the mitral ostium would only admit the tip of the little finger. After each operation, the index finger could be inserted quite easily. From Edler I: Ultrasoundcardiography. Part III: Atrioventricular valve mobility in the living human heart recorded by ultrasound. *Acta Med Scand Suppl* 370:83, 1961.

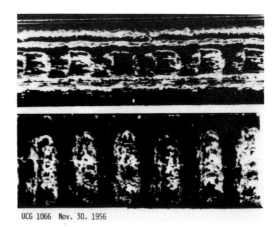

Figure 1.16. Echocardiogram from our first patient with left atrial myxoma. From Edler I, Gustafson A, Karlefurs T, Christensson B: The movements of aortic and mitral valves recorded with ultrasonic echo techniques. Scientific film presented at the Third European Congress of Cardiology, Rome, September 18–24, 1960.

In 1956 the quartz crystal used in the transducer was replaced by barium titanate, a more sensitive echo receiver. With the new transducer, echoes could be recorded from structures that had previously defied inspection. Even in patients with a normal-sized heart, echoes from the anterior atrial wall could usually be recorded. These peaks and valleys were labelled (40) (Fig. 1.17). We now found that, in patients with complete A-V blocks, A-waves on the echocardiogram could be

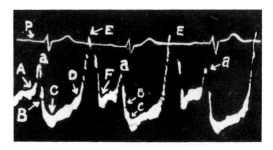

Figure 1.17. Echocardiogram from a healthy person showing movement of the "anterior left atrial wall." The origin of this echo source was unknown at the time it was recorded, but the peaks were labeled. By comparing simultaneously recorded ECG and echo, B-C-D was seen to correspond with ventricular systole. In early diastole, E-F corresponded to the rapid ventricular filling period. From Edler I, Gustafson A: Ultrasonic cardiogram in mitral stenosis. *Acta Med Scand* 159:85, 1957.

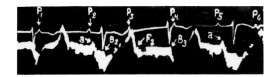

Figure 1.18. Echocardiogram showing movement of the anterior wall of the left atrium in complete atrioventricular block. P1 through P5 represent the P waves on ECG. P2 and P5 occur during ventricular systole and correspond to A-waves on the echocardiogram. From Edler I, Gustafson A: Ultrasonic cardiogram in mitral stenosis. *Acta Med Scand* 159:85, 1957.

correlated with the P-waves on the ECG (Fig. 1.18). However, in atrial fibrillation, A-waves were absent. It became obvious that the a- or A-wave is attributed to atrial systole and B-C-D to ventricular systole. The downstroke E-F coincides with the ventricular filling period (37,40). Simultaneous recordings of the echocardiogram, left atrial pressure and left ventricular pressure confirmed this (Figs. 1.19, 1.20).

Anatomical Studies

The new barium titanate transducer allowed us to record echoes from various areas of the precordium. Figure 1.21 shows recordings from different intercostal spaces. It now seemed possible to record echoes from many different heart structures. In order to establish the exact origin of various echoes, Arne Gustafson, Bo Christensson and I carried out studies on cadavers (53–55). Prior to opening the thoracic cavity, needles were inserted from the interspace and through the chest wall in the direction of the ultrasound beam. In most cases, needles inserted from the left third and fourth intercostal space had crossed the right ventricle, interventricular septum, left ventricular outflow tract, anterior mitral leaflet and left atrium. In some cases the needles passed through both the anterior and posterior mitral leaflets, then through the posterior left ventricular wall (Fig. 1.22, Table 1.1).

In an experimental study in isolated heart preparations, we simulated valve motion (51). We demonstrated that reflected ultrasound could be used to record mitral and aortic valve movement (51,56,57).

The earlier-described echoes with rapid motion, which we believed emanated from the anterior left atrial wall, were now recorded in 77 healthy males. The distance between the anterior chest wall and position E was, on average, 58 mm (Fig. 1.17). The mean value for position C was 83 mm (53,54).

Results from the transfixion studies helped identify echoes from many other structures. These include the leaflets of all four valves, the interventricular septum and left ventricular outflow tract (51,53,54,56) (Figs. 1.23–1.28). In these early studies, echoes from the tricuspid and pulmonary

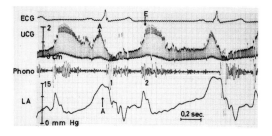

Figure 1.19. Simultaneous recording of ECG, echo of the anterior mitral leaflet (*UCG*), phonocardiogram, and left atrial (*LA*) pressure recorded by suprasternal puncture ad modum Radner in a patient with aortic regurgitation. Atrial systole, indicated as *A* in the pressure curve, is synchronous with peak *A* in the UCG. In the UCG, *E* represents the time when the echo source is closest to the transducer. The echo-producing structure approaches the transducer with rising atrial pressure and recedes with falling pressure. From Edler I: Ultrasoundcardiography. Part III: Atrioventricular valve mobility in the living human heart recorded by ultrasound. *Acta Med Scand Suppl* 370:83, 1961.

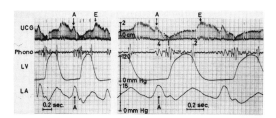

Figure 1.20. Simultaneous recording of anterior mitral leaflet echocardiogram (*UCG*), phonocardiogram, left ventricular (*LV*) pressure and left atrial (*LA*) pressure in a patient with hypertrophic subaortic stenosis. The lowest point on the UCG tracing is reached in early ventricular systole. Immediately after the second heart sound (2), the UCG tracing rises steeply to point *E*. This point is reached 0.10 sec after the second heart sound. From Edler I: Ultrasoundcardiography. Part III: Atrioventricular valve mobility in the living human heart recorded by ultrasound. *Acta Med Scand Suppl* 370:83, 1961.

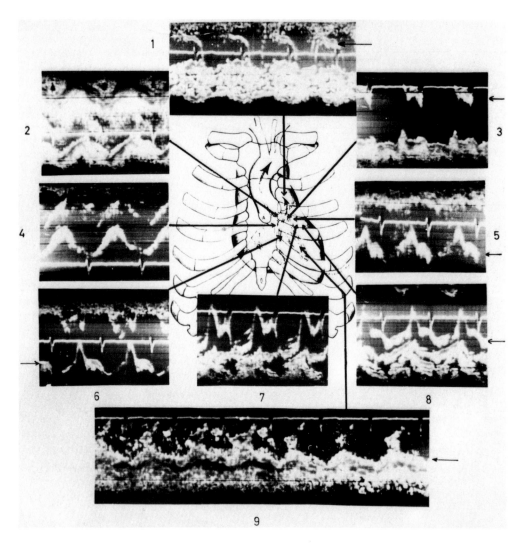

Figure 1.21. Echocardiograms recorded from various areas of the precordium (indicated) in a patient with persistent ductus arteriosus. Tracing *1* is from the medial part of the second left interspace over the pulmonary artery. Tracings *5, 7–8* are taken from the third left interspace with the beam directed antero-posteriorly (AP). Tracings *2* and *4* are from the same position with the beam directed 10°–15° medially. Tracings *6* and *9* are from the fourth left interspace with AP beam direction. Tracings *5–8* show the characteristic motion sequence of large amplitude (*arrows*), at the time believed to emanate from the anterior left atrial wall. In tracings *2* and *4* the sound beam was directed against the left ventricular outflow tract. From Edler I: Ultrasoundcardiography. Part III: Atrioventricular valve mobility in the living human heart recorded by ultrasound. *Acta Med Scand Suppl* 370:83, 1961.

valves could be obtained only in patients with dilatation of the right ventricle (54,56).

As early as the 1950s we had discussed the possibility of using two-dimensional echocardiography. Many of the problems we had encountered, such as echo identification and interpretation of anatomy, were made much easier by two-dimensional images. Ian MacDonald observed that "the techniques of echocardiography has developed back to front." (58)

Two-dimensional cross-sections of biological objects were obtained by Howry et al. in 1952 and 1954 (59,60) and Donald in 1958 (45,46). In the latter investigations the transducer was moved

Table 1.1. Transfixion studies of the heart performed by Edler I, Gustafson A, and Christensson B in 1961.

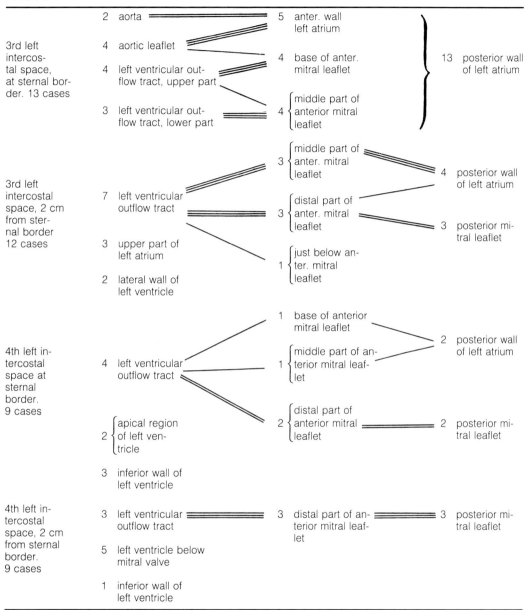

on the area over the organ to be visualized. It is impossible to use this method clinically, since the transducer must be applied only to small acoustic windows on the thoracic wall. Further, in order to follow the movements of the heart structures, many pictures must be produced each second.

In 1960, Hertz and Olofsson built an instrument for two-dimensional imaging of the heart. Using a mechanically oscillating transducer they produced a real-time sector scan of the heart (61–64). Part of the ultrasound not reflected directly back to the transducer was collected by a mirror system. In this manner the transverse resolution of the ultrasonic beam was improved appreciably.

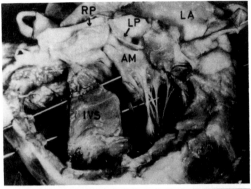

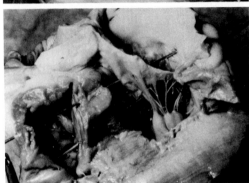

Figure 1.22. Section of a heart with left ventricular hypertrophy. The right ventricular cavity is on the *left* and the left ventricular cavity is on the *right*. *IVS* = interventricular septum; *AM* = anterior mitral leaflet; *RP, LP* = aortic cusps; *LA* = left atrium. From Edler I: Ultrasoundcardiography. Part III: Atrioventricular valve mobility in the living human heart recorded by ultrasound. *Acta Med Scand Suppl* 370:83, 1961.

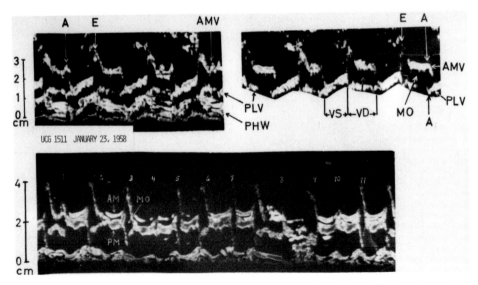

Figure 1.23. Echocardiogram showing movement of the mitral leaflets. *Top left*, Normal case in sinus rhythm. *Top right*, Bisecting the figure, the mitral leaflets are separated from the posterior heart wall. This makes identification of the mitral leaflets easier. *Bottom left*, Mitral leaflets in atrial fibrillation. *AM* and *AMV* = anterior mitral leaflet; *PM* and *PLV* = posterior mitral leaflet; *PHW* = posterior heart wall; *VS* = ventricular systole; *VD* = ventricular diastole; *MO* = mitral ostium; *A* = atrial systole; *E* = the position of maximal opening of the *AMV*. Modified from Edler I, Gustafson A, Karlefors T, Christensson B: The movements of aortic and mitral valves recorded with ultrasonic echo techniques. Scientific film presented at the Third European Congress of Cardiology, Rome, September 18–24, 1960; Edler I: Ultrasoundcardiography. Part III: Atrioventricular valve mobility in the living human heart recorded by ultrasound. *Acta Med Scand Suppl* 370:83, 1961.

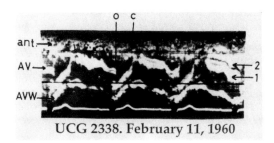

UCG 2338. February 11, 1960

Figure 1.24. Normal echocardiogram from the aortic leaflets. Transducer applied to the third left interspace with the sound beam directed against the aortic ostium. *AV* = aortic valve; *1* and *2* = aortic leaflets; *ANT* = anterior aortic wall; *AVW* = atrioventricular or posterior aortic wall; *O* = rapid opening of aortic leaflets; *C* = rapid closing of the aortic leaflets. From Edler I, Gustafson A, Karlefors T, Christensson B: The movements of aortic and mitral valves recorded with ultrasonic echo techniques. Scientific film presented at the Third European Congress of Cardiology, Rome, September 18–24, 1960.

The transducer and mirror system were placed in a water tank, providing a suitable contact with the anterior chest wall of the patient. Using this method only six frames per second could be recorded (Fig. 1.29). Later Hertz and Lindstrom were able to obtain 16 frames/second using a rotating mirror system (65). However, while this was the first clinically used real-time instrument, it was unwieldy for routine clinical use.

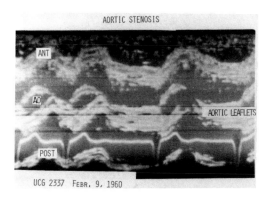

UCG 2337. Febr. 9, 1960

Figure 1.25. Echocardiogram showing the aortic leaflets in aortic stenosis. *ANT* = anterior aortic wall; *POST* = posterior aortic wall; *AO* = aortic ostium during ventricular systole. From Edler I, Gustafson A, Karlefors T, Christensson B: The movements of aortic and mitral valves recorded with ultrasonic echo techniques. Scientific film presented at the Third European Congress of Cardiology, Rome, September 18–24, 1960.

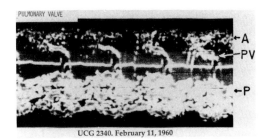

UCG 2340. February 11, 1960

Figure 1.26. Echocardiogram of the pulmonary valve in persistent ductus arteriosus. *A* = anterior wall of the pulmonary artery; *P* = posterior wall of pulmonary artery; *PV* = pulmonary leaflet. From Edler I: Ultrasoundcardiography. Part III: Atrioventricular valve mobility in the living human heart recorded by ultrasound. *Acta Med Scand Suppl* 370:83, 1961.

ECHOCARDIOGRAPHY AS A DIAGNOSTIC TOOL: 1954–1960

At the Third European Congress in Cardiology, held in Rome in 1960, we presented a scientific film describing the echocardiographic technique and the clinical application of the method (51). At this time the most important use of echocardiography was in patients with pericardial effusion or mitral stenosis. By 1960 we had investigated more than 300 patients with mitral valve disease. In pure mitral stenosis the anterior mitral leaflet showed a reduced speed of diastolic downstroke E–F. The degree of reduction was a meas-

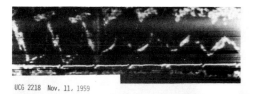

UCG 2218 Nov. 11, 1959

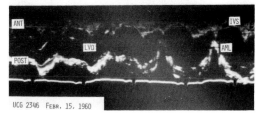

UCG 2346 Febr. 15, 1960

Figure 1.27. M-mode scan from mitral region to the left ventricular outflow tract (*LVO*) and back. *AML* = anterior mitral leaflet; *IVS* = interventricular septum. From Edler I, Gustafson A, Karlefors T, Christensson B: The movements of aortic and mitral valves recorded with ultrasonic echo techniques. Scientific film presented at the Third European Congress of Cardiology, Rome, September 18–24, 1960.

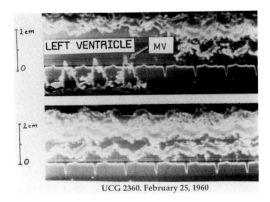

UCG 2360. February 25, 1960

Figure 1.28. M-mode scan from the left ventricle to the aortic root in a patient with subaortic stenosis. The left ventricular outflow tract was very narrow. *MV* = mitral valve. From Edler I: Diagnostic ultrasound. In Donald, Levi (eds): Rotterdam, Kooyker Scientific Publications, 1976, p 128.

ure of the degree of stenosis in cases without calcification of the leaflets. After closed commissurotomy the speed of the diastolic downstroke increased (Fig. 1.15) (53,54,66).

Physiological Studies

In 1959, Effert, Hertz and Bohme described a method that allowed direct recording of an echocardiogram via an electrocardiograph (67). However, this technique only permitted recording the movements of a single echo. That single echo could be correlated with the electrocardiogram, phonocardiogram, and intracardiac pressure.

In this manner we correlated the movement pattern of the anterior mitral leaflet to the apical phonocardiogram (66) (Fig. 1.30). In mitral stenosis the opening snap coincides with point E on the echocardiogram (Fig. 1.31). In right bundle branch block with wide splitting of the first sound,

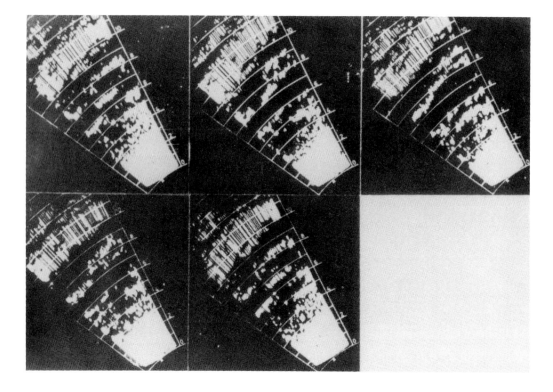

Figure 1.29. Sixteen mm film images of the heart in a healthy person using the mechanical sector scanner developed by Hertz et al. The heart is shown in cross section. The movement of the mitral valve is seen at a depth of 6–8 cm. Only seven pictures/second were produced, which resulted in unsatisfactory scan quality. From Hertz CH: Ultrasonic engineering in heart diagnosis. *Am J Cardiol* 19:6, 1967.

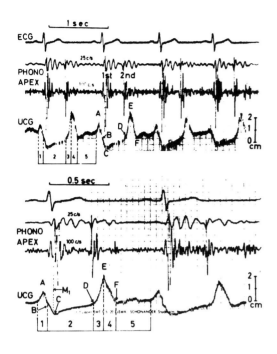

Figure 1.30. Direct recording of a normal echocardiogram (*UCG*) of the anterior mitral leaflet. Paper speed is between 50 and 100 mm/sec. The five main phases of the mitral echocardiogram are shown. The correlation between UCG and simultaneous recordings of the ECG and apical phonocardiogram is demonstrated. *M1* = mitral component of the first heart sound. From Edler I: Mitral valve function studied by the ultrasound echo method. In Grossman CC, Holmes JH, Joyner C, Purnell EW (eds): *Diagnostic Ultrasound: Proceedings of the First International Conference.* New York, Plenum Press, 1966, p 198.

mitral valve closure coincides with the first component and tricuspid closure with the second component of the first heart sound (53) (Fig. 1.32). It had been postulated that intensity of the first heart sound was related to the degree of separation of the mitral leaflets at the beginning of ventricular systole (68,69). This was confirmed by the echocardiogram (66) (Fig. 1.33).

Further, it was shown that the presystolic mur-

mur in pure mitral stenosis coincides with a traction of the leaflet and annulus backwards against the atrial cavity. This is in spite of increasing atrial pressure during atrial systole (66) (Fig. 1.34). This finding supports the observation of Nichols et al. that the presystolic murmur coincides with a late diastolic billowing of the leaflet toward the atrium (70).

In the 1960s Nils Rune Lundstrom started his

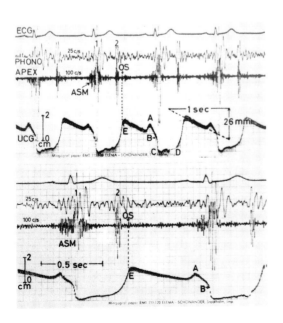

Figure 1.31. Echocardiogram showing the movement of the anterior mitral leaflet in pure mitral stenosis without calcification and in sinus rhythm. The downstroke *A-B* coincides with the atrial systolic murmur (*ASM*). The speed of diastolic downstroke is reduced to 26 mm/sec (normally > 90 mm/sec). The position of maximal opening of the leaflet (*E*) coincides with the opening snap (*O*). From Edler I: Mitral valve function studied by the ultrasound echo method. In Grossman CC, Holmes JH, Joyner C, Purnell EW (eds): *Diagnostic Ultrasound: Proceedings of the First International Conference.* New York, Plenum Press, 1966, p 198.

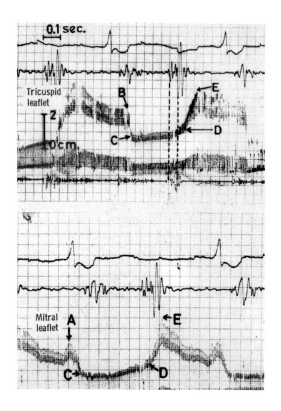

Figure 1.32. Simultaneous recording of the electrocardiogram, apical phonocardiogram, and echocardiogram in a patient with right bundle branch block. *Top*, Echocardiogram from the anterior tricuspid leaflet. Points *C* and *D* coincide with the second component of, respectively, the first and second heart sound. *Bottom*, Echocardiogram from the anterior mitral leaflet. Points *C* and *D* as above. This asynchrony was used in anatomic studies to identify the anterior tricuspid leaflet. From Edler I: Ultrasoundcardiography. Part III: Atrioventricular valve mobility in the living human heart recorded by ultrasound. *Acta Med Scand Suppl* 370:83, 1961.

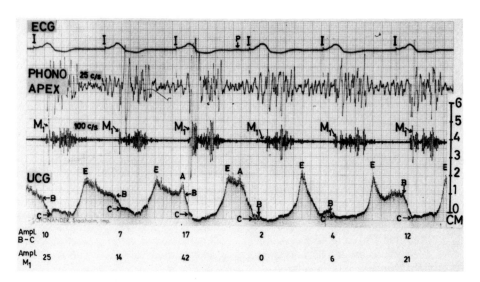

Figure 1.33. Electrocardiogram (ECG), apical phonocardiogram and echocardiogram in a patient with complete A-V block treated by pacemaker. The echo shows movements of the anterior mitral leaflet. On the ECG, I indicates the pacemaker's electrical impulse and *P* is the P wave. The mitral component of the first sound is indicated by *M*. The closing movement of the mitral leaflet in early ventricular systole is indicated by *B-C*. For each heartbeat the distance of movement *B-C* and the amplitude (intensity) of M1 are given below the UCG curve. A large *B-C* distance gives a high-intensity first heart sound. From Edler I: Mitral valve function studied by the ultrasound echo method. In Grossman CC, Holmes JH, Joyner C, Purnell EW (eds): *Diagnostic Ultrasound: Proceedings of the First International Conference.* New York, Plenum Press, 1966, p 198.

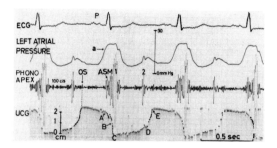

Figure 1.34. Pure mitral stenosis and normal sinus rhythm. Simultaneous recordings of the ECG, left atrial pressure, apical phonocardiogram and echo-cardiogram (*UCG*) showing the movement of the anterior mitral leaflet. The left atrial pressure was recorded by suprasternal puncture ad modum Radner. The atrial systolic pressure (*A-wave*) increases to 21 mm Hg. The downstroke of *A-B* on the *UCG* curve starts when the atrial pressure is 15 mm Hg. The atrial systolic crescendo murmur (*ASM*) with the *A-B* downstroke. The ASM is produced when the anterior mitral leaflet is moving in an opposite direction to the pressure gradient between the left atrium and left ventricle. Edler I: Mitral valve function studied by the ultrasound echo method. In Grossman CC, Holmes JH, Joyner C, Purnell EW (eds): *Diagnostic Ultrasound: Proceedings of the First International Conference.* New York, Plenum Press, 1966, p 198.

pioneering work at Lund in pediatric and congenital heart diseases (71,72).

Echocardiography Outside Lund

Siemens-Reiniger Werke in Erlangen, the manufacturer of our equipment, was interested in introducing echocardiography within West Germany. Three investigative groups began to work with echocardiography.

The first was Sven Effert, who began his investigations in Dusseldorf after studying echocardiography at Lund in 1956. His group's work confirmed our observations (73–75). In 1959 he published the first report on atrial myxoma diagnosed by ultrasound (76).

The other two groups were at Hamburg (Gassler et al.) and Wurzburg (Braun). However, there are only a few publications from these centers (77–79).

Chinese doctors were among the first to use ultrasound for diagnostic purposes. Dr. Hsu Chihchang read my paper in Acta Medica Scandinavica in 1955 (36) and was interested in the method. In 1958, at Chung-shan Hospital, Shanghai First Medical College, he began looking at the heart with a self-designed A-mode device. Beginning

in 1960, animal experiments and observations on cadavers were performed. Our observations, that the interface between the heart walls and water-filled cardiac cavities reflect ultrasound, were reconfirmed (80). In these experiments he showed that echoes obtained from the fourth left interspace emanated from the anterior wall of the left ventricle, anterior mitral leaflet and posterior left atrial wall. Further, he postulated that echoes obtained from the third left interspace represent the pulmonary artery, ascending aorta and left atrium (Fig. 1.35) (81).

Hsu Chih-chang also published preliminary results using an A-scope apparatus to diagnose heart disease (82). In an investigation of 100 healthy persons, he described the normal movement of the anterior mitral leaflet (Fig. 1.36).

An investigation was made in 55 cases of rheumatic heart disease with mitral stenosis. Changes were observed, including enlargement of the en-

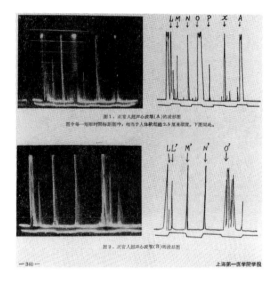

Figure 1.35. *Top,* Ultrasonic cardiogram of normal cardiac *echo group A,* the transducer applied to the fourth left intercostal space. Each square pulse of the time mark corresponds to a depth of 2.5 cm in soft tissue. *L* = chest wall and pleura; *M* = anterior wall of the left ventricle; *N* = anterior mitral valve leaflet; *O* = posterior wall of the left atrium. *Bottom,* Normal cardiac *echo group B,* the transducer applied to the third left intercostal space. *L' – M1'* = pulmonary artery; *M' – N'* = ascending aorta, *N' – O'* = left atrium. From Hsu CC: Preliminary studies on ultrasonics in cardiological diagnosis: II The use of A-scope ultrasound apparatus in the diagnosis of heart diseases. *Acta Academiae Medicinae Primae Shanghai.* 2:335–343, 1964.

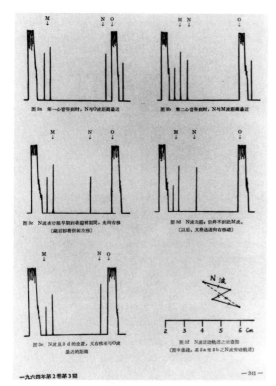

Figure 1.36. *Top left,* Tracing *N* is closest to *O* when the first heart sound is produced. *Top right,* Tracing *N* is closest to *M* when the second heart sound is produced. *Middle left,* Tracing *N* moves to the right during the early phase of diastole and the prephase of systole, then moves back to the left. *Middle right,* Tracing *N* moves to the left, though not close to *M*, then quickly moves to the right. *Bottom left,* Tracing *N* moves close to *O* again from its position in *D*. *Bottom right,* The dotted line shows the movement of *N* from the position shown in the *top left panel* to the position shown in *B*. Hsu CC: Preliminary studies on ultrasonics in cardiological diagnosis: II: The use of A-scope ultrasound apparatus in the diagnosis of heart diseases. *Acta Academiae Medicinae Primae Shanghai* 2:335–343, 1964.

tire outline, dilatation of the right atrium and abnormal diastolic movement of the anterior mitral leaflet. The normally rapid movements of the leaflet changed to slow motion during entire diastole, "denoting diminution of elasticity of the mitral valve" (Fig. 1.37).

In five cases of pericardial effusion, he found an echo-free area between the pericardium and both the anterior and posterior heart wall (Fig. 1.38). Further, he noted a relative decrease in the activity of the anterior mitral leaflet.

In March of 1961, Hsu Chih-chang began to develop an ultrasonic "brilliance-modulation"

scanner, an ultrasonic time-position indicator (83). With this equipment, M-mode recordings became possible (Fig. 1.39).

By 1962 the method was introduced in many cities, including Beijing, Wuhan and Xian. Thus the diagnosis of heart disease using the ultrasonic cardiogram spread throughout the country (84). That same year Dr. Hsu also started a medical electronics group at the Zhong Shen Hospital. In this way they learned about the physics and electronics of ultrasonic techniques, about which so many physicians are ignorant (85,86).

The Shanghai Medical Ultrasonics Group pro-

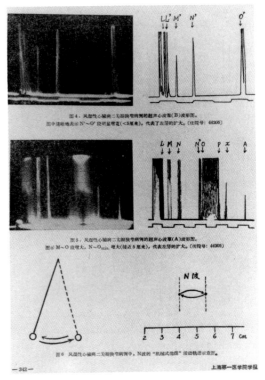

Figure 1.37. *Top,* A patient with rheumatic heart disease (*RHD*) and mitral stenosis (*MS*) from *ultrasonic cardiac echo group B* (transducer on third left interspace). Enlargement of the *N′ – O′* segment is demonstrated, representing dilatation of the left atrium. *Middle,* A patient with *RHD* and *MS* from *ultrasonic cardiac echo group A* (transducer on fourth left interspace). The enlargement of segments *M-O* and *N-O* (approximately 5 cm) is demonstrated, indicating dilatation of the left atrium. *Bottom,* Abnormal swinging of *N* in a patient with *RHD* and *MS*. From Hsu CC: Preliminary studies on the ultrasonics in cardiological diagnosis: II: The use of A-scope ultrasound apparatus in the diagnosis of heart diseases. *Acta Academiae Medicinae Primae Shanghai* 2:335–343, 1964.

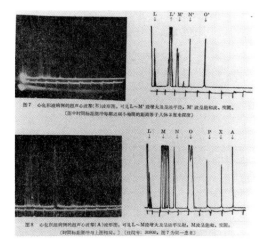

Figure 1.38. *Top*, Pericardial effusion in a patient from *ultrasonic echo group B* (transducer on third left interspace). The increased distance between *L* and *M'* indicates fluid accumulation in the pericardial sac. Tracing *M'* is saturated and enlarged. Two time mark divisions equal a depth of roughly 2 cm in the body. *Bottom*, Pericardial effusion in a patient from *group A* (transducer on the fourth left interspace). The increased distance between *L* and *M* indicates the fluid accumulation in the pericardial sac. Tracing *M* is saturated and enlarged. From Hsu CC: Preliminary studies on ultrasonics in cardiological diagnosis: II: The use of A-scope ultrasound apparatus in the diagnosis of heart diseases. *Acta Academiae Medicinae Primae Shanghai* 2:335–343, 1964.

duced their first book on ultrasonic diagnosis in 1961. An enlarged second edition was published in 1978.

Echocardiography was introduced in the United States by Reid and Joyner in 1961 (87–89). Reid, who in the early 1950s worked with Wild on tissue characterization, read a paper by Hertz on our investigations at Lund (90) and built an echocardiograph. In 1962 he and Claude Joyner, in Philadelphia, began investigating the heart with ultrasound.

During the 1960s echocardiography's main application was to evaluate mitral valve disease. Several investigative groups established a good correlation between reduction in speed of diastolic downstroke E–F and the degree of stenosis (89,91–95). Effert studied 3076 patients with mitral valve disease, of whom 1231 underwent closed commissurotomy. In tight mitral stenosis the speed of diastolic downstroke was less than 10 mm/sec. In moderate stenosis, where the ostium was open for a fingertip, the speed was 10–25 mm/sec (95).

After successful commissurotomy the velocity of diastolic downstroke increased. This finding was confirmed by other investigators (Fig. 1.40).

However, when the mitral valve is calcified, the total amplitude of movement between the closed position, C, and the maximal opening position, E, is reduced to 15 mm or less. Under these conditions, the speed of diastolic downstroke E–F cannot be used as a measure of the mitral valve orifice area (Fig. 1.41) (94).

In 1972 Duchak et al. reported that simultaneous recording of both mitral leaflets is necessary for accurate diagnosis of mitral stenosis (96). In this technique the sound beam impinges upon the tip of the anterior leaflet, which does not move as much as the ballooning portion of the anterior mitral leaflet. Investigators using this technique failed to find a close relationship between E–F slope and the mitral valve area (97–99).

Harvey Feigenbaum became interested in echocardiography in the latter part of 1963. While operating a hemodynamic laboratory, he became frustrated with the limitations of cardiac catheterization and angiography. He borrowed an ultrasonoscope from neurologists and began to look at the posterior wall of the left ventricle. However, it was impossible to record echoes from the mitral valve with this equipment.

A visit to Joyner's laboratory revealed the difference in equipment. Joyner's interest was still limited to the mitral valve, but Feigenbaum concentrated on the posterior left ventricular wall. Feigenbaum et al. found a distinct change in the appearance of posterior wall echoes in patients with pericardial effusion (100). In an experimental study on dogs they showed that an infusion of saline in the pericardial sac separated the posterior wall echo from that of the pericardium. When the fluid was removed, the echoes fused

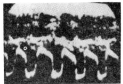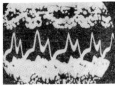

Figure 1.39. *Left*, Ultrasonic cardiogram from the anterior mitral leaflet in a patient with mitral stenosis. *Right*, Ultrasonic cardiogram from the anterior mitral leaflet in a healthy person. From Hsu CC: The application of an ultrasonic brilliance-modulation scanner in the study of ultrasonic cardiogram. *Acta Acoustica Sinica* 1:95–96, 1964.

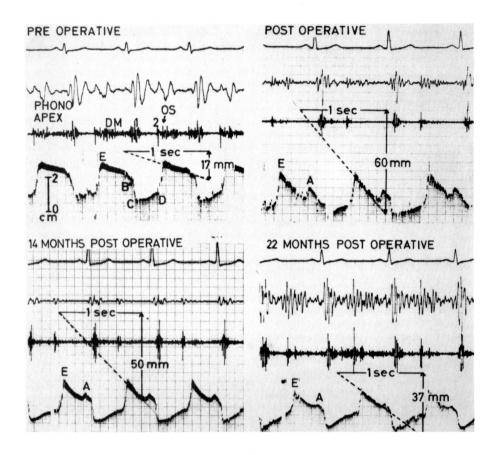

Figure 1.40. Anterior mitral leaflet echograms from a patient with pure mitral stenosis. *Top right,* Before closed commissurotomy in 1963. *Top left,* Echogram a few days after the operation. *Bottom left,* Echo from 14 months after operation. *Bottom right,* Echo 22 months after operation. The speed of diastolic downstroke was 17 mm/sec before the operation, 60 mm/sec shortly after surgery, 50 mm/sec 14 months after surgery, and 37 mm/sec at 22 months postsurgery. This follow-up study shows a slight degree of restenosis. From Edler I: Ultrasoundcardiography in mitral valve stenosis. *Am J Cardiol* 19:18, 1967.

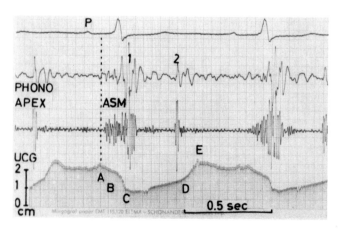

Figure 1.41. Echogram (*UCG*) of the anterior mitral leaflet in a patient with surgically confirmed mitral stenosis and calcification of the mitral valve. The total amplitude of movement between the closed position (*C*) and maximally open position (*E*) is reduced to 15 mm. In this case the diastolic slope cannot be used as a measure of the mitral area.

(Fig. 1.42). In patients it was possible to demonstrate both anterior and posterior pericardial effusion (101,102). Contrary to our experience in Europe, these findings stimulated an interest in echocardiography in the United States and these results were confirmed by many investigators (103–106).

Feigenbaum et al. developed the techniques for measuring posterior left ventricular wall thickness (107), left ventricular internal dimensions (108,109) and left ventricular stroke volume (110–112). Much of the increasing interest in echocardiography during the 1970s depended on this work. He demonstrated the practicality of echocardiography as a noninvasive tool for studying left ventricular function.

Further investigations in the United States reconfirmed our observations in Europe. In addition, the value of a mitral valve echogram was demonstrated in diagnosing hypertrophic subaortic stenosis (113,114), aortic insufficiency (115) and prolapsed mitral valve (116).

The echocardiographic anatomy described earlier in this chapter was confirmed and expanded upon by Gramiak et al. in 1969 (117). They used the contrast method introduced by Joyner, who had observed echoes from within the heart following intracardial injection of saline solution or indocyanine green dye (118). Gramiak et al. used four transducer positions and identified typical movement patterns of the mitral valve, aortic root, tricuspid valve and atrial septum. Cardiac chambers were identified by intracardiac injection of contrast in 32 patients undergoing cardiac catheterization. From the mitral valve position the right ventricular outflow tract, ventricular septum and left ventricular outflow tract were seen in front of the mitral valve. From the aortic root position the right ventricular outflow tract, aortic root and left atrium were identified (Fig. 1.43). In the tricuspid valve position the right atrium was localized just behind the valve, with the right ventricle in front of the valve.

A new transducer position was introduced to record echoes from the atrial septum. The transducer was applied parasternally, at the fourth or fifth intercostal space, and the beam was directed medially and cephalically. The atria were identified on either side of the septum. The contrast method also permitted direct measurements of the intracardiac structures, including leaflet thickness and left ventricular outflow tract width. Gramiak et al. also used the contrast method to diagnose intracardiac shunts and aortic valve regurgitation, as well as to study hypertrophic obstructive cardiomyopathy (117).

Two-Dimensional Echocardiography

In 1960 Hertz introduced the first real-time instrument for two-dimensional echocardiography. However, it could not produce more than 16 frames/second, which was not sufficient. During the 1960s many other methods of two-dimensional echocardiography were presented. In Japan, Ebina et al. described a system called ultrasound cardiotomography in 1967 (119). They used a water tank with a mechanically rotated transducer to obtain sector scans of the heart. Another method for recording two-dimensional echocardiograms, introduced by King, involved an electrocardiographically gated B-scanner of the same type used for abdominal ultrasound (120). The transducer was moved by hand over the precordium and an image of the heart was built up from many cardiac cycles. Images of cardiac anatomy were recorded in different pathological conditions (121–124). However, the cardiac dynamics could not be studied and image quality was poor.

Gramiak et al. developed another method for two-dimensional echocardiography called cine ultrasound cardiography. They combined M-mode echocardiography and compound B-mode scanning to develop a computer-assisted, pseudo real-time cross-sectional echocardiogram (125). How-

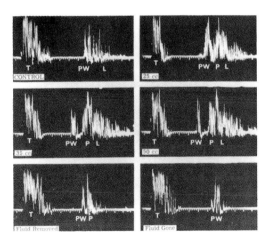

Figure 1.42. Saline infusion into the pericardial sac of a dog. As the fluid is injected, the posterior heart wall (*PW*) is separated by an echo-free space from the pericardium (*P*) and lung (*L*). This space disappears as the saline is removed. From Feigenbaum H, Waldhausen JA, Hyde LP: Ultrasound diagnosis of pericardial effusion. *JAMA* 191:107, 1965.

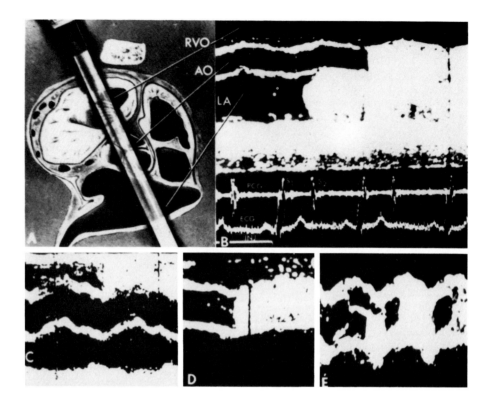

Figure 1.43. Contrast identification of cardiac structures, aortic root recording position. *A*, The position of the transducer to the left of the sternum showing the medial angulation required to direct the ultrasonic beam through the aortic root. *B*, Left atrial contrast injection identifies the left atrium (*LA*) behind the aortic root with the aorta (*AO*) filling during the subsequent systole. *C*, Right ventricular outflow (*RVO*) lies anterior to the aorta. *D* and *E*, Left ventricular and supravalvular injections identify the aortic root. The linear echoes between the root margins in E arise from the aortic valve cusps. The rectangular defects in the contrast pattern are due to ejection of noncontrast blood from the left ventricle and demonstrate the function of the aortic valve. From Gramiak R, Shah PM, Kramer DH: Ultrasoundcardiography: Contrast studies in anatomy and function. *Radiology* 92:939, 1969.

ever, as Hertz asserted in 1960, it was clear that real-time recording was necessary to produce images of sufficient quality.

Unfortunately, Hertz had to interrupt his experiments in two-dimensional echocardiography because he did not receive any research grants. Meanwhile, in Sweden, diagnostic ultrasound was considered to be valueless.

Hugenholtz came to the Department of Cardiology at The Erasmus University in Rotterdam in 1969 and started a group under the direction of Nicholas Bom to work on cardiac ultrasound. During his early work in the United States, Hugenholtz had expressed an interest in cardiac ultrasound. He was told he was crazy.

In 1972 Bom presented the first two-dimensional electronic sector scanner (126,127). The transducer was 8 cm long and 1 cm wide and consisted of 20 piezoelectric elements, 3 mm in diameter (Fig. 1.44). The fixed elements were fired in rapid sequence by electronic switching. The resulting echoes were displayed as B-mode scans along the horizontal axis on the oscilloscope, while the vertical position of each line corresponded to an element. In this manner a linear scan of the heart was obtained, at a repetition rate of approximately 150 frames/second (Fig. 1.45). A Polaroid photograph could be taken directly from the oscilloscope via an electrocardiographically activated trigger device.

The first commercially available two-dimensional system, it was used clinically by many groups (128). The major limitation was the large transducer, which covered a number of interspaces and

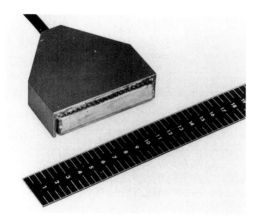

Figure 1.44. Multielement transducer comprising 20 individual piezoelectric elements. Reproduced by permission from Dr. N. Bom.

ribs. Also, the small elements made the near field of the beam very short, while the quality of the frames was not completely acceptable. Bom subsequently developed a dynamic electronically focused system, which today is indispensable in fetal and abdominal ultrasound.

The real-time two-dimensional system introduced by Hertz (65), using a water bath contact for the transducer, was modified by Griffith and Henry (129,130). The previous limitations were overcome by using a conventional transducer moved by a mechanical drive unit. The transducer was applied directly to the interspaces and the sector limited to 30 or 45 degrees. By using many

transducers rotating through a 360 degree arc, the scan sector was increased to 84 degrees. Several years later, Von Ramm and Thurstone described a phased array real-time sector scanner (131).

Both mechanical and phased array sector scanning use transducers that can be angled in different directions and require only one interspace for an acoustic window. These systems are now used for real-time two-dimensional echocardiography. However, the simultaneous recording of two-dimensional images and M-mode is highly desirable.

Doppler Echocardiography

The Doppler effect—named after the Austrian physicist Christian Johann Doppler—was described in 1842. In 1956 and 1957 Satomura et al. developed a technique using the Doppler effect to obtain information about movements of the heart (132–134). They transmitted a continuous sound beam toward the heart from the anterior chest wall. Sound reflected from the moving heart structures undergoes the Doppler effect, so the frequency of the returning sound is altered. The change in frequency is proportional to the velocity of the moving structure in the plane parallel to the sound beam.

Using this method, Yoshida et al. studied the movements of the heart and heart valves (135). The Doppler signals were classified as either low or high frequency. The low frequency signals (< 500 cps) were believed to indicate movements of the heart that coincided with ventricular systole,

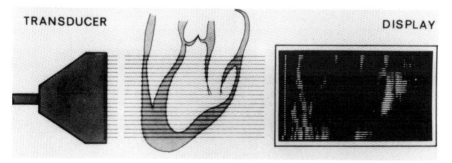

Figure 1.45. Schematic representation of Bom's multielement electronic scanning design. The elements transmit an acoustic pulse, in sequence from *top* to *bottom*, into the thoracic cavity. Echoes are electronically converted to brightness dots (*B-mode*) and displayed along a horizontal line on the oscilloscope screen. The dots' position on the screen represents cardiac dimensions (depth) along that echo beam. On the vertical axis of the screen, each echo line corresponds to the relative position of each element in the transducer. On the oscilloscope screen the heart structures are represented by brightness dots, as indicated on the diagram. Fast electronic switching between elements allows real-time visualization. Reproduced with permission from Dr. N. Bom.

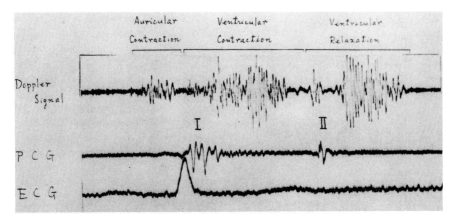

Figure 1.46. Ultrasonic Doppler signals of low frequency, which were believed to show the movement of the heart. Simultaneous recordings of Doppler, phonocardiogram (*pcg*), and ECG. During ventricular systole the Doppler signals appear immediately after the first heart sound and last about 2/3 of ventricular systole. In early diastole, and also at atrial systole, Doppler signals are recorded. From Yoshida T, Mori M, Nimura Y, Hikita G, Takagisha S, Nakanischi K, Satomura S: Analysis of heart motion with ultrasonic Doppler method and its clinical application. *Am Heart J* 61:61, 1961.

early diastole and atrial systole (Fig. 1.46). High frequency signals (> 1000 cps) were believed to indicate the opening and closing of the valves. These signals were recorded as high pitched clicks, which can be timed with a simultaneously recorded ECG and phonocardiogram. The time of closing and opening of the valves determines the duration of isometric contraction and the iso-

metric relaxation of the ventricles. Figure 1.47 shows a prolonged relaxation in a patient with reduced myocardial function. This same method has been used by Kostis et al. (136).

The Doppler ultrasonic flowmeter was described by Franklin in 1961 (137,138). This method has been used extensively for studying peripheral vessels. In 1969 Lindstrom and I used continuous

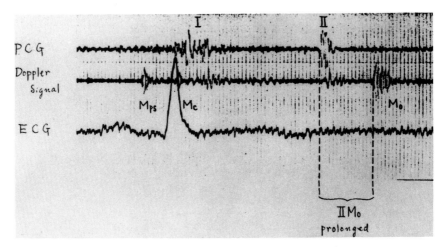

Figure 1.47. Ultrasonic high-frequency Doppler signals emanating from the mitral valve in a patient with myocardial disease. Simultaneous recordings of the phonocardiogram (*pcg*), Doppler, and ECG. Opening of the mitral valve is markedly delayed. The time interval between the second heart sound (*II*) and the opening of the mitral valve (*Mo*) (isometric relaxation period) is 0.14 sec. The normal range is between 0.05 and 0.10 sec. *I* = first heart sound; *Mc* = closing of the mitral valve. From Yoshida T, Mori M, Nimura Y, Hikita G, Takagisha S, Nakanischi K, Satomura S: Analysis of heart motion with ultrasonic Doppler method and its clinical application. *Am Heart J* 61:61, 1961.

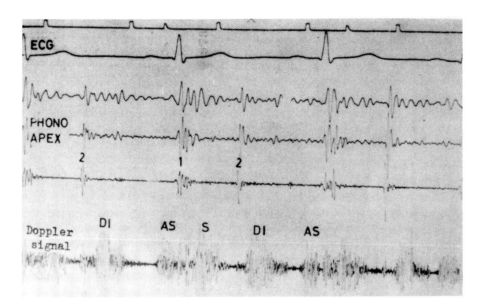

Figure 1.48. Simultaneously recorded Doppler, ECG and apex phonocardiogram in a healthy person. The Doppler transducer was applied to the precordium and the sound beam directed toward the mitral ostium. On the Doppler tracing early rapid diastolic inflow (*DI*) in the left ventricle starts 0.07–0.08 sec after the second heart sound (2). Its maximal amplitude occurs 0.13 sec after *2*, followed by a decrescendo with a duration of approximately 0.15 sec. Consequently, *DI* represents the rapid inflow of blood into the left ventricle. *AS* = atrial systole; *S* = systolic ventricular blood flow. From Edler I, Lindström K: Ultrasonic Doppler technique used in heart disease. II: Clinical application. In Böck J, Ossoinig K (eds): *Proceedings of the First Congress on Ultrasonic Diagnostics in Medicine 1969*. Ultrasono Graphia Medica, Verlag der Wiener Medizinischen Akademie, 1971, p 455.

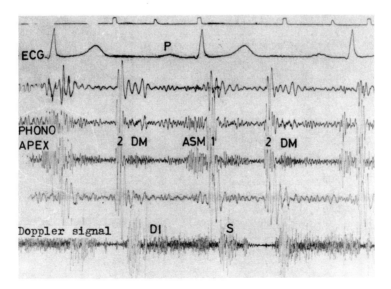

Figure 1.49. Pure mitral stenosis and sinus rhythm. Simultaneous recordings of information as shown in Figure 1.48. The Doppler signal *DI* starts > 0.05 sec after the second heart sound (2) and continues throughout systole. From Edler I, Lindström K: Ultrasonic Doppler technique used in heart disease. II: Clinical application. In Böck J, Ossoinig K (eds): *Proceedings of the First Congress on Ultrasonic Diagnostics in Medicine 1969*. Ultrasono Graphia Medica, Verlag der Wiener Medizinischen Akademie, 1971, p 455.

wave Doppler to examine blood flow in the region of the heart valves (139,140). The transducer was applied to the precordium with the sound beam directed toward the left ventricular outflow tract or the mitral orifice. In this position, regurgitation in the aortic or mitral valve could be demonstrated (Figs. 1.48 to 1.51). Also, Doppler signals in mitral stenosis differed characteristically from normal.

In 1969 Light et al. used continuous Doppler to estimate blood velocity in the aorta (141,142). The transducer was applied to the suprasternal notch with the beam directed toward the aortic notch. In 1974 Boughner used Doppler in aortic valve insufficiency to estimate if flow was directed towards or away from the transducer (143,144).

In 1970 Baker introduced a pulsed ultrasonic Doppler instrument to study velocity in a small range cell (145). In this manner valve areas and velocities in different heart cavities can be studied selectively. Clinically, pulsed Doppler is used to detect and localize stenotic and regurgitant flow

(146,147). Also, intracardiac shunts can be detected. Today, this instrument is combined with a conventional imaging system and a real-time echocardiograph.

In 1976 Holen et al. introduced a Doppler method to estimate pressure drop across a flow obstruction (148,149). Clinical application of this technique was performed by Liv Hatle in Trondheim, Norway (150). Her pioneering work has been of great importance in the advancement of echocardiography (151–154).

In 1982 a new technique was developed for real-time imaging of intracardiac blood flow (155,156). Clinical application of this technique, color flow Doppler echocardiography, was reported by Omoto et al. (157).

When Heinrich Hertz discovered radio waves in 1887, he was asked if the discovery could have any future practical use. "I don't think so," was his response. Perhaps, had they been asked, the Curie brothers' answer would have been the same after their discovery of the piezoelectric effect.

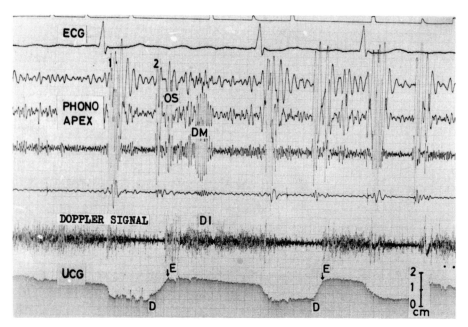

Figure 1.50. Simultaneous recordings as in Figure 1.48 and echocardiogram from the anterior mitral leaflet (*UCG*) in a patient with mitral stenosis and atrial fibrillation. The Doppler detector was applied laterally and below the echocardiographic transducer. The Doppler beam was directed toward the mitral ostium. The Doppler signal *DI* starts at or just before the opening snap (*OS*) on the phonocardiogram and point *E* on the echocardiogram. Doppler signals continue with the same amplitude throughout diastole. From Edler I, Lindström K: Ultrasonic Doppler technique used in heart disease. II: Clinical application. In Böck J, Ossoinig K (eds): *Proceedings of the First Congress on Ultrasonic Diagnostics in Medicine 1969.* Ultrasono Graphia Medica, Verlag der Wiener Medizinischen Akademie, 1971, p 455.

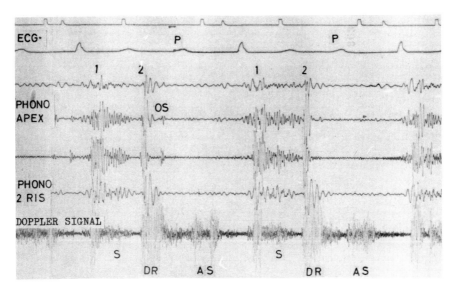

Figure 1.51. Simultaneous recording of Doppler, ECG, apex phonocardiogram, and phonocardiogram from the second right interspace (*phono 2RIS*) in a patient with aortic regurgitation. The Doppler detector was applied laterally to the conventional mitral valve echo recording position, with the sound beam directed to the left ventricular outflow tract. The start of the Doppler signal (*DR*) coincides with the aortic component of the second heart sound and continues over the opening sound (*OS*) on the apex phonocardiogram. This early start was only found in aortic regurgitation and was felt to represent backflow through the aortic ostium. Because of first degree A-V block, the connection between the *P waves* on ECG and *AS* on the Doppler tracing is obvious. From Edler I, Lindström K: Ultrasonic Doppler technique used in heart disease. II: Clinical application. In Böck J, Ossoinig K (eds): *Proceedings of the First Congress on Ultrasonic Diagnostics in Medicine 1969*. Ultrasono Graphia Medica, Verlag der Wiener Medizinischen Akademie, 1971, p 455.

REFERENCES

1. Schober W: *The Lives of Bats*. London, Groom Helm, 1984, pp. 122–137.
2. Richardson MLF: Apparatus for warning a ship for its approach to large objects in a fog. Brit. Patent No. 9423, 1912.
3. Langevin MP: Procédé et appareil d'émission et de réception des ondes élastiques sousmarine à l'aide des propriétés piezoélectrique du quartz. Franz. Patent No. 505703, 1918.
4. Langevin MP, Ishimoto M: Utilisation des phénomenès piezoélectrique pour la measure de l'intensité des sons en valeur absolute. *J Physiol* 4:539–540, 1923.
5. Hehlgans FW: Über Piezoquartzplatten als Sender und Empfänger hochfrequenter akusticher Schwingungen. *Ann Physiol* (Leipzig) 86:587–627, 1928.
6. Langevin MP: Procédé et appareil d'émission et de réception des ondes élastiques sousmarines a l'aide des propriétés piezoélectriques du quartz. Franz, Patent No. 505703, 1918.
7. Wood RW, Loomis AL: Physical and biological effects of high-frequency sound waves of great intensity. *Physiol Rev* 29:373, 1927.
8. Conte E, Delorenzi E: Azioni biologische delgi ultrasuoni. *Atti Congr Radiobiol* 4:195–204, 1940.
9. Pohlman R: Lassen sich durch Ultraschall thera-peutische Wirkungen erzielen? *Forsch Fortschr* 15:187, 1939.
10. Dussik K: Über die Möglichkeit hochfrequente mechanische Schwingungen als diagnostisches Hilfsmittel zu verwenden. *Z Neurol* 174:153, 1942.
11. Dussik K: Ultraschalldiagnostik, insbesondere bei Gehirnerkrankungen, mittels Hyperphonographie. *Z Phys Therapie* (Austria) 1:40, 1948.
12. Ballantine HT Jr, Bolt RH, Hüter TF, Ludwig GD: On the detection of intracranial pathology by ultrasound. *Science* 112:525, 1950.
13. Hüter TF, Bolt BH: An ultrasonic method for outlining the cerebral ventricles. *J Acoust Soc Am* 23:160, 1951.
14. Güttner W, Fiedler G, Pätzold J: Über Ultraschallabbildungen am menschilchen Schädel. *Acoustica* 2:148, 1952.
15. Ballantine HT Jr, Hüter TF, Bolt RH: On use of ultrasound for tumor detection. *J Acoust Soc Am* 26:581, 1954.
16. Denier A: Ultrasonoscope in medicine. Cited by Bergman L in Ballantine HT Jr, Hüter TF, Bolt RH: On use of ultrasound for tumor detection. *J Acoust Soc Am* 26:581, 1954.
17. Denier A: Les ultrasons; leurs applications au di-agnostic: Ultrasonoscopie et à la therapeutique: Ultra-sono-therapie. Cited by: Bergman L in Ballantine HT Jr, Hüter TF, Bolt RH: On use of

ultrasound for tumor detection, *J Acoust Soc Am* 26:581, 1954.

18. Keidel WD: Über eine Methode zur Registrierung der Volmänderungen des Herzens am Menschen. *Z Kreislaufforsch* 39:257, 1950.

19. Firestone FA: Supersonic reflectoscope, an instrument for inspecting interior of solid parts by means of sound waves. *J Acoust Soc Am* 17:287–299, 1945.

20. Gohr H, Widekind TH: Der Ultraschall in der Medizin. *Klin Wochenschr* 19:25, 1940.

21. Sokoloff SJ: Ultraschallwellenmethoden zur Bestimmung innerer Defekte in Metallgegenständern. *Sawodskaja Laboratorija* 4:1468–1473, 1935.

22. Sokoloff SJ: Ultrasonic oscillations and their application. *Technic Physics* (USSR) 2:522–544, 1935.

23. Ludwig GD, Struthers FW: Considerations underlying the use of ultrasound to detect gallstones and foreign bodies in tissue. Project No NM 004 001, Report No 4, United States Naval Medical Research Institute, Bethesda, MD, 1949. Cited by Herrick and Krusen in Nichols HT, Likoff W, Goldberg H, Fuchs M: The genesis of the presystolic murmur in mitral stenosis. *Am Heart J* 52:379, 1956.

24. Ludwig GD: The velocity of sound through tissues and the acoustic impedance of tissues. *J Acoust Soc Am* 22:862, 1950.

25. Wild JJ: The use of ultrasonic pulses for the measurement of biological tissues and the detection of tissue density changes. *Surgery* 27:183, 1950.

26. French LA, Wild JJ, Neal D: Detection of cerebral tumors by ultrasonic pulses: Pilot studies on post mortem material. *Cancer* 3:705, 1950.

27. Wild JJ, Neal D: Use of high frequency ultrasonic waves for detection of changes of texture in living tissues. *Lancet* 260:655, 1951.

28. Wild JJ, Reid JM: Further pilot echocardiographic studies on the histological structure of tumors of living intact human breast. *Am J Pathol* 28:839, 1952.

29. Wild JJ, Reid JM: Application of echo-ranging techniques to the determination of structure of biological tissues. *Science* 115:226, 1952.

30. Howry DH, Stott DA, Bliss WR: The ultrasonic visualization of soft tissue structures of the body. *J Lab Clin Med* 40:579, 1952.

31. Howry DH, Stott DA, Bliss WR: The ultrasonic visualization of carcinoma of the breast and other soft tissue structures. *Cancer* 7:354, 1954.

32. Holmes JH, Howry DH: The ultrasonic visualization of soft tissue structures in the body. *Trans Am Clin Climatol Assoc* 66:208, 1954.

33. Holmes JH, Howry DH: Ultrasonic visualization of edema. *Trans Am Clin Climatol Assoc* 70:235, 1958.

34. Holmes JH, Howry DH: Ultrasonic diagnosis of abdominal diseases. *Am J Dig Dis* 8:12, 1963.

35. Edler I: Ultrasoundcardiogram in Pericardial Effusion: Follow Up of Six Cases. Scientific session, Swedish Society of Internal Medicine, Lund, Sweden, June 4, 1955.

36. Edler I: The diagnostic use of ultrasound in heart diseases. *Acta Med Scand Suppl* 308:32, 1955.

37. Edler I: Ultrasoundcardiogram in mitral valvular diseases. *Acta Chir Scand* 111:230, 1956.

38. Edler I, Hertz CH: Die diagnostische Anwendung von Ultraschallkardiogramm bei Mitralisstenose. Paper read at the IV International Congress on Diseases of the Chest of the American College of Chest Physicians, Köln, 1956.

39. Hertz CH, Edler I: Die Registrierung von Herzwandbewegungen mit Hilfe des Ultraschall-Impulsverfahrens. *Acoustica* 6:361, 1956.

40. Edler I, Gustafson A: Ultrasonic cardiogram in mitral stenosis. *Acta Med Scand* 159:85, 1957.

41. Effert S, Erkens H, Grosse-Brockhoff F: The ultrasonic echo method in cardiological diagnosis. *Ger Med Month* 2:325, 1957.

42. Effert S: Der derzeitlige Stand der Ultraschall-kardiographie. *Arch Kreislaufforsch* 30:213, 1959.

43. Leksell L: Echoencephalography I: Detection of intracranial complications following head injury. *Acta Chir Scand* 110:301, 1955.

44. Leksell L: Echoencephalography II: Midline echo from the pineal body as index of pineal displacement. *Acta Chir Scand* 115:255, 1958.

45. Donald I, MacVicar J, Brown TG: Investigation of abdominal masses by pulsed ultrasound. *Lancet* 1:1188, 1958.

46. Donald I, Brown TG: Demonstration of tissue interfaces within the body by ultrasonic echo sounding. *Br J Radiol* 34:539, 1961.

47. Baum G, Greenwood I: The application of ultrasonic locating techniques to ophthalmology. *Arch Ophthalmol* 60:263, 1958.

48. Baum G, Greenwood I: Ultrasound in ophthalmology. *Am J Ophthalmol* 42:249, 1960.

49. Baum G, Greenwood I: Ultrasonography—An aid in orbital tumor diagnosis. *Arch Ophthalmol* 64:180, 1960.

50. Edler I, Hertz CH: The use of ultrasonic reflectoscope for the continuous recording of movements of heart walls. *Kungl Fysior Sällsk Lund Forhandl* 24:5, 1954.

51. Edler I, Gustafson A, Karlefors T, Christensson B: The movements of aortic and mitral valves recorded with ultrasonic echo techniques. Scientific film presented at the Third European Congress of Cardiology, Rome, September 18–24, 1960.

52. Effert S, Domangi E: The diagnosis of intra-atrial tumour and thrombi by the ultrasonic echo method. *Ger Med Meth* 4:1, 1959.

53. Edler I: Ultrasoundcardiography. Part III: Atrioventricular valve mobility in the living human heart recorded by ultrasound. *Acta Med Scand Suppl* 370:83, 1961.

54. Edler I: The diagnostic use of ultrasound in heart disease. In Kelly E (ed): *Ultrasonic Energy.* Urbana, University of Illinois Press, 1965, p 303.

55. Edler I: Diagnostic ultrasound. In Donald, Levi (eds): Rotterdam, Kooyker Scientific Publications, 1976, p 128.

56. Edler I, Gustafson A, Karlefors T, Christensson B: A dynamic study of the heart valves and ventricular outflow tracts using an ultrasound echo method. Presented at the XXVII Nordisk Kongress for Inre Medicin, Oslo, June 29–July 2, 1960.

57. Edler I. Gustafson A, Karlefors T, Christensson B: Ultrasoundcardiography. Part II: Mitral and aortic valve movements recorded by an ultrasonic

echo-method: An experimental study. *Acta Med Scand Suppl* 370:67, 1961.

58. MacDonald IG: Problems in clinical use of M-mode echocardiography. In Linhart J, Joyner C (eds): *Diagnostic Echocardiography*. CV Mosby, St. Louis, 1982, p 180.

59. Howry DH, Bliss WR: Ultrasonic visualization of soft tissue structures of the body. *J Lab Clin Med* 40:579, 1952.

60. Holmes JH, Howry DH, Posakony GJ, Cushman C: The ultrasonic visualization of soft tissue structures in the human body. *Trans Am Clin Climatol Assoc* 66:208, 1954.

61. Olofsson S: An ultrasonic mirror system. *Acoustica* 13:361, 1963.

62. Hertz CH, Olofsson S: A mirror system for ultrasonic visualization of soft tissues. In Kelly E (ed): Symposium on Ultrasound in Biology and Medicine: Ultrasonic Energy. Chicago, University of Illinois Press, 1962, p 322.

63. Hertz CH: Ultrasonic engineering in heart diagnosis. *Am J Cardiol* 19:6, 1967.

64. Åsberg A: Ultrasonic cinematography of the living heart. *Ultrasonics* 5:113, 1967.

65. Hertz CH, Lindström K: A fast ultrasonic scanning system for heart investigation. Third International Conference on Medical Physics, Gothenburg, Sweden, August 1972.

66. Edler I: Mitral valve function studied by the ultrasound echo method. In Grossman CC, Holmes JH, Joyner C, Purnell EW (eds): *Diagnostic Ultrasound: Proceedings of the First International Conference*. New York, Plenum Press, 1966, p 198.

67. Effert S, Hertz CH, Böhme W: Direkte Registrierung des Ultraschall-Kardiogramms mit dem Elektrokardiographen. *Kreislaufforsch* 48:230, 1959.

68. Dock W: Mode of production of the first sound. *Arch Intern Med* 51:737, 1933.

69. Shearn MA, Tarr E, Rytland DA: The significance of changes in amplitude of the first heart sound in children with A-V block. *Circulation* 7:839, 1953.

70. Nichols HT, Likoff W, Goldberg H, Fuchs M: The genesis of the presystolic murmur in mitral stenosis. *Am Heart J* 52:379, 1956.

71. Lundstrom NR: Reflected ultrasound in the diagnosis of congenital heart disease. In Bock J, Ossoinig K (eds): *Proceedings of the First Congress on Ultrasonic Diagnostics in Medicine 1969*. Ultrasono Graphica Medica, Verlag der Wiener Medizinischem Akademie, 1971, vol III, p 395.

72. Lundstrom NR, Edler I: Ultrasoundcardiography in infants and children. *Acta Paediatr Scand* 60:117, 1971.

73. Effert S, Erkens H, Grossebrockhoff F: Ultrasonic echo method in cardiological diagnosis. *Ger Med Meth* 2:325, 1957.

74. Effert S, Domanig E, Erkens H: Moglichkeiten des Ultraschall-Echoverfahrens in der Herzdiagnostik. *Cardiologica* 34:73, 1959.

75. Effert S: Der derzeitige Stand der Ultraschall-kardiographie. *Arch Kreislaufforsch* 30:213, 1959.

76. Effert S, Domanig E: Diagnostik intraauricularer tumoren und grosser thromben mit dem ultraschall-echoverfahren. *Dtsch Med Wochenschr* 84:6, 1959.

77. Gassler R, Samlert H: Zur Beurteilung des Ultraschallkardiogramms bei Mitralstenosen. *Z Kreislaufforsch* 47:291, 1958.

78. Jacobi J, Gassler R, Samlert H: Neue Ergebnisse mit der Ultraschallkardiographie. *Verh Dtsch Ges Kreislaufforsch* 24:295, 1958.

79. Schmitt W, Braun H: Mitteilungen der mittels ultraschall-kardiographie gewonnen ergebnisse bei mitralvitien und hertzgesunden. *Z Kreislaufforsch* 49:214, 1960.

80. Hsu CC: Ultrasonic diagnostics. *Shang Sci Tech Press* 187, 1961.

81. Hsu CC: Preliminary studies on ultrasonics in cardiological diagnosis: I: Experimental observations on cardiac echo waves. *Acta Academiae Medicinae Primae Shanghai* 2:251–256, 1964.

82. Hsu CC: Preliminary studies on ultrasonics in cardiological diagnosis: II: The use of A-scope ultrasound apparatus in the diagnosis of heart diseases. *Acta Academiae Medicinae Primae Shanghai* 2:335–343, 1964.

83. Hsu CC: The application of an ultrasonic brilliance-modulation scanner in the study of ultrasonic cardiogram. *Acta Acoustica Sinica* 1:95–96, 1964.

84. Hsu CC: Ultrasound cardiogram in the diagnosis of mitral stenosis. *Chinese Med J* 84:475–481, 1965.

85. Hsu CC: Ultrasonic diagnosis of heart disease. In Hsu CC: *Ultrasonic Diagnostics*, 3rd ed. Shanghai, Science and Technology Press, 1978, pp 88–119.

86. White DN: Ultrasound for medical diagnosis in the provinces of Hopei, Shantung, Kiangsu and Shanghai in The People's Republic of China. *Ultrasound Med Biol* 6:87–91, 1980.

87. Joyner CR, Reid JM, Bond JP: Reflected ultrasound in the assessment of mitral valve disease. *Circulation* 27:506, 1963.

88. Joyner CR, Reid JM: Application of ultrasound in cardiology and cardiovascular physiology. *Prog Cardiovasc Dis* 5:482, 1963.

89. Joyner CR, Reid JM: Ultrasound cardiogram in the selection of patients for mitral valve surgery. *Ann NY Acad Sci* 118:512, 1965.

90. Hertz CH, Edler I: Die registrierung von herzwandbewegungen mit hilfe des ultraschall-impulsverfahrens. *Acoustica* 6:361, 1956.

91. Gustafson A: Ultrasound cardiography in mitral stenosis. *Acta Med Scand* 461:82, 1966.

92. Segal BL, Likoff W, Kingsley B: Echocardiography: Clinical application in mitral stenosis. *JAMA* 193:161, 1966.

93. Gustafson A: Correlation between ultrasound-cardiography, haemodynamics and surgical findings in mitral stenosis. *Am J Cardiol* 19:32, 1967.

94. Edler I: Ultrasoundcardiography in mitral valve stenosis. *Am J Cardiol* 19:18, 1967.

95. Effert S: Pre- and post-operative evaluation of mitral stenosis by ultrasound. *Am J Cardiol* 19:59, 1967.

96. Duchak JM, Chang S, Feigenbaum H: The posterior mitral valve echo and the echocardiographic diagnosis of mitral stenosis. *Am J Cardiol* 29:628, 1972.

97. Cope GD, Kisslo JA, Johnson ML, Behar VS: A

reassessment of the echocardiogram in mitral stenosis. *Circulation* 52:664, 1975.

98. Nichol PM, Gilbert BW, Kisslo JA: Two-dimensional echo-cardiographic assessment of mitral stenosis. *Circulation* 55:120, 1977.

99. Henry WL, Kastl DG: Echocardiographic evaluation of patients with mitral stenosis. *Am J Med* 62:813, 1977.

100. Feigenbaum H, Waldhausen JA, Hyde LP: Ultrasound diagnosis of pericardial effusion. *JAMA* 191:107, 1965.

101. Feigenbaum H, Zaky A, Waldhausen JA: Use of ultrasound in the diagnosis of pericardial effusion. *Ann Intern Med* 65:443, 1966.

102. Feigenbaum H, Zaky A, Waldhausen JA: Use of reflected ultrasound in detecting pericardial effusion. *Am J Cardiol* 19:84, 1967.

103. Rothman J, et al.: Ultrasonic diagnosis of pericardial effusion. *Circulation* 35:358, 1967.

104. Pate JW, Gardner HC, Norman RS: Diagnosis of pericardial effusion by echocardiography. *Ann Surg* 165:826, 1967.

105. Goldberg BB, Ostrum BJ, Isard JJ: Ultrasonic determination of pericardial effusion. *JAMA* 202:103, 1967.

106. Klein JJ, Segal BL: Pericardial effusion diagnosed by reflected ultrasound. *Am J Cardiol* 22:57, 1968.

107. Feigenbaum H, Popp RL, Chip JN, Haine CL: Left ventricular wall thickness measured by ultrasound. *Arch Intern Med* 121:391, 1968.

108. Feigenbaum H, Wolfe SB, Popp RL, Haine CL, Dodge HT: Correlation of ultrasound with angiocardiography in measuring left ventricular diastolic volume (Abstr). *Am J Cardiol* 23:111, 1969.

109. Popp RL, Wolfe SB, Hirata T, Feigenbaum H: Estimation of right and left ventricular size by ultrasound: A study of the echoes from the interventricular septum. *Am J Cardiol* 24:523, 1969.

110. Feigenbaum H, Zaky A, Nasser WK: Use of ultrasound to measure left ventricular stoke volume. *Circulation* 35:1092, 1967.

111. Popp RL, Harrison DC: Ultrasonic cardiac echocardiography for determining stroke volume and valvular regurgitation. *Circulation* 41:493, 1970.

112. Feigenbaum H, et al.: Ultrasound measurements of the left ventricle: a correlative study with angiocardiography. *Arch Intern Med* 129:461, 1972.

113. Popp RL, Harrison DC: Ultrasound in the diagnosis and evaluation of therapy of idiopathic hypertrophic subaortic stenosis. *Circulation* 40:905, 1969.

114. Shah PM, Gramiak R, Adelman AG, Wigle ED: Role of echocardiography in diagnostic and hemodynamic assessment of hypertrophic subaortic stenosis. *Circulation* 44:891, 1971.

115. Winsberg F, Gabor GE, Hemberg JG: Fluttering of the mitral valve in aortic insufficiency. *Circulation* 41:225, 1970.

116. Dillon JC, Haine CL, Chang S, Feigenbaum H: Use of echocardiography in patients with prolapsed mitral valve. *Circulation* 43:503, 1971.

117. Gramiak R, Shah PM, Kramer DH: Ultrasound cardiography: Contrast studies in anatomy and function. *Radiology* 92:939, 1969.

118. Joyner CR: Cardiovascular conference: Ultrasound in cardiovascular diagnosis. Scientific sessions, American Heart Association, San Francisco, October 21, 1967.

119. Ebina T, Oka S, Tanaka M, Kosaka S, Teresawa Y, Unno K, Kikuchi D, Uchida R: The ultrasonotomography of the heart and great vessels in living human subjects by means of the ultrasonic reflection technique. *Jpn Heart J* 8:331, 1967.

120. King DL: Cardiac ultrasonography: Cross-sectional ultrasonic imaging of the heart. *Circulation* 47:843, 1973.

121. King DL, Steeg CN, Ellis K: Demonstration of transposition of the great arteries by cardiac ultrasonography. *Radiology* 107:181, 1973.

122. King DL, Steeg CN, Ellis K: Visualization of ventricular septal defects by cardiac ultrasonography. *Circulation* 48:1215, 1973.

123. King JF, DeMaria AN, Reis RL, Bolton MR, Dunn MI, Mason DT: Echocardiographic assessment of idiopathic hypertrophic subaortic stenosis. *Chest* 64:723, 1973.

124. King JF, DeMaria AN, Miller RR, Hilliard GK, Zelis R, Mason DT: Markedly abnormal mitral valve motion without simultaneous intraventricular pressure gradient due to uneven mitral-septal contact in idiopathic hypertrophic subaortic stenosis. *Am J Cardiol* 34:360, 1974.

125. Gramiak R, Waag R, Simon W: Cine ultrasound cardiography. *Radiology* 107:175, 1973.

126. Bom N, Lancee CT, Honkoop J, Hugenholtz PG: Ultrasonic viewer for cross-sectional analyses of moving cardiac structures. *Biomed Eng* 6:500, 1973.

127. Bom N, Lancee CT, VanZweiten G, Kloster FE, Roelandt J: Multiscan echocardiography. I. Technical description. *Circulation* 48:1066, 1973.

128. Bom N, Hugenholtz PG, Kloster FE, Roelandt J, Popp RL, Pridie RB, Sahn DJ: Evaluation of structure recognition with the multiscan echocardiograph: A cooperative study in 580 patients. *Ultrasound Med Biol* 1:243, 1974.

129. Griffith JM, Henry WL, Epstein SE: Real time two-dimensional echocardiography (Abstr). *Circulation* 48:124, 1973.

130. Griffith JM, Henry WL: A sector scanner for real time two-dimensional echocardiography. *Circulation* 49:1147, 1974.

131. Von Ramm OT, Thurstone FL: Cardiac imaging using a phased array ultrasound system. *Circulation* 53:258, 1976.

132. Satomura S: A study on examining the heart with ultrasonics: I principle; II instrument. *Jpn Circ J* 20:227, 1956.

133. Yoshida T, Mori M, Nimura Y, Okimura M, Hikita G, Nakanishi K, Satomura S: Study on examining the heart with ultrasonics: III Kinds of Doppler beats; IV Clinical application. *Jpn Circ J* 20:228, 1956.

134. Satomura S: Ultrasonic Doppler method for the inspection of cardiac functions. *J Acoust Soc Am* 29:1181, 1957.

135. Yoshida T, Mori M, Nimura Y, Hikita G, Takagisha S, Nakanischi K, Satomura S: Analysis of heart motion with ultrasonic Doppler method and its clinical application. *Am Heart J* 61:61, 1961.

136. Kostis JB, Fleishmann D, Bellet S: Use of the

ultrasonic Doppler method for the timing of valvular movement. *Circulation* 40:197, 1969.

137. Franklin DL, Schlegel W, Rushmer RF: Blood flow measured by Doppler frequency shift of backscattered ultrasound. *Science* 134:564, 1961.

138. Franklin DL, Watson NW, Pierson KE, van Citters RL: Technique for radiotelemetry of blood flow from unrestrained animals. *Am J Med Electron* (New York) 5:24, 1966.

139. Lindström K, Edler I: Ultrasonic Doppler technique used in heart disease: An experimental study. In Böck J, Ossoinig K (eds): *Proceedings of the First Congress on Ultrasonic Diagnostics in Medicine 1969.* Ultrasono Graphia Medica, Verlag der Wiener Medizinischen Akademie, 1971, p 447.

140. Edler I, Lindström K: Ultrasonic Doppler technique used in heart disease: II: Clinical application. In Böck J, Ossoinig K (eds): *Proceedings of the First Congress on Ultrasonic Diagnostics in Medicine 1969.* Ultrasono Graphia Medica, Verlag der Wiener Medizinischen Akademie, 1971, p 455.

141. Light LH: Transcutaneous observation of blood velocity in the ascending aorta in man. *Biol Cardiol* 26:214, 1969.

142. Light LH, Gross G, Hansen PL: Non-invasive measurement of blood velocity in the major thoracic vessels. *Proc R Soc Med* 67:142, 1974.

143. Boughner DR: Aortic insufficiency assessed by transcutaneous Doppler ultrasound (Abstr). *Circulation* 50:144, 1974.

144. Boughner DR: Assessment of aortic insufficiency assessed by transcutaneous Doppler ultrasound. *Circulation* 52:874, 1975.

145. Baker DW: Pulsed ultrasonic Doppler blood-flow sensing. *IEEE Trans Sonics Ultrasonics*, Su-17, no 3, July, 1970.

146. Johnson SL, Baker DW, Lute RA, Dodge HT: Doppler echocardiography: The localization of cardiac murmurs. *Circulation* 48:810, 1973.

147. Baker DW, Johnson SL: Doppler echocardiography. In Gramiak R (Ed): *Cardiac Ultrasound.* CV Mosby, St Louis, 1975, p 264.

148. Holen J, Aaslid R, Landmark K, Simonsen S: Determination of pressure gradient in mitral stenosis with a non-invasive ultrasound Doppler technique. *Acta Med Scand* 199:455, 1976.

149. Holen J, Aaslid R, Landmark K, Simonsen S, Östrem T: Determination of effective orifice area in mitral stenosis from non-invasive ultrasound Doppler data and mitral flow rate. *Acta Med Scand* 201:83, 1977.

150. Brubakk AO, Angelsen BAJ, Hatle L: Diagnosis of valvular heart disease using transcutaneous Doppler ultrasound. *Cardiovasc Res* 11:461, 1977.

151. Hatle L, Brubakk A, Tromsdal A, Angelsen B: Non-invasive assessment of pressure drop in mitral stenosis by Doppler ultrasound. *Br Heart J* 40:131, 1978.

152. Hatle L, Brubakk A, Tromsdal A: Non-invasive assessment of aortic stenosis by Doppler ultrasound. *Br Heart J* 43:284, 1980.

153. Skjaerpe T, Hatle L: Diagnosis and assessment of tricuspid regurgitation with Doppler ultrasound. Proceedings of Fourth Symposium on Echocardiography, Rotterdam, The Hague, Martinus Nijhoff, 1981.

154. Hatle L, Rokseth R: Non-invasive diagnosis and assessment of ventricular septum defect by Doppler ultrasound. *Acta Med Scand* 645:47, 1981.

155. Namekawa K, Kasai C, Tsukamoto M, Koyano A: Imaging of blood flow using autocorrelation. *Ultrasound Med Biol* 8:138, 1982.

156. Bommer W, Miller L: Real-time two-dimensional color-flow Doppler: Enhanced Doppler flow imaging in the diagnosis of cardiovascular disease (Abstr). *Am J Cardiol* 49:944, 1982.

157. Omoto R, Yokote Y, Takamoto S, Tamura F, Asano H, Namekawa K, Kasai C, Tsukamoto M, Koyano A: Clinical significance of newly-developed real-time intracardiac two-dimensional blood flow imaging system (2-D Doppler). *Jpn Circ J* 47:974, 1983.

2

Cardiac Ultrasound: Physical Principles and Instrumentation

Mark Durell

THE PHYSICS OF ULTRASOUND

Extraordinary high frequencies are needed to resolve small structures within the body. Consequently, diagnostic ultrasound is generally in the range of 2 to 12 million cycles/sec (megahertz).

The characteristics of ultrasound can be understood better by applying a familiar and simple mathematical model. Figure 2.1 shows a typical sine wave: periodic in nature, it appears as a series of hills and valleys. When applied to ultrasound, the peaks and valleys represent compression and rarefaction of air, tissue, or any other medium as sound energy passes through it.

The vertical distance from the peak (A) to the baseline represents the amplitude or energy level of the sound wave. Amplitude is described in relative rather than absolute terms. The strength of the sound wave is measured in decibels according to the formula

$$db = 20 \log y/x, \tag{2.1}$$

where x is the sound amplitude at one point and y is the amplitude at another.

If y is 10 times stronger than x, it is said to be 20 db above x. A factor of 1000 yields a difference of 60 db. The strength of signals returning from strong mirror-like tissue reflectors such as the pericardium can differ in amplitude by more than 100 db compared to the weak back-scatter from blood cells. Consequently, ultrasound instruments must be able to process a wide range of intensities. This characteristic is referred to as the system's dynamic range.

The distance from B to C is one complete cycle and is described as the wavelength ‡ 1. The wavelength of sound is derived from the formula

$$f = c/l \tag{2.2}$$

where c is the speed of sound in tissue—about 1540 meters/sec.

For audible sound, frequency is equivalent to the tone or pitch we hear. Mathematically, frequency is the number of complete cycles occurring each second. Higher frequency sound has shorter wavelengths and therefore better axial or depth resolution. The shorter the wave or cycle lengths, the better two objects can be resolved in depth (Fig. 2.2).

In nature, single frequency sound waves rarely occur. Most sound waves are a rich combination of individual frequencies. Musical tones are produced by frequencies combined according to the principles of harmonics to form chords. In diagnostic ultrasound, single frequencies are used to describe the characteristics of an emitted sound wave from a transducer. However, the actual emitted signal is composed of a broad range of frequencies (Fig. 2.3).

Single frequency sine waves can be combined to form new waves of varying shapes and frequencies. Phase relationships and destructive and constructive interference among the added waves help determine the outcome of a summation of sine wave components. For example, the sum of the addition of two waves 90° out of phase is zero because of destructive interference (Fig. 2.4). That is, the negative part of one signal cancels the positive part of the second wave.

When two waves are in phase, constructive interference occurs (Fig. 2.5). A square wave, with sharp edges, is created by the addition of high frequency harmonics or multiples of a fundamental base frequency (Fig. 2.6).

The advantage of these sine wave graphics is that they can be described and manipulated mathematically. The sine curve is generated by the familiar sine function. A cosine curve is simply a

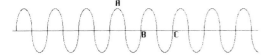

Figure 2.1. A typical sine wave. The distance from the baseline to *A* is amplitude and the distance between *B* and *C* is the cycle length.

sine curve phase shifted 90°. Furthermore, any shape can be described by a unique set of sine wave components with a technique called Fourier analysis. For example, the Fourier analysis of a square wave is a sine wave with the same frequency as the square wave plus an infinite set of sine wave harmonics (Fig. 2.6).

THE SOURCE OF ULTRASOUND

An electrical voltage applied to a piezoelectric element, such as ceramic, will create vibrations. These vibrations create mechanical waves that pass into a coupled medium. While the ceramic can be struck with a single high voltage spike, the emitted sound will have a frequency determined by the resonant characteristics of the element itself. The principles governing resonant characteristics of ultrasound ceramics are the same as for tuning forks, which produce a very narrow band of frequencies symmetrically distributed around the resonant frequency of the fork.

The frequency band produced by ultrasound ceramics is generally broad and the center resonant frequency is determined by the thickness of the ceramic chosen. Higher frequencies require thinner ceramics. Resonance is determined actually by reverberating sound within the element. The thickness of the element determines which waves will add or produce constructive interference. The frequency for which the addition is maximized is the resonant frequency of the transducer.

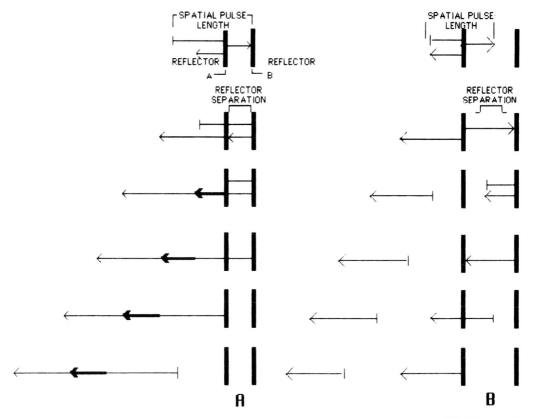

Figure 2.2. *A,* Two reflectors are separated by a distance less than a single pulse width. As a result, echoes from the two structures merge and only a single target will be displayed. *B,* The distance between reflectors is greater than one pulse width. Consequently, two discrete echoes will be detected.

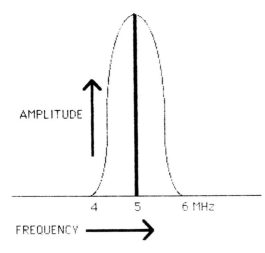

Figure 2.3. The range of frequencies transmitted by a typical ultrasound transducer is graphically displayed. The *bold center line* represents the frequency used to characterize the probe (5 MHz).

Engineers make the simplifying assumption that waves emanate from an infinite number of point sources on the face of the ceramic. This can be visualized as a wave front moving in all directions from the source, similar to ripples created by dropping a stone into water (Fig. 2.7). In reality, the wave front is a three-dimensional sphere surrounding the point source. However, the damping characteristics of the probe ceramic backing material and the transmit focal characteristics of the transducer ensure that most of the sound energy is produced along the desired line propagation. The spacing of point sources and the phase relationships among emitted sound waves are ma-

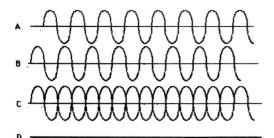

Figure 2.4. An example of destructive interference. *A* and *B* represent sine waves 90° out of phase, cancelling each other. When *A* is positive (above the baseline), *B* is negative and vice versa. The net outcome, *D*, is the sum of *B* and *C*.

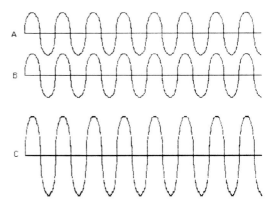

Figure 2.5. An example of constructive interference. Sine waves *A* and *B* are in phase, so their amplitudes are additive (shown in *C*).

nipulated to control the direction of sound energy propagation.

In a fixed focus single element probe, the transmit focal zone and focal length are determined by the transducer aperture size and the radius of curvature of the ceramic or focusing lens (Fig. 2.8). In general, all points on the face of the element are geometrically equidistant from the focal point. The probe frequency and damping characteristics determine axial resolution. Lateral resolution, which is rarely as good as axial resolution, is determined by transducer focal characteristics.

Axial resolution is the system's capability to resolve objects close together in depth. Lateral resolution is the system's ability to resolve two objects which are side by side in the imaging plane (Fig. 2.9).

Lateral resolution is directly related to the narrowness of the transmitted ultrasound beam and the ability of the system to bring the returning signals into focus. These focal characteristics are usually determined by the system probe, electronics, and frequency used. Higher frequencies produce better axial resolution, as well as tighter beam patterns, and therefore, higher lateral resolution.

Recently, phased array technologies have exploited the physical characteristics of ultrasound and innovations in electronics to improve image quality. A typical phased array beam pattern uses phased delays and resulting constructive and destructive interference to propagate a wave in a chosen direction and focus it in depth (Fig. 2.10). This process is often referred to as electronic

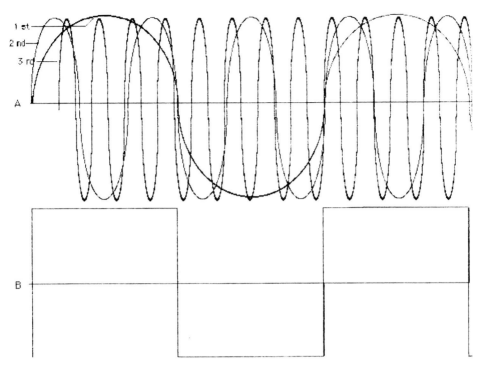

Figure 2.6. A square wave is created by the combination of a base frequency and an infinite series of sine waves in phase. Each successive sine wave is three times the frequency of its predecessor.

steering. These systems use from 48 to 128 elements, or controllable point sources, to create the wave front. Each element can be tied to an independent transmitter and receiver.

These transceivers are programmed to produce small delays on transmission and reception in order to manipulate the ultrasound beam patterns. For cardiology, the number of elements is limited by constraints on aperture size due to tight rib spacing. Elements cannot be made arbitrarily small because of the difficulty in cutting the ceramic.

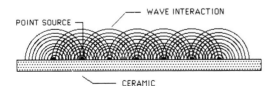

Figure 2.7. The face of a transducer can be modeled as an infinite number of point sources of sound. Sound waves emanate from each point and interact to create a wave front. The characteristics of the wave front depend upon the phase relationships between the emitted waves and the resulting constructive and destructive interference.

Also, a spacing of one-half the emitted wavelength keeps artifacts at a minimum.

A final method for multielement phased array probes involves varying the aperture size by firing the center elements only. This has the potential to improve lateral resolution in the near field. A limitation of phased array technology is that the beam can only be controlled in the lateral plane. In the azimuthal, or z axis, a single focus is predetermined by the placement of an acoustic lens over the ceramic as well as by the length of the elements chosen.

Some manufacturers have divided the imaging elements into rings (Fig. 2.11). This simple arrangement is one way of manipulating the beam focus for enhanced lateral resolution in the near field. With a slightly more sophisticated approach, we could fire both rings but delay the firing of the outer ring. This would have the net effect of flattening the element electronically and extending the focal length even further. A maximum of five to nine rings is practical for cardiac work so that aperture sizes can be kept small. These multiple rings become controllable point sources for focusing the transmit beam. The ad-

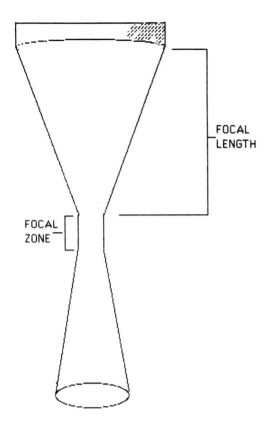

Figure 2.8. Sound emitted from the center of the element lags behind those emitted from the edges. This phase difference produces a waveform with a discrete focal point.

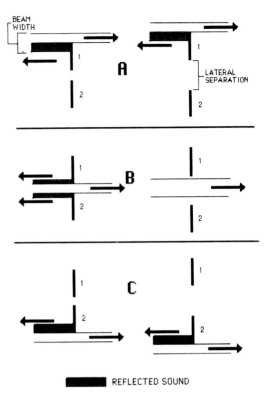

Figure 2.9. Comparing panels, the distance between *targets 1* and *2* is greater in the example on the *right*. In the *right panel*, the distance is greater than the ultrasound beam width. Consequently, the targets will be differentiated. Conversely, the targets on the *left* will not be differentiated since the width between them is less than a single beam width.

vantage is that focusing can be accomplished in all planes. However, the limited number of rings, or electronically controllable elements, does not allow adequate steering of the ultrasound beam. Consequently, the annular array must be moved mechanically through a sector.

THE RETURNING SOUND

Many of the same principles that govern sound transmission apply to the reception of sound as well. A returning echo can be considered to come from a single point source within the body. Sound energy returning from the source will make contact with different parts of the transducer element at different times. A delay circuit holds a returning echo so that it appears to arrive in phase with other echoes, bringing the source of the sound into focus (Fig. 2.12). This can be accomplished by either phased array or annular array technology. Phased array systems, with their larger num-

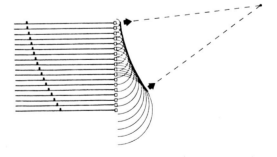

Figure 2.10. Multielement phased array transducers allow complex delay patterns that can produce steered wave fronts focused at any point. In this diagram the lower element is fired first, followed in succession by adjacent elements. This produces steering and focusing of the wave fronts.

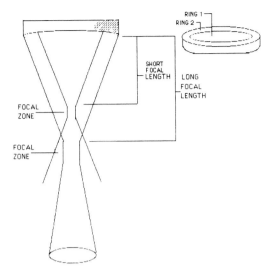

Figure 2.11. Focal points of this transducer will differ, depending on the total transducer aperture. Firing the center ring only will produce a short focal length. Firing both rings together will move the focal length deeper into the body.

ber of channels (48–128) have an advantage over annular arrays, which generally have no more than five to nine channels. A larger number of elements and channels can approximate ideal lenses and produce improved focal characteristics in the lateral plane during the receive cycle (Fig. 2.13).

Transmission of ultrasound occurs in a single instant, with a single pulse, and only one set of delays can be used to determine the direction and focus of the sound energy. On the other hand, detection of returning echoes occurs over a relatively long interval—usually the interval between successive pulses. Since electronics can operate at high speeds and sound moves relatively slowly, the data set or predetermined delays can be changed several times in each receive cycle. This ensures a consistent receive focus throughout the image. The technique is called dynamic focus and is available on several commercial annular and phased array instruments. Using this technique, phased arrays can achieve higher resolution in the lateral plane than annular array systems because of the larger number of elements. On the other hand, annular arrays can achieve equal focal characteristics in both the lateral and azimuthal planes (Fig. 2.14).

In phased and annular array scanning, a high percentage of the sound energy is found at the center of the beam profile. Side lobes of energy also are generated laterally as a result of complexity of the wave front interaction at the ceramic face on transmit. Returning echoes produced by these side lobes are considered artifact and are usually more prevalent on phased array instruments (Fig. 2.15). Side lobes can be eliminated by narrowing the dynamic range of the

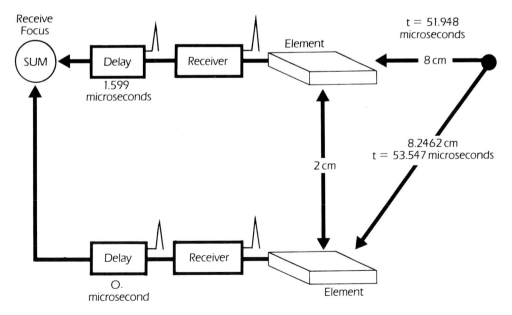

Figure 2.12. Returning signals can be held in delay circuits to bring targets into focus. The echo from a target at an 8-cm depth is held in a delay circuit and later summed with the output of the lower channel.

EFFECT OF NUMBER OF CHANNELS

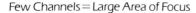

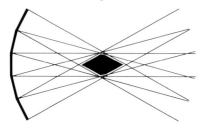

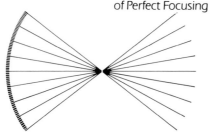

Figure 2.13. An ideal lens is continuously curved. The greater the number of elements and channels used to reconstruct an image, the closer a transducer approximates a perfect lens and the greater the lateral resolution at any point within the image.

displayed image, but this might be at the cost of losing low level anatomic echoes. The problem can also be minimized through additional beam manipulation. One technique for accomplishing this, called apodization, reduces the amplitude of

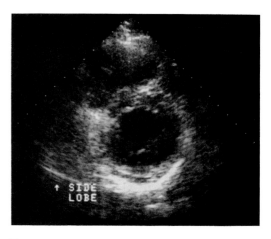

Figure 2.15. The streak-like artifact, called side lobing (*arrow*), is often seen adjacent to bright reflectors. Side lobes exist everywhere in phased array images, but normally go undetected.

the received sound at the outer edges of the array (Fig. 2.16).

Again, as with ultrasound transmission, focus in the azimuthal plane can only be achieved in the receive mode with annular array technology. It is still uncertain which technology will have the advantage in cardiac imaging. Phased array has more controllable point sources for better beam formation in the lateral plane. Phased array probes, having no moving parts, are also easier to handle and are more reliable. The advantage of annular arrays is the ability to focus in all planes, but lateral resolution does not approach that of large multi-channel phased arrays. It is therefore important to note that annular array approaches can

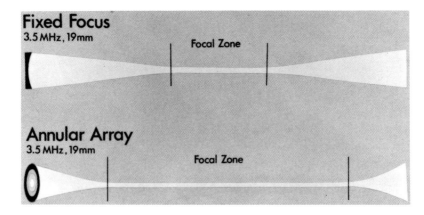

Figure 2.14. Annular array technology allows improved focal characteristics in both the lateral and azimuthal planes by varying the receive delays among the concentric rings.

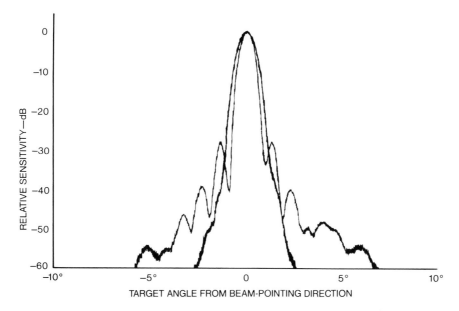

Figure 2.16. The two *curves* represent the amplitude of echoes produced by targets to the left and right of a centered beam. The wider curve indicates that ghost images from these lateral targets will be prominent. The *center narrow curve* shows that apodization signficantly reduces the side lobe response.

only offer azimuthal resolution equal to the lateral resolution obtainable with the concentric ring approach.

Enhancements in lateral resolution have produced the most dramatic improvements in image quality. Azimuthal resolution appears to be a second-order effect. The gains produced by high lateral resolution include improved detail resolution and through apodization, the ability to extend dynamic range and detect subtle differences in tissue texture, sometimes referred to as contrast resolution.

SIGNAL PROCESSING

Considerations for receiver designs are very similar for both single channel mechanical scanners and multichannel phased and annular arrays. Of primary importance is dynamic range. Wide dynamic range receivers have the advantage of being able to detect both strong specular reflections and weak scattered echoes. This is especially useful in the heart, where returns can vary as much as 60 db. Some compression of the echoes can be performed prior to detection by the receivers, reducing demands on receiver design and cost.

A second consideration for receivers is the choice between wide band and narrow band tuning. Both transducer and receiver design determine the system bandwidth. Specifications for system and transducer frequencies usually refer to a center frequency in a range (Fig. 2.3). Also, a broad range of frequencies return from the body. Wide bandwidth systems have the advantage of higher resolving power. Figure 2.6 shows how the sharp edges of a square wave could be reconstructed from a broad range of frequencies, including the base frequency and a series of high frequency harmonics. If the system does not transmit or receive these higher frequencies, the sharp edges, akin to resolution in imaging, cannot be reconstructed.

A short burst of sound, constructed with a broad range of frequencies, is needed to enhance axial resolution (Fig. 2.17). An ideal pulse would look like the square wave in Figure 2.6, with no trailing edges. To generate and detect this shape would require a system bandwidth that included an infinite series of high frequency harmonics. The disadvantage of wide band systems is that they are more sensitive to high frequency systemic noise and therefore limit the dynamic range of the instrument.

The longer bursts used, for example, in Doppler ultrasound, have a narrower spectrum (Fig. 2.17). An infinitely long burst would have a single

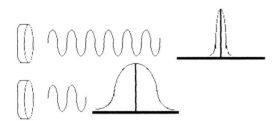

Figure 2.17. Short bursts of transmitted ultrasound require broad band probes (*bottom panel*). An elongated wave contains a narrow band of frequencies in its bandwidth.

frequency spectrum. However, the high resolution required for imaging is not required for Doppler scanning. Therefore, narrow band signal transmission and reception are used to reduce system noise and increase sensitivity. This is necessary to detect the weak Doppler signals.

The most versatile systems operate in both modes and optimize transmission and reception for either Doppler or imaging. Switching between wide and narrow band operation can be achieved electronically or, in part, by changing from wide band to narrow band transducers with different damping characteristics. Dedicated Doppler probes, for example, may be air-backed and have very poor damping characteristics to produce very narrow band operation.

Up to this point the same considerations for beam trasmission and reception apply to both Doppler scanning and anatomical imaging, although less focusing is required during the transmit and receive cycle for Doppler. However, early in the receive signal processing chain the requirements for Doppler and imaging diverge. Information requirements are very different because only amplitude data are needed for imaging, while Doppler analysis requires both amplitude and phase or frequency information.

TWO-DIMENSIONAL SIGNAL PROCESSING

Most manufacturers take the same approach to signal processing of imaging data. There appears to have been very little recent innovation resulting in improved diagnostic quality of images. In signal processing, only the amplitude is of any importance, so the detected waveforms are rectified and enveloped (Fig. 2.18). A variety of manipulations can be performed which might have the net effect of enhancing or suppressing edges. These enveloped samples are taken at a rapid rate but the number rarely exceeds the available number of pixels in the scan converter display.

SCAN CONVERSION

Scan conversion changes data from one form to another. Amplitude imaging data derived from individual scan lines can be described by polar coordinate systems (Fig. 2.19). Hundreds of data points are written on each line. The scan converter transforms the original polar data into a horizontal televison format.

The conversion process usually requires that the polar data be digitized. However, problems arise from this process. Large gaps can exist between data points, especially in the far field. This can create discontinuities in the displayed image. Moreover, this problem is exaggerated in color

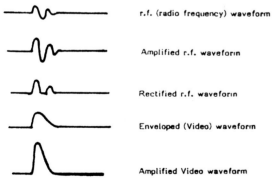

Figure 2.18. An example of how returning ultrasound is analyzed for amplitude information. Returning waves are amplified, rectified, and enveloped. As a result, all phase information is lost and only the amplitude is perceived.

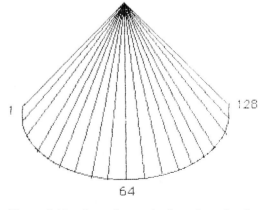

Figure 2.19. A cardiac sector format can be described by a polar coordinate pattern. Each line in the polar system represents an imaging scan line; this example contains 128 scan lines.

flow mapping where line densities may be low. Also data rates can be very rapid, putting demands on the conversion time. This is true for a technique called parallel processing, where line densities are doubled.

Cardiology imaging uses a scan converter in a characteristic way. A stick or line of data is read into a rectilinear memory plane and digitized at a rate which allows for a maximum of 512 samples/line (Fig. 2.20). Lines are read in at a variable rate depending on their location within the sector. The total number of lines formed in this rectilinear plane is equal to the number of lines in the sector image. The data are then read out horizontally and synchronized to the horizontal television rasters or scan lines.

Prior to display, each horizontal line can be placed in an interpolation buffer across 256 or 512 pixels. Since only a maximum of 100 or 120 samples—the number of lines in the sector—may be available, the unfilled pixels can be filled with an average value created by a predetermined interpolation scheme. Less information is required at the apex of the sector. In this case, only the data from the center portion of the memory are used.

The interpolated line is then sent to the television for display. This filling process prevents holes from appearing in the image where a filling scheme has not been used (Fig. 2.21). Holes appear in the far field where the separation between the sector lines is greatest.

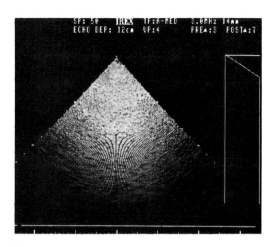

Figure 2.21. An image produced with the scan converter interpolation circuit disengaged. Note the far field dropout of information.

The pixel filling process described above is generally referred to as horizontal filling (Fig. 2.22). Although no holes are seen in the image, there is still a noticeable blockiness, most apparent in the far field. This problem becomes even more pronounced in displays of color flow mapping images, where the line densities can be reduced to less than 50 in a 90° sector image.

In order to improve the smoothness and apparent image quality in two-dimensional displays, manufacturers have developed alternative and more complex techniques for scan conversion and pixel filling. Rather than filling on a horizontal, it is possible to fill on an arc. During horizontal

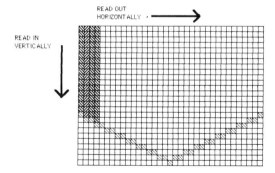

Figure 2.20. An illustration of how each line from the polar coordinate system is read into the rectilinear scan converter plane. Lines are read in vertically from *left* to *right*. Lines in the *center* are expanded over the full length of the plane, and those on the *sides* are compressed. The variable read-in rate insures proper alignment of pixels when converted to television raster lines.

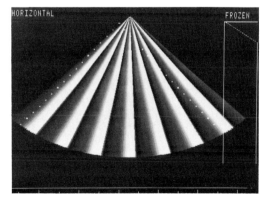

Figure 2.22. Illustration of a simple horizontal pixel filling scheme. Note the blockiness of the test pattern in the far field.

filling, interpolated samples are selected from adjacent points on the television display. In arc filling, adjacent samples are selected along a predetermined curved line (Fig. 2.23). Some blockiness still remains overall but the image is smoother.

The most advanced type of commercially available sector scan conversion is referred to as bilinear. Each pixel is the average of four or more neighboring samples from the polar sector line. No digitization is observed, even in the far field (Fig. 2.24). When bilinear scan conversion is applied to a 50-line image, there is dramatic evidence of the value of this technique (Fig. 2.25).

Another key feature of scan converters used for cardiac applications is time resolution. Displays of cardiac anatomy and blood flow change rapidly, so the scan conversion process must operate in a manner compatible with these rates of change. Two methods are commonly employed to handle rapid data update. The first is a "single plane" scan converter, which displays the image continuously as the image data fill the display in a rotary fashion. With very high frame rates (25 or 30 frames/sec), the eye does not detect this process. As frame rates drop, it appears as if a windshield wiper is moving across the sector.

With the second type, or "dual plane" converter, one complete image is displayed continuously in a memory plane while the second plane is being filled with new data. Here there is no wiper effect, but the presentation of images can appear jarring or discontinuous at very low frame rates (7.5 or 10 frames/sec). The advantage of the single plane system is that it is less expensive because it requires less memory and any frame

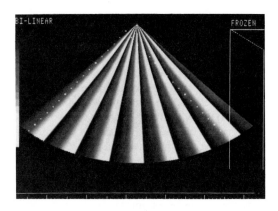

Figure 2.24. The far field has been smoothed by a complex filling algorithm that interpolates data from points surrounding the filled pixel.

rate can be utilized. On the other hand, the dual plane system must operate at predetermined rates such as 15, 20, and 30 frames/sec.

The major disadvantage of the single plane system is that a frozen image may contain data which are discontinuous in time. This is usually not a problem in general anatomical imaging. The frame rates are fast, and any discontinuity in a valve or a wall will be easy to detect. However, in color flow mapping, where frame rates can be slow, the discontinuities are more common. Consequently, juxtaposition of color data between one part of the cardiac cycle and another could be hard to differentiate from similar patterns caused by disease.

Manufacturers can eliminate this problem by completing the filling of the sector image after a

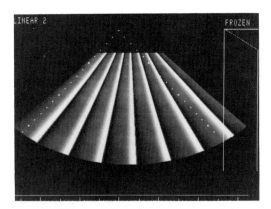

Figure 2.23. Filling pixels in along an arc reduces blockiness.

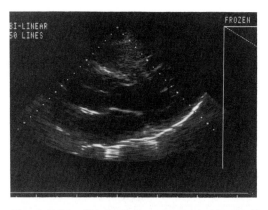

Figure 2.25. This image was created with only 50 scan lines and a bilinear filling technique. There is no evidence of filling or blockiness in the far field.

freeze button is pressed. However, the artifact will still appear on still frames from videotape.

ZOOM OR EXPAND FEATURES

Several systems now allow users to expand an area of interest to many times its original size as shown (Fig. 2.26). The simplest approach is called a read zoom, which doubles the size of an image area as it already exists within the scan converter. Only the area of interest is read out to the video display and each pixel is magnified by the required amount.

On the other hand, write zooms can actually enhance the displayed image. In this case, only the image data within the area of interest are written into the scan converter, so more pixels are available for each image line. Further image enhancements can also be achieved by optimizing the system scan patterns. For example, if the zoom is applied to only a narrow area of interest, all of the transmitted image lines can be compressed into the zoomed area to increase the picture line density (Fig. 2.26). This is especially useful for color Doppler Imaging. Also frame rates can be increased dramatically with this approach.

POST PROCESSING

Gray Scale

All cardiac systems offer the user the ability to modify the gray scale within the image before it is displayed on the system monitor. Low amplitude signals or weak echoes generally are displayed as black or dark gray, and strong reflectors are displayed in white. The relationship between signal strengths and gray tones used can be described graphically (Fig. 2.27). A variety of curves are available for tailoring the gray scale to the

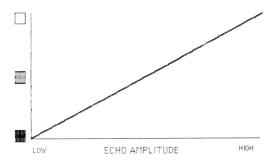

Figure 2.27. The graph illustrates the linear relationship between *echo amplitude* and *gray scale*. Amplitude of returning echoes is shown on the x scale. The *gray scale* level applied to each echo is shown on the y axis.

preferences of the operator or to meet a particular clinical need (Fig. 2.28).

Persistence

Several systems provide a persistence mode which can be used to reduce noise and increase tissue fill-in within the image. Images produced in a persistence mode are averages of old and new data. Persistence works well for slow-moving structures but tends to smear rapidly moving structures, such as valves and dynamically moving chamber walls.

INSTRUMENTATION

Both mechanically and electronically steered sector scanners with triangular formats are used in cardiac scanning. Many believed that phased array or electronically steered systems would predominate quickly. Until now, however, mechanical systems have yielded consistently superior

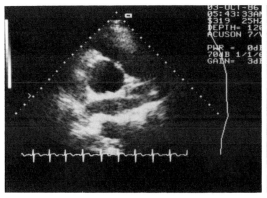
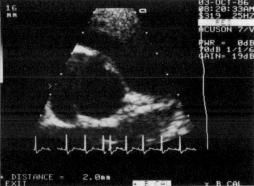

Figure 2.26. The enlarged image (*right*) shows improved detail of the aorta and left main coronary artery.

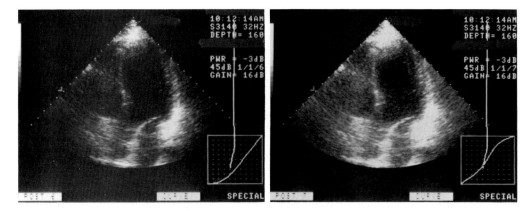

Figure 2.28. Both images are identical except for the postprocessing curves used (*lower right corner* of each image.).

images at a lower cost. Recent advancements in electronically based sector image quality as well as other advantages now appear to give electronic technology a significant edge for cardiac applications.

Phased Array Instruments

The first commercial phased array systems had 32 channels; more recent systems have offered from 48 to 64 channels. The advantage of additional channels appears to be improvement in signal-to-noise ratio and contrast and lateral resolution. Transducer contact area on these newer systems tends to be larger because of the greater number of channels and elements. Further improvements in image quality have been demonstrated with 96- and 128-channel systems.

Transducer fabrication technology has also been evolving over the past few years. Improved ceramics and cutting techniques have led to significant image quality improvements. The advancement of this technology has also permitted the use of high frequency probes, such as 5 and 7 MHz, with phased array units.

As the technical challenges which have limited phased array image quality are met, several significant advantages of phased systems become obvious. Having control over a large number of point sources can improve data acquisition. The beam-forming capability of these systems can be controlled to focus at any user-selected point on transmit, and the receive dynamic focus can improve lateral and contrast resolution throughout the image. Also, the absence of inertia or moving

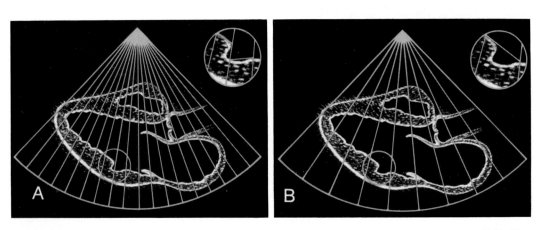

Figure 2.29. A comparison of conventional image acquisition (*right*) and parallel processing (*left*). The number of acquired lines is doubled with parallel processing, producing an apparent improvement in lateral resolution. See this figure in Color Atlas.

parts allows for improved compatibility with M-mode, Doppler, and color flow mapping. With electronically steered systems, switching between modalities can be virtually instantaneous, yielding apparently simultaneous acquisition of two-dimensional and M-mode or Doppler data.

Another unique capability of phased array systems is a technique called parallel processing. Imagine two phased array systems being used to scan a patient's heart. Two probes could be placed on the chest just slightly offset from one another. If only one transmitted, both could still receive. However, the delay schemes for each system would be adjusted to receive adjacent sector lines in an image.

The obvious advantage of this approach is that two display lines can be achieved for every transmitted pulse, thereby cutting the image formation time in half while maintaining the same line density. Parallel processing can be integrated into a phased array system by incorporating two sets of delay lines, which can operate in parallel.

These rapid image acquisition times are rarely required for standard imaging. However, in cases where display times must be shared with another modality (pulsed Doppler) or where image acquisition times are slow (color flow mapping), parallel processing can make a significant contribution (Figure 2.29).

Figure 2.30 shows the apparent simultaneous acquisition of imaging and pulsed wave Doppler data. The two-dimensional image was created in only 20 msec. Since the spectrum is filled in with averaged data during two-dimensional image for-

mation, the image must be created quickly in order to preserve the spectral continuity. The image acquisition time is kept brief by reducing the line density of the image as well as by reducing frame rates so that the spectrum will be interrupted fewer times each second. Parallel processing would be useful here for increasing line densities for simultaneous imaging and Doppler.

Combining two-dimensional and M-mode scanning is a relatively straightforward process with phased array instruments. Time is shared between gathering the two-dimensional information and returning to the selected M-mode cursor line to acquire the M-mode data. The high sampling rates and long interrogation times used in Doppler are not required in M-mode. Therefore, a simple interleave process can be used for simultaneous M-mode and two-dimensional displays. For example, at 20 cm, a system operating at 4 kHz can use 3000 pulses/sec to acquire each image and 1000 pulses/sec for an M-mode, which is more than adequate.

Mechanical Scanners

Until recently it was generally acknowledged that mechanical scanners produced the best two-dimensional images. The single element and single transmitter/receiver construction of these devices were far less complex than phased array scanners. Recent improvements in phased array transducer manufacture have yielded higher quality images. Also, the cost of electronics has plummeted, allowing for the construction of phased array front ends with performance capabilities equal to that of mechanical systems.

Mechanical scanners have also shown recent performance improvements. The cost of these systems has been reduced dramatically, making them ideal for doctors' offices and as secondary units in hospitals. Although M-mode and Doppler scanning can be performed with mechanical systems, they do not have the advantage of simultaneity because of the limitations of a physically moving probe.

Annular Array

Annular array systems are mechanical imaging systems with multiple channels for transmit and receive. The imaging element is an array of concentric rings, each with its own transmitter and receiver. The theoretical advantage of this approach is that point sources of sound can be controlled in two imaging planes, referred to as the

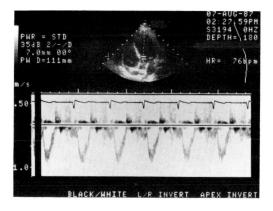

Figure 2.30. Simultaneous Doppler and imaging is accomplished by rapidly switching modes and filling in the missing spectral data with interpolated information during two-dimensional image acquisition.

lateral and azimuthal, or slice thickness, plane (Fig. 2.14).

Annular probes are mechanically complex because multiple leads must be connected to a rapidly moving element. Also, as the number of rings increases, the circle diameter of the element and case must increase as well. This may result in difficulties in patient contact, especially for cardiac scanning. Therefore, it appears that cardiac applications will require the use of smaller apertures with a limited number of rings. This requirement may limit the benefits of annular technology.

DOPPLER

The Doppler effect has been used in medical instruments for more than a decade. Today, there are more Doppler instruments in use than all ultrasound imaging units combined. The most prevalent type of machine is the hand-held Doppler, used to assess peripheral vessel flow and fetal circulation.

There are at least 200,000 hand-held Doppler machines, which are notably inexpensive, in use in the United States. These machines are analogous to a stethoscope, in that detected Doppler shifts are converted to an audio signal from which the diagnosis is made. The results are usually qualitative, and assessments of weak flow or flow disturbance can be easily accomplished.

The hand-held Doppler device employs similar technology to more sophisticated cardiac Doppler instruments. All currently available commercial Doppler systems utilize a single basic circuit design (Fig. 2.31).

Returning ultrasound from the body is composed of the emitted frequency and the positive and negative Doppler shifts produced by blood flow toward and away from the transducer. The graph in Figure 2.32 represents a typical spectral range of returning Doppler shifts produced by a 2 and 3 MHz emitted frequency (f).

Doppler shifts (F) present in signals returning from the body are determined by the equation

$$f_d = 2f_o \frac{V\cos\theta}{C}. \qquad (2.3)$$

Doppler shifts are related to the velocity (v) of the moving blood cells and the angle of incidence of the ultrasound beam (cosine theta) to the detected cells. An angle parallel to flow, where cosine theta equals 1.0, will produce the highest shifts.

Doppler systems usually employ a filter network to eliminate returning frequencies that either deviate widely from the emitted signal or are the result of wall motion. After the receive stage, the composite signal is combined with the original emitted frequency in a component referred to as a mixer (Fig. 2.31). The mathematical result of this process is the sum and the difference of the two input waveforms.

We are interested in the difference result, so the additive waveform is eliminated by low pass filtering. If two mixers are used, directionality can be obtained by summing the base frequency with the returning signal 90° advanced in the second mixer compared to the first. The outputs of the two mixers are called the quadrature components and include both the Doppler shift information

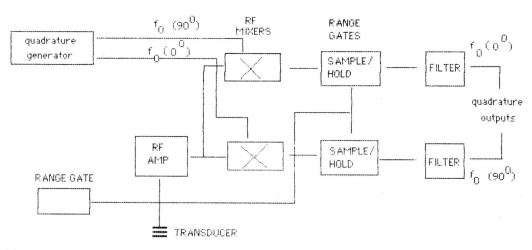

Figure 2.31. Returning echoes are mixed with the emitted frequency and filtered for wall motion artifact. The net results are sine and quadrature components of the Doppler shifts.

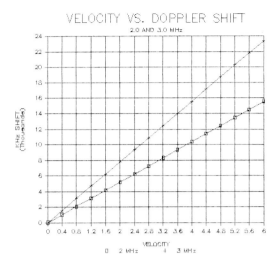

Figure 2.32. Higher velocities and emitted frequencies both produce higher absolute Doppler shifts.

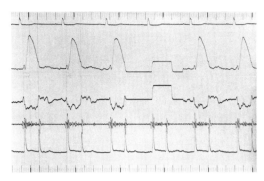

Figure 2.34. The maximum velocity tracing is shown at the *top* of the figure with the mean velocity just below it. A phonocardiogram and Doppler amplitude tracing (*bottom*) are used for timing. The sharp spike on the amplitude tracing corresponds to aortic valve closure. A 3 m/sec flow, typical of aortic stenosis, is shown by the maximum velocity curve. The square waves represent 1 m/sec.

and the sign or direction of flow. Since Doppler shifts are often in the audible range, the outputs can be sent to an audio amplifier.

A characteristic of all Dopplers, of most importance to physicians, is the sensitivity of the receive section of the Doppler. Sensitivity is an important issue for Doppler because the targets, red blood cells, produce very weak back-scattered ultrasound. Anatomical interfaces produce almost 1 million times the power level of returns from red blood cells.

Doppler instruments must possess extraordinary dynamic range to detect weaker signals, which otherwise would be swamped by the high amplitude signals from the heart and vessel walls. The

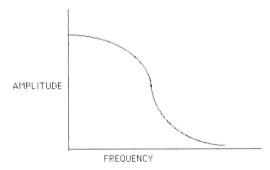

Figure 2.33. Higher velocities are generally lower in amplitude and more difficult to detect than slow velocities. Velocity is shown on the x axis and amplitude on the y axis.

problem is compounded in cardiology where high velocity signals are generally weak in power due to transit time effects. This is because clusters of cells traveling at high velocities spend less time within the ultrasound beam. These cells are sampled for less time and therefore produce less power at the high end of the spectrum (Fig. 2.33).

Several conditions do not require high dynamic range. In peripheral Doppler scanning, there are fewer specular reflectors traveling at high velocities. Also, in the case of pulsed Doppler, blood can be isolated from walls. The most demanding circumstance is in the case of continuous wave Doppler or color flow Doppler, where walls and blood are sampled simultaneously.

Doppler returns are usually complex because a large number of cells are detected simultaneously moving at different speeds. Originally, analog traces were used to represent the mean and maximum of the velocities detected. Several methods were available for obtaining these measurements, such as zero crossing and time interval histogram techniques.

An early cardiac Doppler device employing these calculation techniques was the Vingmed Pedof. This instrument combined both pulsed and continuous wave Doppler capabilities. Velocities were displayed as simple analog traces derived by zero crossing and a peak estimator methods.

Figure 2.34 shows typical analog outputs from the aortic valve area. The amplitude trace at the bottom of the picture shows the presence of valves

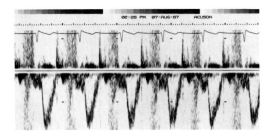

Figure 2.35. The x axis represents time and the y axis velocity or Doppler shift. The *gray scale* represents the amplitude of Doppler shifts or the number of blood cells traveling within each range of displayed velocities.

and the mean velocity trace shows the direction of flow. This approach was the first successful noninvasive technique for quantifying the severity of valvular obstructions.

Spectrum Analysis

Spectrum analysis is a method by which all components of a received Doppler signal can be analyzed and displayed. In the typical Doppler spectrum, the horizontal axis represents time, and the vertical axis represents velocity (Fig. 2.35). The gray scale represents the amplitude of each velocity component. Amplitude is usually related to the volume of cells traveling at a specific velocity. The value of the full frequency spectrum in cardiology is not entirely clear. For the most part, the peak velocity or an envelope around the periphery of the spectrum is all that is necessary for assessing blood flow dynamics.

However, the full frequency spectrum is almost universally accepted for recording velocity data

within the heart. There are several good reasons for this. Peak velocity detectors only display an estimate of peak frequency in an analog trace. Since the rest of the data are not displayed, one is forced to rely on the accuracy of the electronics for the estimation. In addition, the spectrum itself gives some indication of the quality and accuracy of the acquired data.

Several terms are used to describe spectrum analyzer specifications or performance. Since much of the data are not used very often clinically, minimal specifications are adequate. These include the number of velocity bins displayed above and below the 0 baseline (Fig. 2.36), the range of gray scale displayed in each of these bins, the computation time of each spectrum, and the bandwidth of the spectrum analyzer. With the exception of gray scale, these parameters are interdependent.

Oddly enough, the wider the range of Doppler shifts to be analyzed, the less time is necessary for the computation. This is because as the bandwidth of Doppler shifts increases, velocity resolution decreases for a fixed number of bins. This relationship is shown in the formula

$$T = \text{velocity bins/bandwidth.} \quad (2.4)$$

To resolve more bins, the computation takes longer. However, as we increase the computation time we must wait longer to output a spectral line. The resulting spectrum appears coarse and blocky (Fig. 2.37). Some systems combine old and new data so the lines can be generated at a consent rate, regardless of the bandwidth being analyzed. Another scheme is one in which each segment of length T is analyzed and stored in a buffer mem-

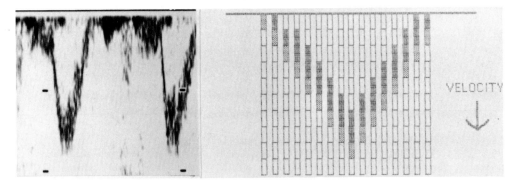

Figure 2.36. Each box on the *right* represents a narrow range of velocities. The box width is determined by spectral update time. The gray level in each box represents the number of blood cells traveling within that velocity range. A spectral line comprises each vertical row of boxes.

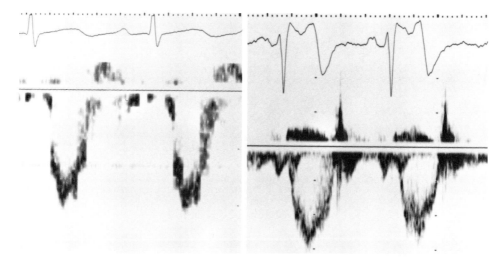

Figure 2.37. The spectral display on the *left* has a slower update time. The broader spectral width gives the spectrum a blocky appearance.

ory. The spectral output is made up of a moving average of several individual computed segments. Each line is output 1000 times/sec, but it can contain data 10 to 15 msec old.

The advantage of this approach is that variance in the estimates of sampled velocities is reduced. It should be understood that any report of velocity detected with Doppler ultrasound is only an estimate of the true instantaneous velocity. Averaging data over time tends to reduce the error of the estimate. Figure 2.38 shows the difference between a signal processed with and without averaging.

Continuous Wave Doppler

The value of continuous wave Doppler (CW) was not generally recognized until the early 1980s. Until that time it was believed that the complexity of the heart would make continuous wave impossible to use. The basic principles of CW involve two elements independently tied to a transmitter and receiver, with both continually operational.

First, in the typical beam profile, all points along the beam are sampled for blood flow velocities (Fig. 2.39). There is no range resolution or accurate localization in depth from which the flow is sampled. Because transvalvular flow is so variable within the heart, many believed it would be impossible to identify the detected flow site. Liv Hatle and others subsequently demonstrated that sampling from the apex and other specific acous-

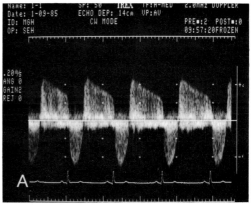

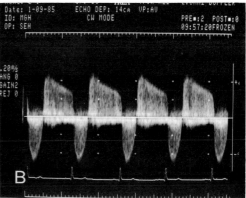

Figure 2.38. *A,* Processed without averaging of spectral lines. Holes are produced by variance of velocity estimates. *B,* Averaging of spectral information improves the display. The borders of this spectrum are better defined and dropout is gone.

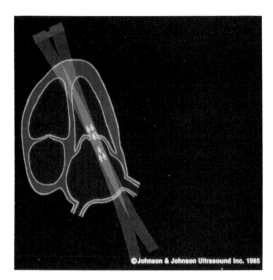

Figure 2.39. A typical continuous wave beam profile. Flow is sampled along the line of sight. One transducer element transmits continuously while the other receives. See this figure in Color Atlas.

tic windows isolated areas of interest and eliminated ambiguities.

The popularity of CW for cardiac diagnosis rapidly increased because of its value in detecting high flow velocities. Sampled pulsed Doppler systems can only detect Doppler shifts up to one-half the value of the pulse repetition frequency. Beyond this point, the system can give ambiguous results (or "alias"). Since stenosed valves can produce velocities as high as 6 meters/sec, CW's advantages are especially important.

Second, pulsed Doppler is less sensitive than CW for the detection of weaker, higher Doppler shifts. This is partly because CW samples flow everywhere along the line of sight, so very little is missed.

One of the key factors leading to the success of CW has been its ability to discriminate between an angle parallel to flow and any other angle. When the CW Doppler beam is aligned to flow, a distinct high-pitched, narrow band tone is heard. At any other angle a less pure signal is heard. With pulsed Doppler techniques one cannot hear dramatic changes in the audio signal as the angle to flow is changed. Many flows, especially stenotic jets, are eccentric to the anatomy. The angle to flow cannot be determined visually, making the audio signal the only dependable criterion.

Pulsed Doppler

Pulsed Doppler requires only a single element to transmit and receive ultrasound signals. Pulsed Doppler differs from CW in that data are acquired from a single finite burst of sound, just as in standard M-mode and two-dimensional imaging. The interval between pulses allows time for the receiving system to gate the returning signal and obtain range information. For adequate range detection the system must wait longer periods of time for echoes returning from greater depths (Fig. 2.40).

If the pulse repetition frequency (PRF) is exceeded for a given depth, it is called a high PRF. This means there will be some uncertainty about the depth from which signals were obtained. For example, if we are interrogating an 8 cm depth with a PRF of 20 kHz, it will be impossible to sort out returns from both 4 cm and 8 cm. There may even be signals from 12 cm if the penetration or sensitivity is good.

High PRF Doppler in the heart permits the user to interrogate abnormally high velocities while maintaining some degree of range resolution (Fig. 2.41). In many situations, the origin of the flow being interrogated can be determined from observing the two-dimensional anatomy, just as in CW. However, the actual clinical value of high PRF has yet to be determined. CW appears to be more sensitive in practice.

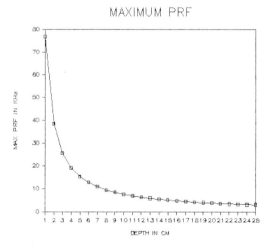

Figure 2.40. The maximum pulse repetition frequency (PRF) for given depths. Exceeding the maximum PRF creates uncertainty about the site of the sampled flow.

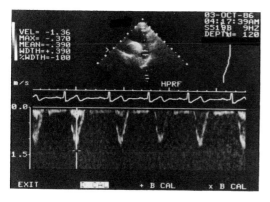

Figure 2.41. The spectral display can represent flow from all three sites shown in this image. However, the origin of the signal can usually be confirmed by examining the two-dimensional image.

Doppler Ultrasound Instrumentation

In the past, manufacturers of mechanical systems found it easier to incorporate high PRF rather than CW. High PRF could be added without changing the probe design, an advantage to both the customer and the manufacturer. Designers of phased array systems have also found it difficult to integrate CW into their systems.

It appears to be even more difficult to produce steerable CW in a phased array system. One major problem is that continually returning echoes create noise, which interferes with the steering of the transmitting elements (Fig. 2.42). New generation phased array products have steered CW capability and the dynamic range necessary to combine imaging and CW Doppler in a single probe. Currently, several phased array systems are also available with a single transmit side element. Returning signals are detected by the imaging elements. This approach allows for some

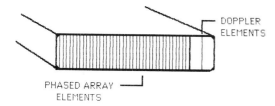

Figure 2.42. Two-dimensional phased array combined with CW Doppler scanning. The two large elements on the *right* are used to transmit and receive CW Doppler. However, the CW Doppler beam cannot be steered.

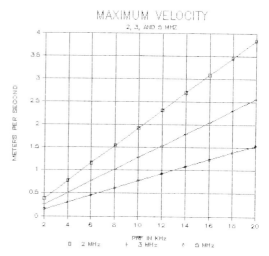

Figure 2.43. Higher pulse repetition frequencies are related linearly to peak detectable velocities. Also, the dependence of the maximal detectable velocity on interrogation frequency is illustrated.

modification of focal zones but without steerability.

There is one more instrumentation issue relevant to the display and recording of high velocity flow, whether it involves high PRF or CW: the bandwidth of the spectral analyzer. Since CW samples continuously, returning signals will not alias. Figure 2.43 shows the peak detectable velocity for a specific PRF. If the PRF is infinite, as in CW, the maximum detectable velocity will also be infinite. High PRF systems can also detect very high Doppler shifts but only up to one-half the transmitted PRF.

Regardless of the system PRF, spectrum analyzers may have limited bandwidths, in the range of 20 to 30 kHz. A 30-kHz system can only detect shifts up to 15 kHz bidirectionally, even in CW mode. A 30 kHz range is usually adequate if the transmitted frequency is in the 2-MHz range (see Doppler equation). However, with high emitted frequencies, high flow can produce shifts outside the analyzer's limits.

Extraordinarily high Doppler shifts—more than one-half the PRF or aliased—also produce signals which can exceed the boundaries of the spectral display. However, if the total shift is still within the spectrum analyzer bandwidth, the Doppler spectrum can be displayed correctly with a feature called movable baseline.

By shifting the baseline up or down, the velocity limit, or bandwidth, can be increased in

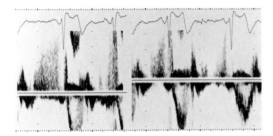

Figure 2.44. An aliased signal (*left*) can be displayed (accurately) by shifting the spectral baseline (*right*). This provides increased spectral bandwidth in one direction and decreased bandwidth in the other direction.

one direction and reduced in the other (Fig. 2.44). One problem inherent to this approach is that the audio signal will still alias and the characteristically narrow band tone used to orient to the flow is no longer available. A few manufacturers are now beginning to offer systems that shift the baseline in the audio signal as well. In summary, the characteristics to evaluate in a Doppler system include the modalities available (i.e., CW, pulsed, or high PRF); the system sensitivity; and the spectral computation time, aesthetics, and bandwidth.

Other Pulsed Doppler Techniques

Several pulsed Doppler techniques have not achieved commercial success. They are probably not important by themselves, but an elaboration

of the techniques form a basis for understanding color flow mapping.

One technique, called multigate Doppler, involves a pulsed Doppler system which can resolve flows at fixed increments of depth in the heart. This is not to be confused with high PRF, which samples from several points but cannot resolve the ambiguity. With multigate Doppler, PRF is determined by the greatest depth under interrogation (Fig. 2.45). Rather than examining a single area, velocities from multiple areas along the line of sight are detected and displayed.

Multisample capability is another interesting feature of some Doppler systems. Here the user can preassign up to nine areas in an image to be sampled for flow. The system can be set to step through each of the areas, perhaps displaying 1 second of a spectral display for each area; or, the user can manually step through each point. In either case, the result is a flow map of the total area sampled (Fig. 2.46). Unfortunately, the long strip of spectral data produced by this method is difficult to interpret.

Color Flow Mapping

Color flow mapping combines the features of multigate and multisample Doppler. Sampling is accomplished in real-time with an extraordinary large number of gates along each scan line. The result is a two-dimensional color map of flow, overlayed on a black-and-white anatomical image

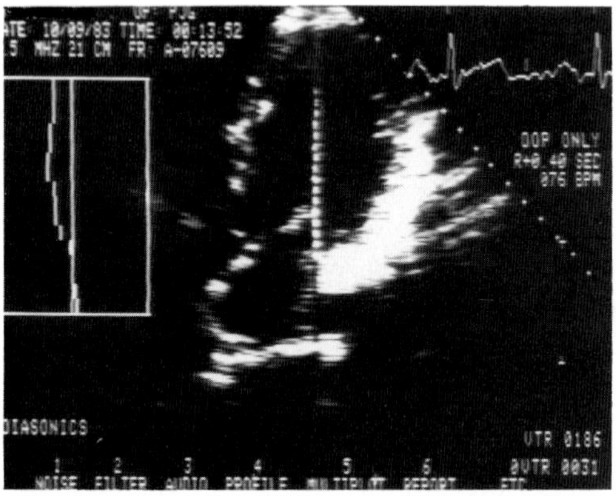

Figure 2.45. *Vertical* dashes in the *center* of the image represent areas sampled simultaneously by the multigate Doppler. The graphic on the *left* indicates sampled velocities from each area. *Leftward* deflection of a *bar* represents flow away from the probe, while *rightward* a deflection indicates flow toward the probe.

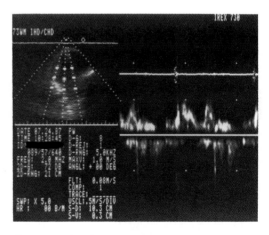

Figure 2.46. Each *box* is a potential sample site for the system Doppler. Each site is automatically sampled in sequence and the spectrum is displayed on a monitor or recorded on a continuous strip.

and displayed at normal imaging frame rates. At a depth of 18 to 20 cm, cardiac flow systems can produce from 200 to 400 sampled gates. These gates can be so close together that often the information in adjacent gates is redundant.

Processing Doppler information normally requires more time than in the case of standard two-dimensional anatomical imaging. This is because the back-scatter from blood cells is far weaker than echoes from anatomical boundaries. Also, more information must be derived, such as flow velocity and direction. For this reason each line of sight is interrogated by multiple pulses. In conventional imaging, only one pulse along each line of sight is used in each frame.

The interrogation times are still far shorter for color than for standard spectral Doppler. For example, if each scan line is pulsed between 8 and 16 times at a PRF of 8 kHz, then interrogation periods will last only 1 to 2 msec. Velocity resolution must be sacrificed to allow for such short observation intervals (Equation 2.4). In most cases, only 8 to 16 velocity bins are resolved with this technique, as opposed to more than 100 bins with conventional Doppler. Because of the brief interrogation times, fast Fourier transforms cannot be used to extract the abundance of velocity information seen in spectral displays.

Most manufacturers are now turning to autocorrelation techniques. With these methods, the entire signal returning from a single pulse is matched or correlated with data from successive pulses. Any movement of blood will produce dis-

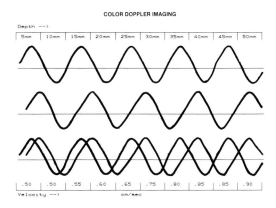

Figure 2.47. The technique of autocorrelation. Returning Doppler shifts are detected, held by the system and compared to subsequent signals. In this case, flow velocities increase as penetration goes from 0 to 6 cm.

crete changes in each successive returning sound wave (Fig. 2.47).

These changes or phase shifts relate directly to the blood velocities that produced them. The resulting velocities are generally close to the mean velocity in the areas sampled. The more correlations that can be made, the more accurate the velocity estimates will be. Sixteen pulses along one vector can produce 15 correlations. The number of samples is limited only by the need for mapping a wide field of view. Increased frequency of sampling along each line also improves system sensitivity. Back-scattered ultrasound from red blood cells is generally very weak and signal-

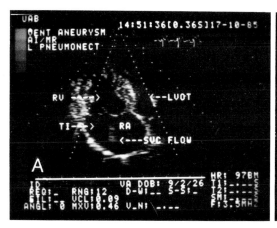
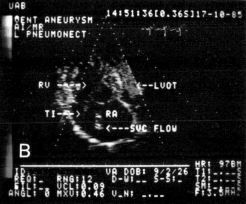

Figure 2.48. *A,* Illustration of flow velocity only. Higher velocities correspond to the bright red or blue. *B,* Green indicates the degree of dispersion of velocities. Regardless of the turbulence of flow, this variance tag produces complex color displays. See this figure in Color Atlas.

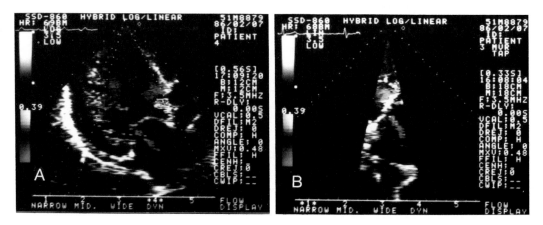

Figure 2.49. *A*, Mitral regurgitation displayed within a 45° color sector. *B*, Narrowing the sector display allows greater concentration of the ultrasound lines. Note the improved definition of the mitral regurgitant jet. See this figure in Color Atlas.

to-noise ratios are poor. Signal-to-noise ratios will improve with the increase in the number of samples.

An estimate of the scatter, or spread, of the estimate can also be derived from the computed correlations. This spread has been termed variance and appears to be related to the degree of turbulence or disorganization within the flow patterns. The computed flow velocities, flow direction, and variance are tagged with colors and displayed as a spatial map (Fig. 2.48).

A key factor in color flow imaging is the PRF (Fig. 2.40). It may be advantageous to set the PRF at a lower level than is necessary. By lowering the range of Doppler shifts, velocity resolution improves, along with the improved detection of low velocities.

COLOR FLOW
FRAMES PER SECOND

NUMBER OF LINES
IN 50 DEGREES

PRF	# SAMPLES	20	30	40
4 KHz	5	40	26.6	20
	10	20	13.3	10
6 KHz	5	60	40	30
	10	30	20	15
8 KHz	5	80	53.3	40
	10	40	26.6	20

Figure 2.50. An illustration of the interdependence of frame rate on PRF, line density, sector width, and flow sample count. The three columns on the *right* indicate possible frame rates with 20, 30, and 40 lines/50° sector image (values are theoretical).

The last variable is line density. Standard two-dimensional imaging usually requires 100 or more lines in a 90° image, or less than 1° between lines. This density is impossible to maintain in color mapping because of the multiple pulses required along each vector. In order to improve line densities, the sector areas can be narrowed (Fig. 2.49). Parallel processing, described earlier in the chapter, could also be used in this application to increase line densities.

The frame rate for the color display is determined by the depth of view and PRF, the number of samples along each vector, and the line densities desired. Figure 2.50 shows the interdependence of these variables with some typical settings for cardiology. High frame rates significantly improve the display of flow within the heart. As rates drop below 15 frames/sec, the natural continuous motion of the blood is lost.

In summary, the ideal color system will have excellent sensitivity and versatility. In order to ensure this sensitivity, the system should allow the user to vary the size of the interrogation area so as to provide maximum samples of each vector and increased line density while maintaining high frame rates.

SUGGESTED READINGS

Feigenbaum H: *Echocardiography*. Philadelphia, Lea & Febiger, 1986.

Hatle L, Angelsen B: *Doppler Ultrasound in Cardiology*. ed 2 Philadelphia, Lea & Febiger, 1985.

Kremkau FW: *Diagnostic Ultrasound*. New York, Grune & Stratton, 1980.

Nanda NC: *Doppler Echocardiography*. New York, Igaku-Shoin, 1985.

3

Standards and Nomenclature: Report of the American Society of Echocardiography

Walter L. Henry, M.D., Chairman, Anthony DeMaria, M.D., Raymond Gramiak, M.D., Donald L. King, M.D., Joseph A. Kisslo, M.D., Richard L. Popp, M.D., David J. Sahn, M.D., Nelson B. Schiller, M.D., Abdul Tajik, M.D., Louis E. Teichholz, M.D., Arthur E. Weyman, M.D.

The Committee on Nomenclature and Standards in Two-dimensional Echocardiography of the American Society of Echocardiography recommends the following nomenclature and image orientations standards.

NOMENCLATURE

Name of Technique

The Committee recommends that the name *Two-dimensional Echocardiography* be used to refer to the technique.

Transducer Location

The nomenclature for transducer location recommended by the Committee is summarized in Figure 3.1. The Committee recommends that when the transducer is placed in the suprasternal notch that it be referred to as in the *suprasternal* location. When the transducer is located near the midline of the body and beneath the lowest ribs, it is recommended that the transducer be referred to as in the *subcostal* location. When the transducer is located over the apex impulse, the Committee recommends that this be referred to as the *apical* location. If the term *apical* is used alone, it will be assumed that this refers to a left-sided apical position. The area bounded superiorly by the left clavicle, medially by the sternum and inferiorly by the apical region will be referred to as the *parasternal* location. If the term *parasternal* is used alone, it will be assumed to be the left parasternal location. In those unusual situations in which the apex impulse is palpated on the right chest, a transducer placed over the right-sided apex impulse will be referred to as in the *right*

apical location. The region bounded superiorly by the right clavicle, medially by the sternum, and inferiorly by the right apical region will be referred to as the *right parasternal* location.

Imaging Planes

Three orthogonal planes will be used to describe the imaging planes used to visualize the heart with two-dimensional echocardiography. The nomenclature recommended by the Committee is not based strictly on the sagittal, transverse and coronal planes used by anatomists to describe body orientation, but rather on the manner in which the two-dimensional echocardiographic imaging planes transect the heart. These imaging planes are illustrated in Figure 3.2. The imaging plane that transects the heart perpendicular to the dorsal and ventral surfaces of the body and parallel to the long axis of the heart will be referred to as the *long-axis* plane. The plane that transects the heart perpendicular to the dorsal and ventral surfaces of the body, but perpendicular to the long axis of the heart will be referred to as the *short-axis* plane. The plane that transects the heart approximately parallel to the dorsal and ventral surfaces of the body will be referred to as the *four-chamber* plane. It should be emphasized that each of these three orthogonal planes should not be thought of as a single plane but rather as a family of planes. For example, the *long-axis* plane is described as being "perpendicular to the dorsal and ventral surfaces of the body." However, any plane that is parallel to the long axis of the heart and is within 45° of the plane perpendicular to

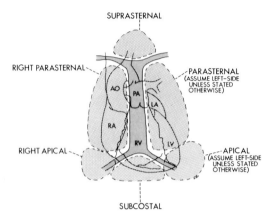

NOMENCLATURE FOR TRANSDUCER LOCATION

Figure 3.1. Diagram indicating the nomenclature to describe the location on the body from which echocardiographic studies can be obtained. *LV* = left ventricle; *RV* = right ventricle; *LA* = left atrium; *RA* = right atrium; *AO* = aorta; *PA* = pulmonary artery.

the dorsal and ventral surfaces of the body should be referred to as a *long-axis* plane.

Identification of Two-Dimensional Images

The Committee recommends that two-dimensional images be identified by referring to the

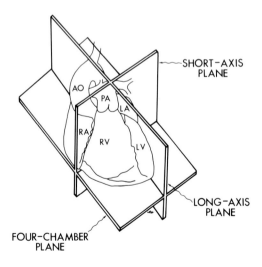

TWO-DIMENSIONAL ECHOCARDIOGRAPHIC IMAGING PLANES

Figure 3.2. Diagram of the three orthogonal imaging planes used to visualize the heart with two-dimensional echocardiography. Abbreviations as in Figure 3.1.

transducer location and the imaging plane. For example, if the transducer is placed in the *parasternal* location and oriented so that the imaging plane transects the heart parallel to the *long-axis* of the heart, the Committee recommends that the resulting image be referred to as a *parasternal long-axis* view. As another example, if the transducer is placed in the *apical* location and oriented so that the *four-chamber* imaging plane is used, the Committee recommends that the resulting image be referred to as an *apical four-chamber* view.

IMAGE ORIENTATION STANDARDS

In considering recommendations for image orientation standards, the Committee attempted to adopt standards that are compatible with image orientations presently used by clinicians. In addition, the Committee was motivated by a desire to develop image orientation standards that result from transducer orientations that are consistent from one view to the next and, therefore, can be easily taught and explained to both experienced and inexperienced users of two-dimensional imaging equipment. With these two considerations in mind, the Committee recommends the following.

Index Mark

It is recommended that an index mark be placed on every two-dimensional imaging transducer. This index mark should be placed on the side of the transducer to indicate the edge of the imaging plane, i.e., the direction in which the ultrasound beam is being angled (Fig. 3.3). The index mark should be located on the transducer to indicate the part of the image plane that will appear on the right side of the image display. For example, if the index mark is pointed in the direction of the aorta in a *parasternal long-axis* view, the aorta will appear on the right side of the image display (Fig. 3.3).

Image Inversion Switch

It is recommended that every ultrasound imaging unit incorporate an image inversion switch. When the switch is in the "off" position, ultrasound signals returning from reflecting structures located *near* the surface of the ultrasound transducer will appear on the *top* of the image display. These signals will be referred to as "near signals." Conversely, ultrasound signals returning from reflecting structures located *far* from the transducer will appear at the *bottom* of the image display.

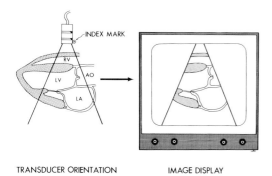

TRANSDUCER ORIENTATION   IMAGE DISPLAY

Figure 3.3. Illustration of the relation between the transducer orientation (as indicated by the direction of the index mark) and the orientation of the resulting image on the display. Abbreviations as in Figure 3.1.

When the image inversion switch is moved to the "on" position, ultrasound signals returning from reflecting structures located *near* the surface of the transducer will appear on the *bottom* of the image display and signals from reflecting structures located *far* from the transducer will appear at the *top* of the image display. Thus, moving the switch from the "off" to the "on" position will invert the "near signals" in the image from the top to the bottom of the display, but will not produce a change in the left-right orientation of the image. This image inversion switch will only be used in conjunction with the *four-chamber* imaging plane. When either the *long-axis* imaging plane or the *short-axis* imaging plane is being used, the image inversion switch will always be in the "off" position.

Transducer Orientation

When orienting the transducer during the performance of a two-dimensional echocardiographic study, it is recommended that the transducer index mark always be pointed either *in the direction of the patient's head or to the left side of the patient*. The image orientations that result from this transducer orientation strategy are summarized below.

Long-axis Views

The long axis of the heart can be viewed from either the apical, the parasternal or the suprasternal locations. Figure 3.4A illustrates long-axis views of the left ventricle obtained from these three transducer locations using the strategy that the index mark is always pointed toward the pa-

tient's head. Figure 3.5A illustrates the image that will appear on the image display when the transducer is oriented in the *apical long-axis* view with the transducer index mark pointing toward the patient's head. In this view, the apex of the heart is visualized at the top of the image display, the aorta at the bottom, the right ventricle to the right and the posterior wall of the left ventricle to the left of the image display. When the *parasternal long-axis* image is obtained, the transducer index mark will also be pointing toward the patient's head. The resulting image display is illustrated in Figure 3.5B. In this image, the right ventricle appears at the top of the image display, the apex of the heart to the left, the aorta to the right and the posterior wall at the bottom of the image display. This image orientation is identical with that previously recommended by the American Society of Echocardiography. When the *suprasternal long-axis* view is obtained, the transducer mark also will be pointing to the patient's head. The resulting image display is illustrated in Figure 3.5C. In this image, the aorta will appear at the top of the image display, the posterior wall of the

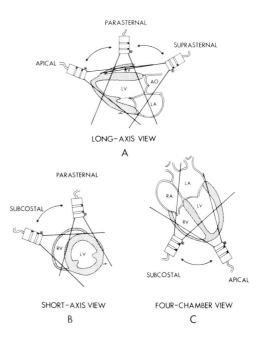

Figure 3.4. Diagram of the transducer orientations used to obtain long-axis views (A), short-axis views (B) and four-chamber views (C) of the heart. Note that the transducer index mark is always pointed either in the direction of the patient's head or the patient's left side. Abbreviations as in Figure 3.1.

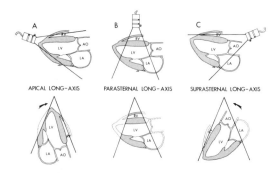

Figure 3.5. Illustration of the long-axis two-dimensional images that result when the transducer is used to visualize the *apical long-axis* view (*A*), *parasternal long-axis view* (*B*), and *suprasternal long-axis* view (*C*). These images were obtained with the transducer index mark pointing to the patient's head as illustrated in Figure 3.4*A*. Abbreviations as in Figure 3.1.

left ventricle on the right side, the apex of the heart in the lower left and the right ventricle on the left side of the image display. By making small changes in transducer orientation, the ascending aorta, transverse aorta (including major arterial branches), descending aorta and pulmonary artery also can be visualized in a *suprasternal long-axis view*. As can be seen from Figure 3.4*A*, the long-axis views of the heart can be obtained from any of the three transducer locations by simply sliding the transducer from one transducer location to the next. Since the transducer index mark is always pointed toward the patient's head, this sliding motion does not result in the transducer being rotated 180° during any portion of the sweep from the apical location to the suprasternal location. In addition, it should be noted that all three long-axis views of the heart are similar to views which would be seen by an operator sitting on the left side of a supine patient and looking at the cross-sectioned heart from the patient's left side.

Short-Axis Views

The short-axis views of the heart (Fig. 3.4*B*) can be obtained from either the parasternal or the subcostal locations. (Short-axis views also can be obtained from the suprasternal location, but will not be discussed in this report.) The *parasternal short-axis* view is obtained with the transducer index mark pointing to the patient's left side (Fig. 3.6*A*). If the heart is viewed in this

manner at the level of the papillary muscles, the ventricular septum will appear at the top of the image display, the lateral papillary muscle will appear to the right, the medial papillary muscle will appear to the left and the posterior left ventricular free wall will appear on the bottom of the image display. This image orientation is identical with that previously recommended by the American Society for Echocardiography. The *subcostal short-axis* view is also obtained with the transducer index mark pointing to the patient's left side (Fig. 3.6*B*). If the heart is being imaged at the level of the papillary muscles, the right ventricle will appear at the top of the image display, the posterior free wall will appear in the lower left, the lateral papillary muscle will appear in the lower right and the anterior free wall will appear on the right side of the image display. As can be seen in Figure 3.4*B*, the short-axis views of the heart can be obtained from either the parasternal location or the subcostal location by simply sliding the transducer from one location to the other. Since the transducer index mark is pointing to the patient's left side in both views, it is not necessary to rotate the transducer 180° in order to go from the *parasternal short-axis* view to the *subcostal*

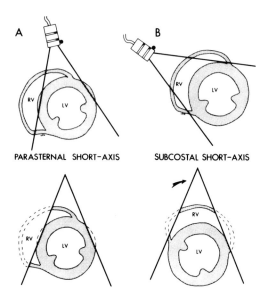

Figure 3.6. Diagram of the short-axis two-dimensional images that result when the transducer is used to visualize the *parasternal short-axis* view (*A*) and the *subcostal short-axis* view (*B*). These images were obtained with the transducer index mark pointing to the patient's left side as illustrated in Figure 3.4*B*. Abbreviations as in Figure 3.1.

short-axis view. In addition, it should be noted that both short-axis views of the heart are similar to views which would be seen by an operator sitting close to the patient's left hip and looking up at the cross-sectioned heart through the cardiac apex.

Four-Chamber Views

The four-chamber views of the heart can be obtained with the transducer located either in the apical or subcostal locations (Fig. 3.4*C*). The *apical four-chamber* view is obtained with the transducer index mark pointing toward the patient's left side. Two options are recommended for displaying the resulting image (Fig. 3.7*A*). Option 1 involves moving the image inversion switch to the "on" position to invert the "near signals" of the image from the top to the bottom of the image display. Doing so will result in an image in which the apex of the heart appears on the bottom of the image display, the left ventricle appears on the right side, the right ventricle appears on the left side and the atria appear at the top of the image display. This image orientation is similar to that which would be seen by an operator sitting close to the patient's left hip and looking directly down at the cross-sectioned heart. Option 2 involves leaving the image inversion switch in the

"off" position so that the "near signals" of the image remain at the top of the image display. The resulting image will have the apex of the heart at the top and the atria at the bottom of the image display. As in option 1, the left ventricle appears on the right side and the right ventricle on the left side of the image. Option 2 results in the cross-sectioned heart being viewed from behind the patient. It should be emphasized that option 1 and option 2 result in the same left-right orientation of the image. The only difference between the two is that in option 1, the "near signals" of the image are located at the bottom of the image display while in option 2, they are located at the top. The *subcostal four-chamber* view is also obtained with the transducer index mark pointing to the patient's left side (Fig. 3.7*B*). As in the *apical four-chamber* view, two options are recommended for displaying the image. In option 1, the "near signals" of the image are placed at the bottom of the image display by using the image inversion switch. In the resulting image, the right ventricle appears at the bottom of the image display, the apex of the heart appears on the right side and the atria appear on the left side of the image display. This view is similar to the one that would be seen by an operator sitting close to the patient's left hip and looking directly down at the cross-sectioned heart. Option 2 involves leaving the "near signals" of the image at the top of the image display. In this image orientation, the right ventricle appears at the top of the image display, the apex of the heart appears on the right side and the atria appear on the left side of the image display. As in the *apical four-chamber* view, option 2 results in the cross-sectioned heart being viewed from behind the patient. It should be emphasized that options 1 and 2 result in the same left-right orientation of the image. Also, both the apical and subcostal four-chamber views are obtained with the transducer index mark pointing to the patient's left side. Therefore, it is possible to simply slide from the *apical four-chamber* view to the *subcostal four-chamber* view without having to rotate the transducer 180°.

The image orientation standards recommended by the Committee are intended as a general framework for describing two-dimensional images. It is realized that not all images can be described without ambiguity by the present system without additional descriptive information. For example, the *two-chamber* view described by Schiller et al. is not precisely described by the image orientation standards alone (11). The *two-*

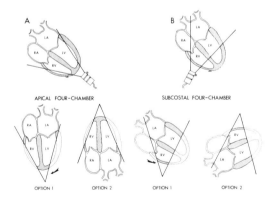

Figure 3.7. Illustration of the four-chamber two-dimensional images that result when the transducer is used to visualize the *apical four-chamber* view (A) and the *subcostal four-chamber* view (B). These images were obtained with the transducer index mark pointing to the patient's left side as illustrated in Figure 4C. Two options are included for each four-chamber view. In each case, option 1 is produced by activation of the image inversion switch which results in the near signals of the image being inverted from the top to the bottom of the display. Abbreviations as in Figure 3.1.

chamber view is a variant of the *apical long-axis* view of the heart in which the transducer is rotated clockwise (when viewed from the handle). By rotating the transducer clockwise, the image plane transects the heart lateral to the junction of the lateral border of the right ventricle and the anterolateral left ventricular free wall. The resulting image does not visualize the right ventricle and, hence, is referred to as the *two-chamber* view. Although the Committee realizes that not all views can be precisely identified by the present nomenclature alone, it does believe that these alternative views can be identified by stating the image plane and transducer location that most closely correspond to the image and by using additional descriptive information in parentheses. For example, the *two-chamber* view could be described as an *apical long-axis view* (*clockwise rotation*). Alternatively, the *two-chamber* view could be described as an *apical long-axis view* (*two-chamber view*).

Because of the complicated anatomy being displayed by two-dimensional imaging of the heart, and the need to easily understand the image orientation, it is important that standard nomenclature and image orientations be adopted. The Committee believes that by adopting nomenclature and image orientation standards, the technique of two-dimensional imaging of the heart will be advanced and communication between laboratories will be improved. In addition, it is hoped that these standards will be of considerable help to individuals who are seeing two-dimensional images of the heart for the first time.

REFERENCE

1. Schiller NB, Acquatella H, Ports TA, Drew D, Goerke J, Ringerty H, Silverman NH, Brundage B, Botvinick EH, Boswell R, Carlsson E, Parmley WW: Left ventricular volume from paired biplane two-dimensional echocardiography. *Circulation 60:* 547, 1979

4

Recommendations for Terminology and Display for Doppler Echocardiography

The Doppler Standards and Nomenclature Committee
American Society of Echocardiography[a,b]

Chairman: David J. Sahn, M.D., San Diego, California
Members: Donald W. Baker
Anthony DeMaria, M.D.
Jim Gessert
Stanley J. Goldberg, M.D.
Howard Gutgesell, M.D.
Walter Henry, M.D.
Randy Martin, M.D.
Richard Popp, M.D.
Norman Silverman, M.D.
Rebecca Snider, M.D.
Geoffrey Stevenson, M.D.

INDUSTRIAL LIAISON: REPRESENTATIVES
Mark Durrell—Irex Corporation
Michael Buchin—Diasonics
Daniel Wade Piraino—Advanced Technology
Laboratories
Nancy McRae—Advanced Technology
Laboratories
Douglas Blagg—Ekoline
Al Langguth—Hewlett-Packard
Marty Rogers—Hewlett-Packard
Allan Schultz—General Electric
Gary Wilson—General Electric
Joe Gentile—Elscint

[a]For ASE information, please write: The American Society of Echocardiography, 1100 Raleigh Building, 5 W. Hargett Street, Raleigh, North Carolina, 27601, or phone (919) 821-1435.
[b]For the AIUM NEMA Standards, see American Institute of Ultrasound in Medicine and National Electrical Manufacturers Association Safety Standard for Diagnostic Ultrasound Equipment, Draft V, January 27, 1981. Copies available from the NEMA Executive Office, 2101 L Street NW, Washington, DC 20037, and from the AIUM Executive Office, 4405 East-West Highway, Suite 504, Bethesda, Maryland 20814.

PREAMBLE

Doppler echocardiography has recently emerged as a major noninvasive technique with many applications in cardiology. To a large extent, this has been based upon a combination of clinical and engineering advances which now make possible the use of quantitative Doppler echocardiography in combination with two-dimensional imaging for measurement of volume flows, transvalve gradients, and other physiologic flow parameters which reflect cardiac function. It was the purpose of this Committee to provide a glossary of terms which could be used in standard fashion for papers and discussions related to Doppler echocardiography. As part of its task, the Committee also undertook an attempt to recommend a standard for display of Doppler information which would be useful, both for manufacturers and for clinicians. The document, therefore, includes: Section I, the Committee's recommendations for Doppler display. Section II, the glossary of Doppler terms, related to engineering and to clinical applications.

SECTION I

This Committee makes the following recommendations for page print outputs of Doppler information related to studies in the cardiovascular system:

Doppler records should contain information related to the area which was interrogated and the type of interrogation performed. This could be an inserted, freeze-frame image, as a spatial locater showing the position of the sample volume and the direction of sampling, or an alphanumeric display designating the structure, the area of the cardiovascular system sampled and the echocardiographic view used, suprasternal notch, apex, etc. The display should denote the depth and the type of sampling whether single pulsed-gate, high pulse repetition frequency, multi-gate or continuous wave Doppler. In addition, to this spatial localization, this Committee suggests that the angle of incidence estimated for the Doppler interrogation be shown either by a cursor or alphanumerically with a statement included "angle corrected" or "uncorrected" to denote whether the calibrations of the Doppler record shown have or have not already been corrected for the angle of interrogation.

With regards to the Doppler content of the record, the Committee recommends that Doppler waveform should be calibrated in centimeters or in meters per second. We believed this to be preferable to kilohertz calibrations since it provides a more physiologic means for communication of Doppler information as a velocity within the circulatory system. The Doppler record should be displayed with flow towards the transducer, shown as positive in direction and upward on the record and flow away from the transducer as negative and downward, regardless of the direction of the beam or area of interrogation. As stated, Doppler records should specify the frequency of interrogation and the type of Doppler interrogation (pulsed, high PRF, or continuous). If a pulsed or high PRF record, the record should show the pulse repetition frequency being used and the Nyquist limit for that pulse repetition frequency, denoted in centimeters per second. The inclusion of this information as to spatial localization and Doppler interrogation parameters, should allow records to be passed between laboratories, and provide a complete documentation of the data obtained during a Doppler examination.

SECTION II: GLOSSARY

The following suggestions are made regarding a standardized Doppler nomenclature for use by physicians, clinicians and engineers. The nomenclature is subdivided into general Doppler terms, Doppler instrumentation and engineering parameters, Doppler display outputs, and hydrodynamic terms relevant to pulsatile blood flow within the circulatory system.

General Doppler Terminology

Doppler echocardiography: Analysis of intracardiac or intravascular flow by ultrasonic techniques involving the Doppler effect with or without a spatial reference by A-mode, M-mode, two-dimensional imaging, or auditory signals for the localization of the site being sampled.

Doppler effect: A shift in frequency and wave length caused by relative motion between transducers and scatterers, such as from motion of targets within the blood stream, when there is a component of relative motion parallel to the direction of ultrasound interrogation.

Doppler frequency shift: The difference in frequencies of transmitted and received sound energy. This difference is directly proportional to the velocity of relative motion between the transducer and reflectors and the interrogation frequency. It is inversely proportional to the velocity of sound in the intervening medium:

$$\Delta F = \frac{V \times 2F_0 \times \cos \Theta}{\text{velocity of sound}}$$

$$V = \frac{\Delta F \times \text{velocity of sound}}{2F_0 \times \cos \Theta}$$

Where V = velocity ΔF = frequency shift
F_0 = frequency of interrogation (mHz)
Θ = Angle of incidence between the direction of motion of the scatterers and the direction of interrogation

Doppler Instrumentation and Engineering Terms:

Aliasing: Ambiguous plotting of velocities which are too high to be determined with certainty due to PRF (Nyquist) sampling limitation in pulsed or ranged gated Doppler. For example, the very high velocity may wrap around and be displayed as negative velocity, or i.e., two different velocities may be displayed as the same velocity.

Continuous wave Doppler: A wave of almost constant amplitude which persists for a large number of cycles and is used for sampling Doppler shifts regardless of distance from the transducer. There is no sampling limitation or inherent limitation on peak detected velocity, as there is for range gated Doppler. This technique can be achieved along a known line of interrogation from within a two-dimensional image. It always uses one transducer or transducer elements for sending and another or others for receiving the back-scattered ultrasound.

Doppler interrogation frequency: The frequency of the transmitted acoustic energy relative to which a Doppler frequency shift is measured. This frequency is usually, but not necessarily, the nominal transducer frequency.

2D Doppler (Duplex) scanner: A real-time two-dimensional ultrasonic imaging device which is capable of simultaneous or sequential Doppler sampling from an area within the planar image.

Pulsed Doppler (range gated Doppler): Doppler interrogation using a pulsed mode of transmission wherein establishment of a temporal gate allows determination of Doppler shift from within a specific axial area or areas at a known distance from the transducer. This area is known as the sample volume and it has axial and lateral dimensions which should be defined.

High PRF Doppler: A method of achieving high sampling rates: multiple pulses, and their return signals from within the heart are present at any one point in time and Doppler shifts along the beam are summed along sample volume depths which are multiples of the initial sample volume depth to give a single output.

Nyquist frequency: One-half the pulse repetition frequency in pulsed/range-gated Doppler. Frequency shifts exceeding this limit cannot be unambiguously displayed unless other information such as the time history of a narrow band flow spectrum is available.

Multigate Doppler: A pulsed/range-gated Doppler interrogation approach in which multiple range gates sample Doppler shift information from multiple, closely spaced depths along the ultrasound beam. As opposed to high PRF Doppler, multigate Doppler is implemented to sample and display separately the information from the individual gates.

Power output in Doppler mode: Manufacturers should be prepared to make available to the user, information relevant to the power output for their instrumentation in its various modes of Doppler interrogation. Power output in Doppler mode, as defined in the AIUM NEMA Standards may be defined as a spatial peak intensity averaged over time.

Pulse repetition frequency: The rate at which pulses of acoustic energy are transmitted in a pulse or range gated Doppler system. This is usually a function of the depth of the (first) sample volume and determines peak velocity limit which can be unambiguously detected by range gated or pulsed Doppler systems.

Sampling angle: The angle of incidence (see Doppler frequency shift) between the direction of flow and the direction of sampling within the imaged plane. This angle may be estimated during the Doppler examination.

Sample volume: The region in space from which Doppler data is collected for analysis in pulsed/range-gated Doppler systems. The size of the sample volume is axially determined by the length of the transmitted acoustic pulse and the length of the range gate. The width is determined by the lateral width of the ultrasound beam.

Wall (thump) filter: A filter in a Doppler system which rejects echo information from low velocity reflectors such as stationary or slow moving tissue. This filtering is needed to keep high amplitude tissue echos from saturating the Doppler receiver, masking very low amplitude echoes from flowing blood.

SECTION III:
DOPPLER SIGNAL PROCESSING AND DISPLAYS

Chirp Z transform: An algorithm which may be used to generate the discrete Fourier transform for spectral analysis. It is commonly used to implement spectrum analysis utilizing primarily analog electronics.

Doppler image (D)-mode flow map (color flow map) (flow image): A display method in which only areas containing moving targets are displayed. It is a Doppler imaging technique in which the flow information can be shown as an overlay on the image to denote areas with flow. A spatial plot of Doppler flow may be superimposed upon the two-dimensional image with the direction and spectral content of flow shown either by color coding or gray scale overlay and the area of flow denoted by specific overlay on the image itself.

At an early stage in this technology, the Committee feels strongly that color flow map color schemes should, in fact, be standardized. Historically, the first published color flow mapping by Brandestini used orange to yellow colors as flow towards the transducer and blue as flow away from the transducer. With this historical perspective, the Committee believes this general color scheme is visually and informationally acceptable and that spectral broadening and disturbances can be shown as variance and mixtures of these colors with an additional hue, probably green.

Discrete Fourier transform: Sampled data representation of the Fourier transform which converts a waveform from the time to the frequency domain.

Fast Fourier transform FFT: An algorithm for efficient rapid computation of the discrete Fourier transform. The FFT is commonly used to implement spectral analysis.

Modal velocity (frequency mode): The mode in the frequency analysis of a signal is the frequency component which contains the most energy. In display of the Doppler frequency spectrum, the mode corresponds to the brightest (or darkest) display points of the individual spectra and represents the velocity component which is most commonly encountered among the various moving reflectors.

M-mode velocity (MQ) display: Doppler shift information along with the M-mode echocardiogram, usually derived along the line of sampling and displayed as a function of time, usually with an accompanying EKG.

Maximal velocity: The highest velocity found with significant amplitude within the sampled area usually for use in Bernoulli type gradient estimations.

Mean spectral velocity of blood flow: A mathematical mean of the spectral shifts in velocity within a given sample volume.

Mean velocity/time: (Mean temporal velocity) (Mean velocity as a function of time as in mean systolic velocity, mean diastolic velocity, or mean velocity for the cardiac cycle). Velocity time integral divided by the time period over which the integral was determined.

Spectral analysis: A method of analyzing waveforms derived from Doppler shift information by separating the waveform into its frequency velocity components.

Multiple frequency components may be derived from a single waveform. A common technique for spectral analysis is the fast Fourier transform.

Spectral width: The spectral width can be defined by a variety of statistical terms including: the standard deviation, full width to half maximal amplitude, or 6dB falloff from the modal velocity within the spectrum.

Velocity (Q)-mode: A display of Doppler velocities as a function of time (or waveform display), usually with an accompanying EKG.

Velocity time (flow velocity) integral: Calculated area under the Doppler curve over a specified period of time.

SECTION IV:
HYDRODYNAMIC TERMS

Bernoulli equation = Relationship between velocity change across an obstruction and the pressure gradient. Neglecting viscous and early phasic accelerational factors, it is commonly *simplified* to: gradient = $4 \times$ maximal velocity^2.

Disturbed flow: A pattern of flow with a disorganized velocity distribution. It is characterized by marked differences in direction and speed of blood cells within a vessel. The term turbulence can be mathematically defined but has been generally used interchangeably with disturbed flow.

Jet: A very high (unphysiologic) velocity area downstream from an obstruction where laminar flow proceeds at high velocity.

Laminar flow: Flow in which most blood cells are moving with a general uniformity of direction and velocity, and in which there is an organized distribution of velocities across the flow area.

Series effect: Extension or propagation of turbulent flow within the circulatory system downstream from an abnormal flow area.

Spatial velocity profile: Plot of velocity distribution across a vessel diameter which may be described as irregular, parabolic or flat, "flat" suggesting that approximately 80–90% of the flow cross-section of the vessel has the same velocity.

Vortex shed distance: The distance distal to a jet orifice after which laminar flow becomes disturbed.

AVAILABLE ASE PUBLICATIONS

"Report of the ASE Committee on Nomenclature and Standards in 2D Echocardiography," August 1980

"Report of the ASE Committee on Education and Training of the Echocardiographer (Cardiac Sonographer)," August 1982

"Report of the ASE Committee on Nomenclature and Standards: Identification of Myocardial Wall Segments," November 1982

"Report of the ASE Committee on Contrast Echocardiography," June 1984

"Report of the ASE Doppler Standards and Nomenclature Committee: Recommendations for Terminology and Display for Doppler Echocardiography," August 1984

"Report of the Standards Committee on Nomenclature of the Society of Pediatric Echocardiography and the American Society of Echocardiography: Nomenclature for Cardiac Septa," January 1986

"Guidelines for Optimal Physician Training in Echocardiography, Recommendations of the American Society of Echocardiography Committee for Physician Training in Echocardiography," July 1987

5

Nomenclature, Image Orientation, and Anatomic-Echocardiographic Correlations with Tomographic Views

James B. Seward, M.D., A. Jamil Tajik, M.D., Donald Hagler, M.D., William D. Edwards, M.D.

In recent years, two-dimensional echocardiography has become widely accepted as a useful technique for the diagnosis and management of various forms of congenital and acquired heart disease. It has gained wide acceptance because of its unique ability to provide spatial information regarding cardiac structure and function in a noninvasive manner. The images are presented in a familiar format, comparable to that of tomographic angiography, and can be correlated directly with cardiac anatomy. Because of the ever-increasing popularity of this imaging modality, it is crucial that the cardiologist remain familiar with the current image orientation, nomenclature, and anatomic details of various ultrasonic tomographic sections of the heart and great vessels. The purpose of this chapter is to discuss the basics of two-dimensional real-time echocardiographic image orientation and to correlate resulting images with normal cardiac anatomy. A detailed discussion of recognized tomographic sections and the frequency with which they are obtainable is reviewed in serial fashion. The chapter concludes with a discussion of the two-dimensional echocardiographic technique of imaging specific cardiac structures (e.g., atrial septum, ventricular septum, thoracic aorta).

METHODS

A commercially available 80° phased-array sector echocardiographic scaner (Varian 3000) was utilized. The two-dimensional echocardiographic images were permanently recorded on videotape. Still frames of sector scans in this chapter were photographed with a 35-mm camera assembly. The desired single-frame image was displayed on an oscilloscope in stop-frame mode and photographed directly. An 8- by 10-inch photographic enlargement was labeled and rephotographed for publication (1).

TECHNIQUES UTILIZED FOR VALIDATION OF TWO-DIMENSIONAL ANATOMY

For better assessment of the various two-dimensional echocardiographic views, multiple techniques are necessary. Initially, most echocardiographers relate the two-dimensional echocardiographic examination to previous M-mode experience. A simultaneous M-mode examination greatly enhances the ease of understanding both techniques. The advantage of two-dimensional echocardiography is that it permits appreciation of spatial anatomic relationships, can utilize multiple ultrasound windows and produces a more easily recognizable image that more closely approximates standard angiography (1). Thus, for the ultimate validation of this new noninvasive imaging modality, contrast echocardiography and standard angiography, in addition to pathologic and surgical anatomic correlation, have also been essential.

M-mode Echocardiography

Usually, only the parasternal long-axis projection of the left ventricle has any relationship to the M-mode examination (1) (Fig. 5.1). Two-dimensional echocardiography facilitates understanding of the M-mode examination. However, certain motion abnormalities and timed events are more easily appreciated by the M-mode technique (e.g., premature valve closure, fluttering of septa and valves and subtle septal motion abnormalities). Presently, the simultaneously obtained M-mode tracing permits more accurate measurement of chamber dimensions; however, it is very much limited to conventional image projections. The advantage of the two-dimensional examination is its versatility and unconventional

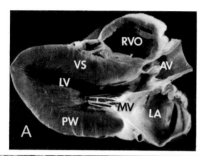

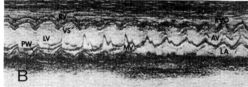

Figure 5.1. M-mode echocardiography in relation to the two-dimensional examination. *A*, pathologic specimen corresponding to a parasternal long-axis projection of the left ventricle. The cardiac chambers and structures sectioned correspond to the structures identified on a simultaneous M-mode sweep from apex to base. *B*, an M-mode echocardiographic sweep from apex (*left*) to base (*right*) obtained during a two-dimensional echocardiographic examination. The right ventricular cavity (*RV*) is located anteriorly. The ventricular septum (*VS*) is continuous with the anterior wall of the aortic root. The visible left ventricular (*LV*) myocardium is the ventricular septum anteriorly and the posterior wall (*PW*) posteriorly. The anterior mitral valve leaflet (*MV*) is continuous with the posterior wall of the aortic root. The aortic valve (*AV*) is visualized within the aortic root and opens with each systole. The left atrium (*LA*) lies posterior to the aorta. *RVO* = right ventricular outflow tract. (*A* modified and *B* from Tajik, AJ, Seward, JB, Hagler, DJ, Mair, DD, Lie, JT: Two-dimensional real-time ultrasonic imaging of the heart and great vessels: technique, image orientation, structure identification, and validation. *Mayo Clin Proc 53:* 271, 1978. By permission.)

viewing angles, which cannot be duplicated or improved upon by M-mode echocardiography.

On-line analysis of video images will ultimately eliminate the need for most M-mode-assisted measurements. The M-mode examination, however, remains an excellent, cost effective diagnostic tool that will remain an integral part of noninvasive cardiac evaluation.

Contrast Echocardiography

Although two-dimensional real-time wide-angle echocardiography allows direct visualization of cardiac defects and provides accurate spatial relationships of various intracardiac structures, blood and its flow pattern cannot be visualized with this technique. The ability to visualize the blood pool and its flow markedly enhances the sensitivity and specificity of the ultrasound examination (2). Blood normally acts as a relatively homogeneous ultrasonic medium. Thus, the cardiac chambers appear echo-free, and blood flow patterns cannot be visualized. Toward achievement of this end, the concept of contrast echocardiography was conceived in the mid-1960s, and it has been widely used in recent years.

Contrast echocardiography involves injection of echo-producing agents such as saline, indocyanine green dye, dextrose and the like into the cardiac chambers (2). These agents produce dense clouds of echoes, thought to represent highly echo-refractile microbubbles, which are readily visualized not only at the site of injection but also in downstream chambers (3) (Fig. 5.2). In our laboratory, we have utilized indocyanine green and saline as the contrast material (i.e., 1 ml of indocyanine green is injected, followed by a manual flush of 5 to 10 ml of normal saline) (4). The dosage of indocyanine green was varied according to the patient's weight.

Contrast echocardiography can be easily performed at bedside with minimal technical assistance. A short 20-gauge polyethylene needle is inserted into a superficial antecubital or hand vein. A three-way stopcock is utilized to occlude the needle between injections and to allow injection of indocyanine green and saline in a double-syringe fashion. The same injection technique used in the invasive laboratory is used for outpatient examinations. Frequently, saline alone will suffice as an echo-producing agent, particularly in younger patients or in the presence of low output, polycythemia, or severe valvular incompetence (3).

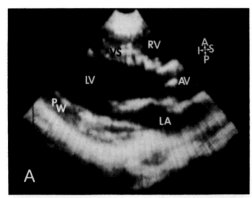

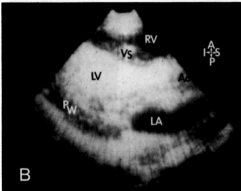

Figure 5.2. Two dimensional contrast echocardiography. *A*, parasternal long-axis projection of the left ventricle of a two-dimensional echocardiogram corresponding to Figure 5.1. At the time of cardiac catheterization, a selective left ventricular injection of indocyanine green and saline was utilized to opacify the left ventricle. *B*, following injection, a dense cloud of echoes opacifies the left ventricle (*LV*) and during systole is ejected into the aorta (*Ao*). The resulting opacified left ventricle, in real-time, is comparable to a standard angiogram. The left atrium (*LA*) remains echo-free; this finding substantiates the absence of mitral regurgitation. The ventricular septum (*VS*) and posterior wall (*PW*) are silhouetted by the opacified left ventricle. The right ventricular cavity (*RV*) remains echo-free. *AV* = aortic valve; *A* = anterior; *S* = superior; *P* = posterior; *I* = inferior. From Seward, JB, Tajik, AJ, Hagler, DJ: Two-dimensional contrast echoangiography. In *Pediatric Echocardiography—Cross-Sectional, M-Mode and Doppler*. pp. 239–255, N-R Lundström, ed. Amsterdam, Elsevier/North-Holland Biomedical Press, 1980. By permission.

Angiography

Because two-dimensional echocardiography in many respects closely approximates a standard angiographic examination of the heart, certain correlations can be made. Substantiation of echocardiographic anatomy by angiographic techniques was necessary for the evaluation of this new image modality. However, as two-dimensional echocardiography becomes more accepted, certain aspects of the invasive examination can be expected to be replaced.

Pathologic and Surgical Correlation

As illustrated in this chapter, there is an ever-increasing need to become more familiar with detailed cardiac anatomy for better understanding of the versatile two-dimensional echocardiographic examination. Two-dimensional echocardiography permits the examiner to look in the heart with unconventional tomographic views. With increasing use of tomographic anatomic assessment of the heart, it is important for the pathologist, the clinician and the surgeon to reassess their knowledge of and approach to cardiac anatomy. The classic "inflow-outflow" approach to cardiac dissection bears little resemblance to the ultrasonic tomographic views. A more in-depth and versatile knowledge of cardiac anatomy is needed for a proper understanding of the tomographic two-dimensional image.

In this report, for the purpose of structure identification and validation, pressure-perfused fixed autopsy hearts were sectioned in the presumed planes of the ultrasonic tomographic section. The tissue sections were photographed in the same orientation as the ultrasound images. For the purposes of labeling, drawings of these same representative sections were made by our medical art department.

NOMENCLATURE

The two-dimensional tomographic views of the heart and great vessels should be described relative to 1) transducer position, 2) plane of section and 3) structure(s) visualized (5) (Fig. 5.3).

Transducer Positions

Four standardized transducer positions are utilized (Fig. 5.4).

Parasternal

The transducer is placed over the anterior precordium (i.e., usually along the left sternal border) in the third or fourth intercostal space and directed posteriorly.

Apical

The transducer is placed at the lower left side of the chest, usually near the point of maximal

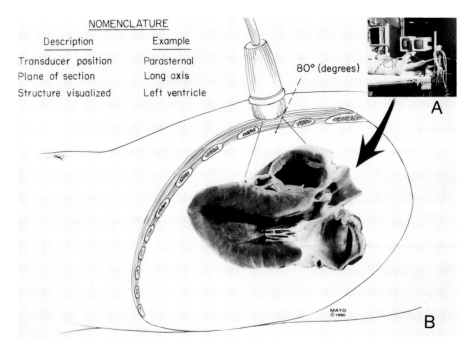

NOMENCLATURE

Description	Example
Transducer position	Parasternal
Plane of section	Long axis
Structure visualized	Left ventricle

80° (degrees)

A

B

MAYO
© 1980

Figure 5.3. Nomenclature. Each tomographic image is described relative to the transducer position, plane of section and structure visualized. *A*, echocardiographer examining the subject from the *left parasternal transducer position. B*, the scan plane extends along the *long axis of the left ventricle* (i.e., apex to base). Thus, this particular view would be described as a *parasternal long-axis projection of the left ventricle. B* from Seward, JB, Tajik, AJ: Two-dimensional echocardiography. *Med Clin North Am 64:* 177, 1980. By permission of WB Saunders Company.

apical impulse, and directed superiorly and to the patient's right.

Subcostal

The transducer is positioned below the xiphoid process or along the lower costal margin and directed superiorly.

Suprasternal

The transducer is positioned in the suprasternal notch and directed inferiorly toward the aortic arch and the base of the heart.

Although each transducer position may not yield diagnostic information for a particular patient, the ability to obtain unique apical, subcostal and suprasternal views makes the two-dimensional technique very adaptable and versatile (6). The apical views in adult patients are the easiest to obtain and the most helpful in the assessment of segmental (coronary) heart disease and congenital heart disease. The subcostal examination often provides a clear ultrasound window to the heart in otherwise technically difficult situations (i.e., in the patient with obstructive lung disease and

chest deformities and in the neonate or younger child). The suprasternal views are most valuable for the assessment of aortic arch and pulmonary artery anomalies in cases of congenital disease.

Plane of Section

Definition of Axes and Planes of Section

The heart and associated structures should be perceived as three-dimensional objects within the thorax. Through these objects, various *axes* (lines) can be drawn, along which *planes* (surfaces) of section can be obtained.

An *axis is a straight line about which a body or geometric figure rotates or may be supposed to rotate.* Thus, the heart (with the left ventricle as the reference object) has two primary axes (Fig. 5.5A): 1) a *long* or *major axis* formed by a line from the base of the heart to the apex and 2) a *short* or *minor axis* formed by a line at right angles to the long axis.

A *plane is a surface extending through or along an axis.* Multiple or a family of planes can po-

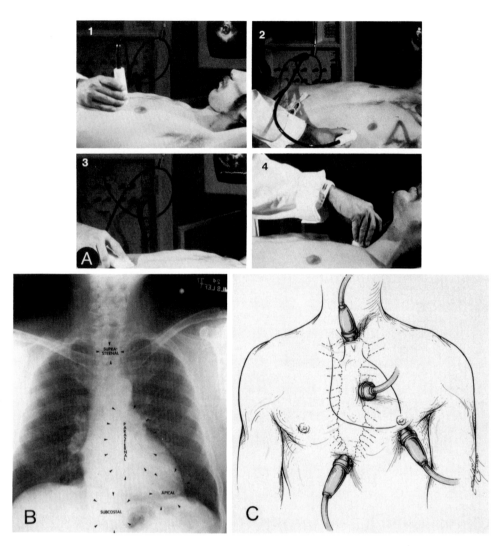

Figure 5.4. Four standardized transducer positions, *A*, the transducer positions utilized during the two-dimensional examination are illustrated: *1*, parasternal; *2*, apical; *3*, subcostal; and *4*, suprasternal. *B* and *C*, the relative transducer positions from a postero-anterior chest x-ray film and a drawing of the anterior chest wall. For the parasternal examination, the transducer is directed posteriorly. From the apical transducer position, the transducer is directed superiorly and to the right. From the subcostal position, the transducer is directed superiorly and to the left. From the suprasternal transducer position, the transducer is directed inferiorly toward the base of the heart. *A* modified from Tajik, AJ, Seward, JB, Hagler, DJ, Mair, DD, Lie, JT: Two-dimensional real-time ultrasonic imaging of the heart and great vessels: Technique, image orientation, structure identification, and validation. *Mayo Clin Proc 53:* 271, 1978. By permission. *C* from Bansal, RC, Tajik, AJ, Seward, JB, Offord, KP: Feasibility of detailed two-dimensional echocardiographic examination in adults: Prospective study of 200 patients. *Mayo Clin Proc 55:* 291, 1980. By permission.

tentially be obtained along any axis. In the case of the heart, this results in two basic groups of tomographic views: (Fig. 5.5*B*)—that is, a short-axis group and a long-axis group of images (1). For the purposes of consistency and ease of understanding, the tomographic images within each group are displayed such that all cavities and structures are oriented in a similar manner, approximating their anatomic position within the thorax regardless of transducer position.

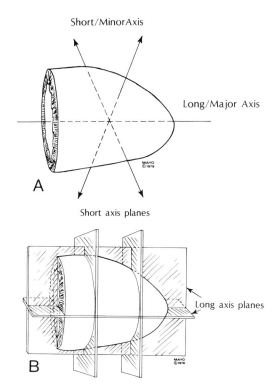

Figure 5.5. Axes and planes of section. *A, axes:* with the left ventricle used as the reference object, two primary axes can be produced. A long or major axis is formed by a line from the base of the heart to the apex, and a short or minor axis is formed by a line at right angles to the long axis. *B, planes of section:* two basic groups of tomographic views or planes can be obtained along the two axes of the heart. Long-axis planes extend from the apex to the base, and short-axis planes are at right angles to the long axis. From Seward, JB, Tajik, AJ: Two-dimensional echocardiography. *Med Clin North Am 64:* 177, 1980. By permission of WB Saunders Company.

Two-Dimensional Echocardiographic Planes of Section

By convention (5), three planes, at right angles to each other (i.e., the short-axis, long-axis, and four-chamber planes), are used to describe all cardiac and extracardiac two-dimensional echocardiographic tomographic views (Fig. 5.6). It should be noted that both the long-axis plane and the four-chamber plane are on the long axis of the heart.

Short-Axis Plane. Tomographic views in the short-axis plane are parallel to the minor axis of the heart. These views are displayed as though

the observer were looking from the abdomen toward the head (Fig. 5.7). Short-axis views of the heart are obtained from the parasternal and subcostal transducer positions. The resulting images, when rotated into the same anatomic position, are all displayed in a similar fashion.

Long-Axis Plane. Tomographic views in the long-axis plane are parallel to the major axis of the heart and perpendicular to the dorsal and ventral surfaces of the chest. These planes of section are displayed as though the observer were looking from the left side of the patient (a left sagittal cut of the left ventricle) (Fig. 5.8). Long-axis views of the heart are obtained from the parasternal and apical transducer positions. This plane is at right angles to the four-chamber plane. When rotated into the same anatomic position, the images are displayed in a consistent fashion regardless of transducer position.

Four-Chamber Plane. Tomographic views in the four-chamber plane are along the major axis of the heart and parallel to the dorsal and ventral surfaces of the chest. These planes of section are displayed as though the observer were looking down upon the heart (i.e., comparable to a fron-

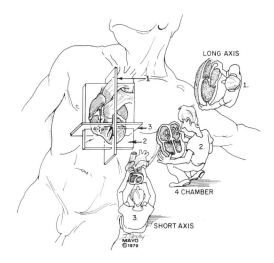

Figure 5.6. Two-dimensional echocardiographic planes of section. *Long-axis planes* are viewed as a left sagittal cut of the left ventricle. The *four-chamber planes* are viewed as though one were examining the heart anterior to posterior. The *short-axis planes* are viewed from the apex toward the base of the heart. From Seward, JB, Tajik, AJ: Two-dimensional echocardiography. *Med Clin North Am 64:* 177, 1980. By permission of WB Saunders Company.

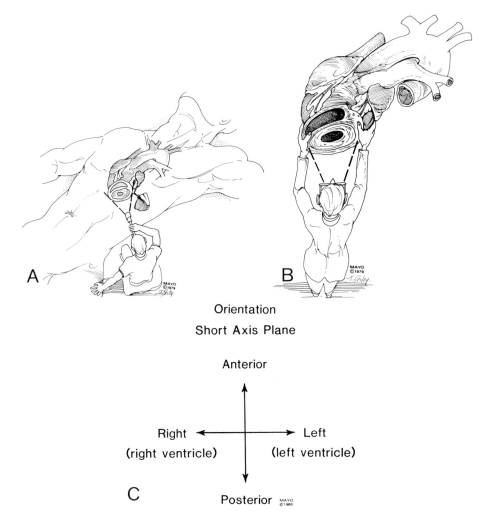

Orientation

Short Axis Plane

Figure 5.7. Short-axis plane. *A* and *B*, short-axis views are displayed as though the observer were looking from the abdomen toward the head. *C*, the display is oriented such that anterior structures are to the top of the screen and posterior structures to the bottom, with left structures to the right and right structures to the left. *A* and *B* from Seward, JB, Tajik, AJ: Two-dimensional echocardiography. *Med Clin North Am 64:* 177, 1980. By permission of WB Saunders Company.

tal projection of the left ventricle) (Fig. 5.9). Four-chamber planes can be obtained from the apical, subcostal and parasternal transducer positions. It is the recommendation of the American Society of Echocardiography Committee on Nomenclature and Standards (5) that this particular plane be displayed with the apex of the heart toward the bottom of the image, which most closely corresponds to the anatomic position within the chest (Fig. 5.10*A*, *bottom*). (See "Apical Transducer Position," p. 70, for details.)

Note that this particular display orientation is comparable to the long-axis group of images (i.e., rotated 90°, apex down).

Many sector echocardiographic machines, however, have a fixed display of the pie-shaped sector scan with the transducer artifact presented at the top of the screen (i.e., the images are inverted 180°, apex up, from the recommended anatomic position) (Fig. 5.10*A*, *top*). For this reason, an optional orientation of the cardiac images has been suggested. With the apex up, the left

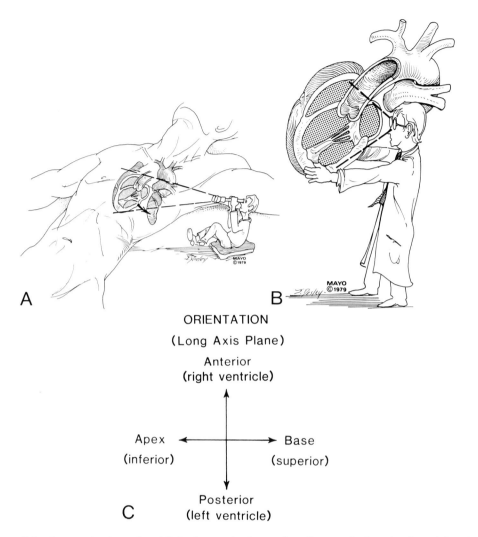

ORIENTATION
(Long Axis Plane)

Anterior
(right ventricle)

Apex ←——→ Base
(inferior)   (superior)

Posterior
(left ventricle)

Figure 5.8. Long-axis plane. *A* and *B*, the long-axis planes of section are displayed as though the observer were looking from the left side of the patient (a left sagittal cut of the left ventricle). *C*, the images are oriented such that anterior structures are to the *top* of the screen and posterior structures are to the bottom; basal structures are to the *right* and the cardiac apex is to the left. From Seward, JB, Tajik, AJ: Two-dimensional echocardiography. *Med Clin North Am 64:* 177, 1980. By permission of WB Saunders Company.

ventricle is displayed to the right, the right ventricle to the left, the right atrium to the left, and the left atrium to the right (Fig. 5.10*A*, *top right*). One must be aware, however, that this is a mirror image of the recommended apex-down orientation. If this image is correlated with cardiac anatomy (Fig. 5.10, *B* and *C*, *top*), the examiner would be looking at the heart from *posterior to anterior* (i.e., as though he were dissecting the heart from posterior to anterior surface). This is in deference to the recommended apex-down orientation (5)

(Fig. 5.10, *B* and *C*, *bottom*) or the previously reported alternate apex-up orientation (1), which views cardiac anatomy anterior to posterior.

Another apex-up orientation (Fig. 5.10*A*, *top left*) of the four-chamber plane places the left ventricle to the left and the right ventricle to the right (1). This particular orientation represents a 180° *rotation* from the recommended apex-down four-chamber plane. If this image is correlated with cardiac anatomy (Fig. 5.10*D*), the examiner would be viewing the heart from *anterior to pos-*

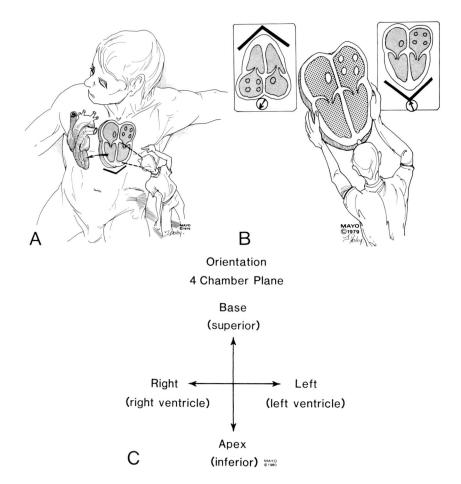

Figure 5.9 Four-chamber plane. *A*, four-chamber views are displayed as though the observer were looking down upon the heart (i.e., comparable to a frontal projection of the left ventricle). *B*, the four-chamber plane is displayed with the apex down (5) (*upper right*), in which the left ventricle is viewed to the right and inferior and the right ventricle is to the left and inferior. Alternate apex-up projections include a mirror image of the apex-down position (not shown) in which the left ventricle is imaged to the right and the right ventricle to the left with the apex up. Note that this is a mirror image of the heart, and thus one would be looking at the heart from posterior to anterior. For maintenance of an anatomic orientation similar to the apex-down position, the left ventricle would be oriented to the left and the right ventricle to the right, as shown in the *upper left* (1). *C*, with an apex-down position, the image is oriented such that the base of the heart is to the top of the screen, apex to the bottom of the screen, left-sided structures to the right and right-sided structures to the left. (*A* and *B* from Seward, JB, Tajik, AJ: Two-dimensional echocardiography. *Med Clin North Am 64:* 177, 1980. By permission of WB Saunders Company.)

terior (i.e., as though he were dissecting the heart from anterior to posterior surface).

In this chapter images in the four-chamber plane (i.e., apical, subcostal and parasternal four-chamber planes) will be presented with the apex down, as recommended by the American Society of Echocardiography (5).

Tomographic Views

The following discussion outlines the standard anatomic projections obtained from the various transducer positions (Table 5.1). The transducer manipulation utilized and the orientation of the plane will be described in each instance. Anatomic correlation will be illustrated with appro-

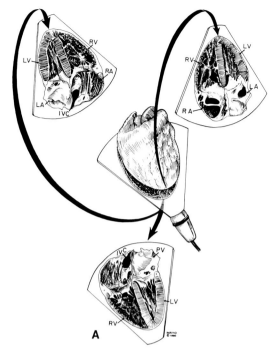

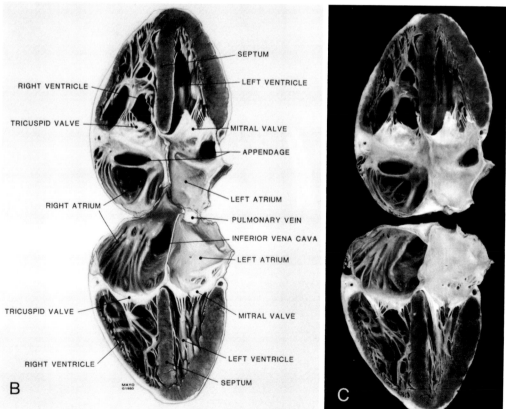

Figure 5.10. Four-chamber plane, anatomic correlation. *A*, illustration showing the variable presentations of the four-chamber plane. *Lower*, the recommended apex-down four-chamber view. The left ventricle (*LV*) is to the *right*, right ventricle (*RV*) to the *left*. Note that the posteriorly located inferior vena cava (*IVC*) is visible in the right atrial cavity. *Right upper*, an alternate apex-up view. This displays the left ventricle to

Table 5.1. Nomenclature of Commonly Obtained Two-Dimensional Tomographic Views

Transducer Position	Plane of Section	Views[a]	Tomographic Section
I. Parasternal	A. Long	Left ventricle	1
		RV inflow tract	2
		RV outflow tract	3
	B. Four-chamber	Foreshortened parasternal four-chamber	4
	C. Short	Apex	5
		Papillary muscles	6
		Mitral valve orifice	7
		LV outflow tract	8
		Aortic valve	9
		Pulmonary bifurcation	10
II. Apical	A. Four-chamber	Four-chamber	11
		Four-chamber coronary sinus	11A
		Four-chamber and aorta	12
	B. Long	Left ventricle (RAO equivalent)	13
		Left ventricle (two-chamber view)	13A
III. Subcostal	A. Abdominal 1. Short 2. Long	Viscera	14A
		Aorta	14B
		Inferior vena cava	14C
		Hepatic veins	14D
	B. Four-chamber	Four-chamber	15
		Four-chamber and aorta	16
		RV outflow tract	16A
	C. Short	Apex	17A
		Papillary muscles	17B
		Mitral valve orifice	17C
		LV outflow tract	17D
		Aortic valve	17E
		Pulmonary bifurcation	17F
IV. Suprasternal	A. Long	Aortic arch	18
	B. Short	Great arteries	19
	C. Frontal	Ascending aorta	20
		Descending aorta	20A

[a]*RV* = right ventricular; *LV* = left ventricular; *RAO* = right anterior oblique.

the *right* and the right ventricle to the *left*. Note that the structures within the atria are the atrial appendages. This section, if correlated with the anatomic specimen, is the anterior half of the cut specimen. *Left upper*, a second alternate view of the apex-up four-chamber view. Note that this is a 180° rotation of the apex-down specimen. The left ventricle is to the *left*, the right ventricle to the *right*. Note that, similar to the apex-down specimen, the inferior vena cava is visible in the right atrial cavity. *LA* = left atrium; *RA* = right atrium; *PV* = pulmonary vein. *B* and *C* anatomic drawing and pathologic specimen of a bisected heart cut in the four-chamber plane. Note that the recommended apex-down orientation views the heart from anterior to posterior. The anterior specimen views the heart from a posterior-to-anterior projection.

priate pathologic specimens and contrast echocardiography. *The anatomic projections are in no way absolute standards but do correspond to accepted anatomic projections of the heart (7) and are utilized to best accomplish a complete anatomic presentation of the cardiac chambers and structures.*

Note: *After each view, plane of section and transducer position, a percentage will appear which is* *the frequency with which each can be expected to be obtained during an adult two-dimensional echocardiographic examination (6).*

IA. Parasternal Long-Axis Plane (97%).

Section 1 (97%) (Parasternal Long-Axis Plane of Left Ventricle) (Fig. 5.11). The transducer is positioned parasternally in the third or fourth left

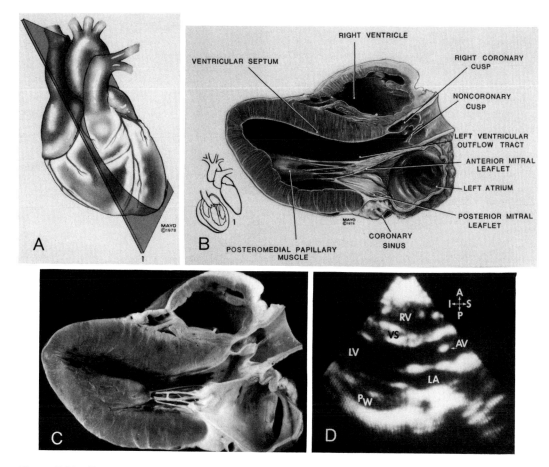

Figure 5.11. Tomographic section 1 (parasternal long-axis plane of left ventricle). *A*, plane of section. *B*, anatomic drawing. *C*, specimen cut to presumed plane of section. *D*, sector echographic image of ventricular septum (*VS*) is continuous with the anterior wall of the aorta. The anterior leaflet of the mitral valve is continuous with the posterior wall of the aorta. Within the aortic root, the aortic valve (*AV*) is visualized. The left atrium (*LA*) lies posterior to the aorta. Posterior to the left atrium, an echo-lucent area represents the descending thoracic aorta. The left ventricle (*LV*) is limited anteriorly by the ventricular septum and posteriorly by the posterior wall (*PW*). The right ventricular outflow tract (*RV*) is located anteriorly. *A* = anterior; *S* = superior; *P* = posterior; *I* = inferior. (*A* and *D* from Seward, JB, Tajik, AJ: Two-dimensional echocardiography. *Med Clin North Am 64:* 177, 1980; WB Saunders Company. *B* and *C* modified from Tajik, AJ, Seward, JB, Hagler, DJ, Maier, DD, Lie, JT: Two-dimensional real-time ultrasonic imaging of the heart and great vessels: technique, image orientation, structure identification, and validation. *Mayo Clin Proc 53:* 271, 1978. By permission.)

intercostal space and directed nearly straight posteriorly. This scan produces a plane extending from the right shoulder toward the left flank (i.e., comparable to the base-to-apex scan obtained during an M-mode examination). This view displays the apex of the heart to the left, the base to the right, the right ventricular outflow anteriorly, and the left ventricle posteriorly. The ventricular septum (i.e., *outflow* ventricular septum) separates the right and left ventricular outflow tracts. The septum is contiguous with the anterior wall of the aortic root. The posterior wall of the aortic root is continuous with the anterior leaflet of the mitral valve. Within the aortic root, the right and usually the noncoronary aortic cusps are visualized. Posterior to the aortic root is the left atrium. Posterior to the left atrium or (mitral) atrioventricular groove, a large echolucent area represents the descending thoracic aorta (8) (Fig. 5.12); and anteriorly, more closely associated with the atrioventricular groove, the coronary sinus can occasionally be visualized. However, the coronary sinus is more readily visualized when dilated, in the presence of anomalous venous return (persistent left superior vena cava or anomalous pulmonary venous connection to coronary sinus) (9) or right atrial hypertension (i.e., tricuspid re-

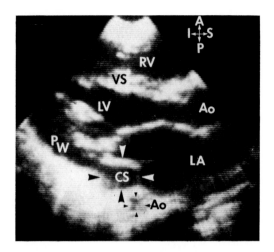

Figure 5.13. Persistent left superior vena cava to coronary sinus. Coronary sinus (*CS*) appears as a large echolucent circle in the left atrioventricular groove. The thoracic aorta (*Ao*) is less well visualized posterior to the coronary sinus. Left-hand vein contrast echocardiographic techniques were utilized to confirm the presence of left superior vena cava to coronary sinus. *RV* = right ventricle; *VS* = ventricular septum; *LV* = left ventricle; *Ao* = aortic root; *LA* = left atrium; *PW* = posterior wall; *A* = anterior; *S* = superior; *P* = posterior; *I* = inferior. From Seward, JB, Tajik, AJ: Two-dimensional echocardiography. *Med Clin North Am 64:* 177, 1980. By permission of WB Saunders Company.

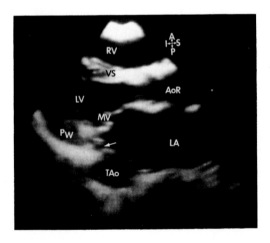

Figure 5.12. Parasternal long-axis plane of left ventricle. Posterior to the left atrium (*LA*) is a large echolucent area representing the descending thoracic aorta (*TAo*) (8). *Small arrow* represents the normal coronary sinus in the posterior left atrioventricular groove. *AoR* = aortic root; *RV* = right ventricle; *VS* = ventricular septum; *LV* = left ventricle; *MV* = mitral valve; *PW* = posterior wall; *A* = anterior; *S* = superior; *I* = inferior.

gurgitation, pulmonary hypertension, and so on) (Fig. 5.13). The posterobasal left ventricular myocardium is visualized inferior to the posterior leaflet of the mitral valve. With a slight medial tilt of the transducer, the posteromedial papillary muscle is visualized and, with a lateral tilt, the anterolateral papillary muscle. The true apex of the left ventricle usually cannot be appreciated from this position.

Section 2 (54%) (Parasternal Long-Axis Plane of Right Ventricular Inflow) (Fig. 5.14). From tomographic section 1, the transducer is tilted medially and slightly inferiorly (i.e., beneath the sternum) (Fig. 5.15). The scan plane is now oriented more or less from the right shoulder to the left hip. To the right of the image is the right atrium and to the left, the inflow portion of the right ventricle. The anterior and septal or posterior leaflets of the tricuspid valve separate the right atrium from the right ventricle. Right atrial anatomic landmarks include, anteriorly, the right atrial appendage, and posteriorly, toward the tri-

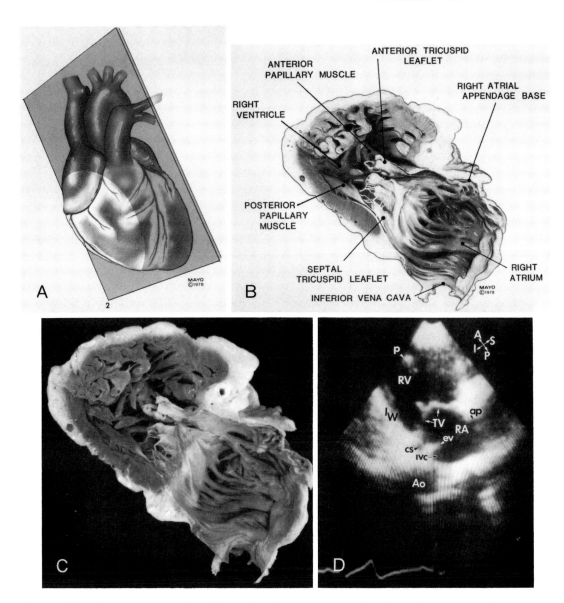

Figure 5.14. Tomographic section 2 (parasternal long-axis plane of right ventricular inflow). *A,* plane of section. *B,* anatomic drawing. *C,* pathologic specimen cut to the presumed plane of section. *D,* two-dimensional echocardiographic image of right ventricular inflow. The tricuspid valve (*TV*) separates the right atrium (*RA*) from the right ventricle (*RV*). A single papillary muscle (*p*) is visualized in the body of the right ventricle. The inferior right ventricular wall (*IW*) is imaged posteriorly to the *left.* Identifiable structures within the right cavity include the orifice of the coronary sinus (*cs*) and the Eustachian valve (*ev*) separating the coronary sinus from the orifice of the inferior vena cava (*ivc*). Anteriorly, portions of the right atrial appendage (*ap*) can be visualized. An echolucent area posterior to the right atrium is an oblique short-axis cut of the descending thoracic aorta (*Ao*). A = anterior; S = superior; P = posterior; I = inferior. *A* and *B* by permission of the Mayo Clinic.

cuspid atrioventricular groove, the orifice of the coronary sinus. The coronary sinus is separated from the inferior vena cava by the Eustachian valve. Portions of the anterior and posterobasal right ventricular myocardium are also visualized. Within the right ventricle, one and occasionally two papillary muscles are also seen.

Section 3 (50%) (Parasternal Long-Axis View

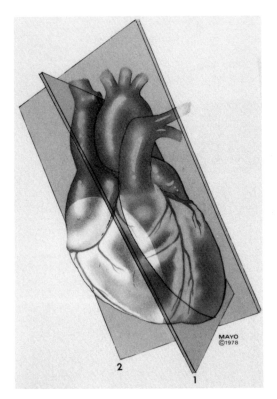

Figure 5.15. Tomographic sections 1 and 2. The right ventricular inflow tract (section 2) is visualized by medial tilting of the transducer from the parasternal long-axis projection of the left ventricle (section 1). By permission of the Mayo Clinic.

of Right Ventricular Outflow Tract) (Fig. 5.16). Tomographic section 3 is obtained by scanning from tomographic section 1 with approximately a 30° clockwise rotation of the transducer and a slight medial and superior tilt. The plane of section extends in a left paravertebral projection, parallel to a true sagittal plane of the thorax. Anteriorly, the long-axis projection of the right ventricular outflow tract is visualized, and posteriorly, an oblique section of left ventricle. The anterior and posterior leaflets of the pulmonary valve are often best displayed from this position, and they separate the right ventricular outflow tract from the proximal pulmonary trunk. An oblique section of the anterior and posterior leaflets of the mitral valve and left ventricle are also visualized. With appropriate adjustment of the posterior gain, the long-axis projection of the descending thoracic aorta is also best imaged from this transducer position (8) (Fig. 5.17).

IB. Parasternal Four-Chamber Plane (65%).

Section 4 (65%) (Parasternal Four-Chamber Plane) (Fig. 5.18). From tomographic section 1, the transducer is rotated 90° to lie perpendicular to the long axis of the left ventricle, displaced slightly laterally and inferiorly by one rib space and directed toward the right shoulder. This view is comparable to an apical four-chamber view (see below); however, the transducer is actually overlying the free wall of the left ventricle and is superior to the true apex of the left ventricle. The scan cuts obliquely through the ventricle toward the atria. The plane of section extends from the left thorax toward the right scapula and is oriented such that the examiner is looking down on the heart in a frontal projection. With the apex displayed at the bottom of the image, the right ventricle is to the left, the left ventricle to the right, and the atria to the top of the screen, with the left atrium to the right and the right atrium to the left. The ventricles are separated by the *inflow ventricular septum*, which separates the two atrioventricular valves. The septal leaflet of the tricuspid valve inserts lower toward the right ventricular cavity than the septal portion of the anterior leaflet of the mitral valve. The constant anatomic relationships of the atrioventricular valves and septa form the crux of the heart and are most useful in elucidating ventricular morphology (i.e., in patients with inverted ventricles, this relationship is reversed). The pulmonary veins can occasionally be visualized entering the left atrium. See tomographic sections 11 and 12 (apical four-chamber view) for other possible views from this parasternal four-chamber transducer position.

IC. Parasternal Short-Axis Plane (92%). Short-axis views of the heart are obtained by rotating the transducer until it assumes a position approximately parallel to the plane extending from the left shoulder to the right flank (90° to the long-axis plane of left ventricle). By an inferior and superior tilt of the transducer, serial short-axis cuts of the left ventricle can be obtained in a bread-loafing fashion (Fig. 5.19). The left ventricle appears as a doughnut-like structure; this view permits assessment of cavity dimensions and left ventricular wall thickness and performance.

Section 5 (52%) (Parasternal Short-Axis Plane of Left Ventricular Apex) (Fig. 5.20). This projection of the left ventricle is obtained frequently from a lower parasternal interspace (i.e., fourth left intercostal space). The plane of section remains parallel to a plane from the left shoulder

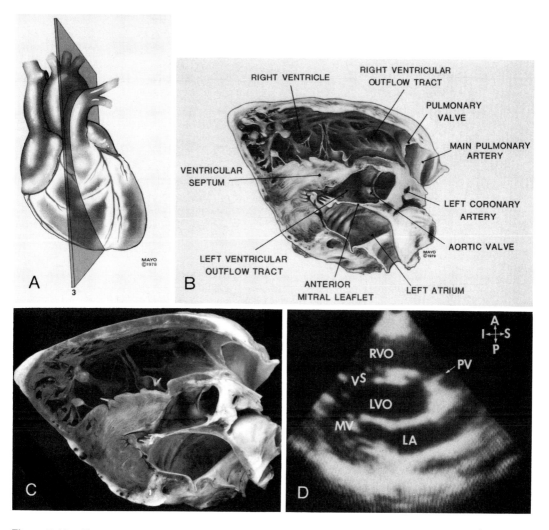

Figure 5.16. Tomographic section 3 (parasternal long-axis view of right ventricular outflow tract). *A,* plane of section. *B,* anatomic drawing. *C,* pathologic specimen cut in the presumed plane of section. *D,* two-dimensional echocardiographic view of right ventricular outflow tract. The right ventricular outflow tract (*RVO*) is viewed in its long projection. The pulmonary valve (*PV*) separates the right ventricular outflow tract from the proximal main pulmonary artery. The left ventricular outflow tract (*LVO*) is cut obliquely. The left atrium (*LA*) is posterior to the anterior leaflet of the mitral valve (*MV*). The left ventricle and ventricular septum (*VS*) are also cut obliquely. *A* = anterior; *S* = superior; *P* = posterior; *I* = inferior. *C* from Seward, JB, Tajik, AJ, Hagler, DJ: Orientation of the great arteries: Normal, complete transposition, and corrected transposition. In *Pediatric Echocardiography — Cross-Sectional M-Mode and Doppler.* pp. 105–120. N-R Lundström (ed) Amsterdam, Elsevier/North-Holland Biomedical Press, 1980. By permission. *D* from Tajik, AJ, Seward, JB, Hagler, DJ, Mair, DD, Lie, JT: Two-dimensional real time ultrasonic imaging of the heart and great vessels: Technique, image orientation, structure identification, and validation. *Mayo Clin Proc 53:* 271, 1978. By permission.

to the right flank. This projection of the left ventricle is helpful in delineating apical pathology (i.e., aneurysm, thrombus and infarct).

Section 6 (78%) (Parasternal Short-Axis Pro-

jection of Left Ventricle and Papillary Muscles) (Fig. 5.21). With the transducer in the standard parasternal position, the plane of section is parallel to a plane from the left shoulder to the right

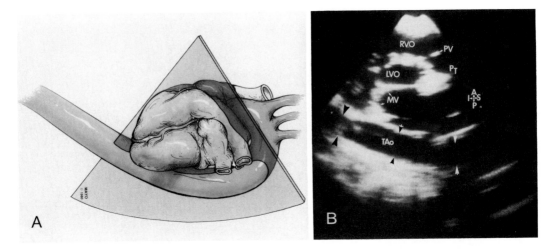

Figure 5.17. Long-axis projection of the descending thoracic aorta. *A*, plane of section across the long axis of the right ventricular outflow tract. The plane is parallel to the long axis of the body (left paravertebral). *B*, with proper posterior gain settings, the long-axis projection of the descending thoracic aorta (*TAo*) is visualized posterior to the cardiac structures. The remainder of the examination is similar to that in Figure 5.16*D*. *RVO* = right ventricular outflow tract; *LVO* = left ventricular outflow tract; *MV* = mitral valve; *PV* = pulmonary valve; *PT* = pulmonary trunk; *A* = anterior; *S* = superior; *P* = posterior; *I* = inferior.

flank. The papillary muscles appear as echo-refractile structures within the left ventricular cavity, usually at 3 and 7 o'clock. The left ventricle appears doughnut-like, and its function and dimensions can be appreciated. The ventricular septum separates the left ventricular cavity from the right ventricle, which lies anterior and to the left on the image. Frequently, with further superior tilting of the transducer, the moderator band of the tricuspid support apparatus can be visualized within the right ventricular cavity (Fig. 5.22).

Section 7 (85%) (Parasternal Short-Axis Plane of Left Ventricle at Mitral Valve) (Fig. 5.22). The scan plane remains parallel to a line from the left shoulder to the right flank. The mitral orifice, formed by the anterior and posterior leaflets, appears ovoid (i.e., like a fish mouth). Anterior to the mitral valve orifice is the left ventricular outflow tract. Midportions of the ventricular septum separate the left and right ventricular cavities. The septal and posterior leaflets of the tricuspid valve are visualized. It is noted that the tricuspid orifice does not lie in the same plane as the mitral valve orifice. Thus, the three cusps of the tricuspid valve are usually not appreciated in short-axis views of the left ventricle. The anterior leaflet of the tricuspid valve inserts much higher in the right ventricular cavity and is seen with a more superior

tilt of the transducer. The right ventricular outflow tract appears as an increasing echolucent area wrapping anteriorly over the left ventricle.

Section 8 (87%) (Parasternal Short-Axis Plane of Left Ventricular Outflow Tract) (Fig. 5.23). Further superior tilt allows more complete visualization of the left ventricular outflow tract lying anterior to the mitral valve orifice. Basal portions of the outflow ventricular septum are visualized anteriorly, separating the right and left ventricular outflow tracts.

Section 9 (88%) (Parasternal Short-Axis Plane at Aortic Valve Level) (Fig. 5.24). The aortic valve and its respective leaflets form the central portion of this particular image. The right, left, and noncoronary cusps are visualized forming a Y configuration during diastole and an inverted triangle (∇) during systole (Fig. 5.25). Posterior to the aortic valve and root is the left atrium. Laterally, the left atrial appendage is viewed, and medially, portions of the atrial septum separate the right and left atria. At the inferior portion of the atrial septum, the orifice of the coronary sinus can occasionally be appreciated along with the orifice of the inferior vena cava. A scan between tomographic sections 8 and 9 will permit visualization of the long axis of the coronary sinus. This particular view of the coronary sinus, however, is less productive than a posteriorly directed ap-

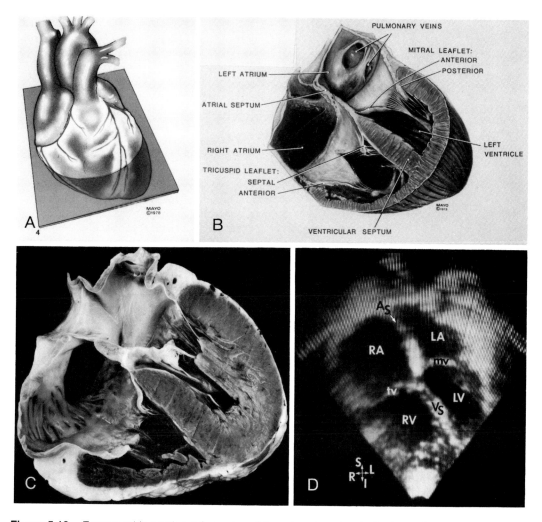

Figure 5.18. Tomographic section 4 (parasternal four-chamber plane). *A*, plane of section. *B*, anatomic drawing. *C*, pathologic specimen cut in the presumed plane of section. *D*, two-dimensional sector echographic image of a foreshortened four-chamber view. The mitral valve (*mv*) separates the left atrium (*LA*) from the left ventricle (*LV*). The tricuspid valve (*tv*) separates the right atrium (*RA*) from the right ventricle (*RV*). The atrial septum (*A$_s$*) is slightly displaced to the left of the long axis of the ventricular septum (*V$_s$*). The septal leaflet of the tricuspid valve inserts lower into the ventricle than the septal portion of the anterior mitral valve leaflet. The above features are typical of the normal crux of the heart. *S* = superior; *L* = left; *I* = inferior; *R* = right. *B* modified from Tajik, AJ, Seward, JB, Hagler, DJ, Mair, DD, Lie, JT: Two-dimensional real-time ultrasonic imaging of the heart and great vessels: Technique, image orientation, structure identification, and validation. From *Mayo Clin Proc 53:* 271, 1978. By permission. *D* from Bansal, RC, Tajik, AJ, Seward, JB, Offord, KP: Feasibility of detailed two-dimensional echocardiographic examination in adults: Prospective study of 200 patients. *Mayo Clin Proc 55:* 291, 1980. By permission.

ical four-chamber view (section 11A, see below). The right atrium is bounded anteriorly by the anterior leaflet of the tricuspid valve. Coursing leftward and anterior to the aortic valve is the right ventricular outflow tract, which produces a sausage-like echolucent area anteriorly. Right-ward of and anterior to the aortic valve, portions of the pulmonary valve are visualized. Beyond the pulmonary valve is the proximal pulmonary trunk. The echolucent area posterior to the left atrium is an oblique view of the descending thoracic aorta.

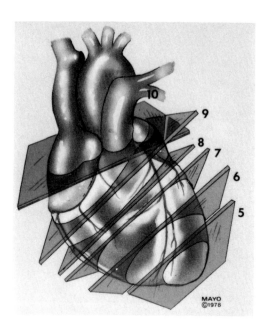

Figure 5.19. Short-axis planes of left ventricle. The left ventricle can be cut in a serial bread-loafing fashion from apex to base utilizing the parasternal transducer position.

Section 10 (25%) (Parasternal Short-Axis Plane of Pulmonary Bifurcation) (Fig. 5.26). By further superior tilt and slight leftward angulation of the transducer, the main pulmonary artery and proximal bifurcation into left and right pulmonary arteries can be visualized. The scanning plane now extends from the left shoulder toward the right scapula. The pulmonary valve is no longer visible, and only the proximal portions of the left pulmonary artery can be visualized. The right pulmonary artery, however, circles beneath the aortic root and can be viewed in its long axis. Portions of the descending thoracic aorta are visualized as an echolucent area beneath the bifurcation of the main right and left pulmonary arteries. The scan plane is superior to the left atrial cavity.

IIA. Apical Transducer Position (99%) Four-Chamber Plane (99%). Images will be oriented according to the recommendations of the American Society of Echocardiography (5), that is, with the apex down. This corresponds to the anatomic view of the heart one would see by looking into the chest from anterior to posterior. Various tomographic projections of the ventricles can be obtained by superior or inferior tilting of the transducer.

Section 11 (99%) (Apical Four-Chamber Plane

of Ventricles) (Fig. 5.27). The transducer is positioned near the left ventricular apical impulse. However, it should be noted that the apical impulse is often formed by the anterior free wall of the left ventricle and does not invariably represent the apex of the ventricle. Thus, the true apical transducer position is usually in close proximity to the apical impulse but not necessarily at the point of maximum impulse. The plane of section is in a frontal projection parallel to the dorsal and ventral surfaces of the chest. The transducer is directed superiorly and toward the right shoulder. The optimal transducer position may be found more laterally in the anterior axillary line or in the midaxillary line in patients with dilated hearts.

The apical transducer position is distinctly different from that utilized for the parasternal foreshortened four-chamber view (section 4). With the apex toward the inferior portion of the screen, the left ventricle is displayed to the right, the right ventricle to the left, the left atrium superiorly to the right and the right atrium superiorly to the left. The crux of the heart is formed by the conjoined ventricular and atrial septa and the septal portions of the atrioventricular valves. In the normal heart, the atrial septum is slightly displaced to the left of the long axis of the ventricular septum. The septal leaflet of the tricuspid valve inserts more inferiorly toward the right ventricular cavity than the septal portion of the anterior leaflet of the mitral valve. These are consistent and predictable anatomic relationships and can be utilized to predict valvular and ventricular morphology.

1. Left Ventricle: The septal portion of the anterior leaflet and the posterior leaflet of the mitral valve separate the left atrium from the left ventricle. The left ventricular cavity appears as a smooth-walled ovoid cavity with no gross trabeculations. However, posterior and anterior tilting of the transducer will permit visualization of the posteromedial and anterolateral papillary muscles, respectively. The portions of the ventricular septum separating the two atrioventricular valves is the *inflow septum* and, from midseptum to apex, the *trabecular septum.*

2. Right Ventricle: Leaflets of the tricuspid valve separate the right atrium from the right ventricular cavity. The right ventricular cavity is more triangular in configuration, and distinctly larger trabeculations and more irregular papillary muscles within the right ventricular cavity are morphologic signates. A linear echo across the middle of the right ventricle, usually seen with a slight

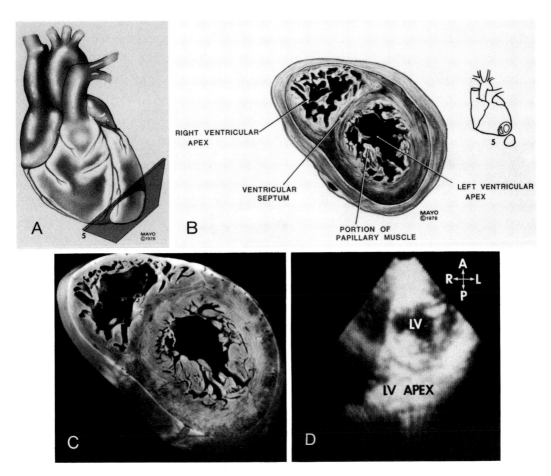

Figure 5.20. Tomographic section 5 (parasternal short-axis plane of left ventricular apex). From a low parasternal intercostal space, a short-axis view of the left ventricle is obtained. *A*, plane of section. *B*, anatomic drawing. *C*, pathologic specimen cut in the presumed plane of section. *D*, sector echographic view of the cardiac apex (*LV APEX*). Only small portions of the apical left ventricular cavity (*LV*) and the right ventricle are visualized. *A* = anterior; *L* = left; *P* = posterior; *R* = right. *B*, *C* and *D* from Tajik, AJ, Seward, JB, Hagler, DJ, Mair, DD, Lie, JT: Two-dimensional real-time ultrasonic imaging of the heart and great vessels: Technique, image orientation, structure identification, and validation. *Mayo Clin Proc 53:* 271, 1978. By permission.

anterior transducer tilt, represents the moderator band of the tricuspid support apparatus (Fig. 5.28).

3. Left Atrium: Pulmonary veins enter the left atrium in the posterosuperior aspect of the left atrial chamber. Superior to the left atrial cavity, the descending thoracic aorta and the more medially positioned vertebral column appear as ovoid echolucent areas.

4. Right Atrium: The right atrium appears equal in dimension to the left atrial cavity. Only with superior (sections 12 and 16) or inferior (section 11A) tilting of the transducer are additional landmarks (i.e., superior vena cava, inferior vena cava, Eustachian valve and coronary sinus) visualized (see below).

The four-chamber view is the easiest to obtain (6) and the most helpful in the assessment of ventricular function, dimension and anatomy. The predictable anatomy of the crux is the single most important two-dimensional echocardiographic landmark in the assessment of atrioventricular valve and ventricular morphology.

Section 11A (66%) (Apical Four-Chamber Plane of Coronary Sinus) (Fig. 5.29). From section 11 (apical four-chamber plane), the transducer is tilted posteriorly. As the beam passes through the left

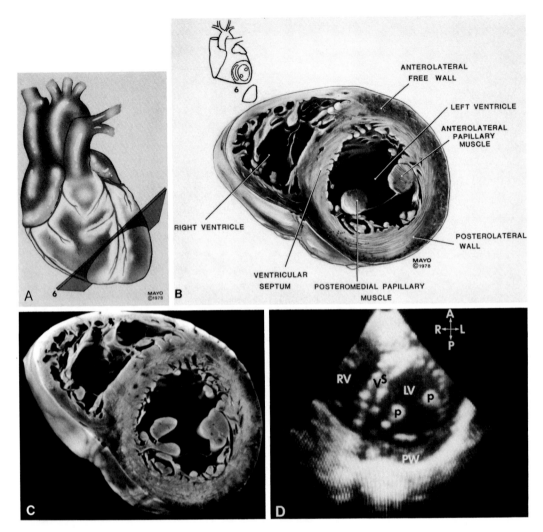

Figure 5.21. Tomographic section 6 (parasternal short-axis projection of left ventricle and papillary muscles). *A,* plane of section. *B,* anatomic drawing. *C,* pathologic specimen cut in the presumed plane of section. *D,* two-dimensional sector echographic short-axis view at papillary muscle level. Two distinct papillary muscles (*p*) are visualized within the left ventricular cavity at 3 and 7 o'clock (anterolateral and posteromedial papillary muscles, respectively). The ventricular septum (*VS*) separates the left ventricular cavity (*LV*) from the right ventricular cavity (*RV*). The posterior left ventricular wall (*PW*) is visualized inferiorly. *A* = anterior; *L* = left; *P* = posterior; *R* = right. *C* and *D* from Tajik, AJ, Seward, JB, Hagler, DJ, Mair, DD, Lie, JT: Two-dimensional real-time ultrasonic imaging of the heart and great vessels: Technique, image orientation, structure identification, and validation. *Mayo Clin Proc 53:* 271, 1978. By permission.

atrioventricular groove, a long-axis view of the coronary sinus can be obtained. As seen on the apex-down image orientation, the coronary sinus crosses from left to right in the left atrioventricular groove, with its orifice entering the right atrium just above the septal leaflet of the tricuspid valve. The orifice is separated from the inferior vena cava—which is often better appreciated with yet

further posterior tilting—by the Eustachian valve. This view of the coronary sinus is obtained in the majority of patients, as opposed to the short-axis (see section 9) or long-axis (see section 1) view of the coronary sinus from the parasternal transducer position.

Section 12 (93%) (Apical Four-Chamber Plane and Aorta) (Fig. 5.30). From tomographic sec-

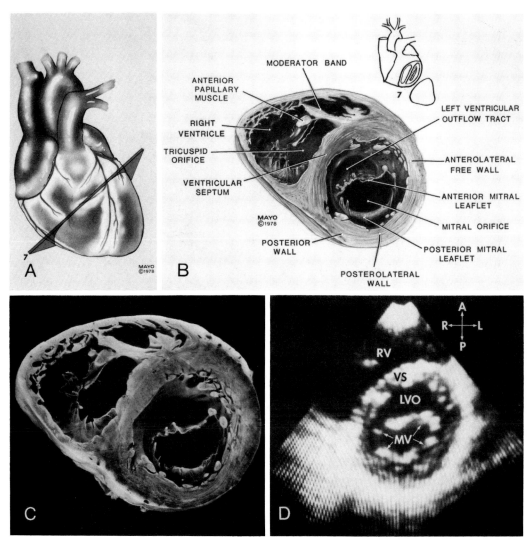

Figure 5.22. Tomographic section 7 (parasternal short-axis plane of left ventricle at mitral valve). *A*, plane of section. *B*, anatomic drawing. *C*, pathologic specimen cut in the presumed plane of section. Note: in the right ventricular cavity, the moderator band is distinctly visible beneath the tricuspid valve orifice. *D*, sector echographic appearance of a short-axis scan at mitral valve level. The mitral valve orifice (*MV*) has a fish-mouth appearance with a large anterior leaflet and a smaller posterior leaflet. The left ventricular outflow tract (*LVO*) lies anterior to the mitral valve. The ventricular septum (*VS*) separates the left ventricular from the right ventricular cavity (*RV*). The right ventricular cavity shows progressive anterior wrapping over the left ventricular cavity to form the right ventricular outflow tract. *A* = anterior; *L* = left; *P* = posterior; *R* = right. *C* and *D* from Tajik, AJ, Seward, JB, Hagler, DJ, Mair, DD, Lie, JT: Two-dimensional real-time ultrasonic imaging of the heart and great vessels: Technique, image orientation, structure identification, and validation. *Mayo Clin Proc 53:* 271, 1978. By permission.

tion 11 (apical four-chamber view), the transducer is tilted anteriorly until the aortic valve comes into view. Because the aortic valve is cut tangentially, the aorta appears as an oval echolucent area above the left ventricular cavity at the crux of the heart. By scanning from tomographic section 11 to tomographic section 12 (apical four-chamber to apical four-chamber plus aorta), the *membranous ventricular septum* is visualized beneath the septal leaflet of the tricuspid valve. A

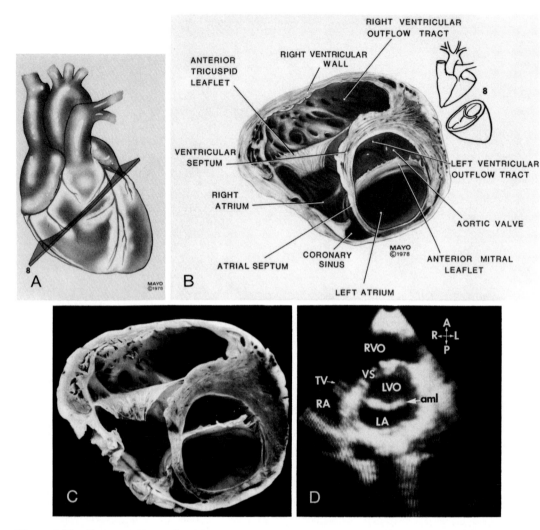

Figure 5.23. Tomographic section 8 (parasternal short-axis plane of left ventricular outflow tract). *A*, plane of section, *B*, anatomic drawing. *C*, pathologic specimen cut in the presumed plane of section. *D*, two-dimensional echographic short-axis view of the left ventricular outflow tract. Anterior mitral valve leaflet (*aml*) separates the left ventricular outflow tract (*LVO*) from the left atrium (*LA*). The basal ventricular septum (*VS*) separates the left ventricular outflow tract from the right ventricular outflow tract (*RVO*); this produces an increasing echolucence anterior to the left ventricle. The tricuspid valve (*TV*) separates the right atrium (*RA*) from the right ventricular outflow tract. A = anterior; L = left; P = posterior; R = right. *C* and *D* from Tajik, AJ, Seward, JB, Hagler, DJ, Mair, DD, Lie, JT: Two-dimensional real-time ultrasonic imaging of the heart and great vessels: Technique, image orientation, structure identification, and validation. *Mayo Clin Proc 53:* 271, 1978. By permission.

membranous ventricular defect can be appreciated with this transducer maneuver or a similar subcostal scan (i.e., sections 15 and 16). Occasionally, the superior vena cava is visualized superior to the right atrium just medial to the aortic root. (A slight clockwise rotation of the trans-ducer will frequently better delineate this structure.)

IIB. Apical Long-Axis Plane (94%).

Section 13 (Apical Long-Axis Plane of Left Ventricle: "Right Anterior Oblique Projection")

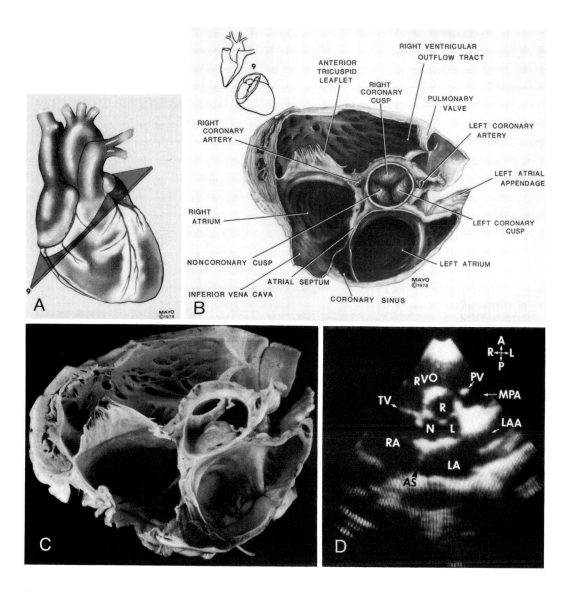

Figure 5.24. Tomographic section 9 (parasternal short-axis plane at aortic valve level). *A*, plane of section, *B*, anatomic drawing. *C*, pathologic specimen cut in the presumed plane of section. *D*, two-dimensional echographic short-axis plane at the aortic valve level. The aorta forms the central portion of this particular view. The right (*R*), left (*L*) and noncoronary (*N*) cusps in diastole form a Y configuration. Posterior to the aorta is the left atrium (*LA*). The left atrial appendage (*LAA*) can often be visualized slightly anterior and to the *right* of the figure. The atrial septum (*AS*) separates right atrium (*RA*) from left atrium. The tricuspid valve (*TV*) separates the right ventricular outflow tract (*RVO*) from the right atrium. The pulmonary valve (*PV*) is located anterior to and to the *right* of the aorta. Proximal portions of the main pulmonary artery (*MPA*) are visualized beyond the pulmonary valve. *A* = anterior; *L* = left; *P* = posterior; *R* = right. *C* and *D* from Tajik, AJ, Seward, JB, Hagler, DJ, Mair, DD, Lie, JT: Two-dimensional real-time ultrasonic imaging of the heart and great vessels: technique, image orientation, structure identification, and validation. *Mayo Clin Proc 53:* 271, 1978. By permission.

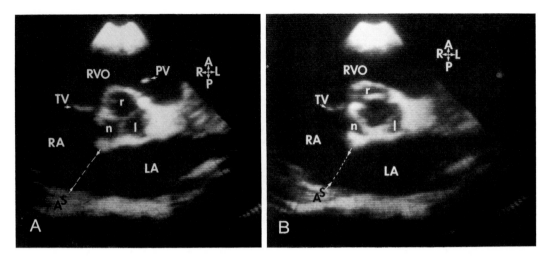

Figure 5.25. Tomographic section 9 illustrating diastolic (A) and systolic (B) frames of the aortic valve leaflet configuration. RVO = right ventricular outflow tract; PV = pulmonary valve; TV = tricuspid valve; RA = right atrium; LA = left atrium; r = right cusp; n = noncoronary cusp; l = left cusp; A = anterior; R = right; L = left; P = posterior.

(Fig. 5.31). From section 11, the transducer is rotated clockwise approximately 90° (Fig. 5.32). This section is produced by a plane from the left flank to the right shoulder. A view similar to the parasternal long-axis view of the left ventricle is obtained. However, from the apical transducer position, the apex of the left ventricle is better delineated. The left atrium lies to the right of and posterior to the aortic root. The inferoposterior left ventricular myocardium forms the right side of the image. At times, this particular image has also been called the "right anterior oblique equivalent" because it is, in some respects, comparable to the right anterior oblique angiographic projection.

Section 13A (Apical Long-Axis Plane of Left Ventricle: "Two-Chamber View") (Fig. 5.33). This view is similar to tomographic section 13 ("Right Anterior Oblique Equivalent") except that the transducer is rotated an additional few degrees clockwise and tilted laterally. Only the left ventricle and left atrium (i.e., two chambers) are visualized. The left atrium and left ventricle are separated by the anterior and posterior leaflets of the mitral valve. The anterior free wall of the left ventricle is to the left of the screen, and the inferior wall is to the right (apex down). In our experience, high quality images of this view are somewhat more difficult to obtain than the "right anterior oblique" apical long-axis view

(section 13). There are no easily recognizable anatomic hallmarks that permit reproduction of myocardial segments. Close attention to scanning technique is necessary to use this view for visualization of comparable wall segments on repeat examination. The echocardiographer must be oriented to his own particular machine and document the orientation of the image for identifying and assessing myocardial walls on serial examination.

III. Subcostal Transducer Position (92%). The subcostal examination can be divided into two categories: 1) upper abdominal great vessels and viscera and 2) the heart and lower thorax. Detailed anatomic descriptions of the upper abdomen will not be attempted in this chapter; however, gross relationships of the great vessels and major viscera will be illustrated.

IIIA. Subcostal Examination of Upper Abdomen (91%).

1. Short-Axis Plane. Section 14A (*Subcostal Short-Axis Projection of Upper Abdominal Viscera and Great Vessels) (Fig. 5.34).* With the transducer positioned in the subxiphoid space and a scanning plane projected perpendicular to the long axis of the body, the transducer orientation is similar to the short-axis views of the heart in which the observer is looking from the patient's abdomen toward the head. The most distinctive

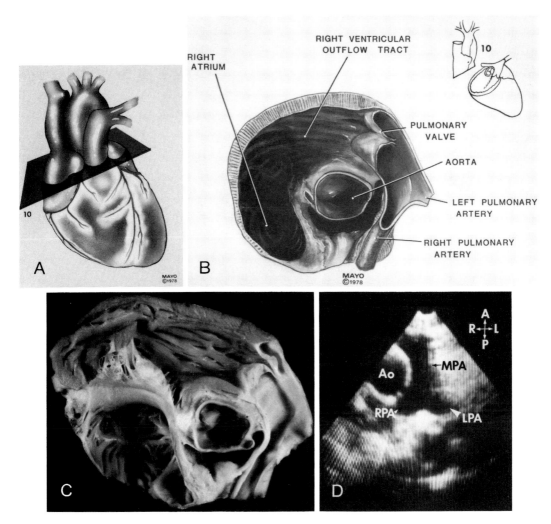

Figure 5.26. Tomographic section 10 (parasternal short-axis plane of pulmonary bifurcation). *A*, plane of section, *B*, anatomic drawing. *C*, pathologic specimen cut in the presumed plane of section. *D*, two-dimensional sector echographic short-axis view of pulmonary bifurcation. The proximal ascending aorta *(Ao)* is imaged to the left of the main pulmonary artery *(MPA)*. The proximal bifurcations of the right pulmonary artery *(RPA)* and the left pulmonary artery *(LPA)* are visualized. The right pulmonary artery will be visualized circling beneath the aortic root. *A* = anterior; *L* = left; *P* = posterior; *R* = right. *D* from Tajik, AJ, Seward, JB, Hagler, DJ, Mair, DD, Lie, JT: Two-dimensional real-time ultrasonic imaging of the heart and great vessels: Technique, image orientation, structure identification, and validation. *Mayo Clin Proc 53:* 271, 1978. By permission.

landmark is the vertebral body and its centrally located neural canal. Anterior to and to the right of the vertebral body is the echolucent short-axis view of the upper abdominal aorta, and to the left is the inferior vena cava. Frequently, the portal vein is viewed anterior to and rightward of the inferior vena cava and is surrounded by more hyper-refractile echoes (i.e., large portal triad).

The liver parenchyma is anterior to and to the left of the image and has a characteristic granular texture.

2. Long-Axis Plane. Section 14B (Subcostal Long-Axis Plane of Upper Abdominal Aorta) (Fig. 5.35). From the short-axis plane (section 14A), the transducer is tilted slightly to the patient's left and rotated 90° counterclockwise. A long-axis

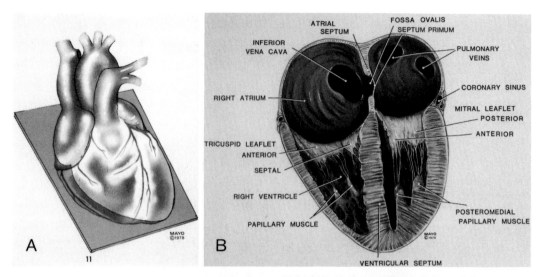

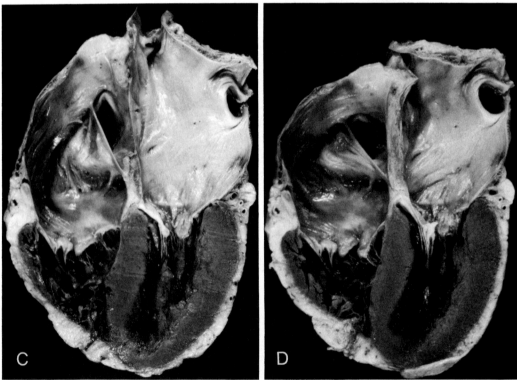

Figure 5.27. Tomographic section 11 (apical four-chamber plane of ventricles). *A*, plane of section, *B*, anatomic drawing. *C* and *D*, pathologic specimen cut in the presumed plane of section. Note that in *C* the atrial septum has been cut in the area of the fossa ovalis. The valve of the fossa ovalis is a thin membrane, which may produce false echo dropout when visualized from the apical transducer position. Note that in *D* (same specimen) the atrial septum has been cut through the limbus of the fossa ovalis, which appears as a thick structure. *E*, two-dimensional examination of the apical four-chamber view. With the apex down, the left atrium (*LA*) and the left ventricle (*LV*) are to the *right* of the image. The right atrium (*RA*) and the right ventricle (*RV*) are to the *left* of the image. The long axis of the atrial septum is displaced slightly to the *right* relative to the long axis of the ventricular septum (*VS*). The septal leaflet of the tricuspid valve inserts more inferiorly than the corresponding septal leaflet of the mitral valve (i.e., the typical anatomic features of the crux of the heart). *AS* = atrial septum; *S* = superior; *L* = left; *I* = inferior; *R* = right. *C* and *D* from and *E* modified from Tajik, AJ, Seward, JB, Hagler, DJ, Mair, DD, Lie, JT: Two-dimensional real-time ultrasonic imaging of the heart and great vessels: Technique, image orientation, structure identification, and validation. *Mayo Clin Proc 53:* 271, 1978. By permission.

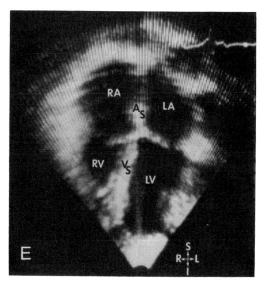

Figure 5.27 (continued).

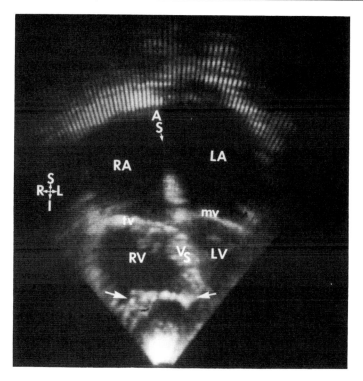

Figure 5.28. Moderator band within the right ventricular chamber. From the standard apical four-chamber view, a slight anterior tilt of the transducer permits visualization of the moderator band within the right ventricular cavity (arrows). This band can occasionally be mistaken for the outer surface of an apical right ventricular thrombus. Note that the tricuspid (tv) and mitral (mv) valves are less distinctly visualized with this more anterior projection. RA = right atrium; LA = left atrium; AS = atrial septum; LV = left ventricle; VS = ventricular septum; RV = right ventricle; S = superior; L = left; I = inferior; R = right. From Seward, JB, Tajik, AJ, Hagler, DJ: Orientation of the great arteries: Normal, complete transposition, corrected transposition. In Pediatric Echocardiography—Cross-Sectional, M-Mode and Doppler. pp 105–120, N-R Lundström, ed. Amsterdam, Elsevier/North-Holland Biomedical Press, 1980. By permission.

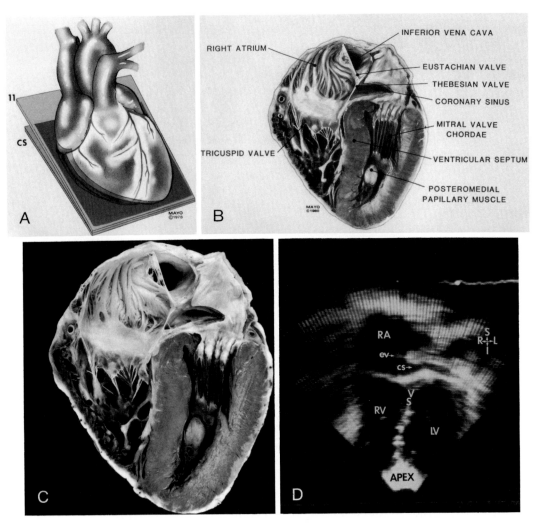

Figure 5.29. Tomographic section 11A (apical four-chamber plane of coronary sinus). *A*, plane of section is obtained with a slight posterior tilt of the transducer from tomographic section 11. *CS* = coronary sinus. *B*, anatomic drawing. *C*, pathologic specimen cut in the plane of section. *D*, sector echocardiographic view of the apical four-chamber plane with visualization of the coronary sinus. The coronary sinus (*cs*) is visualized as a linear echo-free area posterior to the mitral annulus. The orifice of the coronary sinus is bounded by the eustachian valve (*ev*) and the tricuspid valve. *LV* = left ventricle; *VS* = ventricular septum; *RV* = right ventricle; *RA* = right atrium; *APEX* = cardiac apex; *S* = superior; *L* = left; *I* = inferior; *R* = right.

projection of the upper abdominal aorta can be obtained. The scanning plane is a left paravertebral projection parallel to the long axis of the body. By superior and inferior tilting of the transducer, varying portions of the lower thoracic (Fig. 5.35*C*) and upper abdominal aorta (Fig. 5.35*B*) are visualized.

Section 14C (91%) (Subcostal Long-Axis Plane of Inferior Vena Cava) (Fig. 5.36). From tom-

ographic section 14A, the transducer is tilted slightly to the patient's left and rotated 90° counterclockwise to produce a scanning plane in a right paravertebral projection, parallel to the long axis of the body. With superior and inferior tilting of the transducer, varying portions of the inferior vena cava and its major tributaries are visualized. Superiorly, the inferior vena cava enters the right atrium. Just before it does so, a large hepatic vein

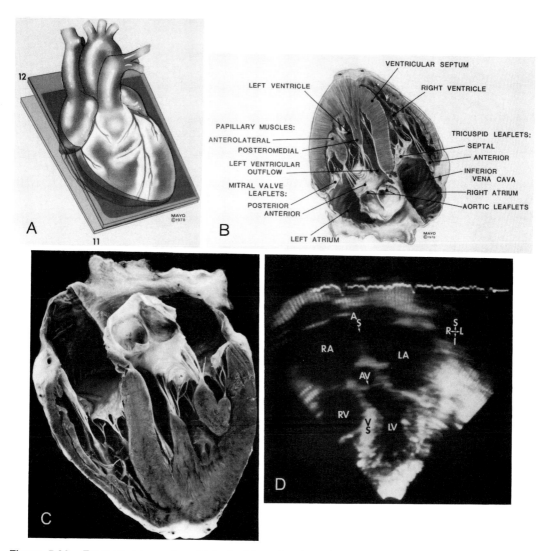

Figure 5.30. Tomographic section 12 (apical four-chamber plane and aorta). *A*, plane of section is produced by a slight anterior tilt of the transducer from tomographic section 11. *B*, anatomic drawing. *C*, pathologic specimen cut in the presumed plane of section. *D*, sector echocardiographic view of the apical four-chamber plane at the aorta. The aortic valve (*AV*) is visualized as a central structure and communicates with the left ventricle (*LV*) across the left ventricular outflow tract. The anterior leaflet of the mitral valve is continuous with the left wall of the aortic root and separates the left atrium (*LA*) from the left ventricle. Portions of the atrial septum (*AS*) remain visible. *RA* = right atrium; *RV* = right ventricle; *VS* = ventricular septum; *S* = superior; *L* = left; *I* = inferior; *R* = right.

can invariably be visualized entering the inferior vena cava. With a slight medial tilt of the transducer, the long-axis projection of the portal vein can also be obtained.

Section 14D (Subcostal Four-Chamber Plane of Hepatic Veins) (Fig. 5.37). With the transducer in the subcostal space and directed to the patient's right (i.e., into the liver parenchyma), a frontal (i.e., four-chamber) projection of the proximal hepatic veins can be imaged. From section 14A the transducer is turned 180° (four-chamber plane) and tilted to the patient's right and anteriorly. The plane of section is parallel to the right abdominal diaphragm. The relationship of the hepatic veins to the inferior vena cava is visualized.

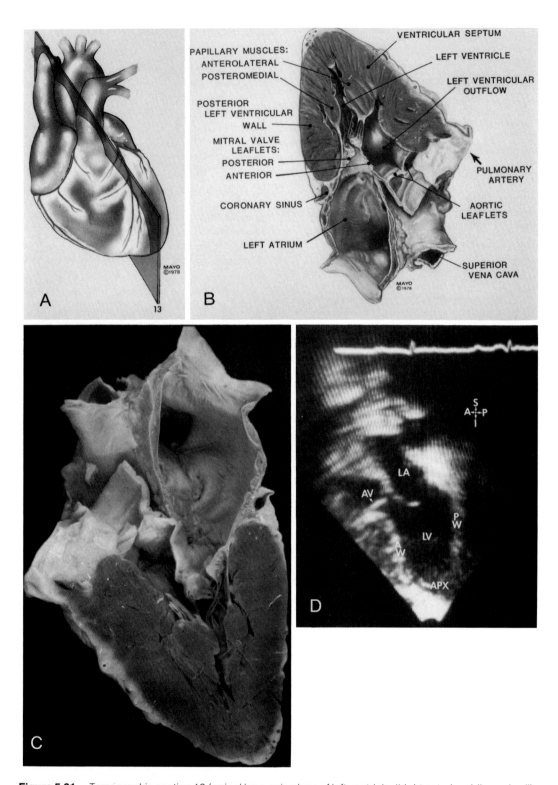

Figure 5.31. Tomographic section 13 (apical long-axis plane of left ventricle: "right anterior oblique view"). *A*, plane of section, *B*, anatomic drawing. *C*, pathologic specimen cut in the presumed plane of section. *D*, sector echocardiographic view of the apical long-axis projection of the left ventricle. This particular projection is comparable to tomographic section 1. The posterior wall of the aorta is continuous with the anterior leaflet of the mitral valve. The mitral valve separates the left atrium (*LA*) from the left ventricle (*LV*).

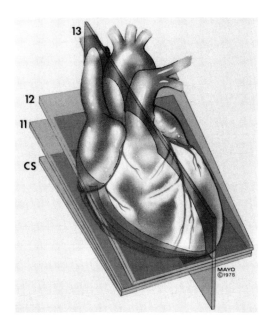

Figure 5.32. Composite planes of section of the apical four-chamber and long-axis projections. The long-axis view is at right angles to the four-chamber plane. *CS* = coronary sinus.

IIIB. Subcostal Cardiac Examination (92%) Four-Chamber Plane (90%).

Section 15 (90%) (Subcostal Four-Chamber Plane) (Fig. 5.38). This view is comparable to the apical four-chamber plane. The transducer is directed toward the left shoulder, and the scanning plane is parallel to the dorsal and ventral surfaces of the chest. This produces a frontal projection of the ventricular and atrial chambers (i.e., four-chamber plane). With the apex-down position (i.e., transducer artifact at bottom of image) the left ventricle appears to the right, the right ventricle to the left, the left atrium superior and to the right, and the right atrium superior and to the left. The *inflow ventricular septum* (i.e., separating the two atrioventricular valves) and *trabecular septum* are visualized. The characteristic insertions of the atrioventricular valves are visualized. With a more superior (i.e., cephalad, toward the left clavicle) direction of the trans-

ducer, the atrial septum is best visualized. The ultrasound beam is perpendicular to the atrial septum, which permits a superior examination of atrial septal anatomy (see below: atrial septum). Centrally, the valve of the fossa ovalis (expected position of a secundum atrial septal defect) appears as a thin membrane. The atrial septum surrounding this valve appears thicker and hyperrefractile, representing the limbus of the fossa ovalis.

Section 16 (89%) (Subcostal Four-Chamber Plane Plus Aorta) (Fig. 5.39). From tomographic section 15, a more anterior tilt of the transducer will bring the aorta into view. That portion of the ventricular septum scanned between sections 15 and 16 is the *membranous ventricular septum.* The transducer remains directed toward the left shoulder, and the scan plane is parallel to the ventral and dorsal surfaces of the chest. It should be noted that, if interpreted incorrectly, the right-sided wall of the aorta may be mistaken for the atrial septum, for both structures lie in the same long-axis plane. The aortic valve cusps and the left ventricular outflow tract are visualized. The lateral aspect of the aortic root is continuous with the anterior leaflet of the mitral valve. With the apex-down orientation, the left ventricle is to the right and the right ventricle to the left. The aorta exits the left ventricular cavity, traversing from right to left on the image. The superior vena cava can be imaged superior to the right atrium, and posterior to and leftward of the ascending aorta (Fig. 5.40).

Section 16A (Subcostal Four-Chamber Plane of Right Ventricular Outflow Tract) (Fig. 5.41). Further anterior tilting of the transducer permits visualization of the right ventricular outflow tract anterior to the aorta. Note that the major axis of the left ventricular outflow tract is from right to left on the image, whereas the major axis of the right ventricular outflow tract is superior or slightly left to right. When scanning from tomographic section 16 to section 16A, the normal orientation of the great arteries can be appreciated. The bifurcation of the pulmonary trunk into right and left pulmonary arteries can be visualized by posterior-anterior scanning. The

---

The left ventricle is bounded by the anterior wall (*AW*), ventricular apex (*APX*) and posterior wall (*PW*). The aortic valve (*AV*) is visualized superiorly. Occasionally, portions of the right ventricular outflow tract are visualized to the left of the image and more closely resemble tomographic section 1. *S* = superior; *P* = posterior; *I* = inferior; *A* = anterior. *D* modified from Tajik, AJ, Seward, JB, Hagler, DJ, Mair, DD, Lie, JT: Two-dimensional real-time ultrasonic imaging of the heart and great vessels: Technique, image orientation, structure identification, and validation. *Mayo Clin Proc 53:* 271, 1978. By permission.

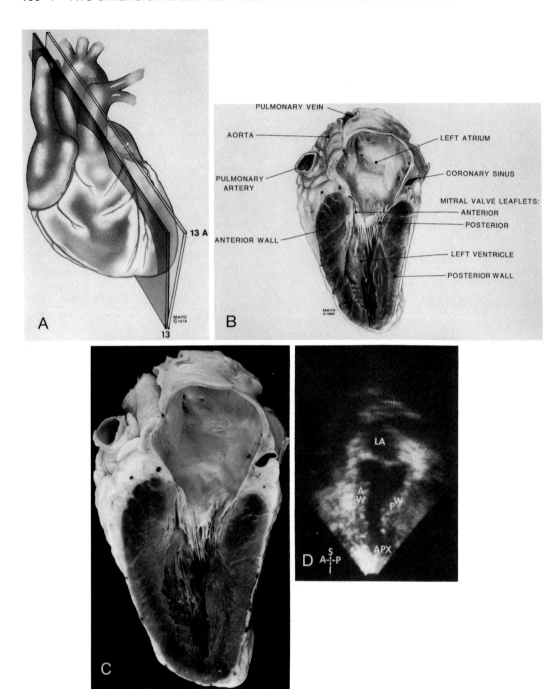

Figure 5.33. Tomographic section 13A (apical long-axis plane of left ventricle: "two-chamber view"). *A,* plane of section is produced by a slight clockwise rotation of the transducer, *B,* anatomic drawing. *C,* pathologic specimen cut in the plane of section. *D,* two-dimensional echocardiographic view of the apical two-chamber projection. Both the aorta and the right ventricular outflow tract are omitted from this particular view. Only the left atrium (*LA*) and the left ventricle are visualized. The left ventricular anterior wall (*AW*), apex (*APX*), and posterior wall (*PW*) are visualized. The mitral valve separates the left ventricle and left atrium. *S* = superior; *P* = posterior; *I* = inferior; *A* = anterior.

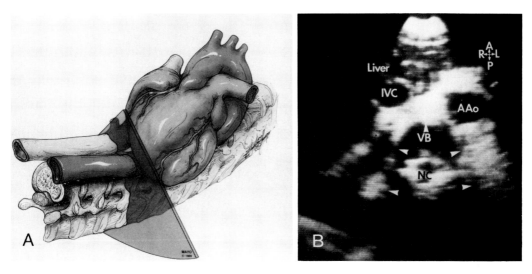

Figure 5.34. Tomographic section 14A (subcostal short-axis projection of upper abdominal viscera and great vessels). *A*, plane of section illustrating the position of the ultrasound beam, which is below the abdominal diaphragm and transects the upper abdominal aorta and vena cava in the short axis. *B*, the vertebral body (*VB*) appears as an echo-free structure posteriorly (*arrowheads*). The neural canal (*NC*) appears echo-lucent and occupies a posterior position in the vertebral body. The inferior vena cava (*IVC*) appears anteriorly and leftward. Characteristically stippled liver parenchyma surrounds the inferior vena cava. The abdominal aorta (*AAo*) appears anterior to and to the right of the vertebral body. *A* = anterior; *L* = left; *P* = posterior; *R* = right.

inflow portion of the right ventricle (i.e., tricuspid valve) is only partly visualized in this tomographic plane.

IIIC. Subxiphoid Short-Axis Plane (67%).

Sections 17A through 17F (67%). From the four-chamber plane (section 15, Fig. 5.42), the transducer is rotated 90° clockwise, such that the scanning plane is perpendicular to the ventral and dorsal surfaces of the chest, and is directed toward the left shoulder (Fig. 5.42). The left ventricle can be cut in short axis in a bread-loafing fashion from apex to base by sweeping the transducer from the apex (transducer directed toward the left flank) toward the base of the heart (transducer directed toward the suprasternal notch). Tomographic cuts of the left ventricle are comparable to cuts obtained from the parasternal transducer position. The left ventricle, however, is cut in a more oblique fashion, particularly near the base of the heart (Fig. 5.43).

IVA. Suprasternal Transducer Position (79%): Long-Axis Plane of Aorta.

Section 18 (76%) (Suprasternal Long-Axis Plane of Aortic Arch) (Fig. 5.44). With the transducer positioned in the suprasternal notch and directed inferiorly, the scan plane, in the presence of a *left aortic arch*, extends from the right nipple toward the left shoulder. Portions of the ascending aorta, aortic arch and upper descending aorta are visualized. This projection is viewed as though one were standing at the left of the patient. Beneath the aortic arch and immediately posterior to the ascending aorta, the echolucent short-axis projection of the right pulmonary artery is visualized. Beneath the right pulmonary artery is the left atrium. The aortic valve and aortic root are invariably out of the scan projection. From the aortic arch, the brachiocephalic vessels, in order from left to right, include the innominate, left common carotid and left subclavian arteries. Anterior to the aortic arch and innominate artery is the innominate vein, which appears as an echo-lucent area. Long-axis projection of a *right aortic arch* produces a scanning plane that extends from the left nipple toward the right shoulder.

Slight leftward tilting of the transducer brings into view the left pulmonary artery, which courses nearly directly posteriorly (see below: pulmonary arteries).

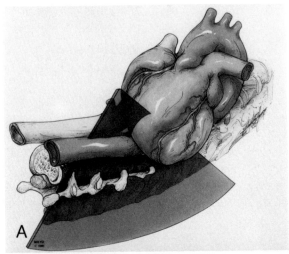

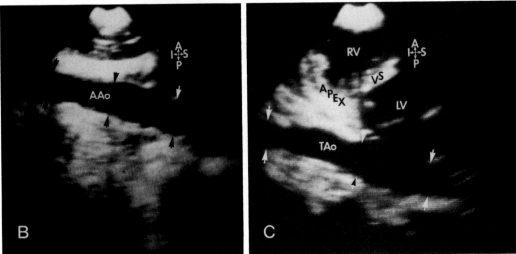

Figure 5.35. Tomographic section 14B (subcostal long-axis plane of upper abdominal aorta). *A*, plane of section in a left paravertebral projection, *B*, two-dimensional echocardiographic visualization of the abdominal aorta (*AAo*) (*arrowheads*). *C*, with a further superior tilt of the transducer the lower thoracic aorta (*TAo*) (*arrowheads*) is visualized. Anteriorly, an oblique projection of the left ventricular apex is visualized. *RV* = right ventricle; *VS* = ventricular septum; *LV* = left ventricle; *APEX* = left ventricular apex; *A* = anterior; *S* = superior; *P* = posterior; *I* = inferior.

IVB. Suprasternal Short-Axis Plane (63%).

Section 19 (63%) (Suprasternal Short-Axis Plane of Aortic Arch) (Fig. 5.45). Starting with the transducer oriented to visualize section 18, the transducer is rotated 90° clockwise, and this produces a scanning plane that extends from the left nipple to the right clavicle. The echolucent short-axis projection of the aortic arch is central in this image. Immediately posterior is the long-axis projection of the right pulmonary artery, and posterior to the right pulmonary artery are the left

atrium and, occasionally, the upper pulmonary veins. To the right of the aortic arch is the superior vena cava. The right subclavian vein enters the superior vena cava from the right of the image; the left innominate vein enters the superior vena cava from the left.

IVC. Suprasternal Frontal Projections of Ascending and Descending Aorta.

Section 20 (Suprasternal Frontal Plane of Ascending Aorta) (Fig. 5.46). From tomographic

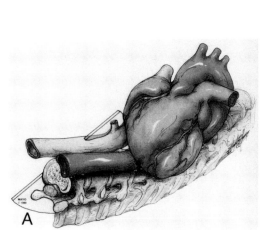 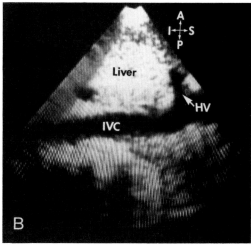

Figure 5.36. Tomographic section 14C (subcostal long-axis plane of inferior vena cava). *A*, plane of section of the long axis of the inferior vena cava. The plane is in a right paravertebral projection. *B*, two-dimensional long-axis projection of the inferior vena cava (*IVC*). Just before the inferior vena cava enters the right atrial cavity, the hepatic vein (*HV*) enters the inferior vena cava anteriorly. The liver is visualized anterior to the inferior vena cava. *A* = anterior; *S* = superior; *P* = posterior; *I* = inferior.

section 19, anterior tilting (i.e., toward the sternum) of the transducer will allow visualization of the ascending aorta, aortic root and aortic valves (Fig. 5.46*C*). To the right of the aorta, the superior vena cava empties into the right atrium.

Section 20A (Suprasternal of Frontal Plane Descending Aorta) (Fig. 5.46D). From tomographic section 19, a posterior tilt of the transducer permits visualization of the upper descending aorta. In the presence of a left aortic arch, the

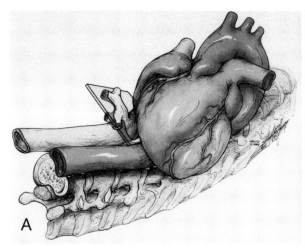 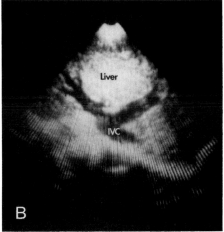

Figure 5.37. Tomographic section 14D (subcostal four-chamber plane of hepatic veins). *A*, plane of section is directed to the patient's right and into the parenchyma of the liver. *B*, two-dimensional echocardiographic long-axis projection of the hepatic veins and their relation to the inferior vena cava (*IVC*). Hepatic parenchyma surrounds the hepatic veins. (*B* from Seward, JB, Tajik, AJ, Hagler, DJ: Two-dimensional contrast echoangiography. In *Pediatric Echocardiography—Cross-Sectional, M-Mode and Doppler.* pp. 239–255, N-R Lundström, ed. Amsterdam, Elsevier/North-Holland Biomedical Press, 1980. By permission.)

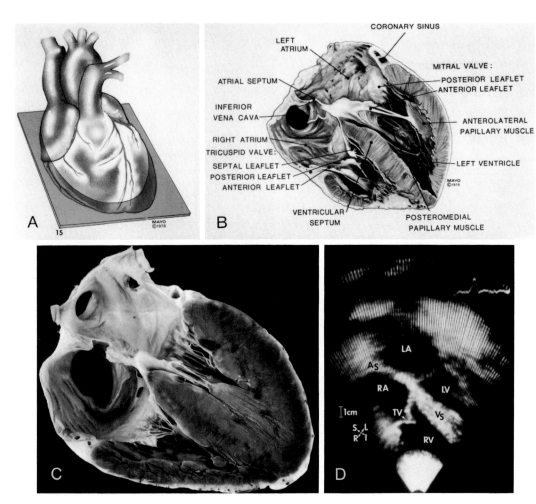

Figure 5.38. Tomographic section 15 (subcostal four-chamber plane). *A*, plane of section, *B*, anatomic drawing. *C*, pathologic specimen cut in the presumed plane of section. Note the thinning of the atrial septum in the area of the foramen ovale. *D*, two-dimensional echocardiogram showing the subcostal four-chamber projection. The ventricular apex is at the *right* of the image, with the ventricular septum (*VS*) separating the rightward-located left ventricle (*LV*) and leftward right ventricle (*RV*). The tricuspid (*TV*) and mitral valves separate the ventricles from their respective atria. *RA* = right atrium; *LA* = left atrium; *AS* = atrial septum. This particular patient has amyloid heart disease. *S* = superior; *L* = left; *I* = inferior; *R* = right. *D* from Seward, JB, Tajik, AJ, Hagler, DJ: Orientation of the great arteries: normal, complete transposition, corrected transposition. In *Pediatric Echocardiography—Cross-Sectional, M-Mode and Doppler.* pp. 105–120, N-R Lundström, ed. Amsterdam, Elsevier/North-Holland Biomedical Press, 1980. By permission.

echolucent structure will project to the right of the image. In the presence of a right aortic arch, the descending aorta will project to the left of the image. This particular maneuver (scanning from section 19 to section 20A) usually is the easiest maneuver for the distinction of a left from a right aortic arch.

IDENTIFICATION OF SPECIFIC STRUCTURES

The two-dimensional echocardiographic examination allows potential visualization of cardiac structures from multiple projections. All possible tomographic sections of the heart and great vessels are not obtainable in each patient

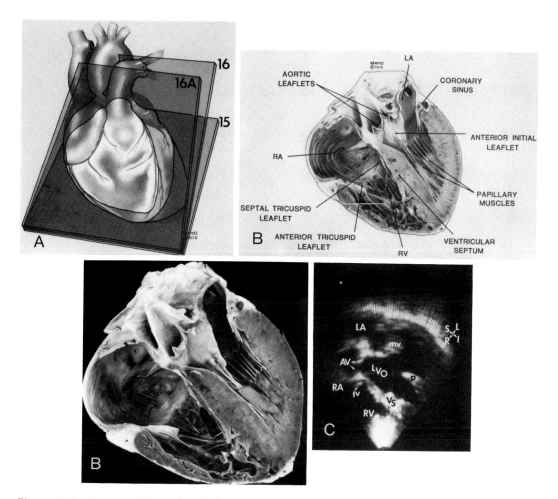

Figure 5.39. Tomographic section 16 (subcostal four-chamber plane plus aorta). *A*, plane of section is obtained by a slight anterior tilt of the transducer from tomographic section 15. *B*, anatomic drawing. *RV* = right ventricle; *RA* = right atrium; *LA* = left atrium. *C*, pathologic specimen cut in the presumed plane of section. *D*, two-dimensional echocardiogram in the subcostal four-chamber plane plus aorta. Portions of the left atrium (*LA*) and left ventricular outflow tract (*LVO*) remain visible. The left-sided border of the aortic root is continuous with the anterior leaflet of mitral valve (*mv*). The aortic valve leaflets (*AV*) separate the left ventricular outflow tract from the proximal aortic root. The ventricular septum (*VS*) separates left ventricle from right ventricle (*RV*). The right wall of the aorta is continuous with the atrial septum. Portions of the tricuspid valve (*tv*) and the right atrium (*RA*) are visualized. *p* = papillary muscle; *L* = left; *I* = inferior; *R* = right; *S* = superior.

because of limited and variable ultrasonic windows, presence of ribs and calcified costal cartilages, variable body habitus, chest deformity, intervening lung parenchyma and occasional lack of patient cooperation (6). However, for optimal appreciation of anatomy or function, it is best to assess the heart and great vessels from multiple projections. Anatomic relationships of specific cardiac structures and pertinent tomographic views are best understood under specific topics. The following general section will cover anatomic features of selected cardiac structures and will also discuss the advantages of certain tomographic views.

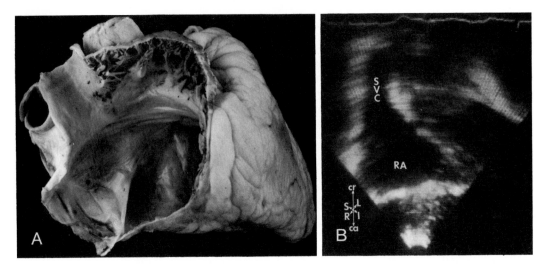

Figure 5.40. Pathologic specimen (*A*) and tomographic section (*B*) illustrating subcostal visualization of the superior vena cava. From section 16, the transducer is tilted slightly superiorly and rotated counterclockwise. In doing so, the superior vena cava (*SVC*) is visualized in its long axis and enters the superior aspect of the right atrium (*RA*). *cr* = cranial; *ca* = caudal; *L* = left; *I* = inferior; *R* = right; *S* = superior.

Atrioventricular Valves

The atrioventricular valves can be visualized from nearly all transducer positions. However, certain aspects of atrioventricular valve function and morphology can be obtained best from selected transducer positions. Atrioventricular morphology is best appreciated from the apical four-chamber plane (section 11, Fig. 5.27). The characteristic lower insertion of the septal leaflet of the tricuspid valve at the crux of the heart is an important morphologic hallmark. In patients with inverted ventricles, this relationship is reversed (10, 11).

Anatomic irregularities of the valve (i.e., vegetations, stenosis, flail leaflet and so on) must be appreciated from multiple positions. However, only the short-axis projection of the respective atrioventricular valve permits calculation of the orifice area. For the mitral valve, this is best obtained from the parasternal or subcostal short-axis projection (section 6, Fig. 5.21, and section 17C). The short-axis projection of the tricuspid orifice is quite difficult, for this valve is large and does not typically lie in an easily accessible plane of section. Tricuspid stenosis is best appreciated from long-axis projections (section 2, Fig. 5.14) and the apical four-chamber view (section 11, Fig. 5.27). Ruptured chordae or prolapsing mitral valve should be studied from multiple projections, including the long-axis (section 1, Fig. 5.11), short-axis (section 7, Fig. 5.22) and apical (section 11, Fig. 5.27) projections.

Semilunar Valves

Spatial orientation of the semilunar valves is best appreciated from the parasternal and subcostal transducer positions (11). From section 1 (long axis of left ventricle, Fig. 5.11), a scan to section 3 (long axis of right ventricular outflow tract, Fig. 5.16) aids in the appreciation of the orientation of the respective outflow tracts (i.e., a crossing relationship). The same relationship can be appreciated from the subcostal transducer position by scanning from section 15 (Fig. 5.38) to section 16A (Figs. 5.41 and 5.47). Short-axis projections of the base of the heart (section 9, Fig. 5.24, and section 10, Fig. 5.26) disclose the typical orientation of the normally related great arteries (i.e., right ventricular outflow wrapping over the aorta and bifurcation of the main pulmonary artery). One must always be certain to visualize the semilunar valves and outflow tracts in order to appreciate the actual spatial relationships of the great arteries (e.g., a high transducer position can cut through the normal main pulmonary artery and ascending aorta and give a false impression of transposition of the great arteries).

The orifice of the aortic valve is best viewed from parasternal or subcostal short-axis projec-

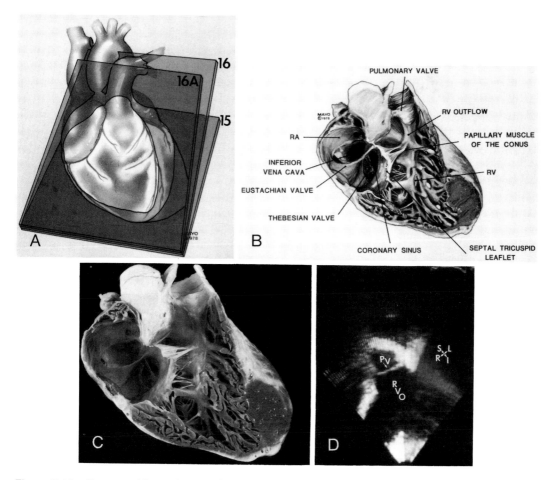

Figure 5.41. Tomographic section 16A (subcostal four-chamber plane of right ventricular outflow tract). *A*, plane of section is obtained by a further anterior tilt of the transducer. *B*, anatomic drawing. *RV* = right ventricle; *RA* = right atrium. *C*, pathologic specimen cut in the presumed plane of section. *D*, echocardiogram of the right ventricular outflow tract (*RVO*) and the pulmonary valve (*PV*). Portions of the right ventricle and main pulmonary artery are visible. *L* = left; *I* = inferior; *R* = right; *S* = superior. (*C* from Seward, JB, Tajik, AJ, Hagler, DJ: Orientation of the great arteries: Normal, complete transposition, corrected transposition. In *Pediatric Echocardiography—Cross-Sectional, M-Mode and Doppler.* pp. 105–120, N-R Lundström, ed. Amsterdam, Elsevier/North-Holland Biomedical Press, 1980. By permission.)

tions (section 9, Fig. 5.24, and section 17E). In diseased states (e.g., calcific aortic stenosis), the aortic valve orifice may be seen. The degree of aortic disease can be assessed by indirect features of ventricular function. However, cusp mobility, amount and distribution of calcification, and orifice, when viewed in both long- and short-axis projections, are only indirect measures of the presence and severity of aortic valvular disease.

Ventricular Septum

The ventricular septum is best visualized from multiple transducer positions. Normal ventricular

septal anatomy must be understood for optimal utilization of the two-dimensional technique for the visualization and understanding of anatomic alterations (i.e., ventricular septal defect, infarct location and so on) (Fig. 5.48). The ventricular septum is divided into four segments: inflow, outflow, trabecular and membranous. The *inflow septum* is posterior at the base of the heart and separates the two atrioventricular valves (i.e., ventricular inflow). This part of the ventricular septum is best appreciated from the apical or subcostal four-chamber projections (section 11, Fig. 5.27, and section 15, Fig. 5.38). The more apical

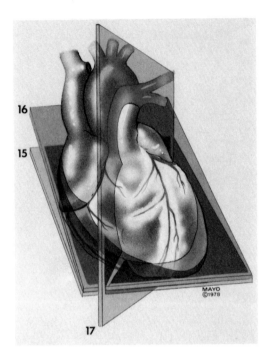

Figure 5.42. Tomographic section 17 (subxiphoid short-axis plane). From the subcostal four-chamber plane (tomographic sections 15 and 16), the transducer is rotated 90° to the short axis of the left ventricle (tomographic section 17). By scanning the transducer in the short-axis plane from apex to base, one can "cut" the left ventricle serially in a bread-loafing fashion.

portion of the ventricular septum, visualized from these same projections, is the *trabecular septum*. The portion of the ventricular septum that is visualized anteriorly in the long-axis projection of the left ventricle (section 1, Fig. 5.11, and section 13, Fig. 5.31) and the long-axis projection of the right ventricular outflow tract (section 3, Fig. 5.16) is the *outflow septum* (separating the ventricular outflow tracts). The *membranous ventricular septum* constitutes only a small portion of the septum and lies beneath the septal leaflet of the tricuspid valve. There is no single tomographic view that delineates the membranous ventricular septum. The membranous septum is best appreciated with two scanning maneuvers. 1) from the parasternal long axis of the left ventricle (section 1, Fig. 5.11), a scan to the long axis of the right ventricular inflow (section 2, Fig. 5.14) will cross the membranous ventricular septum (12). 2) an alternate maneuver is a scan from the subcostal four-cham-

ber plane (section 15, Fig. 5.38) to the four-chamber plus aorta plane (section 16, Fig. 5.39). The scan beam crosses the membranous septum (Fig. 5.47), which lies just beneath the aortic root and septal leaflet of the tricuspid valve.

Atrial Septum

Anatomic landmarks of the atrial septum are equally important in the assessment of atrial pathology (Fig. 5.49). In the midportion of the atrial septum, the valve of the fossa ovalis, a thin, membranous structure, may produce false echo dropout when the ultrasound beam is parallel to this thin structure. Scans along the long-axis plane of the septum—that is, four-chamber projections (section 11, Fig. 5.27, and section 4, (Fig. 5.18) or the parasternal short-axis projection (section 9, Fig. 5.24)—may lead to false-positive interpretation of a *secundum atrial septal defect*. This potential problem is minimized by use of the subcostal examination of the atrial septum. With the subcostal four-chamber projection (section 15, Fig. 5.38), the ultrasound beam is perpendicular to the atrial septum and permits visualization of the thin valve of the fossa ovalis.

Other anatomic landmarks of the atrial septum include the inferior basal portion of the atrial septum, which is a thick structure. This segment of the atrial septum is best viewed from the apical four-chamber plane (section 15, Fig. 5.38). Dropout in the inferior atrial septum (*primum atrial septal defect*) is a highly sensitive observation, and the defect is highlighted by highly refractile margins (13).

Sinus venosus atrial septal defect is located superior and anterior to the fossa ovalis. The subcostal four-chamber plane (section 15, Fig. 5.38) with anterior tilting is utilized to view this segment of the atrial septum (14). However, with extreme anterior transducer tilting, the orifice of the superior vena cava may also give the false impression of a sinus venosus atrial septal defect.

Cavae

Superior Vena Cava

The superior vena cava is consistently visualized from the suprasternal transducer position (section 19, Fig. 5.45). Superiorly, the innominate vein enters from the left over the aortic arch and the right subclavian vein enters from the right. By tilting the transducer anteriorly (section 19

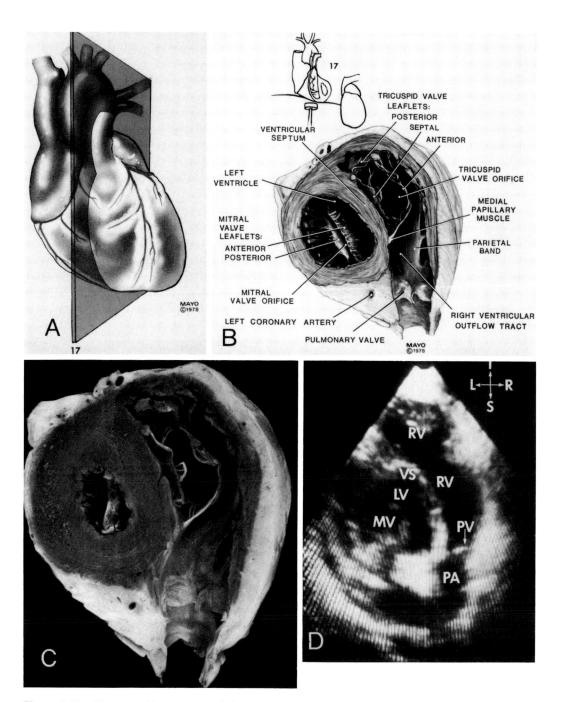

Figure 5.43. Tomographic section 17C (subcostal short-axis projection of left ventricle at mitral valve). *A*, plane of section, *B*, anatomic drawing. *C*, pathologic specimen cut in the presumed plane of section. Note that this section is similar to the parasternal short-axis projection at the mitral valve level or the parasternal short-axis projection at the base of the heart (tomographic sections 7, 8, and 9). *D*, two-dimensional subcostal short-axis projection of the left ventricle at mitral valve level. The image is rotated approximately 90° from a comparable parasternal short-axis projection (tomographic section 7, 8, or 9). The mitral valve orifice (*MV*) is visible within the left ventricular cavity (*LV*). The right ventricle (*RV*) and the right ventricular outflow tract are separated from the proximal main pulmonary artery (*PA*) by the pulmonary valve (*PV*). The outflow ventricular septum (*VS*) is visible. *I* = inferior; *R* = right; *S* = superior; *L* = left. *C* and *D* from Tajik, AJ, Seward, JB, Hagler, DJ, Mair, DD, Lie, JT: Two-dimensional real-time ultrasonic imaging of the heart and great vessels: Technique, image orientation, structure identification, and validation. *Mayo Clin Proc 53:* 271, 1978. By permission.

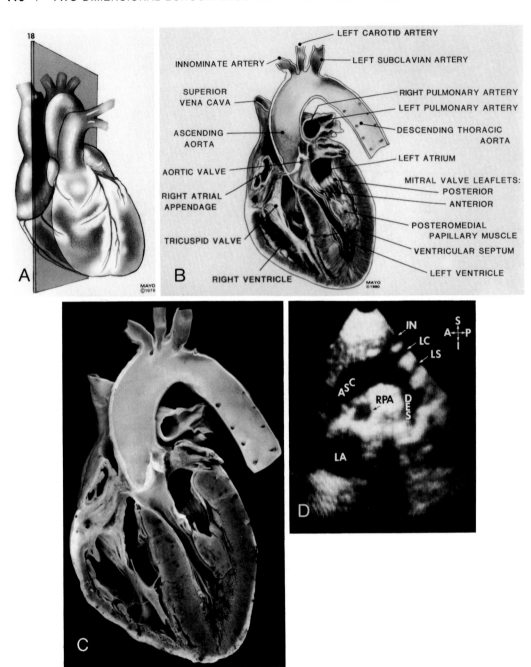

Figure 5.44. Tomographic section 18 (suprasternal long-axis plane of aortic arch). *A*, presumed plane of section, *B*, anatomic drawing of the spatial relationships of the aortic arch and pulmonary arteries. *C*, pathologic specimen. *D*, two-dimensional sector echographic view from the suprasternal transducer position, visualizing the aorta in the long-axis plane. Portions of the ascending (*ASC*) and descending (*DES*) thoracic aorta are visualized. Just posterior to the ascending aorta is the short-axis projection of the right pulmonary artery (*RPA*). Beneath the right pulmonary artery and the ascending aorta is the left atrium (*LA*). Arising from the aortic arch and upper descending aorta are the innominate (*IN*), left carotid (*LC*), and left subclavian (*LS*) arteries. *S* = superior; *P* = posterior; *I* = inferior; *A* = anterior. *C* from Tajik, AJ, Seward, JB, Hagler, DJ, Mair, DD, Lie, JT: Two-dimensional real-time ultrasonic imaging of the heart and great vessels: Technique, image orientation, structure identification, and validation. *Mayo Clin Proc 53:* 271, 1978. By permission.

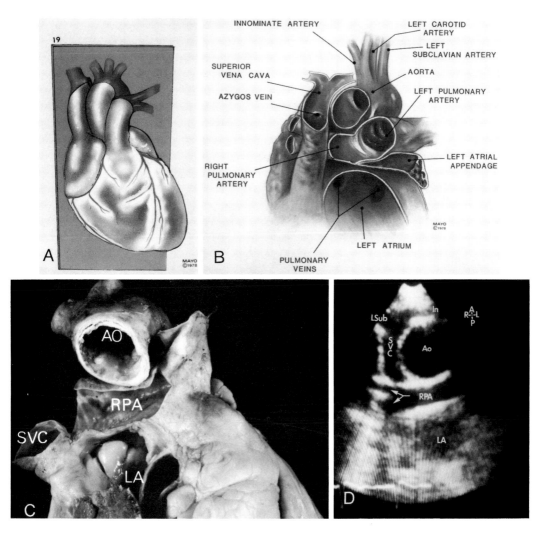

Figure 5.45. Tomographic section 19 (suprasternal short-axis plane of aortic arch). *A,* plane of section, *B,* anatomic drawing. *C,* pathologic specimen showing the anatomic relationships at the base of the heart. *AO* = aorta; *RPA* = right pulmonary artery; *SVC* = superior vena cava; *LA* = left atrium. *D,* two-dimensional sector echocardiogram of the suprasternal short-axis scan of the aortic arch. *Central* to the figure is the short-axis cut of the aortic arch (*Ao*). The long-axis projection of the right pulmonary artery (*RPA*) and its first bifurcation (*arrows*) appears inferior to the aorta. Portions of the superior vena cava (*SVC*) and its tributaries (left subclavian vein (*LSub*) and innominate vein (*In*)) appear to the left of the aortic arch. Posterior to the right pulmonary artery, a small portion of the left atrium (*LA*) is visualized. *A* = anterior; *L* = left; *P* = posterior; *R* = right. *C* from Tajik, AJ, Seward, JB, Hagler, DJ, Mair, DD, Lie, JT: Two-dimensional real-time ultrasonic imaging of the heart and great vessels: Technique, image orientation, structure identification, and validation. *Mayo Clin Proc 53:* 271, 1978. By permission.

and section 19A, Fig. 5.46), entry of the superior vena cava into the right atrium can be visualized. Subcostal transducer scanning of the anterior and superior atrial septum (section 15 and section 16A, Fig. 5.40) will also permit visualization of the distal superior vena cava entering the right atrium.

Occasionally, on parasternal long-axis views of the left ventricle (tomographic section 1), an echolucency superior to the left atrium is visualized (Fig. 5.50). This structure represents an oblique cut of the superior vena cava just before it enters the right atrium. Also from a high par-

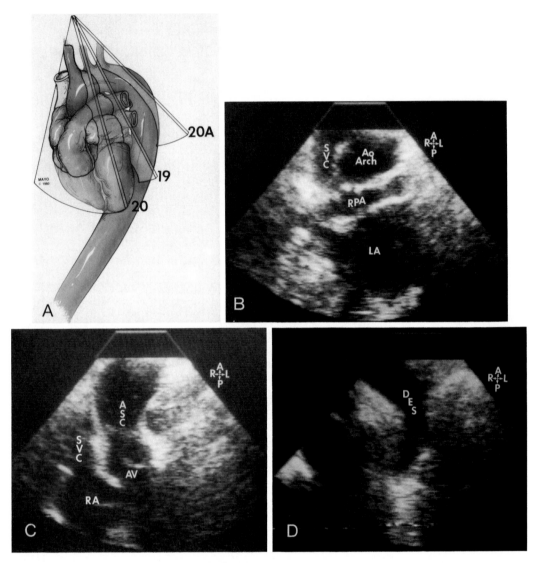

Figure 5.46. Tomographic sections 20 and 20A (suprasternal short-axis projection of ascending and descending thoracic aorta). *A*, from tomographic section 19, an anterior tilt of the transducer will image the ascending aorta (section 20), and a posterior tilt will visualize the descending thoracic aorta (section 20A). *B*, two-dimensional sector echocardiogram illustrating the short-axis scan of the aortic arch (*Ao Arch*) (tomographic section 19). *SVC* = superior vena cava; *RPA* = right pulmonary artery; *LA* = left atrium. *C*, following an anterior tilt of the transducer (section 20), the ascending aorta (*ASC*) and aortic root are visualized. The aortic valve leaflets (*AV*) can occasionally be assessed from this transducer position. To the right of the aortic root is the superior vena cava (*SVC*), which drains to the right atrium (*RA*). *D*, following a posterior tilt of the transducer (section 20A), the descending thoracic aorta is visualized, and in the presence of a normal left aortic arch, the descending thoracic aorta (*DES*) is projected to the right of the screen. *A* = anterior; *L* = left; *P* = posterior; *R* = right.

asternal short-axis projection of the ascending aorta, the superior vena cava is visualized as an echo-lucency posterior and to the right of the aorta (Fig. 5.51).

Inferior Vena Cava

Subcostal views (section 14A, Fig. 5.34, and section 14C, Fig. 5.36) consistently image the upper abdominal course of the inferior vena cava.

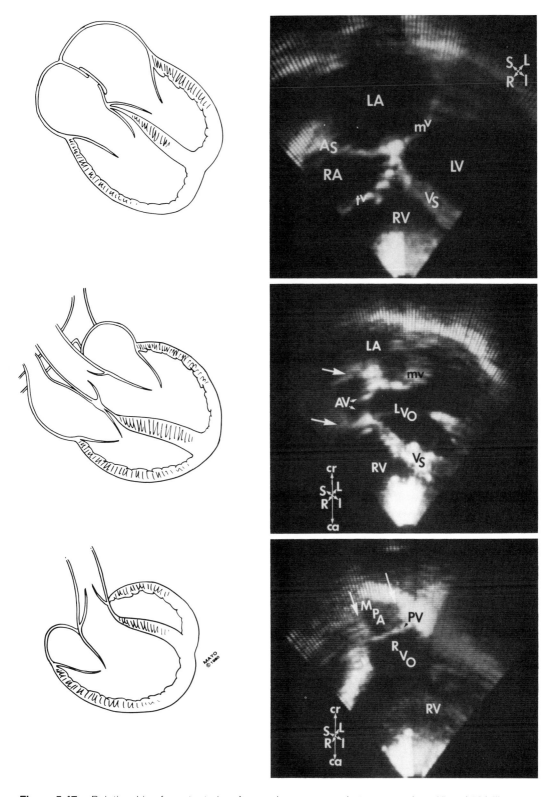

Figure 5.47. Relationship of great arteries. A scanning maneuver between sections 15 and 16A illustrates the technique of recognizing great artery orientation from the subcostal transducer position. With the ultrasound beam in the four-chamber plane, serial "cuts" of the heart from posterior to anterior permit

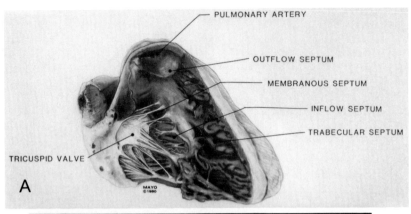

PULMONARY ARTERY

OUTFLOW SEPTUM

MEMBRANOUS SEPTUM

INFLOW SEPTUM

TRABECULAR SEPTUM

TRICUSPID VALVE

A

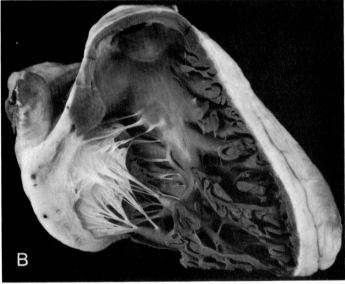

B

Figure 5.48. Anatomic drawing (*A*) and pathologic specimen (*B*) illustrate anatomy of the ventricular septum as viewed from the right ventricle. The lower half of the ventricular septum, designated the "trabecular septum," is characterized by dense myocardial trabeculations (the position of a muscular ventricular septal defect). The posterobasal ventricular septum beneath the septal leaflet of the tricuspid valve represents the inflow ventricular septum (the typical position of an atrioventricular canal septal defect). The superior and anterior septum, which constitutes the floor of the right ventricular outflow tract up to the pulmonary valve, is designated the "outflow septum" (the position of subpulmonic or supracristal ventricular septal defect). The membranous ventricular septum is a small area beneath the superior portion of the septal leaflet of the tricuspid valve (the position of the most commonly encountered membranous ventricular septal defect).

appreciation of great artery orientation. *Line drawings to left* correspond to the sector echocardiographic projections and are utilized to illustrate (*top* to *bottom*) section 15 (subcostal four-chamber view), section 16 (subcostal four-chamber plane plus aorta) and section 16A (subcostal four-chamber plane of right ventricular outflow tract). The *right panels* (*top* to *bottom*) illustrate comparable subcostal four-chamber projections. Note that the aorta lies posterior to the pulmonary artery and crosses from right to left in the image, while the anteriorly located pulmonary artery is directed superiorly. Continuity exists between the anterior leaflet of the mitral valve (*mv*) and the aortic wall. *LA* = left atrium; *LV* = left ventricle; *VS* = ventricular septum; *RV* = right ventricle; *tv* = tricuspid valve; *RA* = right atrium; *AS* = atrial septum; *AV* = aortic valve; *LVO* = left ventricular outflow; *cr* = cranial; *ca* = caudal; *L* = left; *I* = inferior; *R* = right; *S* = superior; *MPA* = main pulmonary artery; *PV* = pulmonary valve; *RVO* = right ventricular outflow. *Right panels, middle* and *bottom*, from Seward, JB, Tajik, AJ, Hagler, DJ: Orientation of the great arteries: normal, complete transposition, corrected transposition. In *Pediatric Echocardiography—Cross-Sectional, M-Mode and Doppler.* pp. 105–120, N-R Lundström, ed. Amsterdam, Elsevier/North-Holland Biomedical Press, 1980. By permission.

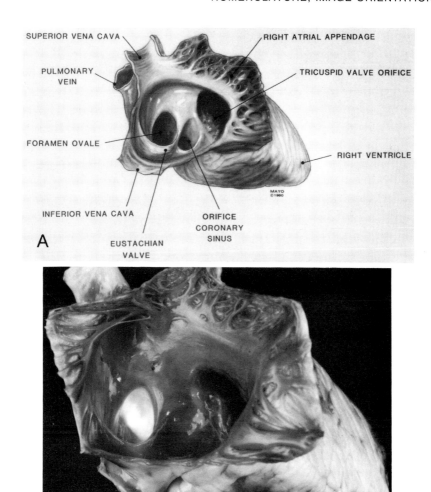

SUPERIOR VENA CAVA

RIGHT ATRIAL APPENDAGE

PULMONARY
VEIN

TRICUSPID VALVE ORIFICE

FORAMEN OVALE

RIGHT VENTRICLE

INFERIOR VENA CAVA

ORIFICE
CORONARY
SINUS

A

EUSTACHIAN
VALVE

B

Figure 5.49. Anatomic drawing (*A*) and pathologic specimen (*B*) illustrate right atrial anatomy. In the midportion of the atrial septum, the thinned foramen ovale is visualized (backlighted on the pathologic specimen). The Eustachian valve separates the orifice of the coronary sinus from the foramen ovale. The coronary sinus enters the right atrium just above the tricuspid valve orifice. The superior vena cava enters the superior and posterior aspect of the right atrium, and the inferior vena cava enters the inferior and posterior aspect of the right atrium. Note that in these figures and in Figure 5.27, *C* and *D*, the atrial septum surrounding the foramen ovale is thick and tends to produce a refractile and invariably easily imaged echo.

Its relationship to the hepatic veins (section 14D, Fig. 5.37) and right atrium (section 14C, Fig. 5.36) can be appreciated. Right atrial relationships to the inferior vena cava are best viewed by utilizing apical four-chamber projections (section 11A, Fig. 5.29, with further posterior tilt) (Fig. 5.52). The Eustachian valve separates the inferior vena cava from the orifice of the coronary sinus and the tricuspid valve.

Medial parasternal scanning to section 2 (right ventricular inflow view, Fig. 5.14) permits visu-

alization of the orifice of the inferior vena cava as it enters the posterobasal aspect of the right atrial cavity (Fig. 5.53).

Internal Crux of the Heart

The internal crux of the heart (section 11, Fig. 5.27) is formed by the basal portions of the atrial and ventricular septa and the septal portions of the mitral and tricuspid atrioventricular valves. This particular portion of the heart has very predictable anatomic relationships, which are im-

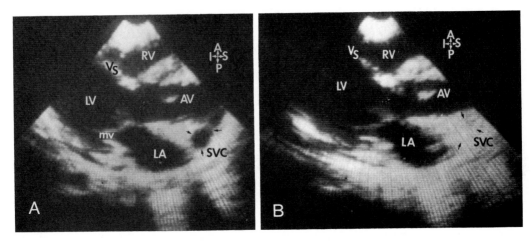

Figure 5.50. Parasternal long-axis projection of left ventricle visualizing the superior vena cava. *A*, with the transducer positioned in a slightly higher intercostal space, an echo-lucency superior to the left atrial cavity represents an oblique cut of the superior vena cava just before it enters the right atrium. *B*, with a catheter positioned in the superior vena cava, selective injection of echo contrast material opacifies the echolucency and confirms the identity of the structure as superior vena cava. *RV* = right ventricle; *AV* = aortic valve; *SVC* = superior vena cava; *LA* = left atrium; *mv* = mitral valve; *LV* = left ventricle; *VS* = ventricular septum; *A* = anterior; *S* = superior; *P* = posterior; *I* = inferior.

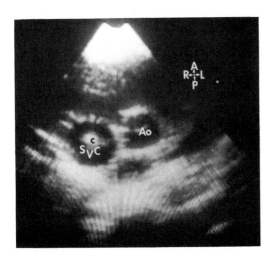

Figure 5.51. High parasternal short-axis projection of the superior vena cava. With the use of a high parasternal short-axis projection of the ascending aorta, an echolucency posterior to and to the right of the aorta represents the superior vena cava (*SVC*). In this particular patient, a catheter (*c*) has been positioned in the superior vena cava to confirm the identity of the structure. *Ao* = ascending aorta; *A* = anterior; *L* = left; *P* = posterior; *R* = right.

portant to the recognition of ventricular and valvular morphology. In the normal heart, the atrial septum is slightly displaced to the left of the ventricular septum, and the septal leaflet of the tricuspid valve inserts further into the right ventricular cavity than the corresponding septal portion of the anterior leaflet of the mitral valve. These relationships are used to predict ventricular morphology (i.e., in patients with inverted ventricles, the relationship of the atrioventricular valves is reversed).

Papillary Muscles

Left ventricular papillary muscle arrangement is consistent and predictable (section 6, Fig. 5.21). The muscles are invariably oriented at 3 and 8 o'clock positions (anterolateral and posteromedial papillary muscles, respectively). The papillary muscle arrangements can also be used to predict ventricular morphology. Calcification, rupture, fibrosis, structural anomalies and size can be appreciated with the two-dimensional technique.

Pulmonary Veins

With the apical four-chamber plane (section 11, Fig. 5.27), entry of the pulmonary veins into the

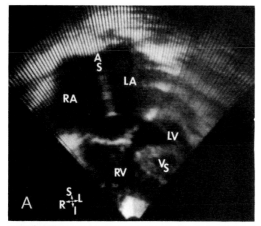

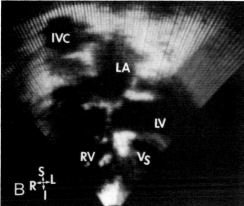

Figure 5.52. Visualization of the inferior vena cava from the apical four-chamber projection. *A,* in a patient with complete atrioventricular canal defect, the modified four-chamber view shows the upper portion of the atrial septum (*AS*) and the right atrial (*RA*) and left atrial (*LA*) cavities. Portions of the left ventricle (*LV*), ventricular septum (*VS*) and right ventricle (*RV*) are also visible. *B,* with further posterior projection of the ultrasound beam (view of the posterobasal right atrial cavity), the inferior vena cava (*IVC*) becomes visible at the superior basal aspect of the right atrial cavity. *S* = superior; *L* = left; *I* = inferior; *R* = right.

left atrium can invariably be visualized. Anomalies of pulmonary venous drainage can occasionally be predicted. Superior pulmonary veins can occasionally be visualized from the suprasternal examination (section 19, Fig. 5.45).

Coronary Sinus

The coronary sinus in the normal heart is best visualized from the apical transducer position (section 11A, Fig. 5.29). The normal coronary

sinus is situated in the left atrioventricular groove and enters the right atrium just above the septal leaflet of the tricuspid valve. The orifice of the coronary sinus is separated from the inferior vena cava by the Eustachian valve. The coronary sinus may be considerably dilated in patients with right atrial hypertension (i.e., tricuspid regurgitation, pulmonary hypertension and so on) and anom-

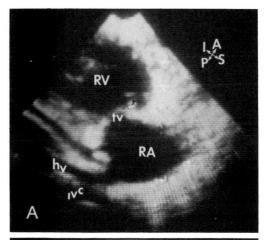

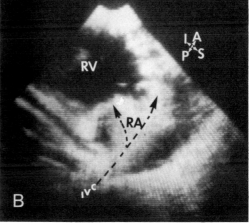

Figure 5.53. Orifice of the inferior vena cava as viewed from the parasternal long-axis projection of the right ventricular inflow (section 2). *A,* the orifice of the inferior vena cava (*ivc*) is visualized in the inferobasal aspect of the right atrial cavity. The hepatic vein (*hv*) is also visible as it enters the inferior vena cava near the cavoatrial junction. *B,* following an injection of echo contrast material into the inferior vena cava, a cloud of echoes appears through the orifice of the inferior vena cava into the right atrial cavity. *RA* = right atrium; *RV* = right ventricle; *tv* = tricuspid valve; *A* = anterior; *S* = superior; *P* = posterior; *I* = inferior.

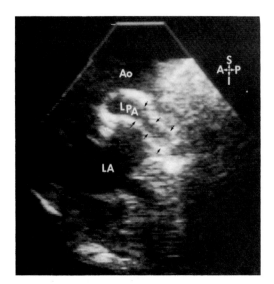

Figure 5.54. Suprasternal visualization of the left pulmonary artery. From tomographic section 18 (suprasternal long axis of the aortic arch), the ultrasound beam is scanned further leftward. The plane of the ultrasound beam would approximate a scan from the sternum to the left clavicle. The left pulmonary artery appears as a posteriorly and inferiorly directed echo-lucency beneath the aortic arch (*small arrows*). *Ao* = aortic arch; *LPA* = left pulmonary artery; *LA* = left atrium; *S* = superior; *P* = posterior; *I* = inferior; *A* = anterior.

alous venous drainage (i.e., persistent left superior vena cava or anomalous pulmonary venous return to coronary sinus). When dilated, the coronary sinus can be visualized easily from the parasternal long-axis view of the right ventricular inflow tract (section 2, Fig. 5.14) and the left ventricle (section 1, Fig. 5.13), and is imaged as a round echolucent area in the atrioventricular groove posterior to the insertion of the posterior leaflet of the mitral valve (9).

Thoracic Aorta

The entire thoracic aorta can be visualized from multiple transducer positions (8). The aortic root, at the base of the heart (section 1, Fig. 5.11), ascending aorta (section 1, Fig. 5.11; section 18, Fig. 5.44; section 19, Fig. 5.45; and section 20, Fig. 5.46), aortic arch (section 18, Fig. 5.44; section 19, Fig. 5.45; and sections 20 and 20A, Fig. 5.46), descending thoracic aorta (section 3, Fig. 5.16; sections 5 through 9, Figs. 5.20 through 5.25) and upper abdominal aorta (section 14A, Fig. 5.34, and section 14B, Fig. 5.35) can be appre-

ciated from variable transducer positions. Multiple short- and long-axis projections of the aorta are required for complete assessment of aortic dimensions and pathology. A complete under-

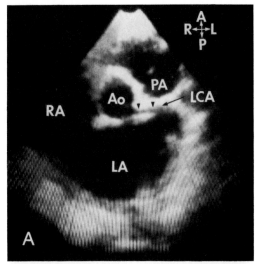

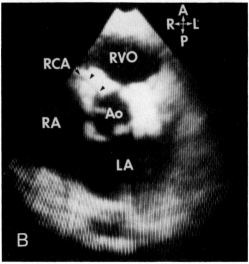

Figure 5.55. Two-dimensional echocardiographic visualization of the proximal coronary arteries. *A,* the proximal left main pulmonary artery (*PA*) is visualized just cephalad to the left coronary cusp of the aortic valve. A linear echolucent coronary artery can be visualized (*LCA*) (*arrowheads*). *B,* in a similar fashion, just above the right coronary cusp of the aortic valve, the proximal portion of the right coronary artery may be visualized (*RCA*) (*arrowheads*). *Ao* = aorta; *RVO* = right ventricular outflow tract; *RA* = right atrium; *LA* = left atrium; *A* = anterior; *L* = left; *P* = posterior; *R* = right.

standing of extracardiac relationships is most important in assessing related pathology.

Pulmonary Artery

The main pulmonary artery can be visualized from parasternal transducer positions (section 3, Fig. 5.16; section 9, Fig. 5.24; section 10, Fig. 5.26) and from the subcostal position (section 16A; Fig. 5.51). However, more often it is the proximal portions of the main right and left pulmonary arteries which are of clinical interest. From the suprasternal transducer position, short-axis (section 19; Fig. 5.45) and long-axis (section 18, Fig. 5.44) projections of the right pulmonary artery are consistently obtained. The right pulmonary artery swings beneath the aortic arch superior to the left atrium and posterior to the superior vena cava.

The left pulmonary artery is more difficult to visualize but is best seen with a slight leftward scan of the transducer from section 18 (suprasternal long-axis view of the aortic arch) (Fig. 5.54). The left pulmonary artery courses nearly directly posteriorly and lies lateral to the descending thoracic aorta.

Occasionally, with the use of section 3 (parasternal long-axis view of the right ventricular outflow tract, Fig. 5.16), the proximal left pulmonary artery can be visualized coursing directly posteriorly as a continuation of the main pulmonary artery.

Examination of the pulmonary arteries is helpful in assessing the size, presence and distribution of the proximal pulmonary arterial tree. This is particularly helpful in certain types of congenital heart defects (e.g., pulmonary valve atresia).

Coronary Arteries

The proximal portions of the left and right coronary arteries can be visualized from parasternal (section 9, Fig. 5.55) and apical (sections 11 and 12) transducer positions. With higher resolution machines and special echo techniques, the examination of the coronary arteries is becoming more feasible.

SUMMARY

With the advent of two-dimensional real-time echocardiographic techniques, many of the limitations of the M-mode examination have been eliminated. The prime advantages include: 1) greater versatility with the use of the parasternal, apical, subcostal and suprasternal ultrasound windows and reduction in the number of nondiagnostic examinations; 2) lateral resolution, which permits appreciation of spatial anatomic relationships; and 3) realization of more conventional images, comparable to those of tomographic angiography. A complete understanding of tomographic anatomy as it relates to this imaging modality is most important. Conventional, standardized and logical imaging orientation and nomenclature are most important for the best understanding of the tomographic relationships. With increasing use of this imaging modality, it becomes ever more important to revive an interest in detailed cardiac anatomy. Only with an in-depth understanding of normal tomographic anatomy will abnormal anatomic relationships become evident.

REFERENCES

1. Tajik AJ, Seward JB, Hagler DJ, Mair DD, Lie JT: Two-dimensional real-time ultrasonic imaging of the heart and great vessels: technique, image orientation, structure identification, and validation. *Mayo Clin Proc 53:* 271, 1978.
2. Tajik AJ, Seward JB, Hagler DJ, Mair DD: Experience with real-time two-dimensional sector angiography. *Am J Cardiol 41:* 353 (Abstr), 1978.
3. Seward JB, Tajik AJ, Spangler JG, Ritter DG: Echocardiographic contrast studies: Initial experience. *Mayo Clin Proc 50:* 163, 1975.
4. Seward JB, Tajik AJ, Hagler DJ, Ritter DG: Peripheral venous contrast echocardiography. *Am J Cardiol 39:* 202, 1977.
5. Report of the American Society of Echocardiography Committee on Nomenclature and Standards in Two-Dimensional Echocardiography. *Circulation 62:* 212, 1980.
6. Bansal RC, Tajik AJ, Seward JB, Offord KP: Feasibility of detailed two-dimensional echocardiographic examination in adults: prospective study of 200 patients. *Mayo Clin Proc 55:* 291, 1980.
7. McAlpine WA: *Heart and Coronary Arteries: An Anatomical Atlas for Clinical Diagnosis, Radiological Investigation, and Surgical Treatment.* New York, Springer-Verlag, 1975.
8. Seward JB, Tajik AJ: Noninvasive visualization of the entire thoracic aorta: A new application of wide-angle two-dimensional sector echocardiographic technique. *Am J Cardiol 43:* 387 (Abstr), 1979.
9. Snider AR, Ports TA, Silverman NH: Venous anomalies of the coronary sinus: Detection by M-mode, two-dimensional and contrast echocardiography. *Circulation 60:* 721, 1979.
10. Hagler DJ, Tajik AJ, Seward JB, Edwards WD, Mair DD, Ritter DG: Atrioventricular and ventriculoarterial discordance (corrected transposition of the great arteries): Wide-angle two-dimensional echocardiographic assessment of ventricular morphology. *Mayo Clin Proc 56:* 591, 1981.
11. Seward JB, Tajik AJ, Hagler DJ: Orientation of

the great arteries: Normal, complete transposition, corrected transposition. In *Pediatric Echocardiography—Cross-Sectional, M-Mode and Dopler.* pp. 105–120, N-R Lundström (ed): Amsterdam, Elsevier/North-Holland Biomedical Press, 1980.

12. Seward JB, Tajik AJ, Hagler DJ, Maier DD: Visualization of isolated ventricular septal defect with wide-angle two-dimensional sector echocardiography. *Circulation 58:* II-202 (Abstr), 1978.

13. Hagler DJ, Tajik AJ, Seward JB, Mair DD, Ritter DG: Real-time wide-angle sector echocardiography: atrioventricular canal defects. *Circulation 59:* 140, 1979.

14. Nasser FN, Tajik AJ, Seward JB, Hagler DJ: Diagnosis of sinus venosus atrial septal defect by two-dimensional echocardiography. *Mayo Clin Proc 56:* 568, 1981.

6

Doppler Echocardiography

John G. Harold, M.D.
Eugenio Carmo, M.D.
Jay N. Schapira, M.D.

INTRODUCTION

Doppler echocardiography noninvasively provides direct information on the velocity and direction of blood flow within the cardiovascular system (1–4). Doppler ultrasound can be used to study valvular stenosis and regurgitation, as well as other abnormal flows (5–9), can assess left ventricular systolic function, and provides complementary information to two-dimensional echocardiography (10, 11). Doppler ultrasound also can be used to assess left ventricular diastolic function through measurements of transmitral blood flow (12).

HISTORICAL ASPECTS

Doppler echocardiography is based on an application of the principle stated in 1842 by the Austrian physicist and astronomer, Christian Johann Doppler. In a paper entitled "On the Coloured Light of Double Stars and Some Other Heavenly Bodies," he postulated that stars emit a pure-spectrum white light and observed that different colors were proportional to the speed at which the star was moving toward (blue color) or away (red color) from the earth (13). Changes in light from stars were used to track the motion of these celestial objects. This principle was termed the "Doppler effect," which states that there is a change in the observed frequency of a wave because of relative motion between the observer and the source of the wave front. The Doppler effect can in fact be applied to any wave in which the source and the receiver are moving in relation to each other. The resultant frequency shift is thus proportional to the relative velocity between the source and the receiver. A typical example of the Doppler effect involves a moving train. As the train (sound source) approaches a stationary observer, sound wavelengths are compressed and the pitch of the train seems to increase. As the train travels away from the observer, the sound wavelengths become elongated and the pitch seems to decrease. Thus, the stationary observer hears an apparent change in frequency from higher to lower as the train passes.

In 1956, Shigeo Satomura from Osaka University in Japan applied the Doppler principle to detect blood velocity (14). He showed that when ultrasound is backscattered from moving red blood cells, there is a change in the frequency of the ultrasound: the larger the frequency shift, the higher the velocity. Using the ultrasonic Doppler cardiograph, Satomura was able to study the movements of the mitral, aortic, and pulmonic valves through analysis of their particular Doppler signals (15). Doppler echocardiography is now a clinically useful diagnostic technique. The remainder of this chapter reviews the applications of Doppler echocardiography to clinical cardiology.

BLOOD FLOW PATTERNS

In order to understand Doppler flow patterns in the cardiovascular system the concept of laminar and disturbed flow must be understood. Laminar flow occurs along smooth parallel lines so that all the red blood cells in a given area are moving at the same velocity. Flow is slightly slower near blood vessel walls due to the effects of viscous drag at the interface of blood and the vessel wall. Blood flow through the heart and great vessels is normally laminar and rarely exceeds a maximum velocity of 1.5 m/sec (5). Disturbed flow occurs when some obstruction disrupts normal laminar flow. Disturbed flow is characterized by disordered whirls and eddies of differing velocities and directions. These abnormal flow patterns are characterized generally by turbulence and an increase in velocity. The term turbulence can be defined mathematically, but generally has been used interchangeably with disturbed flow.

CALCULATIONS AND INSTRUMENTATION

Frequency is a fundamental characteristic of any wave phenomenon, and refers to the number of waves that pass a given point in 1 second. Frequency is usually described in units of cycles per second or Hertz (Hz). Doppler echocardiography depends on the measurement of the relative change between the transmitted ultrasound frequency and the reflected frequency. The difference between the reflected frequency and the transmitted frequency is termed the Doppler shift $(F_r - F_t)$ which is expressed in Hertz. The Doppler shift depends on the velocity of blood flow (v), the transmitted ultrasound frequency (F_t), the frequency of the returning ultrasound (F_r), the speed of sound in blood (c), and the cosine of the angle (Θ) between the ultrasound beam and the direction of blood flow. Solved for blood flow velocity, the Doppler equation becomes

$$v = \frac{c(F_r - F_t)}{2F_t(\cos \Theta)}. \qquad (6.1)$$

Commercially available Doppler systems compare the transmitted waveform with the received waveform for change in frequency. These "phase shifts" are then extrapolated to give velocity data. Since the Doppler equation contains the cosine of the angle between the ultrasound beam and the blood flow, frequency shift will be maximal at zero angle (ultrasound beam parallel to the direction of blood flow) and decrease as the angle increases. Marked decreases in the frequency shift will only occur at angles of more than 25°. For best results the ultrasound beam should be parallel to the direction of blood flow. Fortunately, the frequency shift from blood flow is mostly within audible range, and the audio signal can be used to find the position and direction where the highest frequency shifts can be obtained. As sound wave frequency increases, the pitch gets higher. As the frequency decreases, the pitch declines. Thus, high-pitched sounds result from large Doppler shifts, while low-pitched sounds result from smaller Doppler shifts. Flow relative to the Doppler probe is provided by a stereo audio output in which flow toward the transducer comes out one speaker and flow away from the Doppler probe comes out of the other.

Two-dimensional echocardiography and Doppler echocardiography differ in that the best echocardiographic images are obtained when the ultrasound beam is perpendicular to the heart, whereas the best Doppler signals are obtained when the ultrasound beam is parallel to blood flow. In clinical practice, the two-dimensional image is used to position the ultrasound beam within the heart. Then, with the aid of the audio signal and spectral display, the position and angle of the transducer are adjusted until the best Doppler signals are obtained. A variety of examining windows may be required to detect regions of flow disturbance.

For most ultrasonic imaging and measurement systems, the speed of sound within body tissues is assumed to be a constant 1560 m/sec at normal body temperature (16). The transmitted frequency is constant for a particular transducer. Most current instrumentation incorporates spectral analysis by fast Fourier transform (FFT) of the ultrasound signal, with the frequency shift displayed as a function of time. This digital method permits the simultaneous analysis of the various frequency components within the sample volume. A related method, Chirp-Z transform, provides similar information using analog electronics. With FFT, the various frequency components in the Doppler signal are converted to units of velocity using the Doppler equation and are then visually displayed. Real-time spectral analysis by FFT permits reproducible quantitation of Doppler frequency shifts and timing of flow events, and can provide quantitative estimates of flow velocity (17).

Pulsed and continuous wave Doppler form the two basic types of instrumentation. With conventional pulsed Doppler, velocities from a localized area can be recorded, but the upper limit to the velocities that can be recorded is fairly low. The highest velocity than can be detected with pulsed Doppler is a function of the depth from which the velocity was sampled, the intercept angle, and the transmitting frequency (18). With continuous wave Doppler, velocities from all along the ultrasound beam are recorded, but there is no limit to the velocities that can be recorded. Each modality may be used independently or in combination with simultaneous or interrupted two-dimensional imaging (19).

Doppler signals are processed to provide both audible and visual output. The audio output corresponds to the spectrum of the Doppler frequency shifts recorded and can be appreciated by using stereo headphones or speakers. The Doppler velocity shift usually is displayed using a spectral analysis graphic display (20). Velocity is usually displayed on the y axis, and time is displayed on the x axis. By convention, a positive signal indicates flow toward the transducer, and a negative signal indicates flow away from the transducer. A gray scale typically is used to indicate the intensity of each velocity. The border of the velocity profile is termed the "envelope."

As stated previously, normal blood flow in the heart and great vessels is laminar, with red blood cells moving at relatively similar velocities and direction. Disturbed flow is characterized by red blood cells moving in multiple directions and at multiple velocities simultaneously. Laminar blood flow will produce a "bordered envelope" with well-defined borders and a uniform spectral display. Disturbed flow typically will produce multiple velocity vectors and is displayed as a broad band of Doppler signals, known as spectral broadening. The audio characteristic of laminar flow is one of pure tones. Disturbed flow sounds much rougher and is composed of a number of different frequencies which are heard simultaneously.

PULSED DOPPLER

With pulsed (range-gated) Doppler, a single piezoelectric crystal is used to transmit the ultrasound burst and then receive the reflected signal. A brief burst of ultrasound is emitted by the crystal, which then functions in receive mode until signals from the area of interest have returned to the crystal. To derive the Doppler frequency with pulsed Doppler, the frequencies of the reflected and transmitted ultrasound are subtracted. The pulse repetition frequency (time interval of transmit/receive cycle) determines the "sample volume" from which the Doppler shift is measured. The location of the sample volume is controlled by the operator. The ultrasound reflected from moving red blood cells is received during the time interval between the transmitted pulses.

By combining two-dimensional imaging with the Doppler examination, the exact location of the sample volume within the heart can be displayed. The size of the sample volume can be varied, depending on the duration of the transmitted pulse and ultrasound beam width. Its length is determined by the length of each transmitted ultrasound pulse. The further into the heart the sample volume is moved, the larger it becomes. This results from divergence of the ultrasound beam as it moves further away from the transducer.

Pulsed Doppler has velocity measurement limitations. High blood velocities may be encountered in valvular heart disease and other pathologic conditions. The maximum frequency shift that can be measured by pulsed Doppler is called the "Nyquist limit." This maximal frequency shift is equal to one-half of the pulse repetition frequency.

$$\text{Nyquist limit} = \frac{\text{Number of pulses/second}}{2} \quad (6.2)$$

The Nyquist limit results in a phenomenon termed aliasing, which limits the maximum velocity that can be measured with standard pulsed Doppler (21, 22). Aliasing is simply the inability to measure a Doppler frequency shift that exceeds one-half of the pulse repetition frequency. At any frequency shift higher than the Nyquist limit, the signal will begin to alias, or wrap around upon itself. Stenotic and regurgitant lesions frequently are associated with high velocity flows that exceed the Nyquist limit and are difficult to quantitate with pulsed Doppler systems. The maximum recordable velocities in any jet relate to the frequency of the transducer used. For example, aliasing will be encountered at lower velocities with a 5.0 MHz Doppler probe than with a 2.5 MHz transducer. Extended range (high pulse repetition frequency) pulsed Doppler systems are available which allow higher velocities to be measured. Extended range Doppler can use multiples of the pulse repetition frequency corresponding to the Nyquist limit at a given depth (23). This approach can result in "range ambiguity," where the ability to localize the depth of origin of the high velocity jet may be lost. The "baseline shift" method also can be used to help overcome aliasing. This method takes advantage of the range of velocity available in the opposite channel by moving the baseline to the top or bottom of the display. Use of the baseline shift doubles the Nyquist limit at any given depth. However, continuous wave Doppler remains the technique of choice for measuring valvular lesions with high velocities.

CONTINUOUS WAVE DOPPLER

Continuous wave Doppler transducers are available with or without imaging capabilities. The smaller nonimaging Doppler transducer is useful for assessing valvular lesions, as it is accessible to additional ultrasonic windows, such as the suprasternal notch or narrow intercostal spaces. With continuous wave ultrasound, the ultrasound beam is transmitted continuously by one piezo-electric crystal, and the other continuously records the reflected ultrasound signals (11). Because the pulse repetition frequency is extremely high, the Nyquist limit is not reached and aliasing does not occur. As ultrasound is being transmitted and received continuously, velocities along the entire length of the beam are recorded simultaneously. Thus, the ability to localize the depth of origin of the flow signal is lost, introducing range ambiguity.

In clinical practice, pulsed and continuous wave Doppler modalities complement each other. Continuous wave Doppler measures the high velocities, and pulsed Doppler shows where the changes in velocity occur. Doppler ultrasound can be used together with two-dimensional imaging for localization of flow signals. It can also be used without imaging, because the flow signals from various parts of the heart are characteristic enough to allow pattern recognition. In addition, valve movements and the electrocardiogram can aid in timing and localization.

THE BERNOULLI EQUATION AND MEASUREMENT OF PRESSURE GRADIENT

The ability to measure pressure gradients non-invasively across stenotic valves is one of the most important clinical applications of Doppler echocardiography (8, 24). This application is based on the Bernoulli equation, which can be used to measure the relationship between velocity change across an obstruction and the pressure gradient. Daniel Bernoulli was a Dutch mathematician who, in 1738, showed that the pressure of a moving fluid depends on its velocity, with the pressure within the fluid decreasing as the velocity increases. The complete Bernoulli equation (6.3) is written as shown below, in Equation 6.3, where P_1 = pressure before stenosis, P_2 = pressure after stenosis, ρ = mass density of blood, V_1 = velocity of blood before stenosis, V_2 = velocity of blood after stenosis, $d\vec{v}$ = change in velocity during opening of the valve, dt = time for open-

ing of the valve, $d\vec{s}$ = distance over which the decrease in pressure is measured, R = viscous resistance in a vessel, and $\vec{v}$ = velocity of blood flow.

The contribution of flow acceleration and viscous friction is negligible in most clinical applications and the Bernoulli equation is commonly simplified to

$$P_1 - P_2 = 1/2\,\rho\,(V_2^2 - V_1^2). \qquad (6.4)$$

V_1, the velocity proximal to the stenotic area, is usually less than 1 m/sec and can usually be ignored. For blood, $\frac{1}{2}\rho$ is approximately 4; hence, insertion of 4 into the equation will convert velocity (in meters per second) to the pressure gradient (in millimeters of mercury). Thus, the simplified Bernoulli equation becomes

$$P_1 - P_2 = 4V^2. \qquad (6.5)$$

The modified Bernoulli equation allows the noninvasive determination of the pressure drop across stenotic valves as well as other obstructions, congenital lesions, and prosthetic valves.

The maximal velocity in a regurgitant jet depends on the pressure difference between the two chambers, and the Bernoulli equation can be used to calculate this pressure gradient. There is usually close agreement between pressure gradients predicted by Doppler echocardiography and those determined at cardiac catheterization (25).

Doppler echocardiography can be used to estimate cardiac output if volumetric flow and blood vessel area are measured. This topic is discussed elsewhere in this book by Bryg and Labovitz. (Chapter 17).

THE DOPPLER EXAMINATION

Doppler echocardiography is an integral part of the cardiac ultrasound examination. Whereas M-mode and two-dimensional echocardiography utilize ultrasound to assess cardiac anatomy, the Doppler technique uses ultrasound to assess velocity and blood flow information. Doppler color flow mapping can further complement the ultrasound examination (26, 27).

The patient usually is positioned in the left lateral decubitus position for the examination. Proper

$$P_1 - P_2 = \underbrace{1/2\rho(V_2^2 - V_1^2)}_{\substack{\text{Convective} \\ \text{acceleration}}} + \underbrace{\rho\int_1^2 \frac{d\vec{v}}{dt}}_{\substack{\text{flow} \\ \text{acceleration}}} \times d\vec{s} + \underbrace{R\,(\vec{v})}_{\substack{\text{viscous} \\ \text{friction}}} \qquad (6.3)$$

$$\text{Pressure decrease} = \text{Convective acceleration} + \text{flow acceleration} + \text{viscous friction}$$

transducer positioning will depend upon the information sought. The normal Doppler examination emphasizes those examining windows likely to align the direction of the Doppler ultrasound beam with that of blood flow (1). The four transducer positions routinely used during the Doppler examination include the left parasternal, apical, subcostal, and suprasternal notch. The right lateral decubitus position frequently is used to detect aortic stenosis jets. Doppler and two-dimensional examinations can be recorded simultaneously or sequentially, depending on the available equipment. As stated, two-dimensional echocardiography and Doppler echocardiography differ in that the best echocardiographic images are obtained when the ultrasound beam is perpendicular to the heart, whereas the best Doppler signals are obtained when the ultrasound beam is parallel to blood flow. The two-dimensional image is used to position the ultrasound beam within the heart. Then, with the aid of the audio signal and spectral display, the position and angle of the transducer are adjusted until the best Doppler signals are obtained. The direction of blood flow in three-dimensional space cannot be routinely "imaged" by available equipment. Therefore, the sonographer must look for the highest apparent blood flow velocities.

The routine Doppler examination usually begins with the apical window. As seen from the apical window, flow through the mitral, aortic, and tricuspid valves is nearly parallel to the transducer, and good quality Doppler recordings usually are obtainable.

Normal Aortic Valve

To assess left ventricular outflow, the sample volume usually is placed in the left ventricular outflow tract below the aortic valve and away from the mitral leaflets guided by a five-chamber apical view (28). Left ventricular outflow will appear as a uniform band of systolic velocities that accelerate briskly, peak, and then decelerate. Little waveform is seen in diastole unless mitral inflow velocities also are recorded. From the apex, this flow will be directed away from the transducer and, by convention, will be plotted as shift below the baseline (Fig. 6.1).

The aortic flow has the same characteristics as the left ventricular outflow and is obtained by placing the sample volume on the ascending aorta immediately after the aortic valve (Fig. 6.2). Beside the five-chamber apical view, the supraster-

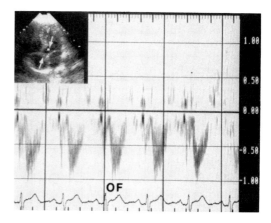

Figure 6.1. Normal flow through the outflow tract of the left ventricle. A simultaneous five-chamber apical view is used to place the sample volume (*upper arrow*) of the pulsed Doppler in the outflow tract of the left ventricle, behind the aortic valve (*lower arrow*). The spectral analysis demonstrates the normal systolic flow (*OF*) away from the transducer, so below the baseline. Peak velocity is approximately 1.0 m/sec.

nal and a high right parasternal approach may be used. In these cases the flow will be toward the transducer and will be plotted as a shift above the baseline (Fig. 6.3). The descending aorta also can be evaluated from a suprasternal approach. In this case the flow will be displayed below the

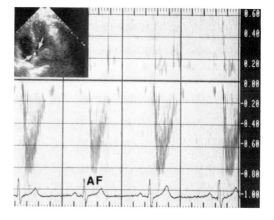

Figure 6.2. Normal aortic flow. The sample volume is placed in the ascending aorta (*lower arrow*) immediately above the aortic valve (*upper arrow*) guided by simultaneous five-chamber apical view. The spectral analysis shows the normal systolic aortic flow (*AF*) below the baseline, because flow is away from the transducer.

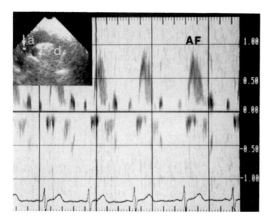

Figure 6.3. Normal aortic flow from a suprasternal view. The sample volume (*arrow*) is placed in the ascending aorta above the aortic valve guided by the two-dimensional image. The spectral analysis shows the normal systolic aortic flow (*AF*) above the baseline, because from the suprasternal window flow in the ascending aorta (*a*) is toward the transducer. The descending aorta (*d*) is also visualized.

baseline because flow moves away from the transducer (Fig. 6.4).

Aortic Stenosis

Doppler echocardiography has revolutionized the noninvasive assessment of patients with aortic stenosis (25). Aortic stenosis is diagnosed by recording a high velocity jet in the ascending aorta or across the aortic valve. Disturbed flow in the ascending aorta is usually a sign of obstruction at the aortic valve and can be recorded with pulsed wave or continuous wave Doppler. Aortic stenosis usually is associated with spectral broadening of the Doppler signal because of multiple velocity vectors in the area of disturbed flow. Continuous wave Doppler remains the best ultrasonic technique for quantifying aortic stenosis. By aligning the ultrasound beam to the high velocity jet, the peak velocity can be obtained (29). Using the simplified Bernoulli equation it is possible to measure the instantaneous pressure gradient across the aortic valve. However, there are some inherent limitations in using Doppler peak gradient estimates. Doppler is used to define the highest velocity of flow across a stenotic valve, which is referred frequently to as "peak instantaneous gradient."

Hemodynamic transvalvular gradients measured at cardiac catheterization are usually "peak-to-peak" or mean pressure gradients. The mean pressure gradient is estimated by summing the gradients measured at sequential time intervals and dividing by the number of measurements. In aortic stenosis, the peak-to-peak gradient is the difference between the peak left ventricular pressure and the peak aortic pressure (30). The peak instantaneous pressure gradient measured by Doppler is invariably larger than hemodynamically measured peak-to-peak or mean gradients. Thus "maximum" pressure gradients measured by Doppler when compared to "maximum" pressure gradients by catheterization may not be measuring the same quantity. Pressure gradients also change with volume flow, and they do not always indicate the degree of valvular obstruction. A patient with a low cardiac output because of poor left ventricular function may have a low pressure gradient as measured by Doppler and cardiac catheterization, despite severe valvular stenosis.

It is critical that the maximal velocity be recorded and that the ultrasonic beam be parallel to the aortic stenotic jet. Obtaining the highest velocity across the aortic valve is often the most technically difficult aspect of the Doppler examination. Failure to obtain the highest velocity may lead to underestimation of the degree of aortic stenosis. Various ultrasound windows must be tried to make certain that the highest velocity is located. The direction of the jet varies widely from patient to patient. The most common win-

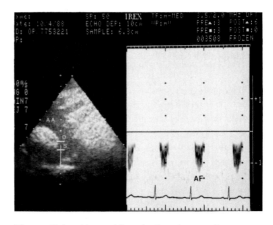

Figure 6.4. Normal flow in the descending aorta. The sample volume (*s*) is placed in the descending aorta (*D*) guided by a simultaneous suprasternal view. The normal systolic aortic flow (*AF*) in this case is recorded below the baseline because flow is away from the transducer. The aortic arch (*AA*) is also visualized.

dows utilized for recording peak aortic systolic velocity are the apical, suprasternal, and right parasternal windows. Considerable operator skill is necessary to obtain adequate Doppler spectral tracings for measurement of aortic peak velocity. Color flow Doppler may assist in localizing the forward jet of aortic stenosis (31).

An occasional patient may be found to have Doppler-predicted aortic valve gradient but no gradient at cardiac catheterization (32). Use of the simplified Bernoulli equation in these patients may be the reason. The complete Bernoulli equation takes into account blood velocity on both sides of the stenotic valve, whereas the simplified form only uses peak velocity after the flow crosses the valve. Patients with hyperdynamic circulatory states, such as those with aortic insufficiency, may have a significant velocity profile below the valve. Use of the simplified Bernoulli equation in these patients may lead to overestimation of the aortic gradient. Other conditions that may be associated with overestimation of aortic gradient include anemia, thyrotoxicosis, and exercise.

The pressure drop across the valve in aortic stenosis is only one indication of the severity of obstruction, because it varies greatly with flow across the valve. A similar pressure drop may occur in moderate obstruction with high flow across the valve and in severe obstruction with reduced flow. Several recent studies described the measure of stenotic valve area by use of the continuity equation (33, 34). This equation applies the law of conservation of mass to hydrodynamic systems. The principle is simple: Forward volume flow on the ventricular side of the valve is the same as forward flow on the aortic side. Whether or not an obstruction is present, these two flows must always be equal. The product of the peak flow velocity (or flow velocity integral) distal to the site of obstruction times the area of the valvular obstruction should equal the product of the peak velocity (or flow velocity integral) proximal to the valve times the area of the left ventricular outflow tract just proximal to the valvular narrowing. The continuity equation as applied to aortic stenosis is written:

$$\text{Flow}_2 = \text{Flow}_1$$
$$A_2 \times V_2 = A_1 \times V_1 \qquad (6.6)$$
$$A_2 = \frac{A_1 \times V_1}{V_2}$$

where A_1 and V_1 represent the cross-sectional area and the mean velocity at the nonstenotic portion

in the left ventricular outflow tract, and A_2 and V_2 represent the cross-sectional area and the mean velocity at the aortic valve. V_1 is measured in the left ventricular outflow tract using pulsed Doppler, and V_2 is measured using continuous wave Doppler. The proximal area is best calculated using the parasternal long-axis view, measuring the dimensions of the left ventricular outflow tract at the level of the aortic annulus. The aortic valve area is then calculated by multiplying peak velocity (or flow velocity integral) proximal to the valve times the area of the left ventricular outflow tract at the level of the aortic annulus and dividing that by the peak flow velocity (or flow velocity integral) distal to the valve.

The severity of aortic stenosis also may be judged by time from onset of systole to peak velocity divided by the ejection time (35). A value of 0.50 or greater has been found to correlate with significant aortic stenosis. Some investigators have used Doppler-derived measures of volume flow and pressure gradient and applied them to the Gorlin formula to assess stenotic valve area (36, 37).

Further details and clinical examples of aortic stenosis are reviewed in Chapter 8.

Aortic Insufficiency

Doppler echocardiography is the examination of choice for assessing aortic insufficiency (38). The best window for the evaluation of aortic insufficiency is the apical long-axis view. In this view the left ventricular outflow tract is directly parallel to the Doppler signal. Using continuous wave Doppler, aortic insufficiency appears as a holodiastolic, high frequency turbulent jet, with spectral broadening and flow toward the transducer. When pulsed wave Doppler is used the sample volume should be placed in the left ventricular outflow tract below the aortic valve. Color flow Doppler is of value in locating eccentric aortic insufficiency jets, particularly those associated with periprosthetic leaks (39). Care should be taken to distinguish aortic insufficiency from mitral valve diastolic inflow, particularly when mitral stenosis is present.

Pulsed wave Doppler has been reported to have a sensitivity of between 86% and 100% for the detection of aortic insufficiency. Pulsed wave Doppler can help assess the severity of aortic insufficiency by mapping the regurgitant flow into the left ventricle. Continuous wave Doppler also has been used for quantitative evaluation of aortic insufficiency (40).

Left ventricular end-diastolic pressure may be estimated in patients with aortic insufficiency by use of the modified Bernoulli equation (41). The velocity of the aortic insufficiency jet at end-diastole can be substituted into the modified Bernoulli equation to solve for the pressure gradient between the aorta and left ventricle. Subtracting this pressure from diastolic blood pressure provides an estimate of left ventricular end-diastolic pressure (LVEDP). For example, if diastolic blood pressure = 50 mm Hg and aortic insufficiency jet velocity = 3 m/sec, then LVEDP = $50 - 4(3)^2$ = $50 - 36 = 14$ mm Hg.

Quantitation of aortic insufficiency has also been attempted by examining the flow pattern within the aorta. Patients with severe aortic insufficiency have been shown to have a higher retrograde diastolic velocity in porportion to the forward systolic velocity (42). The regurgitant volume in aortic insufficiency also can be assessed by Doppler echocardiography (43).

Further details and clinical examples of aortic insufficiency are reviewed in Chapter 8.

Normal Mitral Valve

To assess left ventricular inflow the transducer is placed at the cardiac apex and is angulated superiorly, posteriorly, and toward the right. Mitral valve flow is recorded by placing the sample volume at the tip of the mitral valve leaflets in the left ventricular inflow tract. Mitral flow is typically laminar and biphasic, consisting of a low velocity diastolic flow toward the transducer with two peaks resembling an M-mode echocardiographic recording of the mitral valve (Fig. 6.5). The initial peak occurs during the rapid filling phase of diastole. The second peak, due to atrial contraction, occurs in late diastole. Loss of atrial contraction will result in absence of the second peak. The Doppler audio output consists of "clicking" sounds that coincide with valve opening and closure as a low frequency diastolic flow signal. The normal mitral valve peak diastolic velocity is less than 1.4 m/sec. A negative systolic deflection after aortic valve opening usually represents left ventricular outflow velocity.

Mitral Stenosis

Doppler echocardiography can be used to quantitate the severity of mitral stenosis. Mitral stenosis causes a high diastolic velocity which usually exceeds 1.5 m/sec. Using continuous wave Doppler, the spectral recording of mitral stenosis demonstrates spectral broadening in diastole, with

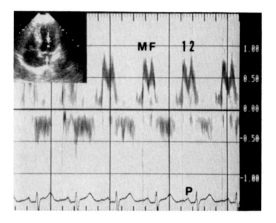

Figure 6.5. Normal mitral flow. The sample volume (*upper arrow*) is placed in the left ventricle inflow tract immediately after the mitral valve (*lower arrow*) guided by simultaneous four-chamber apical view. The normal diastolic mitral flow (*MF*) is recorded above the baseline (flow toward the transducer) and has two peaks like an M-mode recording of the mitral valve. The first peak (*1*) represents the rapid filling phase of diastole, and the second peak (*2*) follows atrial contraction represented by the P wave of the electrocardiogram (*P*).

peak flow early in diastole and a progressive but slowed diastolic descent. In addition, disturbed blood flow can be detected in the left ventricle. The biphasic quality of the recording is absent in patients with atrial fibrillation due to the loss of effective atrial contraction. The pressure gradient across the mitral valve can be measured with Doppler echocardiography using the modified Bernoulli equation (8, 9). For patients in atrial fibrillation, at least 10 cardiac cycles should be measured and then averaged to obtain a mean pressure gradient across the mitral valve.

An estimate of mitral valve area can be obtained noninvasively using the pressure half-time (44). The rate at which the left atrial-left ventricular pressure gradient falls during diastole is determined by the rate of left atrial emptying, which decreases as the mitral orifice size decreases. The pressure half-time is defined as the time (in milliseconds) necessary for the initial diastolic pressure gradient to decline by 50% (Fig. 6.6). The velocity equivalent to the pressure half-time is obtained by dividing the initial peak velocity by the square root of two. The point at which the mitral velocity decreases to this value is located, and a vertical line is drawn through

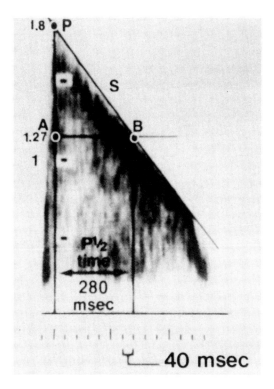

Figure 6.6. Calculation of pressure half-time. The peak velocity (*P*) is marked on the diastolic mitral flow as well as the diastolic slope (*S*). *Point A* is obtained dividing the peak velocity by the square root of 2 (1.41). From *point A* a *horizontal line* is drawn toward the diastolic slope, and *point B* is obtained. The time measured from *A* to *B* represents the pressure half-time, i.e., the time necessary for the mitral diastolic pressure gradient to decline by 50%.

the point at which the diastolic slope intersects this value. The time interval (in milliseconds) between this point and the initial peak velocity is the pressure half-time. The normal pressure half-time is 20–60 msec.

In mitral stenosis, the pressure half-time may range from 100 to 400 msec, depending on the severity of the stenosis. A pressure half-time of 220 msec has been found to correlate with a mitral valve area of 1.0 cm². Thus, the mitral valve area can be derived by dividing the measured pressure half-time (in milliseconds) into 220 msec/cm²:

$$\text{Mitral valve area} = \frac{220}{\text{pressure half-time.}} \quad (6.7)$$

The pressure half-time is much less influenced by flow across the mitral valve and by heart rate than is the pressure drop. The pressure half-time becomes longer with increasing obstruction and can be used to obtain a noninvasive estimate of mitral valve area. In cases of mitral stenosis associated with severe aortic regurgitation, the pressure half-time method is likely to overestimate the true mitral valve area (45).

The continuity equation also can be applied to the assessment of valve area in mitral stenosis. As discussed, the continuity equation states that when there is a constant flow in a flow channel with stenosis, a flow volume at the stenotic portion equals that of the nonstenotic portion. In mitral stenosis, a flow volume through the mitral valve during one cardiac cycle should be equal to stroke volume. Mitral valve area can then be determined as a ratio of stroke volume to the transmitral flow velocity integral over one cardiac cycle. Mitral valve area determined by the continuity equation has been shown to correlate with that determined by cardiac catheterization and the pressure half-time method.

Further details and clinical examples of mitral stenosis are reviewed in Chapter 8.

Mitral Insufficiency

Mitral insufficiency can be diagnosed by recording reversed flow at the mitral orifice during systole and following this back into the left atrium. The severity of the insufficiency is assessed by mapping the distance from the valve orifice to the point where the jet no longer can be detected (46). The regurgitant jet is three-dimensional; therefore, mapping must be done in more than one imaging plane. Using pulsed wave Doppler, most cases of mitral insufficiency can be detected using the apical window with the sample volume placed in the left atrium just behind the mitral valve. Normally, no systolic signals are detected at this level except for the "clicks" produced by opening and closing of the mitral valve. Further details and clinical examples of mitral insufficiency are reviewed in Chapter 8. Color flow Doppler has simplified the assessment of mitral insufficiency and avoids the time-consuming pulsed Doppler mapping technique (47). Color flow transesophageal echocardiography is especially helpful in assessing the severity of mitral insufficiency (48).

Intraoperative color flow mapping has been used to assess the efficacy of mitral valve repair. This topic is discussed elsewhere in this book by Maurer and Czer (Chapter 8).

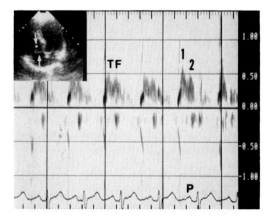

Figure 6.7. Normal tricuspid flow. The sample volume (*upper arrow*) is placed in the right ventricle inflow tract in front of the tricuspid valve (*lower arrow*) guided by simultaneous four-chamber apical view (a parasternal view could also be used). The normal diastolic tricuspid flow (*TF*) is represented above the baseline, and flow moves toward the transducer. Like the mitral valve flow, tricuspid flow has two peaks (*1* + *2*) where the second follows atrial contraction represented by the P wave (*P*) of the electrocardiogram.

Normal Tricuspid Valve

Tricuspid valve flow is also well recorded from the apex by use of both pulsed wave and continuous wave Doppler. Slight medial angulation of the transducer will align the ultrasound beam with right ventricular inflow. The sample volume is placed just distal to the tricuspid valve leaflets. A velocity profile similar to mitral flow will be recorded (Fig. 6.7). The first peak represents rapid diastolic filling, and the second peak is due to atrial contraction. Higher velocities will occur with inspiration, and lower ones, with expiration. Tricuspid valve velocities are usually lower than mitral valve velocities.

Tricuspid Stenosis

The presence of tricuspid stenosis is determined easily by Doppler echocardiography (49). The Doppler findings in tricuspid stenosis are similar to Doppler findings in mitral stenosis (50). However, tricuspid stenosis is an exceedingly rare condition, and the published experience with Doppler echocardiography is limited. Peak velocities in early diastole are increased and show a slow rate of decline throughout diastole (51).

Peak velocities are less than those seen in mitral stenosis.

The pressure half-time also can be used to calculate the severity of the valvular obstruction. Further details and clinical examples of tricuspid stenosis are reviewed in Chapter 8.

Tricuspid Insufficiency

Tricuspid insufficiency is best evaluated from the apical window and is identified as a holosystolic signal. For pulsed Doppler assessment, the sample volume should be placed behind the tricuspid valve leaflets in the right atrium (52). The width and depth of the regurgitant flow can then be mapped by moving the sample volume from side to side and toward the right atrial posterior wall. The spectral profile of tricuspid insufficiency is similar to that seen with mitral insufficiency. Trace tricuspid insufficiency is found frequently in normal individuals (53). Because of this, many laboratories will not report tricuspid regurgitation if it is localized just behind the tricuspid valve leaflets.

Respiratory variations are observed frequently in patients with tricuspid insufficiency. This finding is helpful in distinguishing mitral insufficiency from tricuspid insufficiency when a nonimaging Doppler probe is used (54). In severe tricuspid insufficiency, pulsed Doppler sampling in the hepatic vein may show retrograde or positive flow during systole. The presence of reverse systolic flow in the jugular veins is a highly sensitive marker for the presence of tricuspid insufficiency (55, 56). Doppler color flow imaging has further simplified the echocardiographic assessment of tricuspid regurgitation (57).

Continuous wave Doppler assessment of tricuspid insufficiency has been useful in the noninvasive assessment of right ventricular pressure and pulmonary hypertension (58). The peak systolic velocity of tricuspid insufficiency correlates with the gradient between the right ventricular systolic pressure and the mean right atrial pressure. This method, like all Doppler pressure measurements, is based on the modified Bernoulli equation (59, 60). Thus, the right ventricular pressure (RV_p) minus the right atrial pressure (RA_p) equals four times the regurgitant velocity squared:

$$\text{Gradient} = RV_p - RA_p. \qquad (6.8)$$

The mean right atrial pressure in centimeters H_2O is first estimated from examination of the jugular venous pulse (JVP) with the patient at 45°. Right atrial pressure (RA$_p$) is then estimated by adding 5 cm (approximates distance from right atrium to clavicle) to the venous pressure measurement and then converting this to millimeters of mercury by dividing it by 1.3. The normal mean right atrial pressure may be assumed to be 10 mm Hg in adults. A measure of the right ventricular systolic pressure can then be obtained:

$$RV_p = (\text{gradient}) + \frac{JVP + 5}{1.3} \quad (6.9)$$

where the RV − RA gradient = (4) (peak systolic velocity)^2.

In the absence of pulmonic stenosis, right ventricular systolic pressure will reflect pulmonary artery systolic pressure. Noninvasive assessment of pulmonary artery systolic pressure by these methods closely approximates right ventricular or pulmonary artery systolic pressure measurements obtained at cardiac catheterization.

Right ventricular function and pulmonary hypertension is discussed in further detail elsewhere in this book by Foale (Chapter 19).

Normal Pulmonic Valve

The short-axis parasternal view obtained at the level of the aortic valve will show the right ventricular outflow tract wrapping around the aorta, pulmonic valve, and pulmonary artery. In this position, the ultrasound beam will be parallel to flow in the right ventricular outflow tract and pulmonary artery. Pulmonic flow is obtained by placing the sample volume in the pulmonary artery just distal to the pulmonic valve (Fig. 6.8). Using the nonimaging Doppler probe, the pulmonic valve is best evaluated by placing the transducer in the second or third left intercostal space and directing the beam posteriorly. The spectral tracing of normal pulmonic flow will consist of systolic laminar flow directed away from the transducer and displayed below the baseline. The velocity of pulmonic flow is usually less than aortic flow and does not normally exceed 1.0–1.2 m/sec.

Pulmonic Stenosis

Pulmonic stenosis has Doppler findings similar to aortic stenosis. These include an increased velocity across the valve and spectral broadening related to turbulent flow (61). The severity of pulmonic stenosis can be assessed with continuous wave Doppler applying the modified Ber-

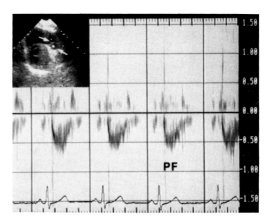

Figure 6.8. Normal pulmonic flow. The sample volume of the pulsed Doppler (*lower arrow*) is placed in the pulmonary artery immediately after the pulmonic valve (*upper arrow*). The normal systolic pulmonic flow (*PF*) is displayed below the baseline following the QRS complex of the electrocardiogram, because flow is away from the transducer.

noulli equation (62). There is good correlation between noninvasive predictions of pulmonic valve gradient and findings at catheterization. Further details and clinical examples of pulmonic stenosis are reviewed in Chapter 8.

Pulmonic Insufficiency

The diastolic pattern of pulmonic insufficiency resembles that seen in aortic insufficiency (63, 64). Pulmonic insufficiency is best assessed from the left parasternal window with angulation of the ultrasound beam toward the patient's left shoulder (65). As with tricuspid insufficiency, pulmonic insufficiency is found in a large number of otherwise normal patients. If the sample volume is close to the pulmonary valve, a normal low frequency early diastolic flow may be recorded. Pathologic pulmonic insufficiency is associated with a higher frequency pansystolic flow and is recorded more proximal to the pulmonic valve.

The most common cause of pulmonic insufficiency is pulmonary hypertension. Using the modified Bernoulli equation, the diastolic gradient between the right ventricle and the pulmonary artery can be measured if pulmonic insufficiency is present: pulmonary artery diastolic pressure = diastolic gradient across the pulmonic valve + assumed diastolic pressure in the right ventricle (5 mm Hg). The diastolic gradient reflects the severity of the pulmonary hypertension.

The severity of the pulmonic insufficiency may be estimated by mapping the jet down the right ventricular outflow tract. Further details and clinical examples of pulmonic insufficiency are reviewed in Chapter 8. Color flow mapping is a useful adjunct in the Doppler assessment of pulmonic insufficiency.

CONCLUSION

Doppler echocardiography has revolutionized the noninvasive assessment of cardiac function in health and disease. By recording the velocity of flow across normal as well as diseased valves, Doppler provides complementary information to the echocardiographic assessment of structure and function. Doppler echocardiography is now a quantitative clinical diagnostic technique. It reduces the need for invasive studies and can help differentiate patients with significant valvular lesions from those with mild lesions.

REFERENCES

1. Nishimura RA, Miller FA, Callahan MJ, Benassi RC, Seward JB, Tajik AJ: Doppler echocardiography: Theory, instrumentation, technique, and application. *Mayo Clin Proc* 60:321–343, 1985.
2. Pearlman AS, Stevenson JG, Baker DW: Doppler echocardiography: Applications, limitations and future directions. *Am J Cardiol* 46:1256–1269, 1980.
3. Berger M (ed): *Doppler Echocardiography in Heart Disease, Basic and Clinical Cardiology.* New York, Marcel Dekker, 1987, vol 10.
4. Goldberg SJ, Allen HD, Marx GR, Flinn CJ: *Doppler Echocardiography.* Philadelphia, Lea & Febiger, 1988.
5. Hatle L, Angelsen B: *Doppler Ultrasound in Cardiology.* ed 2. Philadelphia, Lea & Febiger, 1985.
6. Jaffee WM, Roche AHG, Coverdale HA, McAlister HF, Ormiston JA, Greene ER: Clinical evaluation versus Doppler echocardiography in the quantitative assessment of valvular heart disease. *Circulation* 78:267–275, 1988.
7. Otto CM, Pearlman AS, Comes KA, Reamer RP, Janko CL, Huntsman LL: Determination of the stenotic aortic valve area in adults using Doppler echocardiography. *J Am Coll Cardiol* 7:509–517, 1986.
8. Skjaerpe T, Hegrenaes L, Hatle L: Noninvasive estimation of valve area in patients with aortic stenosis by Doppler ultrasound and two-dimensional echocardiography. *Circulation* 72:810–818, 1985.
9. Richards KL: Doppler echocardiographic quantification of stenotic valvular lesions. *Echocardiography* 4:289–303, 1987.
10. Magnin PA, Stewart JA, Myers S, Von Ramm O, Kisslo JA: Combined Doppler and phased-array echocardiographic estimation of cardiac output. *Circulation* 63:388–392, 1981.
11. Nishimura RA, Callahan MJ, Schaff HV, Ilstrup DM, Miller FA, Tajik AJ: Noninvasive measurement of cardiac output by continuous-wave Doppler echocardiography: Initial experience and review of the literature. *Mayo Clin Proc* 59:484–489, 1984.
12. Spirito P, Maron BJ: Doppler echocardiography for assessing left ventricular diastolic function. *Ann Int Med* 109:122–126, 1988.
13. Doppler CJ: Ueber das farbige Licht der Doppelsterne und einiger anderer Gestirne des Himmels. *Abhandlungen der Koniglishen Bohmischen Gesellschaft der Wissenschaften.* II:465, 1842.
14. Satomura S: A study on examining the heart with ultrasonics. I. Principles; II. Strumentation. *Jap Circ J* 20:227, 1956.
15. Yoshida T, Mori M, Nimura Y, Hikita G, Takagisha S, Nakanischi K, Satomura S: Analysis of heart motion with ultrasonic Doppler method and its clinical application. *Am Heart J* 61: 61, 1961.
16. Spencer MP, Reid JM: Physics for ultrasonic diagnosis. In Spencer MP (ed): *Cardiac Doppler Diagnosis.* The Netherlands, Martinus Nijhoff Publishers, 2:15–38, 1986, vol 2.
17. Klepper JR: The physics of Doppler ultrasound and its measurement instrumentation. In Spencer MP (ed): *Cardiac Doppler Diagnosis.* The Netherlands, Martinus Nijhoff Publishers, 1984, vol I, 3:19–31.
18. Baker DW, Rubenstein SA, Lorch GS: Pulsed Doppler echocardiography: Principles and applications. *Am J Med* 63:69–80, 1977.
19. Durell M. Doppler instrumentation. In Nanda NC (ed): *Doppler Echocardiography.* New York, Igaku-Shoin, 1985, pp 51–74.
20. Bommer WJ, Miller LR, Mason DT, De Maria AN: Enhancement of pulse Doppler echocardiography in the evaluation of aortic valve disease by development of computerized spectral frequency analysis. *Circulation* 58 (Suppl II):II–187, 1978.
21. Stamm RB, Martin RP: Quantification of pressure gradients across stenotic valves by Doppler ultrasound. *J Am Coll Cardiol* 2:707–718, 1983.
22. Bom K, deBoo J, Rijsterborgh H: On the aliasing problem in pulsed Doppler cardiac studies. *J Clin Ultrasound* 12:559–567, 1984.
23. Stewart WJ, Galvin KA, Gilliam LD, Guyer DE, Weyman AE. Comparison of high pulse repetition frequency and continuous wave Doppler echocardiography in the assessment of high flow velocity in patients with valvular stenosis and regurgitation. *J Am Coll Cardiol* 6:565–571, 1985.
24. Hegrenaes L, Hatle L: Aortic stenosis in adults. Non-invasive estimation of pressure differences by continuous wave Doppler echocardiography. *Br Heart J* 54:396–404, 1985.
25. Currie PJ, Seward JB, Reeder GS, Vliestra RE, Bresnahan DR, Bresnahan JF, Smith HC, Hagler DJ, Tajik AJ: Continuous-wave Doppler echocardiographic assessment of severity of calcific aortic stenosis: A simultaneous Doppler-catheter correlative study in 100 adult patients. *Circulation* 71:1162–1169, 1985.
26. Omoto R: *Color Atlas of Real-Time Two-Dimensional Doppler Echocardiography.* Tokyo, Shindan-To-Chiryo, 1984.
27. Sahn DJ: Real-time two-dimensional Doppler echocardiographic flow mapping. *Circulation* 71:849–853, 1985.

28. Loeber CP, Goldberg SJ, Allen HD: Doppler echocardiographic comparison of flows distal to the four cardiac valves. *J Am Coll Cardiol* 4:268–272, 1984.
29. Kosturakis D, Allen HD, Goldberg SJ, Sahn DJ, Valdes-Cruz LM: Noninvasive quantification of stenotic semilunar valve areas by Doppler echocardiography. *J Am Coll Cardiol* 3:1256–1262, 1984.
30. Yeager M, Yock PG, Popp RL: Comparison of Doppler-derived pressure gradient to that determined at cardiac catheterization in adults with aortic valve stenosis: Implications for management. *Am J Cardiol* 57:644–648, 1986.
31. Po-Hoey F, Kapur KK, Nanda NC: Color-guided Doppler echocardiographic assessment of aortic valve stenosis. *J Am Coll Cardiol* 12:441–449, 1988.
32. Panidis IP, Mintz GS, Ross J: Value and limitations of Doppler ultrasound in evaluation of aortic stenosis: A statistical analysis of 70 consecutive patients. *Am Heart J* 12:150–158, 1986.
33. Zoghbi WA, Farmer KL, Soto JG, Nelson JG, Quinones MA: Accurate noninvasive quantification of stenotic aortic valve area by Doppler echocardiography. *Circulation* 73:452–459, 1986.
34. Richards KL, Cannon SR, Miller JF, Crawford MH: Calculation of aortic valve area by Doppler echocardiography: A direct application of the continuity equation. *Circulation* 73:964–969, 1986.
35. Hatle L: Noninvasive assessment and differentiation of left ventricular outflow obstruction with Doppler ultrasound. *Circulation* 64:381–387, 1981.
36. Warth DC, Stewart WJ, Block PC, Weyman AE: A new method to calculate aortic valve area without left heart catheterization. *Circulation* 70:978–983, 1984.
37. Teirstein P, Yeager M, Yock P, Popp RL: Doppler echocardiographic measurement of aortic valve area in aortic stenosis: A noninvasive application of the Gorlin formula. *J Am Coll Cardiol* 8:1059–1065, 1986.
38. Grayburn PA, Smith MD, Handshoe R, Friedman BJ, DeMaria AN: Detection of aortic insufficiency by standard echocardiography, pulse Doppler echocardiography, and auscultation. *Ann Int Med* 104:599–605, 1986.
39. Perry GJ, Helmcke F, Nanda NC, Byard C, Soto B: Evaluation of aortic insufficiency by Doppler color flow mapping. *J Am Coll Cardiol* 9:952–959, 1987.
40. Labovitz AJ, Ferrara RP, Kern MJ, Bryg RJ, Mrosek DG, Williams GA. Quantitative evaluation of aortic insufficiency by continuous wave Doppler echocardiography. *JACC* 8:1341–1347, 1986.
41. Nishimura RA, Tajik AJ: Determination of left-sided pressure gradients by utilizing Doppler aortic and mitral regurgitant signals: Validation by simultaneous dual catheter and Doppler studies. *J Am Coll Cardiol* 11:317–321, 1988.
42. Masuyama T, Kodama K, Kitabatake A, Nanto S, Sato H, Uematsu M, Inoue M, Kamada T: Noninvasive evaluation of aortic regurgitation by continuous wave Doppler echocardiography. *Circulation* 73:460–466, 1986.
43. Kitabatake A, Ito H, Inoue M, Tanouchi J, Ishihara K, Morita T, Fujii K, Yoshida Y, Masuyama T, Yoshima H, Hori M, Kamada T: A new approach to noninvasive evaluation of aortic regurgitant fraction by two-dimensional Doppler echocardiography. *Circulation* 72:523–529, 1985.
44. Hatle L, Angelsen B, Tromsdal A: Noninvasive assessment of atrioventricular pressure half-time by Doppler ultrasound. *Circulation* 60:1097–1104, 1979.
45. Nakatani S, Masuyama T, Kodama K, Kitabatake A, Fujii K, Kamada T: Value and limitations of Doppler echocardiography in the quantification of stenotic mitral valve area: comparison of the pressure half-time and the continuity equation methods: *Circulation* 77:78–85, 1988.
46. Ascah KJ, Stewart WJ, Jiang L, Guerrero JL, Newell JB, Gillam LD, Weyman AE: A Doppler two-dimensional echocardiographic method for quantitation of mitral regurgitation. *Circulation* 72:377–383, 1985.
47. Miyatake K, Izumi S, Okamoto M, Kinoshita N, Asonuma H, Nakagawa H, Yamamoto K, Takamiya M, Sakakibara H, Nimura Y: Semiquantitative grading of severity of mitral regurgitation by real-time two-dimensional Doppler flow imaging technique. *J Am Coll Cardiol* 7:82–88, 1986.
48. Seward JB, Khandheria BK, Oh JK, Abel MD, Hughes RW, Edwards WD, Nichols BA, Freeman WK, Tajik AJ: Transesophageal echocardiography: Technique, anatomic correlations, implementation, and clinical applications. *Mayo Clin Proc* 63:649–680, 1988.
49. Guyer DE, Gillam LD, Foale RA, Clark MC, Dinsmore R, Palacios I, Block P, King ME, Weyman AE: Comparison of the echocardiographic and hemodynamic diagnosis of rheumatic tricuspid stenosis. *J Am Coll Cardiol* 3:1135–1144, 1984.
50. Veyrat C, Kalmanson D, Farjon M, Manin JP, Abitol G: Noninvasive diagnosis and assessment of tricuspid regurgitation and stenosis using one and two dimensional echo-pulsed Doppler. *Br Heart J* 47:596–605, 1982.
51. Perez JE, Ludbrook PA, Ahumada GG: Usefulness of Doppler echocardiography in detecting tricuspid stenosis. *Am J Cardiol* 55:601–603, 1985.
52. Miyatake K, Okamoto M, Kinoshita N, Ohta M, Kozuka T, Sakakibara H, Nimura Y: Evaluation of tricuspid regurgitation by pulsed Doppler and two-dimensional echocardiography. *Circulation* 66:777–784, 1982.
53. Missri J, Agnarsson U, Sverrisson J: The clinical spectrum of tricuspid regurgitation detected by pulsed Doppler echocardiography. *Angiology* 36:746–753, 1985.
54. Benchimol A, Harris CL, Desser KB: Noninvasive diagnosis of tricuspid insufficiency utilizing the external Doppler flowmeter probe. *Am J Cardiol* 32:868–873, 1973.
55. Benchimol A, Desser KB, Gartlan J: Bidirectional blood flow velocity in the cardiac chambers and great vessels studied with the Doppler ultrasonic flowmeter. *Am J Med* 52:467–473, 1972.
56. Scheck-Krejca H, Zulstra F, Roelandt J, Vletter-McGhie J: Diagnosis of tricuspid regurgitation: Comparison of jugular venous and liver pulse tracings with combined two-dimensional and Doppler echocardiography. *Eur Heart J* 7:973–978, 1986.
57. Suzuki Y, Kambara H, Kadota K, Tamaki S, Ya-

mazato A, Nohara R, Osakada G, Kawai C, Kubo S, Karaguchi T: Detection and evaluation of tricuspid regurgitation using a real-time, two-dimensional, color-coded, Doppler flow imaging system: Comparison with contrast two-dimensional echocardiography and right ventriculography. *Am J Cardiol* 57:811–815, 1986.

58. Yock PG, Popp RL: Non-invasive estimation of right ventricular systolic pressure by Doppler ultrasound in patients with tricuspid regurgitation. *Circulation* 70:657–662, 1984.

59. Berger M, Haimowitz A, Van Tosh A, Berdoff RL, Goldberg E: Quantitative assessment of pulmonary hypertension in patients with tricuspid regurgitation using continuous wave Doppler ultrasound. *J Am Coll Cardiol* 6:359–365, 1985.

60. Hatle L, Angelsen BAJ, Tromsdal A: Non-invasive estimation of pulmonary artery systolic pressure with Doppler ultrasound. *Br Heart J* 45:157–165, 1981.

61. Snider AR, Stevenson JG, French GW, Rocchini AP, Dick M, Rosenthal A, Crowley DC, Beekman RH, Peters J: Comparison of high pulse repetition frequency and continuous-wave Doppler for velocity measurement and gradient prediction in children with valvular and congenital heart disease. *J Am Coll Cardiol* 7:873–879, 1986.

62. Lima CO, Sahn DJ, Valdes-Cruz LM, Goldberg SJ, Barron JV, Allen HD, Grenadier E: Noninvasive of transvalvular pressure gradient in patients with pulmonary stenosis by quantitative two-dimensional echocardiographic studies. *Circulation* 67:866–871, 1983.

63. Patel AK, Rowe GG, Dhanani SP, Kosolcharsen P, Lyle LEW, Thomsen JH: Pulsed Doppler echocardiography in diagnosis of pulmonary regurgitation: Its value and limitations. *Am J Cardiol* 49:1801–1805, 1982.

64. Miyatake K, Okamoto M, Kinoshita N, Matsuhisa M, Nagata S, Beppu S, Park YD, Sakikabara H, Nimura Y: Pulmonary regurgitation studied with the ultrasonic pulsed Doppler technique. *Circulation* 65:969–976, 1982.

65. Goldberg SJ, Allen HD: Quantitative assessment by Doppler echocardiography of pulmonary or aortic regurgitation. *Am J Cardiol* 56:131–135, 1985.

7

Real-Time Color Flow Imaging

Ryozo Omoto, M.D.

PART 1.
Color Doppler Images in a Normal Heart

This section deals with examining blood flow patterns in the left side of the heart in normal adult subjects through color Doppler flow mapping studies (color flow studies). Limitations of space preclude discussing patterns of blood flow on the right side of the heart, although they have as great an importance as those on the left. Other sources should be consulted for normal blood flow patterns in children (1) and infants.

When imaging blood flow patterns in the left side of the heart, the transducer is most commonly positioned to provide either a parasternal or apical view. The findings obtainable with these and other approaches are discussed below.

PARASTERNAL APPROACH

The left ventricular outflow tract is occupied by outflow blood in both diastole and systole. In the parasternal view in flow mapping M-mode, the blood entering the left ventricle during diastole (inflow blood) and the blood leaving the left ventricle during systole (outflow blood) are clearly separated by the anterior mitral leaflet into a lower and upper stream. These are further differentiated by being displayed in red and blue, respectively (Fig. 7.1). Frequency analysis of blood flow in the left ventricular outflow and inflow tracts indicates that the directions of pulsed wave Doppler signals are completely in accord with the blood flow color coding. In other words, when the pulsed wave Doppler sample volume is in the

inflow tract, the waveform points upward ("toward"), consistent with a red color in the color Doppler display. When it is in the outflow tract, the waves are directed downward, consistent with a blue color in the display (Fig. 7.1F and G.

Ejection blood flow from the aortic root appears blue during systole. In flow mapping M-mode, the orifice of the aortic valve exhibits a box-like image representing ejection flow.

APICAL APPROACH

In the apical long-axis view, color Doppler findings of left ventricular inflow and outflow are consistent with findings from the parasternal view (Fig. 7.2). However, there are considerable differences between the two views in the direction of the blood flow and the beam direction. Specifically, in the apical long-axis view the beam direction is more closely parallel to the direction of blood flow (so that θ is approximately equal to 0), and the frequency of the Doppler signals (f_d) is high (cosine of θ is approximately equal to 1).

$$f_d = 2f_0 \times \frac{v (\cos \theta)}{c} \tag{7.1}$$

where f_d = frequency of Doppler signals, f_0 = frequency of ultrasound, v = velocity of blood flow, c = velocity of sound, and θ = angle between blood flow and beam direction.

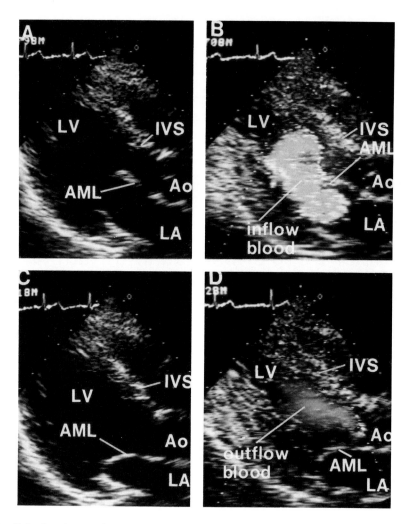

Figure 7.1. Color flow images in a normal heart—parasternal approach in a 25-year-old male. *A*, B-mode in the long-axis view during diastole. *B*, Color flow image in the same view during diastole. *C*, B-mode, same view, systole. *D*, Color flow image, same view, systole. *E*, Flow mapping M-mode at the level of the mitral valve. *F*, Simultaneous display of flow mapping M-mode and pulsed wave Doppler (*PWD*). Sample volume (s) is located in the left ventricular outflow tract (*LVOT*). *G*, Same as *F*. Sample volume is located in the left ventricular inflow tract. *H*, B-mode in the long-axis view during systole. The aortic valve (*AoV*) is clearly imaged. *I*, Flow mapping M-mode at the level of the aortic valve. The orifice of the aortic valve exhibits a box-like image representing ejection flow. *J*, Simultaneous display of flow mapping M-mode and pulsed wave Doppler. Sample volume is located in the aortic orifice. *AML* = anterior mitral leaflet. *LA* = left atrium, *LV* = left ventricle, *IVS* = interventricular septum, *AO* = aorta. See this figure in Color Atlas.

Thus, the apical approach is a better choice for measuring maximum velocities of left ventricular inflow and outflow. This is because correction of the angle θ is unnecessary or less necessary. Use of continuous wave Doppler technique, which is free of aliasing, is preferable when maximum velocities are being determined. Analysis of the flow pattern of diastolic inflow to the left ventricle is important for assessment of left ventricular func-

tion, particularly its characteristics during diastole. The amplitudes of the E and A waves of the left ventricular inflow pattern, which, respectively, correspond to rapid filling and and atrial contraction, as well as the A/E ratio, are of special interest.

The most important fact shown by the apical four-chamber view is that the side of the ventricular septum within the left ventricle corresponds

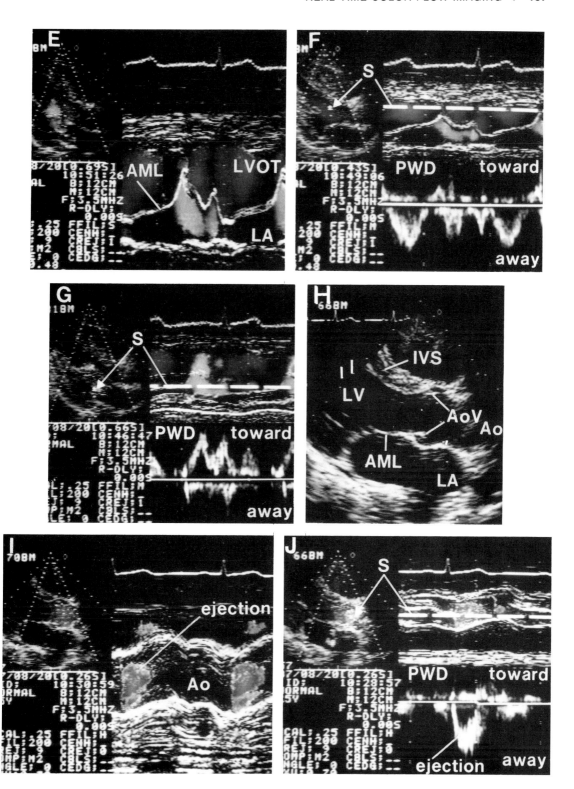

Figure 7.1. (*continued*).

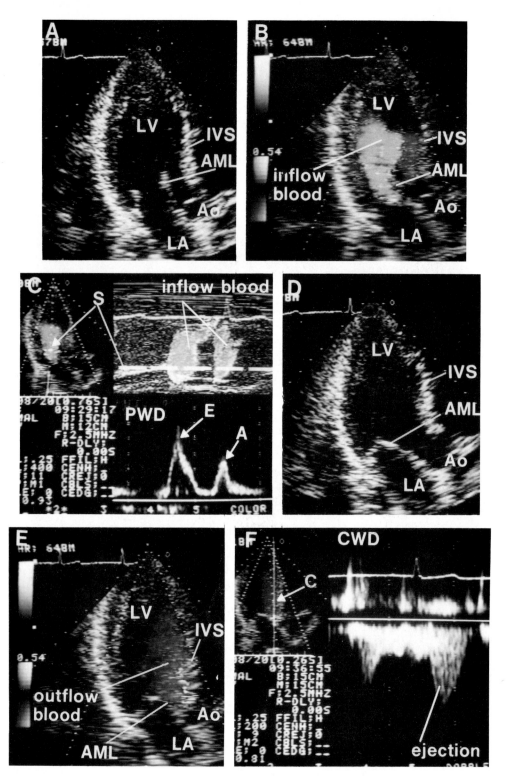

Figure 7.2. Color flow images in a normal heart—apical approach, long-axis view, in a 29-year-old male. *A*, B-mode in the apical long-axis view during diastole. *B*, Color flow image, same view, diastole. *C*, Simultaneous display of flow mapping M-mode and pulsed wave Doppler (*PWD*). Sample volume (*s*) is located in the left ventricular inflow tract (*LVOT*). *D*, B-mode in the apical long-axis view during systole. *E*, E wave = 75 cm/sec, A wave = 62.5 cm/sec. In this measure, "baseline shift" of the system is working. *F*, Continuous wave Doppler (*CWD*). Maximum velocity of ejection = 75 cm/sec. In this case the cursor line (*c*) may not be set optimally. Normally, in a young adult, mitral diastolic velocity spectra consist of E and A waves, with the E wave predominant. *E wave* = early diastolic velocity, *A wave* = late velocity following atrial contraction, *MV* = mitral valve. See this figure in Color Atlas.

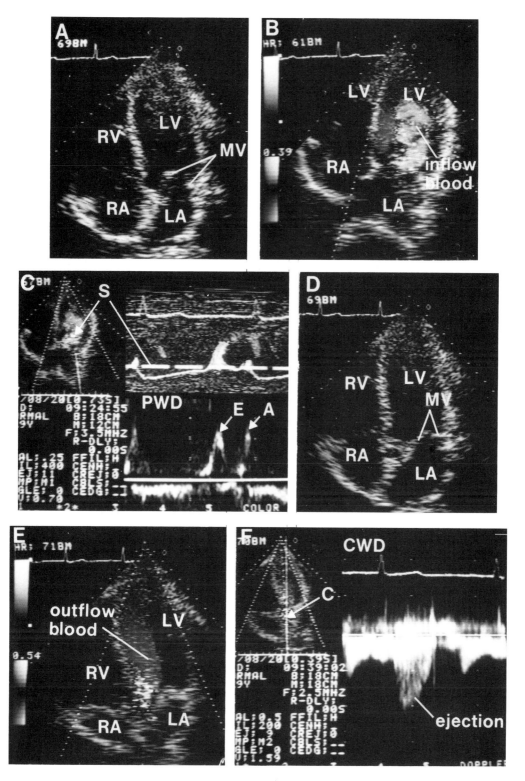

Figure 7.3. Color images in a normal heart—apical approach, four-chamber view, in a 29-year-old male. *A*, B-mode in the apical four-chamber view during diastole. *B*, Color flow image, same view, diastole. *C*, Simultaneous display of flow mapping M-mode and pulsed wave Doppler (*PWD*). Sample volume is located in the left ventricular inflow tract. E = 58 cm/sec, A = 58 cm/sec. *D*, B-mode in the apical four-chamber view during systole. *E*, Color flow image, same view, systole. *F*, Continuous wave Doppler (*CWD*) recording. Maximum velocity of ejection = 105 cm/sec, *MV* = mitral valve. See this figure in Color Atlas.

with the left ventricular outflow tract (Fig. 7.3). With only a minor adjustment in the position of the transducer used for this view, a five-chamber view can be obtained. The five-chamber view is employed with continuous wave Doppler to determine the maximum velocity of blood flow through the aortic valve.

Parasternal short-axis and suprasternal aortic arch views in normal subjects are discussed in detail elsewhere (1, 2).

REFERENCES

1. Omoto R: 2-D Doppler images in normal heart. In: Omoto R (ed): *Color Atlas of Real-Time Two-Dimensional Doppler Echocardiography*, 2nd ed. Tokyo, Shindan-To-Chiryosha (distributed by Lea & Febiger, Philadelphia), 1987, pp 65–68, 81–87.
2. Harrison MR, Smith MD, Grayburn PA, Kwan OL, DeMaria. AN: Normal blood flow patterns by color Doppler flow imaging. *Echocardiography* 4:485–493, 1987.

PART 2.
Pitfalls in Reading Color Flow Images

When interpreting color flow images, it is necessary to recognize from the outset that there are a number of limitations to the technique. Some of these limitations are not confined to color Doppler flow mapping but apply to all types of diagnostic ultrasound. However, color Doppler flow mapping differs from conventional echocardiography in two important ways which require special attention (1).

Primarily, color flow mapping involves superimposition of a colored display of intracardiac blood flow, obtained through Doppler technology, on an ordinary echocardiogram. Also, the levels of detected Doppler signals that carry intracardiac blood flow data are extremely low. The levels of these signals from the blood are less than one-hundredth of the usual echo signals reflected from the heart wall and valve structures. Therefore, in modern color flow mapping equipment, many measures have been taken to improve the signal-to-noise (S/N) ratio. To obtain one raster of the sector scan, anywhere from 8 to 16 ultrasound beams are superposed as a means of improving the S/N ratio. As a result, it is necessary to reduce the angle and depth of the blood flow image field of view and use a slower frame rate.

Pitfalls arise when special attention is not paid to these points during interpretation of color flow mapping images. The following pitfalls are often encountered in clinical practice (2).

The optimum transducer position and cross-sectional plane for obtaining clear, good quality, two-dimensional echocardiograms do not necessarily correspond with the transducer position and cross-sectional plane required for producing the clearest color flow images.

Even when there are no blood flow signals from within the heart, it does not indicate the absence of any blood flow. In principle, color flow mapping is a form of velocity mapping. Consequently, no blood flow images can be obtained when the velocity of the flow is below a certain level. The theoretical values of the Doppler signals from the blood flow within the heart f_d are calculated from the following formula:

$$f_d = 2f_0 \frac{v \times \cos \theta}{c} \qquad (7.2)$$

where v = velocity of blood flow, f_0 = frequency of ultrasound, and c = velocity of ultrasound.

When f_d is large, it is easy to obtain a good image of blood flow by color flow mapping. According to the equation, when the blood velocity is high, θ is small, and f_0 is large, a large value for f_d can be obtained. One point that must be strongly emphasized is that, with x-ray angiography, images obtained depend on the density of contrast medium in the heart, whereas images obtained by color flow mapping depend on velocity of blood.

Another point is that frequently a variety of abnormalities can be recorded on the photograph of a single frozen image. However, in order to make the correct diagnosis, the optimum fields of view must be selected one by one to produce

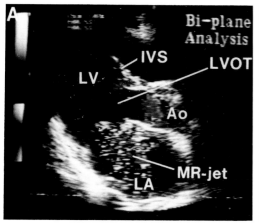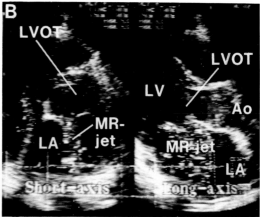

Figure 7.4. Conceptual reconstruction of three-dimensional intracardiac blood flow dynamics. Biplane analysis of color flow images in a 60-year-old male patient with mitral regurgitation (Sellers' grade 3). *A,* Color flow image in the long-axis view during systole. A regurgitant jet flow in mosaic patterns (*MR-jet*) is demonstrated in the left atrium during systole. *B,* Simultaneous display of biplane color flow images in short-axis and long-axis views at the same point in systole. *Left:* Mitral regurgitant image in short-axis view. *Right:* Mitral regurgitant image in long-axis view, same image as *A.* A three-dimensional concept of the mitral regurgitation may be obtained from "biplane analysis." See this figure in Color Atlas.

the best image of each individual lesion. For example, in a case where both mitral stenosis and mitral regurgitation are present, different views should be used to obtain the most accurate image of each lesion. In such circumstances, minimal alterations of the transducer position and Doppler beam direction need to be made in seeking the optimal flood flow image.

A three-dimensional reconstruction of intracardiac blood flow dynamics should be made using images from a wide variety of cross-sectional planes. Also, the echocardiographer must not make inferences about three-dimensional blood flow dynamics from a single two-dimensional blood flow image. Figure 7.4B presents biplane images, recorded during systole, of mitral regurgitation. The image on the left is a short-axis view, and that on the right is a long-axis view. In the former, the regurgitant flow (MR-jet) presents a mosaic pattern and a narrow, rod-like form. However, the long-axis view shows a large, circular image of the same jet. It may be deduced from this evidence that the MR-jet has a disk-like shape.

Intracardiac blood flow images vary with the change in hemodynamics. For example, where regurgitation is present, an elevation of blood pressure increases the size of the regurgitant jet. Therefore, when mitral regurgitation is being assessed by means of color flow mapping, it is essential to take the blood pressure into account.

The same phenomenon no doubt also occurs during x-ray cineangiography. However, unlike color flow mapping, angiography cannot be repeated several times, hence this phenomenon can only be imagined as a result of changes in heart murmurs. Color flow mapping has made it possible to observe that mitral regurgitation is aggravated by the blood pressure increase caused merely by hand-grip exercise (Fig. 7.5).

Color flow images of blood flow vary greatly according to the frame rate, pulse repetition frequency (PRF) and the ultrasound frequency f_0. The maximum detectable velocity without aliasing is determined by f_0 and PRF (Table 7.1). The PRF, in turn, influences the diagnostic depth and the frame rate. For instance, with the Aloka-870 system at frame rates of 15 frames/sec, 20 frames/sec, and 30 frames/sec, the PRFs are 4 kHz, 6 kHz, and 8 kHz, respectively. The maximum detectable velocities are 32 cm/sec, 48 cm/sec, and 64 cm/sec, respectively (Table 7.2). The frame rate, PRF, depth, and maximum detectable velocity without aliasing are usually not independent variables. Without a high PRF, a high maximum detectable velocity cannot be achieved. Without a good system S/N ratio, a high frame rate cannot be realized. In general, a low frame rate causes a decrease in time resolution of real-time two-dimensional images and may produce a distorted color flow image with many artifacts.

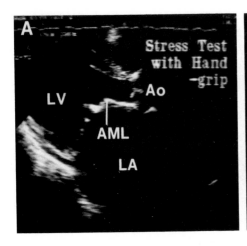
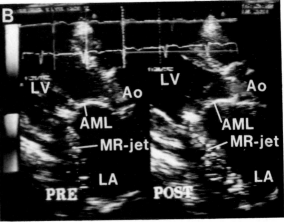

Figure 7.5. Relationship between the size of a mitral regurgitant jet and change in afterload—the effect of hand-grip on mitral regurgitant jet patterns in a 60-year-old male with mitral regurgitation (Sellers' grade 3). *A,* B-mode in long-axis view during diastole. *B,* Color flow images, in the same view, at the same point in systole. *Left:* Before exercise (*PRE*): heart rate = 77/min, blood pressure = 128/82 mm Hg. *Right:* After 3 min exercise (*POST*): heart rate = 88/min, blood pressure = 160/92 mm Hg. The increase in blood pressure after 3 min of hand-grip caused a remarkable increase in size of the regurgitant jet pattern (*MR-jet*). *AML* = anterior mitral leaflet. See this figure in Color Atlas.

When the heart rate is fast, the frame rate and the PRF have major effects on the blood flow images.

Figure 7.6 shows color Doppler images from a 6-day-old infant with a VSD and a heart rate of 153/min. The left ventricular inflow and outflow

Table 7.1. Detectable Maximum Velocity without Aliasing (m/sec)[a]

Frequency of transducer	PRF 4 kHz	6 kHz	8 kHz	12 kHz
2.5 MHz	0.64	0.93	1.23	1.91
3.5 MHz	0.48	0.70	0.93	1.43
5.0 MHz	0.32	0.47	0.62	0.96

[a]$\cos \theta = 1$; PRF, pulse repetition frequency; θ, angle of incidence.

Table 7.2. An Example of Relation between Frame Rate and Detectable Maximum Velocity without Aliasing and Pulse Repetition Frequency (PRF)[a]

	Frame Rate 15 f/sec	20 f/sec	30 f/sec
Detectable maximum velocity	32 cm/sec	48 cm/sec	64 cm/sec
PRF	4 kHz	6 kHz	8 kHz

[a]Frequency of ultrasound, 5 MHz; depth, 6 cm; system, SSD–870.

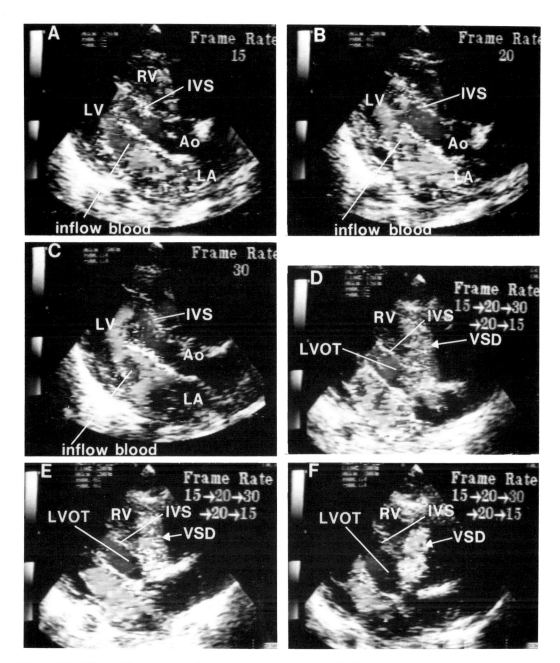

Figure 7.6. Effect of frame rate and pulse repetition frequency (PRF) on color flow images demonstrated in a 6-day-old female with a ventricular septal defect (VSD). Frequency of ultrasound = 5 MHz, depth = 6 cm, HR = 153/min. *A,* Color flow images of the left ventricular inflow and outflow tracts in diastole, long-axis view. Frame rate = 15/sec, PRF = 4 kHz, maximum velocity = 32 cm/sec. *B,* Same images as in *A.* Frame rate = 20/sec, PRF = 6 kHz, maximum velocity = 48 cm/sec. *C,* Same images with a frame rate = 30/sec, PRF = 8 kHz, maximum velocity = 64 cm/sec. *D,* Color flow images of shunt flow of a VSD in the long-axis view. Frame rate = 15/sec, PRF = 4 kHz, maximum velocity = 32 cm/sec. *E,* Same images with a frame rate = 20/sec, PRF = 6 kHz, maximum velocity = 48 cm/sec. *F,* Same images with a frame rate = 30/sec, PRF = 8 kHz, maximum velocity = 64 cm/sec. The increase in both frame rate and PRF resulted in clear color flow images by decreasing artifacts and aliasing. With a lower PRF, the inflow blood and outflow blood, which seems to be almost laminar flow, is imaged in mosaic patterns by "aliasing." See this figure in Color Atlas.

blood can also be seen. At frame rates of 15 frames/sec, with PRF of 4 kHz, and 20 frames/sec, with PRF of 6 kHz, both of these color flow images are displayed in a mosaic pattern, owing to the occurrence of aliasing phenomenon. Using a frame rate of 30 frames/sec with a PRF of 8 kHz, the aliasing has disappeared almost completely, and the left intraventricular blood flow patterns are easier to comprehend with fewer artifacts. It should be noted carefully that a mosaic pattern sometimes is displayed even in laminar flow when the maximum detectable velocity is low. Figure 7.6 D–F shows the shunt flow due to the VSD in the same case. This shunt flow is displayed at its clearest with the frame rate at 30 frames/sec and a PRF of 8 kHz. The frame rate and the PRF are the most important parameters, but it can hardly be emphasized too strongly that their importance is particularly high when the heart rate is fast.

Present-day color Doppler systems are manufactured by almost all companies that produce echocardiographic equipment. However, since changes in equipment appear extremely frequently, a caution should be observed in interpreting the output of these devices. When a specific case is being discussed with reference to a frozen image, at the very least the patient's heart rate and blood pressure, must be known. Also, the f_0, PRF, frame rate, depth, and other particulars related to the equipment in use should be specified to all concerned.

REFERENCES

1. Omoto R, Kasai C: Physics and instrumentation of Doppler color flow mapping. *Echocardiography* 4:467–483, 1987.
2. Takamoto S: Pitfalls and artifacts. In Omoto R (ed): *Color Atlas of Real-Time Two-Dimensional Doppler Echocardiography*, 2nd ed. Tokyo, Shindan-To-Chiryo (distributed by Lea & Febiger), 1987, pp 41–48, 60–64.

PART 3.
Color Flow and Acquired Valvular Heart Disease

Equipment designed for color flow mapping allows selection of different modes, according to need: conventional M-mode, two-dimensional echocardiography, pulsed wave Doppler (PWD), continuous wave Doppler (CWD), and real-time blood flow imaging (Table 7.3). With the employment of color flow mapping in the diagnosis of acquired valvular disease, the imaging of anatomical changes, the measurement of the pressure gradient across a stenotic valve, the semiquantitative assessment of valvular regurgitation can now be carried out more accurately. In assessing valvular stenosis, the actual blood flow through the stenotic valve is imaged and the pressure gradient is calculated by using Bernoulli's equation (1–4). Additionally, in mitral stenosis, the valve area is obtained from the pressure half-time (5).

A semiquantitative assessment of regurgitation is made on the basis of the distance covered by the regurgitant jet, as displayed by color flow mapping, and the area of the jet. A fairly good correlation is found so far between these data and angiographic grading by Sellers' technique or surgical findings. In cases in which tricuspid regurgitation is present, the right ventricular systolic pressure can be estimated through the combined use of color flow imaging and continuous wave Doppler (6, 7). If coronary heart disease has been ruled out, it is felt that color flow imaging, without cardiac catheterization or x-ray angiography, provides a possible approach to the definitive preoperative diagnosis of acquired valvular disease.

ASSESSMENT OF VALVULAR STENOSIS WITH COLOR FLOW MAPPING

The morphologic changes associated with valvular stenosis have been diagnosed with considerable degree of detail using the conventional B-mode technique. The diagnosis of mitral stenosis and aortic stenosis is possible to a certain extent by recognizing morphologic changes. For example, diagnosis can be made possible through the degree of calcification, the size of the valvular

Table 7.3. Color Doppler Flow Mapping System: Available Modes and Applications

Modes	Examples of Applications
M-mode	Measurement of dimensions
B-mode	Segmental wall motion analysis
Color flow imaging	Real-time imaging of regurgitant or shunt flows
Pulsed wave Doppler	Spectral analysis of aortic, mitral or tricuspid flows
Continuous wave Doppler	Measurement of velocity and estimation of pressure gradients across stenotic valves

orifice, the wall thickness of the left ventricle, and other dimensions of the heart. The drawback of conventional echocardiography for assessing valvular stenosis has been that the pressure gradient across the stenotic valve is not known. By the combined use of continuous wave Doppler and Doppler color flow imaging, it has been possible to bridge this gap.

In the modified Bernoulli's equation,

$$\Delta P = 4V^2$$
$$\Delta P = \text{Pressure gradient}$$
$$\text{(millimeters of mercury)} \quad (7.3)$$
$$= \text{maximum velocity}$$
$$\text{(meters per second)},$$

It should be noted that ΔP, obtained from the formula $\Delta P = 4V^2$, is the maximum pressure gradient. Of course, the peak-to-peak pressure gradient and the maximum pressure gradient are not identical. In many cases the value of the latter is greater than that of the former. However, the peak-to-peak pressure gradient across the stenotic valve, obtained by catheterization of the heart, has been found to correlate well with the maximum pressure gradient determined by continuous wave Doppler [8].

The most common Doppler color flow findings related to stenotic lesions are seen in mitral stenosis. With either the parasternal or the apical approach, a jet-like inflow of blood into the left ventricle can be seen coming from the orifice of the stenotic valve, closely resembling the flaring up of a flame (Fig. 7.7). The incidence of tricuspid stenosis is low, but this condition is also accompanied by a clearly visible jet of blood through the stenotic valve. In aortic stenosis, the positioning of the transducer is critical.

In color flow imaging of stenotic blood flows, it is important to select the most appropriate location and orientation of the transducer (Fig. 7.8). In the authors' experience, the right parasternal approach at the second intercostal space is the most commonly used [9]. This is followed by the apical and suprasternal approaches, in that order. These three approaches should all be tried in order to select the most appropriate and sensitive one for the case in hand. In many severe cases of aortic stenosis, conglomerations of calcified deposits are found around the valve structure. Since these deposits cause deterioration of the S/N ratio of Doppler signals received from the blood flow at the orifice of the valve, it is often difficult to obtain good images of the aortic stenosis blood flow using the parasternal approach. To determine the maximum velocity of the blood flow through the valvular stenosis by continuous wave Doppler, it is extremely useful to use color flow imaging also [10]. With this combination of techniques, the continuous wave Doppler cursor line easily can be set to the most appropriate stenotic blood flow obtained with color flow imaging. Rather than using continuous wave Doppler alone to obtain the maximum blood flow velocity by means of audio signals, it is combined with color flow imaging to yield the required results with far less difficulty [11].

ASSESSMENT OF VALVULAR REGURGITATION WITH COLOR FLOW MAPPING

Doppler findings in valvular regurgitation are generally common to all types, but have two distinct characteristics: Almost all blood flows that show regurgitation have both a disturbed flow pattern and a high flow velocity. To be specific, regurgitation is displayed with a mixture of red and bluish colors that resembles a mosaic pattern. These patterns may be analyzed by a combination of flow mapping M-mode and special analysis.

Many criteria have been proposed for the semiquantitative assessment of valvular regurgitation in a Doppler color flow image. From the outset of our present research, the authors employed the maximum distance covered by the mosaic pattern of the regurgitant jet, or jet length, for this

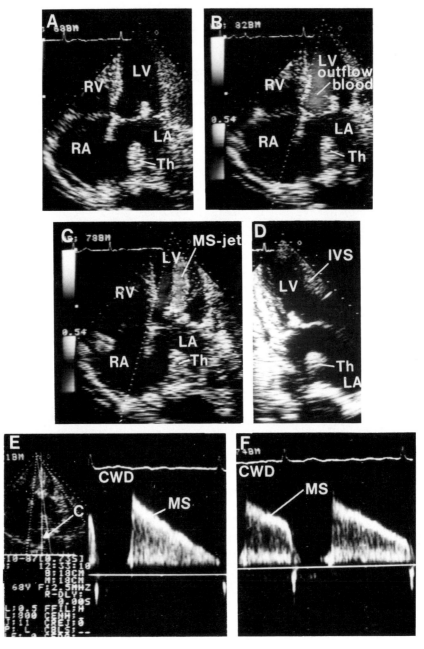

Figure 7.7. Color flow images in a 68-year-old male patient with mitral stenosis (*MS*) and left atrial thrombus. *A,* B-mode, apical four-chamber view, in systole. A thrombus (*Th*) is seen in the left atrium. *B,* Color flow image, same view, in systole. *C,* Color flow image, same view, in diastole. Flame-shaped jet of inflow blood with mosaic pattern passes through the stenotic mitral valve into the left ventricle (*MS-jet*). *D,* B-mode, apical long-axis view, in systole. *E–F,* Continuous wave Doppler (*CWD*) of mitral valve flow (*Beamline: c*). Evaluation of mitral stenosis: maximum velocity = 1.74 m/sec, mean velocity = 0.98 m/sec, maximum pressure gradient = 12.7 mm Hg, mean pressure gradient = 4.4 mm Hg, pressure half-time = 0.222 sec, mitral valve area = 0.99 cm.[2] See this figure in Color Atlas.

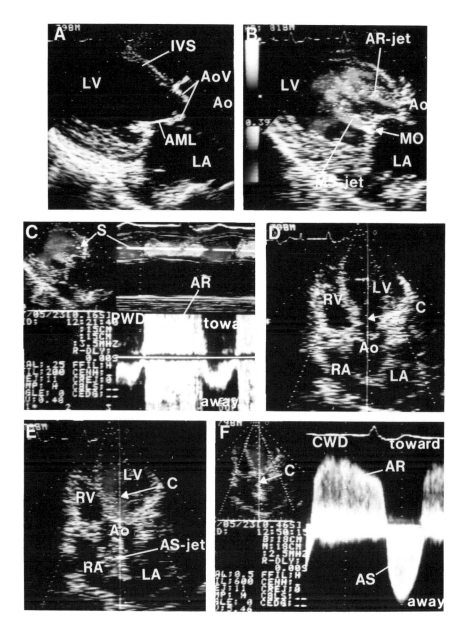

Figure 7.8. Color flow images in a 59-year-old female patient with aortic stenosis and regurgitation (Sellers' grade 2) associated with mitral stenosis and regurgitation (Sellers' grade 3) and tricuspid regurgitation. *A*, B-mode, long-axis view, in systole. *B*, Color flow image, same view, in diastole. A regurgitant jet from the aortic valve (*AR-jet*) as well as the mitral valve (*MR-jet*) is seen. *C*, Simultaneous display of flow mapping M-mode and pulsed wave Doppler (sample volume: *s*). The regurgitant jet is characterized as broadband and bidirectional signals in *PWD* recording. *D*, B-mode in the apical five-chamber view in diastole. *E*, Color flow image, same view, in systole. A cursor line of *CWD* (*c*) is set optimally along the "best jet" of aortic stenosis (*AS-jet*). *F*, Continuous wave Doppler of aortic valve flow. Both aortic regurgitant and aortic stenotic flows are recorded. Evaluation of aortic stenosis: maximum velocity = 4.3 m/sec, maximum pressure gradient = 74 mm Hg; *Ao* = aorta; *AoV* = aortic valve; *MO* = mitral valve orifice; *toward* = flow toward transducer; *away* = flow away from transducer; *AML* = anterior mitral leaflet. See this figure in Color Atlas.

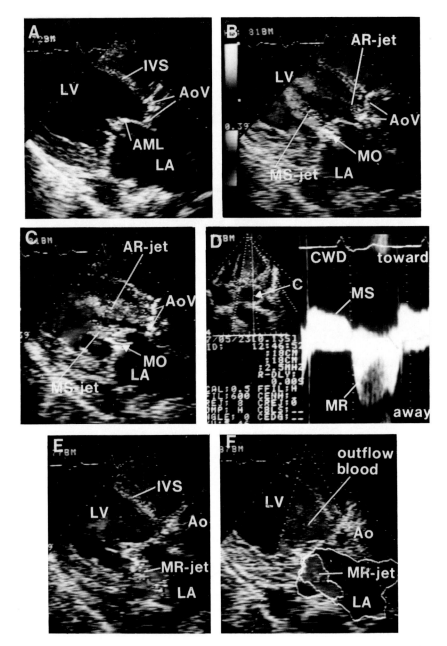

Figure 7.9. Color flow images in a 59-year-old female with aortic stenosis and regurgitation (Sellers' grade 2) associated with mitral stenosis and regurgitation (Sellers' grade 3) and tricuspid regurgitation. *A*, B-mode, long-axis view, in diastole. *B*, Color flow image, same view, in diastole. Both *AR-jet* (Sellers' grade 2) and *MS-jet* are demonstrated. In this cross-sectional plane, however, the image of *AR-jet* is not optimal. *C*, Color flow image in the almost same view with minimal alteration of the beam direction in diastole. In this plane, *AR-jet* is imaged optimally. *D*, Continuous wave Doppler of mitral valve flow from the apical four-chamber view. Doppler signals by mitral regurgitation and mitral stenosis are recorded. *E*, Color flow image, long-axis, in systole. *F*, The same image with planimeter tracing for measurement of area of mitral regurgitant jet (*MR-jet*) and area of the left atrium. The ratio of *MR-jet* area to the area of the left atrium has been shown to be highly correlated with the severity of mitral regurgitation (16). *G*, Color flow image, apical four-chamber view, in systole. Tricuspid regurgitation (grade 1) is imaged in systole. *H*, Color flow image in short-axis view in diastole at the level of the aortic root. Pulmonary regurgitation is demonstrated in the right ventricular outflow tract in diastole. *I*, Continuous wave Doppler of pulmonary valve flow (*beam-line; c*). *RVOT* = right ventricular outflow tract. See this figure in Color Atlas.

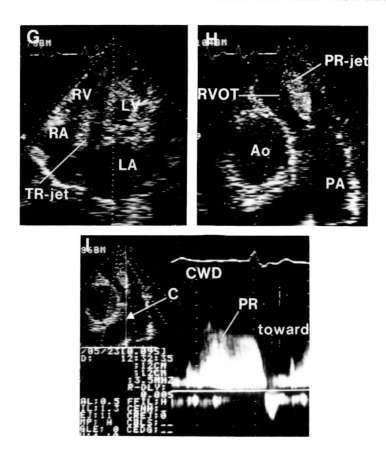

Figure 7.9 *(continued).*

purpose (12, 13) (Figs. 7.9 and 7.10). Assessment of valvular regurgitation by this method not only is the most simple technique, but also shows fairly good correspondence with angiographic and surgical findings. From a practical viewpoint, this makes the method all the more difficult to abandon at this stage. However, the inconvenient fact is that some jets may be narrow and long and others may be broad and short. Consequently, the degree of severity of the former type may be one grade lower, and the latter, one grade higher, than they appear using the maximum distance criterion. This question is at present under study.

It has been pointed out that there are various shortcomings to the assessment of regurgitation flow by this criterion. A number of reports have been published using 2 cm steps, 1.5 cm steps and others for the jet length criterion in mitral regurgitation (14). It has also been reported that in aortic regurgitation, the ratio between the area of the jet, obtained from the short-axis image immediately below the aortic valve, and the cross-sectional area of the valve ring of the aortic valve correlates well with the regurgitant ratio (15). The recent study of Helmcke et al. in mitral regurgitation appears to be the most convincing. Their report describes the use of a ratio between the regurgitant jet area (RJA) and the cross-sectional area of the left atrium (LAA). These were derived from long-axis, short-axis, and apical four-chamber views. Helmcke et al. stated that the maximum RJA/LAA yields the best correlation with angiographic assessment of mitral regurgitation (16) (Fig. 7.11). Further research is now necessary for the quantitative assessment of valvular regurgitation (17).

For tricuspid regurgitation, since angiography of the right ventricle is not carried out as a routine procedure at the authors' institution, three stages of criteria based on the intraoperative findings are used to arrive at a definitive diagnosis (Fig. 7.12). In the authors' experience, the use of color flow mapping in tricuspid regurgitation tends to lead to assessments that are one stage too severe.

(A) AR,MR

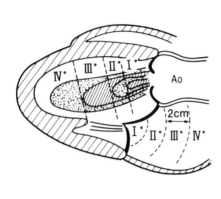

parasternal long-axis view

(B) TR

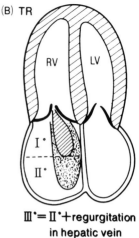

III˙= II˙+regurgitation
in hepatic vein

Apical four-chamber view

Figure 7.10. Diagrams demonstrating how Doppler color flow findings can be used to quantitate the severity of valvular regurgitation on a four-grade scale. Severity of valvular regurgitation by color Doppler flow mapping is determined mainly from the farthest distance reached by the regurgitant jets (13). In the case of aortic regurgitation, grade 1 (I˙), regurgitant flow reaches halfway to the tip of the mitral valve from the aortic ring in long-axis view; grade 2 (II˙), to the tip of the mitral valve; grade 3 (III˙), to the level of the papillary muscle; and grade 4 (IV˙) over the level of the papillary muscle. In the case of mitral regurgitation, in grade 1 (I˙) the regurgitant flow is within half the distance from the mitral orifice to the mitral ring in long-axis view; in grade 2 (II˙) the flow extends to the mitral ring; in grade 3 (III˙) it is within 2 cm of the level of the mitral ring; and in grade 4 (IV˙) flow is more than 2 cm from the level of the mitral ring. In grade 1 (I˙) tricuspid regurgitation the flow reaches within half of the long axis of the right atrium in apical four-chamber view; in grade 2 (II˙) the flow has passed the halfway point but without significant regurgitation in the hepatic vein; and in grade 3 (III˙) the regurgitant flow extends beyond the halfway point of the long axis of the right atrium, occasionally occupying the entire right atrium, with significant regurgitation in the hepatic vein. (Reprinted with permission from Shindan-To-Chiryo Co., Ltd., and from Omoto R (ed): *Color Atlas of Real-Time Two-Dimensional Doppler Echocardiography*, 2nd ed. Tokyo, Shindan-To-Chiryo (distributed by Lea & Febiger), 1987, p 69.

It is necessary to take into account the changes that take place between the time of the Doppler color flow examination and surgery, the efficacy of medical treatment before surgery, and the reduction of cardiac output that takes place during thoracotomy. This is to compensate for the tendency of color flow mapping to lead to oversensitive assessments in tricuspid regurgitation cases.

Quantitative assessments of regurgitation from the aortic valve and the mitral valve according to Sellers' classification do not entirely correspond with the color flow Doppler findings. However, a fully acceptable degree of correlation from the clinical point of view can be found between angiography and color flow imaging. It should be borne in mind that the angiographic assessment of regurgitation cannot necessarily be taken as a gold standard. A number of variables are in-

volved during an angiographic examination, as, for example, cardiac function, heart rate, catheter position, and timing of contrast medium injection. Also, disagreement sometimes occurs among the physicians interpreting the data.

PROSTHETIC VALVES

Color flow mapping is a particularly important procedure in the follow-up of patients after valve replacement surgery. Noninvasive examination is especially desirable for following up such patients. In particular, contrast angiography of the left ventricle is generally avoided in cases where the aortic valve has been replaced with a mechanical prosthetic valve because of the dangers of damaging the cusps of the mechanical valve or displacing it. Under such circumstances, color flow mapping is an extremely useful method for de-

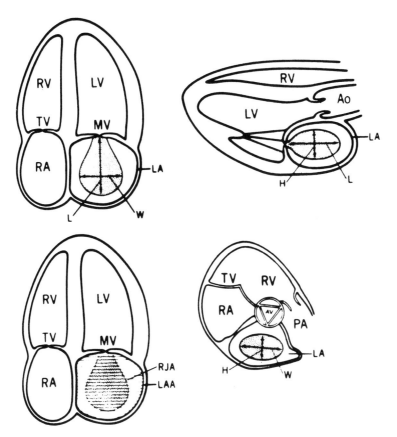

Figure 7.11. Diagrammatic representation of the variables assessed by color Doppler. *Top left*, apical four-chamber view; *top right*, parasternal long-axis view. *Bottom left*, apical four-chamber view (the technique for measurement of the RJA and the LAA is shown); *Bottom right*, parasternal short-axis view. *RV* = right ventricle, *TV* = tricuspid valve, *RA* = right atrium, *LV* = left ventricle, *MV* = mitral valve, *L* = maximal length of the regurgitant jet, *H* = maximum length of the regurgitant jet, *W* = maximum width of the regurgitant jet, *H* = maximum height of the regurgitant jet, *LA* = left atrium, *Ao* = aorta, *AV* = aortic valve. The *dotted area* represents the abnormal color Doppler signals produced by mitral regurgitation (Reprinted with permission from American Heart Association and from Helmcke F, Nanda N, Hsiung MC, Sato B, Adey CK, Goyal RG, Gatewood RP Jr: Color Doppler assessment of mitral regurgitation with orthogonal planes. *Circulation* 75:176, 1987).

tecting and assessing paravalvular leaks around prosthetic valves and functional failure in such prostheses, at the time of postoperative follow-up in valve replacement patients (18–20).

The authors have found that if a prosthetic valve used to replace the mitral valve is functioning normally, the maximum velocity through it is not more than 2 m/sec, be it a mechanical valve or a tissue valve. However, when a prosthetic valve fails mechanically, the maximum velocity through it is over 2 m/sec for both valve types (21) (Fig. 7.13 and Table 7.4). Whether the aortic or mitral valve is replaced with a prosthesis, care must be taken to select a view that will not be affected by artifacts caused by the mechanical prosthesis.

INFECTIVE ENDOCARDITIS AND VEGETATION

Conventional two-dimensional echocardiography generally occupies an unrivaled position in the diagnosis of infective endocarditis during the acute stage. Surgery can already be suggested by the discovery of vegetation in the echocardiographic findings alone and from indirect evidence of regurgitation. However, color flow mapping

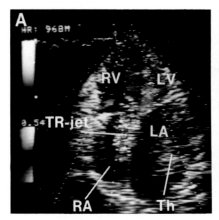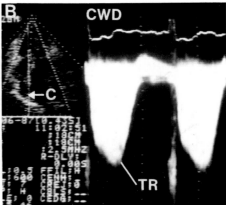

Figure 7.12. Color flow image in a 51-year-old female with mitral stenosis associated with tricuspid regurgitation (*TR*) and left atrial thrombus. *A*, Color flow image, apical four-chamber view, in systole. A large clot (*Th*) is demonstrated in the left atrium, and tricuspid regurgitation (*TR-jet*) is imaged in the right atrium in systole (grade 2). *B*, Continuous wave Doppler of tricuspid valve flow (*beam line; c*). Evaluation of right ventricular systolic pressure (RVP): maximum velocity of tricuspid regurgitation = 5.2 m/sec, maximum pressure gradient = 108 mm Hg, RVP = 108 + 10 = 118 mm Hg (assuming that right atrial pressure is 10 mm Hg). See this figure in Color Atlas.

represents an improvement on these methods. Color flow mapping allows direct visualization of valvular regurgitation and semiquantitative assessment of its degree (Fig. 7.14). Another major merit of this technique is that detection of subclinical lesions in other valves is also possible.

COLOR FLOW MAPPING AND INTRACARDIAC MASSES

Intracardiac masses—intracardiac thrombi and myxomas—are objects of clinical interest and importance. Since both types of masses have a close relationship to valvular diseases as far as diagnostic approach is concerned, they are included in this section on valvular disorders (also see Chapter 25). The most common of these masses, left atrial thrombi and left atrial myxomas, are discussed below.

Left atrial thrombi can occur as complications of all types of valvular disease, but are often found in mitral valve disorders (Figs. 7.7 and 7.12). When atrial fibrillation, giant left atrium, and mitral stenosis are all present concurrently in a patient, the likelihood that there will be a thrombus in the left atrium is high. Color flow mapping is useful for visualization of valvular diseases themselves. It is rare for the presence of a left atrial thrombus to affect the intracardiac blood flow pattern as such.

Left atrial myxoma is the most frequent primary cardiac tumor. Its clinical symptoms and blood flow dynamics very closely resemble those of mitral stenosis. Thanks to the development of echocardiography, diagnosis of this myxoma from its characteristic features is generally very simple. In addition, its differential diagnosis from mitral

Table 7.4. Maximum Transprosthetic Mitral Flow Velocities from Continuous Wave Doppler Recordings and Pressure Gradients after the Mitral Valve Replacement

	Control Normal (n = 10)	Normally Functioning		Malfunctioning Prosthesis (n = 4)
		St. Jude valve (n = 42)	Porcine valve (n = 28)	
Measured max V^a (m/sec)		0.74 ± 0.18	1.41 ± 0.34	2.25 ± 0.25
Calculated ΔP^b (mm Hg)		2.19	10.1	20.3

^{a}max V, maximum velocity.
$^b\Delta P$, pressure gradient.

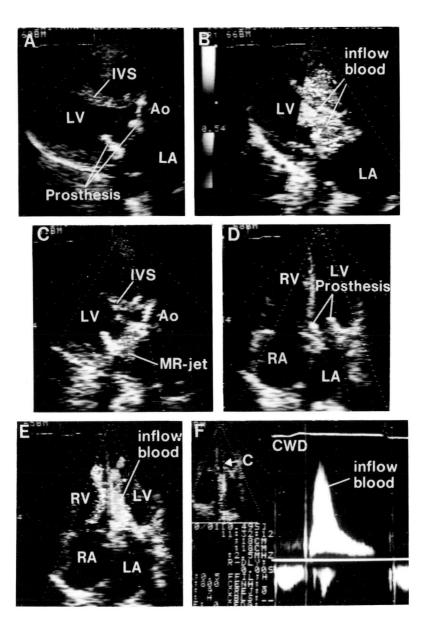

Figure 7.13. Color flow image in a 46-year-old female patient with prosthetic valves in the mitral (Carpentier-Edwards valve) and aortic position (Bjork-Shiley valve): prosthetic valve failure in the mitral position. *A*, B-mode in long-axis view in diastole. *B*, Color flow image, same view, in diastole. During diastole, mitral inflow is directed toward the interventricular septum, occupying the left ventricular outflow tract while ventricular outflow velocities are directed posteriorly toward the inflow tract. In other words, the ventricular diastolic flow patterns are reversed anteroposteriorly from normal. *C*, Color flow image, same view, in systole. Mild mitral regurgitation is demonstrated in mosaic patterns just behind the prosthesis in the left atrium in systole (*MR-jet*). *D*, B-mode, apical four-chamber view, in systole. *E*, Color flow image, same view, in systole. Mitral inflow blood is directed toward the septum as described above. *F*, Continuous wave Doppler of mitral inflow through prosthesis. Maximum velocity of mitral inflow = 2.4 m/sec. See this figure in Color Atlas.

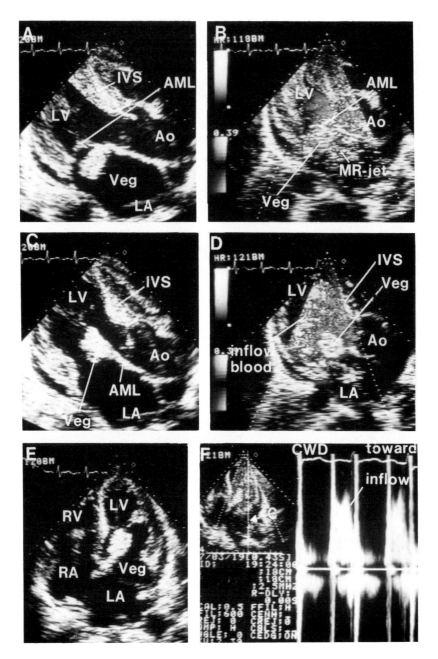

Figure 7.14. Color flow images in a 46-year-old male patient with mitral regurgitation (Sellers' grade 2) due to infectious endocarditis: vegetation on the anterior mitral leaflet. *A*, B-mode, long-axis view, in systole. A large vegetation (*Veg*) is on the anterior mitral leaflet (*AML*) *B*, Color flow image, same view, in systole. A mild mitral regurgitation (Sellers' grade 2) is demonstrated in the left atrium in systole (*MR-jet*). *C*, B-mode, same view, in diastole. *D*, Color flow image, same view, in diastole. Mitral inflow blood is imaged in mosaic patterns in diastole, similar to inflow patterns in mitral stenosis. *E*, B-mode, apical four-chamber view, in diastole. *F*, Continuous wave Doppler of mitral valve flow. Doppler signals are similar to those for mild mitral stenosis; maximum velocity through mitral valve = 1.8 m/sec, maximum pressure gradient = 13 mm Hg. See this figure in Color Atlas.

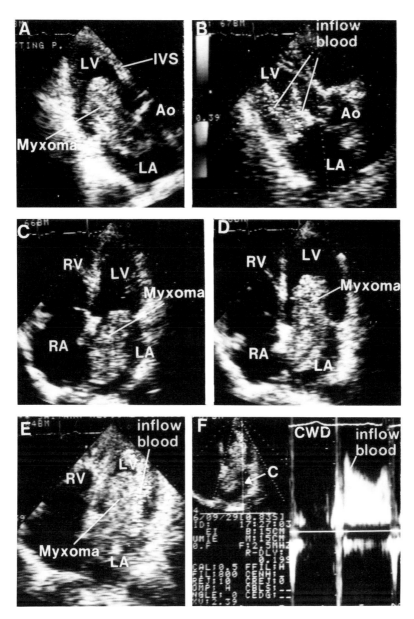

Figure 7.15. Color flow images in a 50-year-old female patient with a left atrial myxoma. *A,* B-mode, apical long-axis view, in diastole. The left atrial myxoma appears obstructing mitral valve orifice in diastole. *B,* Color flow image, same view, in diastole. Mitral inflow blood appears to be forming two streams, anteroposterior to the myxoma. *C,* B-mode, apical four-chamber view, in systole. *D,* B-mode, same view, in diastole. *E,* Color flow image, same view, in diastole. Mitral inflow blood appears mainly posterior to the myxoma in mosaic patterns. *F,* Continuous wave Doppler (*CWD*) of mitral valve flow. Mitral inflow recording from *CWD* is similar to mild mitral stenosis: maximum velocity of mitral inflow = 1.7 m/sec, maximal pressure gradient = 11.7 mm Hg. See this figure in Color Atlas.

stenosis has also become easier. When a left atrial myxoma is pedunculated and exhibits a pendular motion, it intrudes into the mitral valve in diastole, and a characteristic blood flow pattern can be detected. Examination of such a case with color flow mapping reveals a jet of blood spurting from the left atrium into the left ventricle during diastole (Fig. 7.15). Measurements of the mitral valve inflow obtained with continuous wave Doppler can be used to calculate the functional area of the mitral valve in diastole.

REFERENCES

1. Holen J, Aaslid R, Landmark K, Simonsen S: Determination of pressure gradient in mitral stenosis with a noninvasive ultrasound Doppler technique. *Acta Med Scand* 199:455–460, 1976.
2. Hatle L, Brubakk A, Tromsdal A, Angelsen B: Noninvasive assessment of pressure drop in mitral stenosis by Doppler ultrasound. *Br Heart J* 40:131–140, 1978.
3. Hatle L, Angelsen BA, Tromsdal A: Noninvasive assessment of aortic stenosis by Doppler ultrasound. *Br Heart J* 43:284–292, 1980.
4. Berger M, Berdoff RL, Gallerstein PE, Goldberg E: Evaluation of aortic stenosis by continuous wave Doppler ultrasound. *J Am Coll Cardiol* 3:150–156, 1984.
5. Hatle L, Angelsen B, Tromsdal A: Noninvasive assessment of atrioventricular pressure half-time by Doppler ultrasound. *Circulation* 60:1096–1104, 1979.
6. Yock PG, Popp RL: Noninvasive estimation of right ventricular systolic pressure by Doppler ultrasound in patients with tricuspid regurgitation. *Circulation* 70:657–662, 1984.
7. Tei C, Kisanuki A, Arima S, Arikawa K, Otsuji Y, Tanaka H: Quantitative assessment of right ventricular pressure in patients with tricuspid regurgitation by continuous wave Doppler echocardiogram (Abstr). Proceeding of 44th Meeting of the Japan Society of Ultrasonics in Medicine. 1984, pp 533–534.
8. Currie PJ, Seward JB, Reeder GS, Vlietstra RE, Bresnahan DR, Bresnahan JF, Smith HC, Hagler DJ, Tajik AJ: Continuous-wave Doppler echocardiographic assessment of severity of calcific aortic stenosis: A simultaneous Doppler catheter correlative study in 100 adult patients. *Circulation* 71:1162–1169, 1985.
9. Morris AM, Roitman DI, Nanda NC, Shah MR: Color Doppler assessment of stenotic valve area (Abstr). *Circulation* 72:III–100, 1985.
10. Helmcke F, Perry GJ, Nanda NC: Combined color Doppler and continuous wave Doppler in the evaluation of aortic stenosis (Abstr). *J Am Coll Cardiol* 7:101, 1986.
11. Pandian NG, Thanikachalam S, Elangovan D, Calderia ME, Salem DN: Color Doppler flow imaging in valvular stenosis. *Echocardiography* 4:515–526, 1987.
12. Omoto R, Yokote Y, Takamoto S, Kyo S, Ueda K, Asano H, Namekawa K, Kasai C, Kondo Y, Koyono A: The development of real-time two-dimensional Doppler echocardiography and its clinical significance in acquired valvular disease with specific reference to the evaluation of valvular regurgitation. *Jap Heart J* 25:325–340, 1984.
13. Omoto R: 2-D Doppler findings in valvular regurgitation. In Omoto R (ed): *Color Atlas of Real-Time Two-Dimensional Doppler Echocardiography, 2nd ed.* Tokyo, Shindan-To-Chiryo, (distributed by Lea & Febiger), 1987, pp 69–71.
14. Miyatake K, Izumi S, Okamoto M, Kinoshita N, Asanuma H, Nakagawa H, Yamanoto K, Takamiya M, Sakakibara H, Nimura Y: Semi-quantitative grading of severity of mitral regurgitation by real-time two-dimensional Doppler flow imaging technique. *J Am Coll Cardiol* 7:82–88, 1986.
15. Kitabatake A, Nakatani S, Ito H, Tanouchi J, Ishihara K, Fujii K, Uematsu M, Yoshida Y, Tominaga N, Inoue M, Kamada T: Cross-sectional area of aortic regurgitant jet as an estimate of the severity of aortic regurgitation: A study with real-time two-dimensional Doppler flow mapping technique (Abstr). Proceedings of the 47th Meeting of the Japan Society of Ultrasonics in Medicine. 1985, pp 225–226.
16. Helmcke F, Nanda N, Hsiung MC, Sato B, Adey CK, Goyal RG, Gatewood RP, Jr: Color Doppler assessment of mitral regurgitation with orthogonal planes. *Circulation* 75:175–183, 1987.
17. Perry GJ, Nanda NC: Recent advances in Color Doppler Evaluation of valvular regurgitation. *Echocardiography* 4:503–513, 1987.
18. Okumachi F, Yoshikawa J, Yoshida K, Asaka T, Takao S, Shiratori K: Diagnostic value and limitations of two-dimensional Doppler color flow mapping in the evaluation of prosthetic valve dysfunction (Abstr). *Circulation* 72:III–101, 1985.
19. Grube E, Kuhnen R, Becher H: Combined use of 2-D color flow mapping (CFM) and continuous Doppler echocardiography (CWD) to determine flow parameters in prosthetic valves (ABSTR). *Circulation* 74:II–389, 1986.
20. Yamagishi M, Miyatake K, Izumi S, Nagata S, Park Y, Sakakibara H, Nimura Y: Bioprosthetic valve dysfunction studied by two-dimensional color flow imaging: Efficacies and pitfalls (Abstr). *Circulation* 74:II–389, 1986.
21. Omoto R, Matsumura M, Asano H, Kyo S, Takamoto S, Yokote Y, Wong M: Doppler ultrasound examination of prosthetic function and ventricular blood flow after mitral valve replacement. *Herz* 11:346–350, 1986.

8

Intraoperative Doppler Color Flow Mapping for Assessment of Valvuloplasty and Repair of Congenital Heart Disease

Gerald Maurer, M.D.
Lawrence S. C. Czer, M.D.

SUMMARY

Intraoperative Doppler color flow mapping was performed in 60 patients to assess its usefulness in evaluating the adequacy of cardiac surgical repair prior to chest closure. A total of 79 procedures were studied: 13 mitral valve repairs, 5 tricuspid valve repairs, 14 atrial septal and 6 ventricular septal defect closures, 3 operations for redirection of atrial blood flow, 27 prosthetic valve replacements, and 11 control patients who underwent coronary artery bypass grafting only. Imaging was performed before and after cardiopulmonary bypass with the transducer placed directly on the epicardium. In addition, closed-chest pre- and postoperative color Doppler was performed. Grading of mitral and tricuspid regurgitation by open-chest color Doppler correlated well with both angiography and closed-chest color Doppler (κ 0.71–0.92), with good interobserver reproducibility (κ 0.69–0.88). All atrial and ventricular shunts were detected. Intraoperative color flow mapping demonstrated reduction of regurgitation following 11 of the 13 mitral valve repairs and all 5 tricuspid repairs. Increased regurgitation was detected after repair of a cleft mitral valve. It was also noted after a mitral commisurotomy, resulting in prosthetic replacement during the same operation. Sequential postoperative closed-chest color Doppler follow-up of up to 25 weeks demonstrated that there was no change or only one grade change in mitral and tricuspid regurgitation score, compared to the open-chest studies performed after repair. In St. Jude prosthetic valves,

three antegrade flow jets and mild regurgitation were seen. Bioprosthetic valves had single antegrade flow jets and no regurgitation. The adequacy of all atrial and ventricular shunt closures was confirmed, although in three ventricular septal defects small residual shunts were noted near the edges of the patch on open-chest study, but were not seen on subsequent follow-up. Redirection of atrial blood flow and unimpeded venous return were visualized in three cases.

Intraoperative color flow mapping provides immediate evaluation of the adequacy of mitral and tricuspid valvuloplasty prior to chest closure and may also be able to predict long-term outcome. This technique offers information about prosthetic valve flow and may help evaluate shunt repair as well as other operations for correction of complex congenital heart disease. Intraoperative color flow mapping ultimately may allow for valve repair procedures to be performed in greater numbers of patients with better control over outcome and lower reoperation rates, and may also contribute to improving the outcome of other complex cardiac surgical procedures.

INTRODUCTION

Increasingly complex cardiac surgical procedures are being performed for correction of acquired and congenital heart disease. Thus, there has been an increase of interest in operations that attempt to preserve, rather than replace, the patient's own native heart valves, as well as in more sophisticated forms of repair of congenital heart disease. Because the outcome of these procedures can be uncertain at times, there is a greater need to obtain accurate information about intracardiac blood flow at the time of surgery. A new imaging modality, Doppler color flow mapping, is capable of providing high quality, real-time tomographic images of cardiac morphology and blood flow (1–4), and thus appears uniquely suited to provide immediate information about the adequacy of cardiac surgical repair procedures (5, 6).

The purpose of our work was to evaluate the ability of intraoperative Doppler color flow mapping to:

1. Estimate severity of mitral and tricuspid valve regurgitation;
2. Evaluate the adequacy of mitral and tricuspid valve repair prior to chest closure and to predict their long-term outcome;
3. Assess repair of congenital heart disease and acquired shunt lesion;
4. Illustrate flow patterns in prosthetic valves.

METHODS

Patient Population

We studied 79 cardiac surgical procedures in 60 patients (Table 8.1). There were 33 males and 27 females ranging in age from 8 months to 88 years (mean 50 + 26 years). Patients were included in the study if they underwent repair of the mitral or tricuspid valve, prosthetic valve replacement, correction of congenital heart disease, or closure of acquired shunt lesions. Patients undergoing coronary bypass grafting were included as controls.

Eighteen valve repair procedures were studied in 17 patients. Thirteen involved the mitral valve. Ten of these were mitral suture annuloplasties usig the Kay-Zubiate method (7) and were performed for repair of ischemic regurgitation. Two were suture repairs of cleft mitral valves associated with ostium primum atrial septal defect. The remaining procedure was an attempted open commissurotomy for rheumatic mitral stenosis. Five tricuspid valve repairs were studied. Four were annuloplasty procedures (8) using a Carpentier-Edwards ring and were performed in patients with annular dilatation secondary to chronic pulmonary hypertension. One was a suture repair of a cleft tricuspid valve in a patient who also underwent repair of a cleft mitral valve.

Fourteen defects of the atrial septum were closed (eight ostium secundum, two ostium primum, one

Table 8.1. Patient Population[a]

Procedures Studied	Patients
MV repair (ischemic MR)[a]	9
MV repair (ischemic MR) + AVR	1
MV repair (cleft) + ASD (primum) + PFO	1
MV repair (cleft) + ASD (primum) + TV repair	1
MV commissurotomy + subsequent MVR	1
TV repair + MVR	3
TV repair + MVR + AVR	1
ASD (secundum)	7
ASD (secundum) + TAPVR	1
ASD (sinus venosus) + PAPVR	1
VSD	5
VSD + PFO	1
Mustard (d-TGV) + balloon septostomy closure	1
MVR	7
AVR	5
MVR + TVR	1
MVR + AVR	3
CABG only	11
Total	60

[a]ASD, atrial septal defect; AVR, aortic valve replacement; CABG, coronary artery bypass grafting; MR, mitral regurgitation; MV, mitral valve; MVR, mitral valve replacement; PAPVR, partial anomalous pulmonary venous return; PFO, patent foramen ovale; TAPVR, total anomalous pulmonary venous return; IV, tricuspid valve; TVR, tricuspid valve replacement; VSD, ventricular septal defect.

sinus venosus defect, two patent foramen ovale, and one defect after balloon septostomy). There were three operations for redirection of atrial blood flow (one Mustard procedure for dextrotransposition of the great vessels, one repair of total, and one of partial anomalous pulmonary venous return). We studied six closures of ventricular septal defects (two perimembranous, one supracristal, two postmyocardial infarction, and one traumatic).

A total of 27 prosthetic valve replacements were performed. Twenty-five were St. Jude valves placed in the mitral, aortic, or tricuspid position; two were mitral Carpentier-Edwards valves.

Eleven patients underwent only coronary artery bypass grafting.

Color Doppler Imaging

Both open- and closed-chest Doppler color flow mapping were performed using an Irex-Aloka 880 system. This device superimposes real-time flow information on a two-dimensional echocardiographic image (9), and thus offers simultaneous dynamic display of cardiac morphology and intracavitary blood flow. The flow information is obtained by performing simultaneous high speed analysis of Doppler shift in a multitude of sample regions (10) using the autocorrelation technique (11). Flow toward the transducer is displayed in eight shades of red, flow away from the transducer is displayed in eight shades of blue. Each shade corresponds to a specified velocity range. A third color, green, is added as a measure of flow variance. Doppler pulse repetition frequencies can be set at 4, 6, and 8 kHz, allowing for measurements of flow velocities up to 92 cm/sec with a 3.5 MHz transducer and up to 122 cm/sec with a 2 MHz transducer. As with conventional pulsed Doppler, color flow mapping is subject to "aliasing" whenever the Nyquist limit is exceeded (12) resulting in reversal of the displayed colors.

We used a 3.5 MHz transducer for intraoperative imaging and always performed two-dimensional echo imaging in addition to flow mapping. We primarily used a setting that offers a movable 45° color Doppler sector superimposed on a 90° two-dimensional echo sector. In this particular mode, images are displayed at 14 frames/sec. When higher temporal resolution was needed, we sampled at 30 frames/sec, using a 30° sector for both echo and Doppler. For wide-angle display of flow we imaged using a 90° sector for both modalities, although this setting only allowed sampling at 7.5 frames/sec. All studies were recorded on ½-inch videotape.

Study Protocol

After obtaining the patient's history and performing a physical examination, the majority of patients underwent cardiac catheterization and angiography.

A closed-chest, preoperative study was performed 24–48 hs prior to surgery and consisted of both a complete two-dimensional echocardiographic and a color Doppler examination. Imaging was performed from the parasternal, apical, and subcostal windows in multiple planes to inspect each cardiac valve for the presence and severity of regurgitation and to evaluate for presence of shunt flow across the atrial and ventricular septum. The examiner was blinded to the findings obtained at cardiac catheterization.

The initial intraoperative color Doppler study was performed after opening the chest and pericardium. The transducer was covered with a sterile plastic sheet and placed directly on the epicardial surface of the heart. Images were acquired in multiple long- and short-axis planes to visualize the maximum regurgitant flow or shunting. The electrocardiogram, arterial blood pressure, and right atrial, pulmonary arterial, pulmonary capillary wedge pressure, and cardiac output were recorded simultaneously. For assessment of mitral regurgitation, systolic blood pressure was raised to preoperative levels with intravenous phenylephrine whenever the intraoperative pressure was 15 mm or more below this control value.

The adequacy of mitral or tricuspid valvuloplasty was judged by the surgeon intraoperatively using conventional methods (13, 14), which included fluid filling of the arrested ventricle and visual inspection for valve leakage as well as, in the beating heart, measurement of atrial pressures and height of V waves and external palpation of the atria for systolic thrills.

A second intraoperative color Doppler study was performed after cardiopulmonary bypass and rewarming in the manner described above. Phenylephrine was again administered whenever systolic blood pressure was 15 mm Hg or more below the control value. Postoperative, closed-chest color flow mapping was performed prior to discharge and repeated at 3–6 month intervals.

Color flow mapping assessment of both mitral and tricuspid regurgitation was semiquantitative, using a grading system similar to previous descriptions for conventional pulsed Doppler echocardiography (15–17) and color Doppler (2, 18, 19). Valvular insufficiency was graded as 1+ if the regurgitant flow was only present immediately below the valve, 2+ if it extended into up to ⅓ of the atrial cavity, 3+ if it extended into up to ⅔ of the atrial cavity, and 4+ if it extended into more than ⅔ of the atrial cavity. Furthermore, we evaluated for presence or absence of atrial and ventricular shunts. Angiographic estimation of mitral and tricuspid regurgitation was performed by semiquantitative grading on a scale ranging from 0 to 4+ (20). Both angiography and color Doppler studies were read independently by blinded observers.

Since the significance of intraoperative color Doppler findings and their accuracy in estimating the severity of valvular regurgitation had not been established prior to our study, the initial protocol called for merely observing effects of repair procedures without influencing surgical decisions. When good correlations with angiography, closed-chest color flow mapping, and clinical findings became evident after the first 40 patients, we began to inform the surgeon of our intraoperative results, which were incorporated in the decision making process.

Data Analysis

Correspondence of scoring of valvular regurgitation was evaluated using the unweighted κ test (21) as a measure of agreement. The values of continuous variables are summarized as mean ± standard deviation.

RESULTS

No infections or other adverse effects were noted from our intraoperative studies. Pump time was not prolonged, since color flow mapping was performed before and after cardiopulmonar bypass. Pre- and postpump imaging required 5–10 min each.

Assessment of Mitral Regurgitation

Grading of mitral regurgitation by open-chest color flow mapping performed before cardiopul-

monary bypass was compared to left ventricular angiography in 44 of the 60 cases (Fig. 8.1, *top left*) and the closed-chest, preoperative color Doppler study in 53 (Fig. 8.1, *top right*). In addition, grading of mitral regurgitation by preoperative, closed-chest color flow mapping was compared to angiography in 39 patients (Fig. 8.1, *bottom left*). The κ values for these correlations ranged from 0.84 to 0.91 (perfect agreement being a κ of 1.00).

The three comparisons above included all patients in whom the two studies being compared were available. Excluded from the respective correlations were 11 patients who had been operated without left ventricular angiography, one who underwent neither angiography nor preoperative Doppler, one who underwent neither angiography nor prepump Doppler, and five who did not

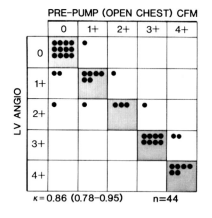

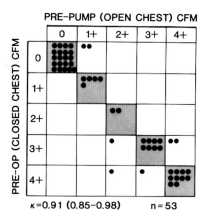

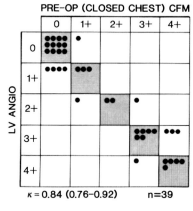

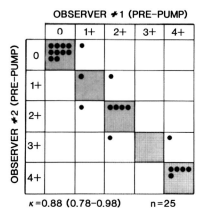

Figure 8.1. Assessment of mitral regurgitation: comparisons between open- and closed-chest color flow mapping and left ventricular angiography, as well as interobserver variability of open-chest color flow mapping. Results are expressed as κ values and 95% confidence limits. *CFM* = color flow mapping; *LV Angio* = left ventricular angiography; *Pre-op* = closed-chest imaging before surgery; Prepump = open-chest imaging before institution of cardiopulmonary bypass.

undergo preoperative Doppler studies. In three additional patients the angiogram was felt not to be usable prospectively for assessment of mitral insufficiency (poor x-ray penetration of the left atrial region in one, antegrade crossing of a common atrioventricular valve by two catheters in one, development of new mitral regurgitation as a consequence of myocardial infarction occurring after cardiac catheterization in one).

Interobserver reproducibility of mitral regurgitation assessed by open-chest color Doppler performed prior to cardiopulmonary bypass (Fig. 8.1, *bottom right*) was studied in 25 patients selected from our study population by a random number generator computer program. Two observers graded these studies independently in a blinded fashion.

A good correlation between them was obtained, yielding a κ of 0.8. Thus, assessment of mitral regurgitation by intraoperative color Dop-

pler correlated well with angiography and closed-chest color Doppler and had good interobserver reproducibility.

Assessment of Tricuspid Regurgitation

Grading of tricuspid regurgitation by open-chest color flow mapping performed before cardiopulmonary bypass could be compared to right ventricular angiography in only 8 patients (Fig. 8.2, *top left*), and to closed-chest, preoperative color Doppler in 51 (Figure 8.2, *top right*). In addition, grading of tricuspid regurgitation by preoperative, closed-chest color Doppler was also compared to right ventricular angiography in eight patients (Figure 8.2, *bottom left*). The Kappa values for these correlations ranged from 0.71 to 0.92.

The three comparisons above also included all patients in whom the two studies being compared were available. Excluded from the respective cor-

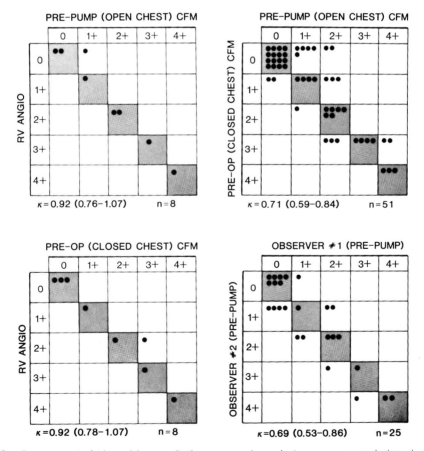

Figure 8.2. Assessment of tricuspid regurgitation: comparisons between open- and closed-chest color flow mapping and right ventricular angiography, as well as interobserver variability of open-chest color flow mapping. *RV Angio* = right ventricular angiography; other abbreviations are as in Figure 8.1. κ = kappa.

relations were 52 patients in whom no right ventricular angiography was performed; 6 of these 52 also had no preoperative Doppler studies. In two the preoperative studies were not interpretable for assessment of tricuspid regurgitation, and one patient had no prepump Doppler study.

Interobserver reproducibility of tricuspid regurgitation assessed by open-chest color flow mapping performed before cardiopulmonary bypass (Fig. 8.2, *bottom right*) was studied in the same 25 patients randomly selected for interobserver reproducibility of mitral regurgitation. The κ value was 0.69.

Thus, assessment of tricuspid regurgitation by intraoperative color Doppler correlated well with angiography in the small number of cases where angiography was available, correlated well with closed-chest color Doppler, and had good interobserver reproducibility.

Valve Repair Procedures

By conventional surgical evaluation, the outcome of all valvuloplasty procedures was judged to be successful. Results of intraoperative color Doppler assessment of mitral valve repairs in 13 patients studied after discontinuation of cardiopulmonary bypass and rewarming are summarized in Figure 8.3.

In all 10 cases of ischemic mitral regurgitation, Kay-Zubiate suture annuloplasty resulted in reduction in regurgitation score (by two grades or more in seven, by one grade in three), even when performing a phenylephrine challenge to increase left ventricular systolic pressure to the preoperative level (Fig. 8.4). In nine patients the residual regurgitation was 2+ or less after the repair. In one patient, operated on during the initial validation phase of our study, 3+ regurgitation persisted after repair.

Suture repair of two cleft mitral valves resulted in no change in regurgitation grade in one patient and in an increase from 0 to 3+ in the other (Fig. 8.5). The greater degree of regurgitation was felt to be due to the inability to perform complete closure of the cleft and also reflects the increase in left-sided flow following repair of the ostium primum defect.

In one patient, open-chest color Doppler after open commisurotomy for repair of rheumatic mitral stenosis displayed an increase of mitral regurgitation score from 1+ to 3+. This necessitated reinstitution of cardiopulmonary bypass and prosthetic valve replacement.

Predischarge closed-chest color flow mapping studies, as well as subsequent follow-up studies up to 25 weeks, revealed no change or only one

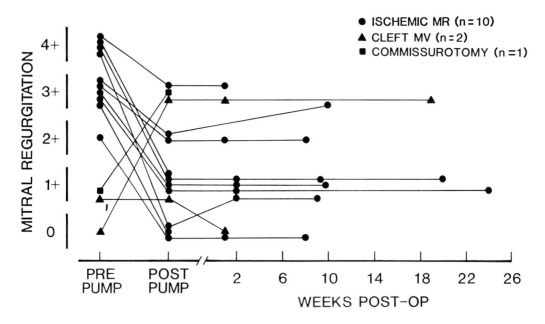

Figure 8.3. Effects of mitral valve repair in 13 patients: severity of regurgitation before and after cardiopulmonary bypass and on subsequent closed-chest follow-up studies. *MR* = mitral regurgitation; *MV* = mitral valve; *Prepump* = before cardiopulmonary bypass; *Postpump* = after cardiopulmonary bypass.

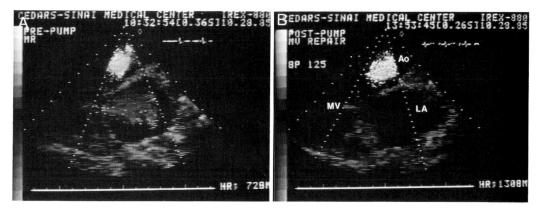

Figure 8.4. Intraoperative CFM (systolic frames) before and after mitral valvuloplasty. *A*, Before repair, severe mitral regurgitation is seen (blue jet in the left atrium). The red color represents normal left ventricular outflow into the aortic root. *B*, After repair, mitral regurgitation is no longer present, in spite of pressor challenge with phenylephrine and comparable blood pressure. *Ao* = aortic root; *LA* = left atrium; *MV* = mitral valve. (From Maurer G, Czer LSC, Chaux A, et al: Intraoperative Doppler color flow mapping for assessment of valve repair for mitral regurgitation. *Am J Cardiol* 60:333–337, 1987. Reproduced with permission of Yorke Medical Journals.) See this figure in Color Atlas.

grade change in regurgitation score, compared to open-chest color Doppler performed after cardiopulmonary bypass. In a patient with cleft mitral valve repair the degree of insufficiency appeared to decrease by one grade on the closed-chest, postoperative study. In two repairs of ischemic regurgitation it increased by one grade, so that in one the severity of regurgitation actually returned to the level before repair. Tricuspid valve repair procedures were performed in five patients and are summarized in Figure 8.6.

Four patients with severe tricuspid regurgitation secondary to long-standing pulmonary hypertension associated with mitral valve disease underwent tricuspid annuloplasty with Carpentier-Edwards rings. In two patients tricuspid re-

gurgitation disappeared (Fig. 8.7). The others continued to have mild (1+ or 2+) regurgitation. One patient underwent suture repair of a cleft tricuspid valve, which resulted in decrease in regurgitation score from 2+ to 1+.

Predischarge closed-chest color flow mapping and subsequent follow-up studies revealed that there was no change or only one grade change in regurgitation score, compared to open-chest studies performed after cardiopulmonary bypass.

Valve Replacements

In all St. Jude valves, normal antegrade flow was visualized on open-chest, postpump color Doppler, and three separate jets could be distinguished (Fig. 8.8). Twenty-four of the 25 St. Jude

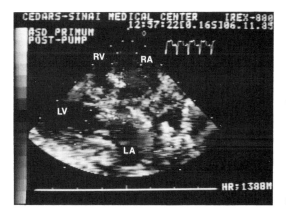

Figure 8.5. Intraoperative color Doppler study after repair of cleft mitral valve and closure of ostium primum atrial septal defect. Mitral regurgitation is seen (blue jet in left atrium) and originates at the base of the anterior leaflet, suggesting a residual cleft. The red color at the origin of the regurgitant jet represents aliasing due to high flow velocity. Tricuspid regurgitation is also present. *LA* = left atrium; *LV* = left ventricle; *RA* = right atrium; *RV* = right ventricle. (From Maurer G, Czer LSC, Chaux, A, Matloff J: Intraoperative color flow Doppler in evaluating valvuloplasty and correction of congenital heart disease. *Am J Cardiac Imag* 1:234–241, 1987. Reproduced with permission of Grune & Stratton.) See this figure in Color Atlas.

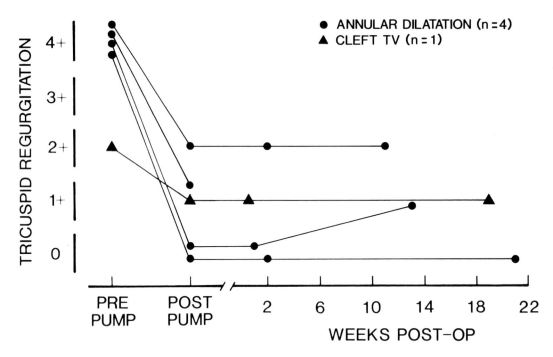

Figure 8.6. Effects of valve repair on tricuspid regurgitation in five patients. *TV* = tricuspid valve; other abbreviations are as in Figure 8.3.

valves were found to have a mild degree of regurgitation which appeared to be greater for larger valve sizes (Figure 8.7*B*). One patient who underwent aortic valve replacement for endocarditis

exhibited more severe regurgitation on open-chest, postpump color Doppler, which filled out most of the outflow tract and extended to the tip of the mitral leaflets. On subsequent follow-up, this

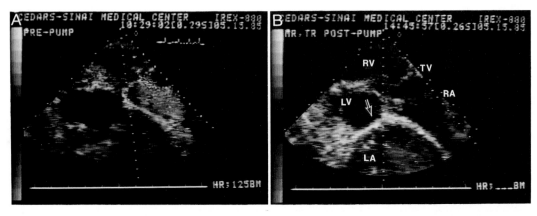

Figure 8.7. Intraoperative CFM (systolic frames) before and after tricuspid annuloplasty with Carpentier ring and prosthetic mitral valve replacements. *A*, Before repair, severe tricuspid regurgitation is seen (blue jet in the right atrium). *B*, After annuloplasty, tricuspid regurgitation is no longer present. Regurgitant flow across a large (# 33) St. Jude mitral prosthesis (*arrow*) is seen and represents a normal finding. *LA* = left atrium; *LV* = left ventricle; *RA* = right atrium; *RV* = right ventricle; *TV* = tricuspid valve. (From Maurer G, Czer LSC, Chaux, A, Matloff J: Intraoperative color flow Doppler in evaluating valvuloplasty and correction of congenital heart disease. *Am J Cardiac Imag* 1:234–241, 1987. Reproduced with permission of Grune & Stratton.) See this figure in Color Atlas.

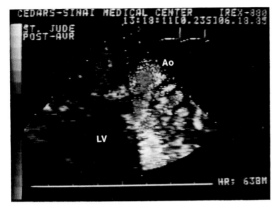

Figure 8.8. Aortic valve prosthesis (St. Jude), in open position: Three distinct jets are identified during systole, representing antegrade flow through the three orifices of this prosthetic valve. The transducer was placed on the aortic root and pointed toward the prosthetic valve. *Ao* = aortic root; *LV* = left ventricular outflow tract. (From Maurer G, Czer LSC, Chaux A, Matloff J: Intraoperative color flow Doppler in evaluating valvuloplasty and correction of congenital heart disease. *Am J Cardiac Imag* 1:234–241, 1987. Reproduced with permission of Grune & Stratton.) See this figure in Color Atlas.

patient was found to have a blowing diastolic murmur of aortic insufficiency and exhibited a similar degree of regurgitation on postoperative closed-chest color Doppler.

The two Carpentier-Edwards bioprosthetic valves had single antegrade flow jets and no regurgitation.

Repair of Congenital Heart Disease

All atrial and ventricular shunts detected by cardiac catherization could be visualized preoperatively and intraoperatively (Fig. 8.9A). In addition, an unsuspected widely patent foramen ovale, which coexisted with a perimembranous ventricular septal defect, was found during the open-chest, prepump color Doppler study (Fig. 8.10). Adequate patch closure of all atrial septal defects was verified on the open-chest, postpump study (Fig. 8.9). In all three congenital ventricular septal defects, minimal residual shunt flow was seen after repair, evidenced by small systolic flow jets near the edges of the patch. In all three patients these jets were most prominent near the septal leaflet of the tricuspid valve, although in two they were also seen in the area of insertion of the patch into the muscular septum. No such leakage was seen on the closed-chest, postoperative examination.

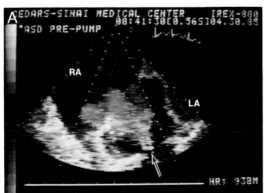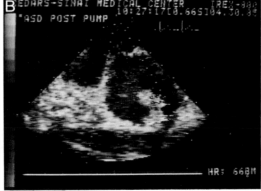

Figure 8.9. Intraoperative CFM before and after closure of a large ostium secundum atrial septal defect. These images were obtained by placing the transducer directly on the right atrium. *A*, Before repair, flow (*red*), which originates from a pulmonic vein (*arrow*), can be seen crossing the atrial septal defect. The blue color within the left atrium probably represents flow deflected by the septum primum. *B*, After closure of the defect with a pericardial patch, the left atrium has increased and the right atrium has decreased in size. No flow crosses the atrial septum; pulmonic vein flow is still seen. *LA*, left atrium; *RA*, right atrium. (From Maurer G, Czer LSC, Chaux A, Matloff J: Intraoperative color flow Doppler in evaluating valvuloplasty and correction of congenital heart disease. *Am J Cardiac Imag* 1:234–241, 1987. Reproduced with permission of Grune & Stratton.) See this figure in Color Atlas.

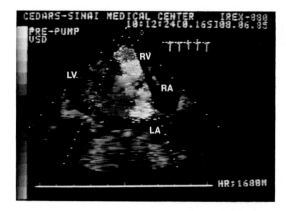

Figure 8.10. Coexisting atrial and ventricular left to right shunts. The intraoperative study demonstrates flow across a known perimembranous ventricular septal defect, as well as unsuspected atrial shunting across a stretched patent foramen ovale. *LA* = left atrium; *LV* = left ventricle; *RA* = right atrium; *RV* = right ventricle. (From Maurer G, Czer LSC, Chaux A, Matloff J: *Am J Cardiac Imag* 1:234–241, 1987. Reproduced with permission of Grune & Stratton.) See this figure in Color Atlas.

Redirection of blood flow could be visualized at the atrial level following correction of total anomalous pulmonary venous return (Fig. 8.11). Redirection could also be seen after baffle repair of partial anomalous pulmonary venous return and Mustard procedure for dextrotransposition of the great vessels. No impediment to venous return was seen in any of these cases.

DISCUSSION

Currently few methods are available to assess the outcome of cardiac surgical repair procedures before chest closure. Intraoperative evaluation is particularly important when performing reconstructive valve surgery, where residual regurgitation may require reoperation. However, it may also be valuable for repair of congenital heart disease and for other complex operations.

Doppler Color Flow Mapping

This technology offers real-time imaging of cardiac structures and blood flow. In addition to displaying the velocity vector of flow toward or away from the transducer, as with conventional Doppler, it also displays the direction of flow within the two-dimensional image plane. Therefore, it offers superior spatial information about

intracardiac flow patterns that previously were unavailable.

The limitations of this new method are currently being investigated (22–24). Among them are problems with the signal-to-noise ratio (especially at greater depth ranges), axial and lateral resolution, gain dependence, ghosting, and wall motion artifacts. Other current limitations include low frame rates, aliasing at relatively low velocities, narrow sector angles, and poor representation of the lower velocity ranges. Furthermore, color flow mapping rapidly displays a wealth of information, which can be difficult to comprehend by visual inspection and ultimately may require computerized image processing (25) for better understanding, as well as for quantitative analysis.

Nevertheless, good correlations between color flow mapping and angiography in the grading of atrioventricular valve regurgitation have previously been reported (2, 18, 19). We also obtained good correlations using a similar simple grading system, which involves measuring the length of the regurgitant jet in relation to the atrial dimension. In addition, we found good correlation between open- and closed-chest imaging.

Other methods to estimate the severity of regurgitation by color flow mapping, such as measuring jet width (26) and regurgitant area on single still frames, are being studied. However, attempts to planimeter the regurgitant area did not appear to improve correlations with angiography when compared to simple length measurements (18). None of the currently used methods accounts for the complexity of jets, which are four-dimensional phenomena (three spatial dimensions and time). These simple grading methods are therefore not volumetric measurements, but only rough semiquantitative estimates. They are nevertheless important, since they do seem to correlate well with angiography, which is also only semiquantitative, but has proven clinical utility. In vitro attempts to measure jet volume and energy are encouraging, but still at an early stage (25).

Color flow mapping has also been shown to be capable of detecting shunts associated with atrial and ventricular septal defects (1, 3), as confirmed by our results. As with regurgitant lesions, true quantification of shunt magnitude using this technique is currently not possible.

Evaluation of Valve Repair Surgery

Mitral valve repair is perhaps performed most commonly for ischemic mitral regurgitation, but

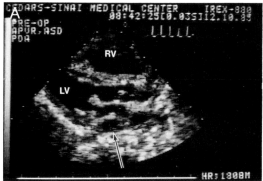
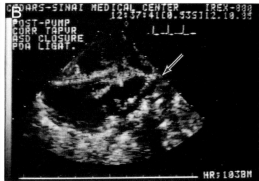
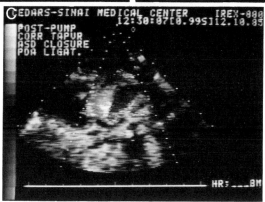

Figure 8.11. Redirection of total anomalous pulmonary venous return in a patient in whom all four pulmonary veins drain into the coronary sinus. *A,* Two-dimensional echocardiogram before repair. A large, dilated coronary sinus (*arrow*) is seen, which presents as a circular structure in the left atrium. *B,* Two-dimensional echocardiogram after repair. The newly created opening of the coronary sinus to the left atrium is seen, and anomalous drainage of a pulmonary vein (*arrow*) into the coronary sinus is apparent. In addition, the orifice of the coronary sinus to the right atrium was closed, and an ostium secundum atrial septal defect was repaired. *C,* Color flow mapping demonstrates the newly created drainage from the coronary sinus to the left atrium (*red*). Flow in the anomalous pulmonary vein to the coronary sinus is seen (*blue*). LV = left ventricle; RV = right ventricle. (From Maurer G, Czer LSC, Chaux A, Matloff J: *Am J Cardiac Imag* 1:234–241, 1987. Reproduced with permission of Grune & Stratton.) See this figure in Color Atlas.

is being done also for prolapsing myxomatous valves, regurgitant rheumatic valves, and congenital valve disorders, and there is renewed interest in commissurotomy procedures for mitral stenosis.

Repair procedures that preserve the patient's native valve offer a number of advantages over prosthetic valve replacement. A recent large series (27) reports that mitral valvuloplasty was associated with significantly fewer valve-related complications than prosthetic replacement, a lower perioperative and 7-year mortality, and a lower incidence of thromboembolic events. Better preservation of left ventricular function with mitral repair has been suggested than with prosthetic

replacement (28, 29), presumably because the continuity between left ventricular wall, mitral apparatus, and mitral anulus is not disrupted (30), and because (at least with suture annuloplasty) there is no rigid ring-impairing contraction of the basal left ventricular segments.

Similarly, tricuspid valve repair is being performed with increasing frequency. This is perhaps done most commonly for regurgitation with annular dilatation secondary to pulmonary hypertension, but is also popular for myxomatous and congenital tricuspid valve disease.

Valve repair operations have been performed in relatively few centers in the past because regurgitation frequently persists after repair (31,

32), and because the adequacy of repair can be difficult to evaluate at the time of surgery (33). Although mild residual regurgitation may be considered acceptable, severe regurgitation can lead to hemodynamic complications and may require subsequent reoperation. Traditional procedures for intraoperative assessment of the adequacy of repair offer only limited information and are frequently poor predictors of outcome. Such methods include fluid injection into the arrested ventricle for assessment of valve leakage (13, 14). However, both the geometry and chamber pressure of the nonbeating heart are different from the physiologic state, potentially leading to both under- and overestimation of the degree of the regurgitation that will subsequently occur. Measurement of atrial pressure and height of V waves in the beating heart after discontinuation of cardiopulmonary bypass may also be misleading, since they are very dependent on atrial size and compliance, as well as on pre- and afterload conditions (34).

A useful newer technique for the intraoperative assessment of valvular regurgitation is contrast echocardiography (33, 35, 36). However, color flow mapping offers a number of advantages over contrast echocardiography. It allows continuous beat-to-beat evaluation and offers simultaneous additional information about coexisting, and at times unsuspected, flow disturbances such as incompetence of other valves and intracardiac shunts. Doppler does not require invasion of the ventricle by needles or catheters or injection of echocardiographic contrast agents, which can lead to complications in rare instances (37, 38). Color flow mapping also can be used for subsequent follow-up and offers information directly comparable to the intraoperative study. Contrast echocardiography, on the other hand, has the advantage that it can be performed with equipment that is cheaper and at present more widely available.

Our results suggest that intraoperative color flow mapping is a safe procedure that does not prolong time on cardiopulmonary bypass and is capable of providing instantaneous information about the degree of valvular regurgitation. We observed a significant decrease in regurgitation on the immediate open-chest, postpump study in the majority of our repair procedures.

In two cases, mitral regurgitation actually increased after repair. One was an open commissurotomy for rheumatic mitral stenosis. Because of the new onset of 3+ insufficiency, demonstrated by color Doppler prior to chest closure, the heart was reopened and a prosthetic valve was inserted. The other was an infant with an ostium primum atrial septal defect in whom the greater degree of regurgitation was attributed to the inability to perform complete closure of the mitral cleft. The increased regurgitation also reflects the increase in left-sided flow after atrial shunt repair. Because of the patient's size the valve was not replaced and a decision was made to follow the clinical course. In one case of ischemic mitral insufficiency, valve repair only decreased the regurgitation from 4+ to 3+. Because this patient was operated in the initial validation phase of our study, when it was our aim to observe the effects of procedures rather than influence their outcome, the surgeon did not perform additional correction.

We did not encounter any evidence of left ventricular outflow tract obstruction after mitral valve repair. This apparently occurs in some cases of valvuloplasty with Carpentier rings (39, 40), but has not been reported with the suture annuloplasty technique employed in this study.

The natural history of regurgitation following valve repair procedures is not well documented. Previous studies only report findings on physical examination, such as the persistence of systolic murmurs in up to 40% of patients (32), or occasional angiographic follow-up. Doppler technology—in particular, color flow mapping—now offers the ability to perform serial noninvasive studies for longitudinal evaluation. Our current follow-up of up to several months in a limited number of patients demonstrates that the degree of postoperative regurgitation, assessed by closed-chest color Doppler, remains identical with or similar to the intraoperative postpump study. This finding suggests that intraoperative color flow mapping may be able to evaluate the adequacy of repair procedures immediately and that it may be capable of predicting their long-term outcome. However, a greater number of cases and longer follow-up are needed to confirm this.

Evaluation of Other Surgical Repair Procedures

Intraoperative evaluation is probably less important after valve replacement than after repair procedures, since immediate prosthetic valve dehiscence or malfunction are uncommon. It may nevertheless have significance in selected cases, such as in patients with recent endocarditis, as illustrated by our case of perivalvular leakage at the time of the immediate postpump study, and could also be of value in patients with connective tissue disorders. Our study illustrates the normal intraoperative flow patterns of St. Jude valves and may thus help establish a baseline for such application.

The closure of simple atrial and ventricular septal defects is usually uncomplicated, although residual patch incompetence can occur. Mild early leakage, which is thought to take place through the suture lines, is commonly present after repair of ventricular septal defects, and generally appears to be self-limiting (41). Our findings corroborate this observation, as evidenced by short, narrow flow jets near the margin of the patch, which were most prominent at the insertion near the septal leaflet of the tricuspid valve. We did not see them on our predischarge studies, either because the small leaks had sealed off or because they were too subtle to be visualized through the chest wall. No such leaks were observed with closure of atrial septal defects, possibly because the small pressure difference between the atria only generates small amounts of flow. Intraoperative color flow mapping may be particularly useful when problems with residual patch leakage can be anticipated, particularly in ventricular septal defects with straddling tricuspid valves, or other tricuspid valve abnormalities that can interfere with repair. An additional important application may be the examination for residual muscular ventricular septal defects of the "Swiss cheese" type, which are notoriously difficult to detect by visual inspection.

In operations for redirection of atrial blood flow, baffle leakage as well as obstruction of venous inflow can occur and may be detected and corrected before chest closure, although no such complications occurred in our limited series.

Primary Diagnostic Evaluation by Closed- and Open-Chest Color Flow Mapping

By combining two-dimensional echocardiography for assessment of chamber size and wall motion and color Doppler for assessment of mitral regurgitation, left ventricular angiography can be avoided in patients who are at high risk for dye-related complications (42). In our series, surgery was performed without any cardiac catheterization in five patients, without left ventricular angiography in eight, and with technically poor angiograms that did not allow for evaluation of mitral regurgitation in three. Thus in 16 patients (26%),

decisions about mitral valve interventions were based on preoperative as well as intraoperative color Doppler evaluation.

In some patients with valvular insufficiency, the open-chest, prepump study may serve as an adjunct to angiography and closed-chest Doppler. This is because it readily allows one to study the effects of different hemodynamic states on regurgitation, using volume loading and pharmacologic interventions. It may thus contribute to the decision regarding the need for valve surgery and whether to perform repair or replacement. In addition, it may offer clarification in cases where the angiogram or closed-chest Doppler study is difficult to interpret because of technical problems or is unavailable in an emergency setting.

Color flow mapping may be of particular significance in deciding whether to approach the tricuspid valve surgically, since regurgitation is difficult to evaluate by other means, including right ventricular angiography. Most of our decisions involving the tricuspid valve were based on color Doppler, since only 8 of the 60 patients underwent right ventricular angiography.

In repair of congenital heart disease, the open-chest, prepump color Doppler study may also offer information that is complementary to the conventional preoperative evaluation. As demonstrated by our case of unexpected atrial shunting in a patient undergoing ventricular septal defect repair, multiple shunts are sometimes missed with the standard evaluation.

Conclusion

Intraoperative color flow mapping is a feasible and safe procedure that offers accurate information about the severity of mitral and tricuspid regurgitation and the presence of intracardiac shunts. Our initial results suggest that it is capable of providing instantaneous evaluation of the adequacy of mitral and tricuspid valvuloplasty prior to chest closure and it may be able to predict their long-term outcome. In addition, it offers information about prosthetic valve flow and may help evaluate shunt repair, as well as other operations for correction of complex congenital heart disease.

Intraoperative color flow mapping ultimately may allow for valve repair procedures to be performed in greater numbers of patients with better control over outcome and lower reoperation rates and also may contribute to improving the outcome of other complex cardiac surgical procedures.

REFERENCES

1. Omoto R, Yokote Y, Takamoto S, et al: Diagnostic significance of real-time two-dimensional Doppler echocardiography in congenital heart diseases, acquired valvular diseases, and dissecting aortic aneurysms. *J Cardiogr* 14 (Suppl V):103–107, 1984.

2. Omoto R, Yokote Y, Takamoto S, et al: The development of real-time two-dimensional Doppler echocardiography and its clinical significance in acquired valvular diseases: With specific reference to the evaluation of valvular regurgitation. *Jap Heart J* 25:325–340, 1984.

3. Miyatake K, Okamoto M, Kinoshita N, et al: Clinical applications of a new type of real-time two-dimensional Doppler flow imaging system. *Am J Cardiol* 54:857–868, 1984.

4. Sahn DJ: Real-time two-dimensional Doppler echocardiographic flow mapping. *Circulation* 71:849–853, 1985.

5. Takamoto S, Kyo S, Adachi H, Matsumura M, Yokote Y, Omoto R: Intraoperative color flow mapping by real-time two-dimensional Doppler echocardiography for evaluation of valvular and congenital heart diseases and vascular disease. *J Thorac Cardiovasc Surg* 90:802–812, 1985.

6. Maurer G, Czer L, DeRobertis M, Kass R, Lee M, Chaux A, Gray R, Matloff J: Intraoperative Doppler color flow mapping in valvular and congenital heart disease (Abstr). *Circulation* 72 (Suppl II):206, 1985.

7. Kay JH, Zubiate P, Mendez AM, Dunne EF: Myocardial revascularization and mitral repair or replacement for mitral insufficiency due to coronary artery disease. *Circulation* 54 (Suppl III):94–96, 1976.

8. Carpentier A, Deloche A, Hanania G, et al: Surgical management of acquired tricuspid valve disease. *J Thorac Cardiovasc Surg* 67:53–65, 1974.

9. Omoto R (ed): *Color Atlas of Real-Time Two-Dimensional Echocardiography.* Tokyo, Shindan-To-Chiryo, pp 9–22, 1984.

10. Bommer WJ, Miller L: Real-time two-dimensional color flow Doppler: Enhanced Doppler flow imaging in the diagnosis of cardiovascular disease (Abstr). *Am J Cardiol* 49:944, 1982.

11. Namekawa K, Kasai C, Tsukamoto M, Koyano A: Imaging of blood flow using autocorrelation (Abstr). *Ultrasound Med Biol* 8 (Suppl):138, 1982.

12. Hatle L, Angelsen B: *Doppler Ultrasound in Cardiology: Physical Principles and Clinical Applications.* Philadelphia: Lea & Febiger, pp 63–69, 1985.

13. Pagliero KM, Yates AK: Peroperative assessment of mitral valve function. *J Thorac Cadiovasc Surg* 63:458–460, 1972.

14. King H, Csicsko J, Leshnower A: Intraoperative assessment of the mitral valve following reconstructive procedures. *Ann Thorac Surg* 29:81–83, 1980.

15. Abbasi AS, Allen MW, DeCristofaro D, Ungar I: Detection and estimation of the degree of mitral regurgitation by range-gated pulsed Doppler echocardiography. *Circulation* 61:143–147, 1980.

16. Nishimura RA, Miller FA, Callahan MJ, Benassi RC, Seward JB, Tajik AJ: Doppler echocardiography: Theory, instrumentation, technique and application. *Mayo Clin Proc* 60:321–343, 1985.

17. Miyatake K, Okamoto M, Kinoshita N, Ohta M, Kozuka T, Sakakibara H, Nimura Y: Evaluation of tricuspid regurgitation by pulsed Doppler and two-dimensional echocardiography. *Circulation* 66:777–784, 1982.

18. Miyatake K, Izumi S, Okamoto M, et al: Semiquantitative grading of severity of mitral regurgitation by real-time two-dimensional Doppler flow imaging technique. *J Am Coll Cardiol* 7:82–88, 1986.

19. Suzuki Y, Kambara H, Kadota K, et al: Detection and evaluation of tricuspid regurgitation using a real-time, two-dimensional color-coded Doppler flow imaging system: Comparison with contrast two-dimensional echocardiography and right ventriculography. *Am J Cardiol* 57:811–815, 1986.

20. Sellers RD, Levy MJ, Amplatz K, Lillehei CW: Left retrograde cardioangiography in acquired cardiac disease: Technic, indications and interpretations in 700 cases. *Am J. Cardiol* 14:437–447, 1964.

21. Fleiss UL: *Statistical Methods for Rates and Proportions.* New York, John Wiley & Sons, 217–225, 1981.

22. Sahn DJ, Tamura T, Valdes-Cruz L, Woo R, Yoganathan A: Color flow mapping Doppler underestimates jet width when compared to laser Doppler anemometry in an in-vitro model of adult aortic stenosis (Abstr). *J Am Coll Cardiol* 7:59A, 1986.

23. Tamura T, Valdes-Cruz L, Sahn DJ: In vitro studies of the accuracy of velocity determination and spatial resolution of a color flow mapping Doppler system (abstr). *J Am Coll Cardiol* 7:59A 1986.

24. Stewart WJ, Schiavone WA, From JA, Castle T, Salcedo EE: In vitro studies of Doppler color flow mapping: Dependence of spatial distribution on instrument settings (Abstr). *Circulation* 72 (Suppl III):98, 1985.

25. Bolger A, Eigler N, Pfaff JM, Maurer G: Computer analysis of color Doppler images for quantitative assessment of flow jets in a phantom model (Abstr). *J Am Coll Cardiol* 7:59A, 1986.

26. Perry GJ, Helmcke F, Nanda NC: Color Doppler assessment of aortic insufficiency in two orthogonal planes (Abstr). *J Am Coll Cardiol* 7:101A, 1986.

27. Perier P, Deloche A, Chauvaud S, et al: Comparative evaluation of mitral valve repair and replacement with Starr, Bjork, and porcine valve prostheses. *Circulation* 70 (Suppl I):187–192, 1984.

28. Bonchek LI: Correction of mitral valve disease without mitral valve replacement. *Am Heart J* 104:865–868, 1982.

29. Goldman ME, Mora F, Fuster V, Guarino T, Mindich BP: Is mitral valvuloplasty superior to mitral valve replacement for preservation of left ventricular function? An intraoperative two-dimensional echocardiographic study (Abstr). *J Am Coll Cardiol* 7:161A, 1986.

30. David TE, Uden DE, Strauss HD: The importance of the mitral apparatus in left ventricular function after correction of mitral regurgitation. *Circulation* 68 (Suppl II):76–82, 1983.

31. Antunes MJ, Colsen PR, Kinsley RH: Mitral valvuloplasty: A learning curve. *Circulation* 68 (Suppl II):70–75, 1983.

32. Carpentier A, Chauvaud S, Fabiani JN, Deloche A, Relland J, Lessana A, D'Allaines C, Blondeau P, Piwnica A, Dubost P: Reconstructive surgery of

mitral valve imcompetence. Ten year appraisal. *J Thorac Cardiovasc Surg* 79:338–348, 1980.

33. Mindich BP, Goldman ME, Fuster V, Burgess N, Litwak R: Improved intraoperative evaluation of mitral valve operations utilizing two-dimensional contrast echocardiography. *J Thorac Cardiovasc Surg* 90:112–118, 1985.
34. Fuchs RM, Heuser RR, Yin FC, Brinker JA: Limitations of pulmonary wedge V-waves in diagnosing mitral regurgitation. *Am J Cardiol* 49:849–854, 1982.
35. Goldman ME, Mindich BP, Teichholz LE, Burgess N, Staville K, Fuster V: Intraoperative contrast echocardiography to evaluate mitral valve operations. *J Am Coll Cardiol* 4:1035–1040, 1984.
36. Eguaras MG, Pasalodos J, Gonzalez V, et al: Intraoperative contrast two-dimensional echocardiography: Evaluation of the presence and severity of aortic and mitral regurgitation during cardiac operations. *J Thorac Cardiovasc Surg* 89:573–579, 1985.
37. Bommer W, Shah PM, Allen H, Meltzer R, Kisslo J: The safety of contrast echocardiography: Report of the Committee on Contrast Echocardiography for the American Society of Echocardiography. *J Am Coll Cardiol* 3:6–13, 1984.
38. Lee F, Ginzton L: A central nervous system complication of contrast echocardiography. *JCU* 11:292–294, 1983.
39. Kronzon IK, Cohen ML, Winer HE, Colvin SB: Left ventricular outflow obstruction: A complication of mitral valvuloplasty. *J Am Coll Cardiol* 4:825–828, 1984.
40. Kreindel MS, Schiavone WA, Lever HM, Cosgrove D: Systolic anterior motion of the mitral valve after Carpentier ring valvuloplasty. *Am J Cardiol* 57:408–412, 1986.
41. Stevenson JG, Kawabori I, Stamm SS, et al: Pulsed Doppler echocardiographic evaluation of ventricular septal defect patches. *Circulation* 70 (Suppl I):38–46, 1984.
42. Taliercio CP, Vlietstra RE, Fisher LD, Burnett JC: Risks for renal dysfunction with cardiac angiography. *Ann Intern Med* 104:501–504, 1986.

9

Valvular Heart Disease

Eugenio Carmo, M.D.
Jay N. Schapira, M.D.
John G. Harold, M.D.

PART 1
The Mitral Valve

The mitral valve has been studied by two-dimensional echocardiography (2DE) more extensively than any other cardiac structure. In addition to being a primary object of study, the mitral valve is also used frequently as an echocardiographic point of reference from which a study is begun. This chapter addresses the common disorders of the mitral valve to which 2DE and cardiac Doppler are clinically applicable and offer a diagnostic advantage.

RHEUMATIC MITRAL STENOSIS

The first clinical use of M-mode echocardiography was to diagnose rheumatic mitral stenosis. Echocardiographers soon established an echocardiographic hallmark for mitral stenosis: thickening and/or calcification of the mitral apparatus and reduction of leaflet motion. Also, in most cases the posterior leaflet moved anteriorly in the initial portion of diastole along with the anterior leaflet due to cuspal fusion (1, 2) (Fig. 9.1). Although these M-mode signs are reliable in diagnosing mitral stenosis, measurement of the reduction of the E-F slope (closing velocity of the mitral valve) (Fig. 9.2) has not proven reliable in determining the severity of mitral stenosis (3). Two-dimensional echocardiography has made it possible to obtain a more reliable quantitation of the severity of mitral stenosis for clinical purposes.

The added spatial information of 2DE allows visualization of the mitral valve orifice in the parasternal short-axis view in diastole. From this view the mitral valve orifice area can be planimetered, either from a frozen frame or by a digitizing microprocessor system (4) (Fig. 9.3). A comparison of mitral valve area determined by both 2DE and direct measurement at surgery by Henry et al. (5) demonstrated a good correlation between the techniques. Nichol et al. (2) found good agreement between mitral orifice area derived by catheterization and by 2DE in patients with pure mitral stenosis ($r = 0.95$) (Fig. 9.4). In a similar study by Wann et al. (6), the accuracy of 2DE estimation of mitral valve orifice area was documented in both patients with pure mitral stenosis and patients with mitral stenosis plus mitral regurgitation.

These studies suggested possible sources of disagreement between 2DE and other techniques in estimating mitral valve orifice area. Primarily, the standard Gorlin formula (7) may overestimate the severity of mitral stenosis in the presence of mitral regurgitation when only the mitral valve orifice itself is visualized by 2DE without regard to mitral regurgitation. Also, the Gorlin formula uses a gradient that is affected not only by the mitral valve orifice area, but also by the effects of the rheumatic process on the entire mitral valve apparatus, such as chordae thickening with subvalvular fusion and bunching of the mitral apparatus.

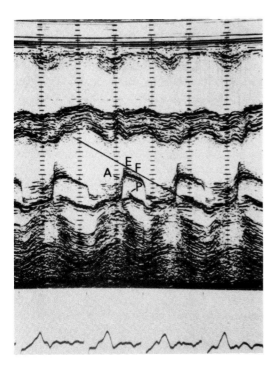

Figure 9.1. M-mode echocardiogram of the mitral valve showing the posterior leaflet (*P*) moving anteriorly with the anterior leaflet (*A*) during diastole due to cuspal fusion. A diminished mitral valve *E-F* slope is also noted.

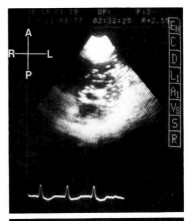

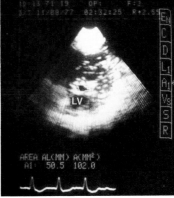

Figure 9.3. Short-axis view at the apex of the mitral valve funnel (see text). The *lower panel* demonstrates the use of the light-pen for determination of the mitral valve orifice area, which in this case was 102 mm² (1.02 cm²). This patient had pure mitral stenosis at cardiac catheterization and a Gorlin formula mitral valve orifice area of 1.0 cm². *A* = anterior, *P* = posterior, *R* = right, *L* = left, *LV* = left ventricle, *small A (lower panel)* = area.

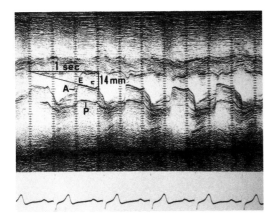

Figure 9.2. M-mode echocardiogram of the mitral valve showing the measurement of the E-F slope in a patient with mitral stenosis. In this patient the E-F slope measures 14 mm (the normal value is 70 mm or more). Anterior motion of the posterior leaflet (*P*) along with the anterior leaflet (*A*) during diastole can also be observed.

Errors that affect echocardiographic valve area can occur when planimetering the irregular borders of the 2DE mitral valve orifice image, due to anatomic and echocardiographic irregularities present in the borders of the orifice. In view of the varying degrees of valvular calcification, thickening, and fibrosis, proper echocardiographic gain settings become critical, as discussed by Martin et al. (8). Inappropriately low gain settings can result in dropouts, creating falsely large orifice areas, while gain settings that are too high can cause blending and blooming of edge irregularities, creating falsely small orifice areas.

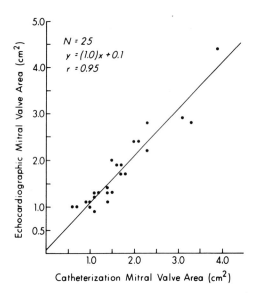

Figure 9.4. The relationship between the mitral valve area measured by cardiac catheterization (*horizontal axis*) and the mitral valve orifice area measured by 2DE (*vertical axis*). (From Nichol PM, Gilbert BW, Kisslo JA, Two-dimensional echocardiographic assessment of mitral stenosis. *Circulation* 55:120, 1977. With permission of the American Heart Association, Inc.)

Improper attention to transducer angle during a 2DE study can create a false mitral valve orifice. The false orifice is bordered by the proximal and distal portions of the arched anterior mitral leaflet instead of the true border, the leaflet edge (Fig. 9.5). This phenomenon is created by the commissure fusion at the tip of the anterior mitral leaflet. To avoid this pitfall, when performing the short-axis examination, the ultrasonic beam should be swept progressively caudally through the mitral apparatus until the apex of the mitral valve funnel is reached. The apex of the funnel represents the true minimal mitral valve orifice, and this area correlates best with the Gorlin-derived orifice areas. Martin et al. (8) suggested that the ideal point of diastole for orifice measurement is the initial portion of the diastole. He also suggested the best place to draw the line for planimetry of the mitral valve orifice is at the black-white interface, after assuring proper gain control settings. It is very important to remember that patients with low cardiac output have a reduced mitral valve leaflet opening and, therefore, a reduced measured mitral valve orifice area.

In addition to mitral valve orifice area, other aspects of rheumatic mitral valve disease can be appreciated by 2DE Figure 9.6A demonstrates

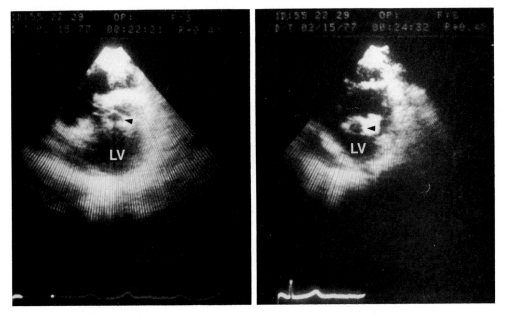

Figure 9.5. *Left*, Short axis view showing the false mitral valve orifice (*arrow*) created by the anterior arching of the anterior mitral leaflet. *Right*, True mitral valve orifice (*arrow*) located by sweeping the transducer slightly toward the apex. *LV* = left ventricle.

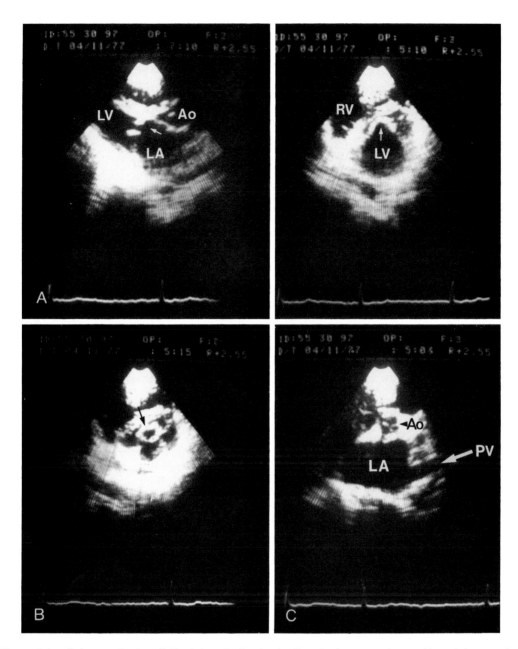

Figure 9.6. *A*, Long-axis view (*left*) of the mitral valve in diastole demonstrating arching of the anterior mitral leaflet (*arrow*). The same arching of the anterior leaflet can be seen in the short-axis view (*right, arrow*). *B*, Short-axis view of a patient with critical mitral stenosis (mitral valve orifice area = 0.8 cm²). *Black arrow* points to the stenotic mitral orifice. *C*, Short-axis view at the base showing a normal tricuspid aortic valve (*Ao*). Because of the severe mitral stenosis, the left atrium (*LA*) is enlarged and the pulmonary veins (*PV*) are very prominent. *LV* = left ventricle, *RV* = right ventricle.

anterior arching or doming of the anterior mitral leaflet, created by commissural tethering in diastole, in both the short- and long-axis views in a patient with critical mitral stenosis. Figure 9.6*B* demonstrates the mitral valve orifice area of 0.8 cm² measured by both 2DE and cardiac catheterization. With 2DE, the size of the left atrium can be assessed accurately, dilated pulmonary veins can be identified frequently, and the other valves can be examined (Fig. 9.6*C*). Figure 9.7 also demonstrates anterior leaflet arching (doming) as well as the thickening and anterior arching (doming) of the posterior mitral leaflet.

When evaluating the mitral valve in consideration of commissurotomy, the pliability of the valve, degree of thickening, fibrosis, calcification of the valve, and dense fibrosis of the subvalvular apparatus (chordae plus papillary muscles) are of extreme importance. The degree of pliability (maximum mitral valve amplitude of 20 mm or greater is considered pliable), calcification, fibrosis, and thickening vary greatly in patients with rheumatic mitral stenosis. The relative preoperative suitability for mitral commissurotomy can be judged accurately by 2DE (9).

Complications of rheumatic mitral stenosis, such as left atrial thrombus and pulmonary hypertension, can be identified clearly by echocardiography (10). Also, 2DE is very useful in the differential diagnosis of other cardiac conditions that can mimic mitral stenosis clinically. An excellent example of this is a large left atrial myxoma (Fig. 9.8).

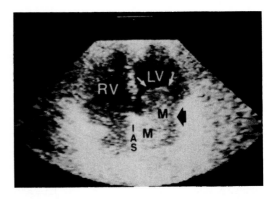

Figure 9.8. Four-chamber apical view showing a large left atrial myxoma (*M*) prolapsing during diastole into the left ventricle (*LV*). This patient was referred for the two-dimensional study with a diagnosis of mitral stenosis. *RV* = right ventricle. *AS* = interatrial septum.

Two-dimensional echocardiography is used widely in evaluating mitral stenosis, although it has not replaced cardiac catheterization. To be effective, 2DE studies must meet three criteria: (*a*) the true commissural edge in early diastole must be located; (*b*) the appropriate gain settings must be used, and (*c*) the images of the orifice must be drawn correctly. Under these circumstances, 2DE can provide reliable qualitative and semiquantitative assessment of mitral stenosis.

The development of sensitive pulsed and continuous wave Doppler, along with simultaneous 2DE imaging and the addition of color flow mapping, provides useful techniques to fill informational gaps and correct pitfalls of the echocardiographic examination of rheumatic mitral stenosis (11, 12). In technically difficult patients with heavily calcified mitral valves, patients with concomitant significant mitral regurgitation or patients with involvement of the aortic valve, Doppler echocardiography permits accurate assessment of even the worst examples of these difficult cases. Presently the great majority of patients with pure rheumatic valvular disease and no suspicion of coronary artery disease can be accurately evaluated preoperatively both anatomically and hemodynamically by 2DE and Doppler echocardiography. This becomes especially useful in patients in whom cardiac catheterization is contraindicated and who require an accurate, reliable preoperative assessment of their anatomy and physiology to direct any surgical intervention (9).

However, as with any technique, there are technical limitations. The optimal Doppler signal

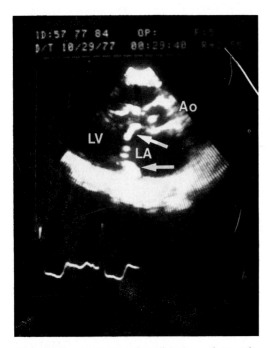

Figure 9.7. Long-axis view demonstrating arching of the anterior leaflet (*upper arrow*) and a thickened, deformed, and heavily calcified posterior leaflet (*lower arrow*). Ao = aorta, *LA* = left atrium, *LV* = left ventricle.

should be obtained with the Doppler beam parallel to the flow of, or "inside," the abnormal jet. Since these jets cannot be visualized, with each patient there is a moderate learning curve for the operator to direct the Doppler beam properly and, recognizing the audio signal, print an adequate spectral analysis. Very often the best 2DE window is not necessarily the best Doppler window, and a slight angulation of the transducer may give an optimal flow velocity profile.

The velocity of mitral flow usually is recorded best from the apical window. In almost all patients, a skilled operator will be able to listen carefully to the audio signal and recognize the highest frequency while performing fine adjustment on the angle and position of the transducer, using the original 2DE image as a reference point. This position represents the direction with the smallest angle to the jet and will give the most accurate assessment of the maximum flow velocities.

In general, the best type of Doppler to use in mitral stenosis is continuous wave, since it is able to record higher velocities than pulsed wave Doppler (Fig. 9.9A and B). After the best spectral analysis of the diastolic flow through the mitral valve is recorded by guiding it with the audio signal, there are four main parameters to be analyzed. Primarily, peak velocity will be considerably higher than normal (Fig. 9.10). The more severe the mitral stenosis, the higher the peak velocity, but since the peak velocity represents flow across the valve, it is heart rate and cardiac output dependent. The next parameter is the diastolic slope of the velocity profile or the rate of decrease in diastolic flow following the initial peak velocity. This slope will be decreased in mitral stenosis, becoming increasingly more flat as the mitral stenosis becomes more severe (Fig. 9.11). The third parameter is pressure half-time, or the time it takes for the initial pressure to drop by half (11). This index can be obtained by dividing the mitral peak velocity by the square root of 2 (approximately 1.4) and measuring the time from peak velocity to the point on the diastolic slope at which this decreased velocity is found. Values of 60 msec or less are considered normal, with values of more than 100 msec being found in mitral stenosis. Since pressure half-time is not influenced by heart rate and cardiac output, it gives a better evaluation of the degree of stenosis (Fig. 9.12). The fourth parameter, mitral valve orifice area, is estimated by dividing 220 by the pressure half-time. Pressure half-time correlates well with true mitral valve orifice area and varies less with flow across the valve.

The pressure half-time method of estimating mitral valve orifice area is especially useful in patients with associated mitral regurgitation and in patients with severe mitral stenosis and low cardiac output. In patients with mitral commissurotomy, 2DE estimation of valve orifice area is inaccurate because the valve is distorted. However, Doppler can estimate the degree of stenosis and define the presence of mitral regurgitation accurately. In these patients, Doppler echocardiography will be the best technique for follow-up studies to assess progression of the mitral stenosis. Also, in patients where suboptimal 2DE images are obtained, Doppler will be the only approach for quantitating the stenosis and following the patient serially.

The Doppler signal in mitral stenosis is one of the easiest signals to obtain, even for operators with little expertise. The use of 2DE and Doppler color flow mapping for the diagnosis of mitral stenosis is presented in the chapter on color flow mapping and presents yet another method of accumulating the same information described above.

MITRAL REGURGITATION

Competence of the mitral valve depends upon the normal, integrated function of the mitral apparatus, comprising the mitral valve anulus, leaflets, chordae tendineae, papillary muscles, and left ventricular myocardium. In a study by Mintz et al. (13), 2DE was shown reliably to differentiate mitral insufficiency secondary to valvular disease from insufficiency secondary to left ventricular or papillary muscle dysfunction, mitral annular calcification, idiopathic hypertrophic subaortic stenosis, cleft mitral leaflet, or atrial myxoma. This was done by analyzing the different anatomical features of the mitral apparatus and left ventricle in each of these conditions.

Another study by Mintz et al. (14) found that 2DE was very useful in evaluating patients with a new systolic murmur or congestive heart failure after acute myocardial infarction. Two-dimensional echocardiography also proved useful in detecting surgically correctable defects of the mitral valve apparatus (papillary muscle rupture) or ventricular septal defects. Wann et al. (15) further studied rheumatic mitral regurgitation with 2DE and found that significant mitral regurgitation could be inferred by qualitative analysis of short-axis views of mitral leaflet coaptation. As with M-mode echocardiography, an enlarged left

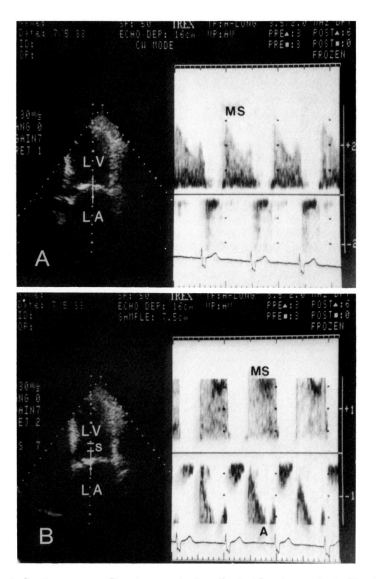

Figure 9.9. *A,* Continuous wave Doppler examination of mitral flow in a patient with mitral stenosis. The simultaneous two-dimensional apical view shows the proper orientation of the Doppler CW beam through the left atrium (*LA*) and left ventricle (*LV*). Spectral analysis shows a diastolic flow above the baseline (toward the transducer), reaching a peak velocity of 2.9 m/sec. *MS* = mitral stenosis. *B,* Pulsed Doppler examination of mitral flow in the same patient with mitral stenosis. The simultaneous two-dimensional apical view shows the sample volume (*s*) positioned in the left ventricle (*LV*), just in front of the mitral valve. Spectral analysis demonstrates an ambiguous direction of the flow during diastole. This phenomenon, called "aliasing" (*A*), occurs because the high velocity flow through the stenotic mitral valve during diastole (in this case, 2.9 m/sec) exceeds the limits of the pulsed Doppler technique (1 m/sec in each direction), and the flow is displayed on both sides of the baseline. *LA* = left atrium.

atrium indicates more significant mitral regurgitation is the dominant lesion.

However, the use of M-mode and 2DE in the diagnosis of mitral regurgitation or any other valvular insufficiency is quite limited. It can help to differentiate the etiology of mitral regurgitation already identified by clinical means. Also, echocardiography can give indirect data, such as left

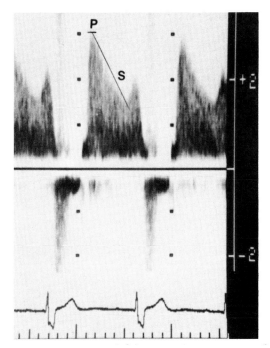

Figure 9.10. Continuous wave Doppler examination in a patient with mitral stenosis. The high peak velocity (P) of the diastolic flow toward the transducer (above the baseline) as well as the diastolic slope (S) can be obtained easily.

atrial size, or suggest pulmonary hypertension in a patient where the diagnosis was obtained by other techniques or by physical examination.

The 2DE findings in mitral regurgitation in-

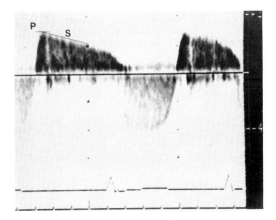

Figure 9.11. Continuous wave Doppler examination in a patient with mitral stenosis. A marked decreased diastolic slope (S) and a high peak diastolic velocity (P) are consistent with severe mitral stenosis.

clude systolic expansion of the left atrial posterior wall, incomplete or improper closure of the valve in systole, a characteristic pattern of aortic valve closure, and a characteristic pattern of interventricular septal motion. However, these signs have little value in the diagnosis and/or quantification of mitral regurgitation. The quantification of valvular insufficiency is the area of cardiac evaluation that has benefited the most by cardiac Doppler and its ability to detect reverse flow velocities (16, 17). Doppler echocardiography is able to detect flow velocities in the chamber behind a diseased valve during the period of the cardiac cycle when that valve should be closed and there should not be any reverse flow.

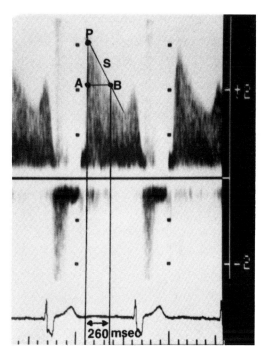

Figure 9.12. Continuous wave Doppler in a patient with mitral stenosis illustrating the measurement of the pressure half-time. The initial peak velocity (P = 3.1 m/sec) is divided by the square root of 2 (approximately 1.41). This result (2.19 m/sec) is located on the *vertical axis* of the peak diastolic velocity (A). *Point B* is the point where a *horizontal line* from *point A* crosses the diastolic slope (S). Since the *horizontal axis* of the graph is time, the measurement between *points A* and *B* is the pressure half-time (260 msec). The mitral valve orifice area is obtained by dividing 220 by the pressure half-time. In this specific case the mitral valve orifice area is 0.85 cm² (220 ÷ 260).

The apical view usually provides the best window for directing the beam in mitral regurgitation. The use of continuous wave and pulsed wave Doppler is helpful in both detecting regurgitation and mapping the three-dimensional orientation of the jet. Once the direction of the jet is identified, pulsed Doppler is used to find the width and extension of the regurgitant jet. This information provides a semiquantitative indication of the severity of the mitral regurgitation.

For the purpose of mapping the mitral regurgitation, a left parasternal window or a window between the left parasternal region and the apical region may be useful. In some patients with marked cardiomegaly, the 16 cm depth limit of pulsed Doppler restricts its ability to map regurgitation to the area of the left atrium adjacent to the mitral valve when the apical view is used. However, in this situation, secondary views will permit the echocardiographer to investigate the more posterior reaches of the left atrium and the pulmonary veins with the sample volume of pulsed wave Doppler.

Using this semiquantitative technique, the degree of mitral regurgitation is related essentially to the width of the jet and how far posterior to the valve orifice it can be detected. Consequently, mitral regurgitation can be classified in four categories:

1. Mild regurgitation (grade 1+), when the regurgitant flow is only recorded immediately adjacent to the posterior aspect of the mitral valve and does not extend as far back as the proximal third of the atrium (Fig. 9.13);
2. Moderate regurgitation, (grade 2+), in which the regurgitant flow is recorded up to the proximal third of the atrium posterior to the valve (Fig. 9.14);
3. Moderately severe regurgitation (grade 3+), in which the regurgitant flow is identified halfway between the mitral valve and the posterior left atrial wall.
4. Severe regurgitation (grade 4+), in which the regurgitant jet is detected more distal than the mid left atrial level and includes the pulmonary veins (Fig. 9.15).

The major limitations of this technique are related to the quality of the equipment used and the expertise of the operator.

The pulsed Doppler is focused at the mitral annular level, the sample volume of which is guided by a simultaneous 2DE apical four-chamber view. At this level, mapping needs to be performed in three dimensions by sweeping from one side to the other of the mitral ring and also more posteriorly and anteriorly. The beam direction may or may not be the same for the forward flow velocity. Usually the regurgitation is recorded best with a more postero-inferior orientation. Sometimes switching back and forth from pulsed to continuous wave Doppler will help detect the direction of the regurgitant flow.

Regurgitant flow needs to be recognized first

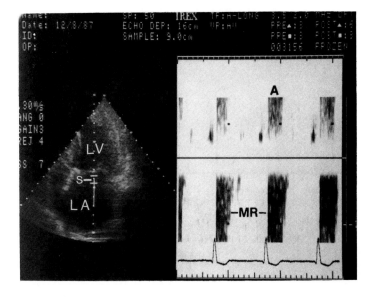

Figure 9.13. Pulsed Doppler in a patient with mild mitral regurgitation (*MR*). The sample volume (*s*) is placed in the left atrium (*LA*) behind the mitral valve. Spectral analysis shows a high velocity turbulent flow during systole (*MR*). Aliasing (*A*) occurs with display on both sides of the baseline because the high velocity of the jet exceeds the limits of pulsed Doppler. The *MR* was graded as mild, as the jet was isolated to the area just below the mitral annulus in the *LA. LV* = left ventricle.

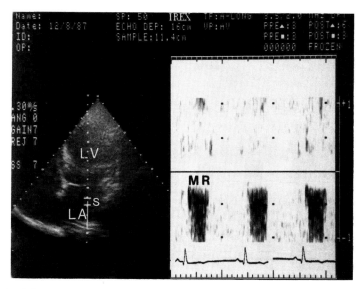

Figure 9.14. Pulsed Doppler in a patient with moderate mitral regurgitation. The high velocity turbulent flow away from the transducer during systole (*MR*) is recorded with the sample volume (*s*) placed in the proximal third of the left atrium *LA*. *LV* = left ventricle.

by the audio signal (intensity and frequency), which will help establish the optimal position of the Doppler beam. Spectral analysis will show a high velocity turbulent flow during systole. With pulsed Doppler, the high velocities will exceed the limits of the technique. When this happens. ambiguity in the direction of flow will occur due to "aliasing" (Figs. 9.13–9.15). The use of continuous wave Doppler will then permit determination of peak velocity, the true direction and delineation of the "systolic envelope" with marked spectral broadening (Fig. 9.16). With severe regurgitation

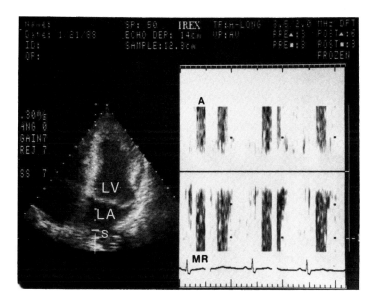

Figure 9.15. Pulsed Doppler in a patient with severe mitral regurgitation. The strong regurgitant jet (*MR*) with aliasing (*A*) is still recorded with the sample volume (*s*) placed at the back wall of the left atrium (*LA*). *LV* = left ventricle.

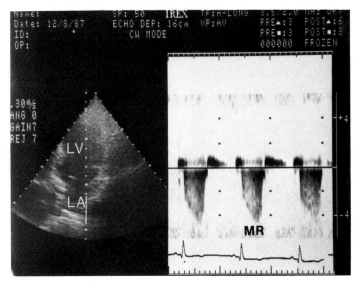

Figure 9.16. Continuous wave (CW) Doppler in a patient with mitral regurgitation. The high velocity turbulent jet moving away from the transducer during systole (*MR*) is obtained from an apical view. The simultaneous two-dimensional image helps to guide the CW beam to find the direction of the regurgitant jet. With the beam parallel to the jet the best audio signal will be obtained and spectral analysis will display a well-defined "envelope" of the regurgitant jet. Analysis of the peak velocity especially when it is reached during the cardiac cycle is important to evaluate the severity of the *MR. LA* = left atrium, *LV* = left ventricle.

there is an earlier decrease in systolic velocity due to an increase in left atrial pressure, which can be demonstrated only by continuous wave Doppler. Usually patients with significant mitral regurgitation will have increased forward mitral flow velocities; however, in contrast with mitral stenosis, this increase is of short duration (Fig. 9.17).

Once the direction of the regurgitant jet is identified at the mitral annular level, the sample volume of the pulsed Doppler can be moved slowly inside the left atrium. With each change in depth settings, fine movements of the transducer are necessary to maintain the sample volume inside the jet. When the strongest audio signal is detected, the sample volume can be moved one step ahead. This technique is repeated step by step until the maximum extension is reached where the regurgitant flow can be detected.

In the vast majority of cases, this approach will be the most accurate. However, some patients will need a lower parasternal window or a window in between the parasternal and apical windows, following the same steps used for the apical window to detect the direction of the flow.

Color flow mapping is especially useful in de-

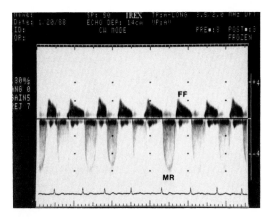

Figure 9.17. Continuous wave Doppler in a patient with severe mitral regurgitation (*MR*). The peak velocity is reached earlier in systole. The contour of the "envelope" (*MR*) is clearly different from the one in Figure 9.16, reaching the peak velocity much earlier in systole. An early increase of the velocity of the forward mitral flow (*FF*) is noted in the presence of significant mitral regurgitation (2.2 m/sec) but decreases fast. When there is obstruction to flow (mitral stenosis), this increased velocity lasts longer (increased pressure half-time).

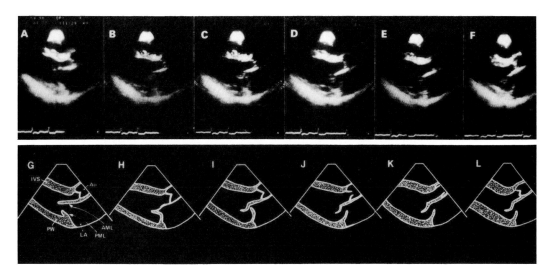

Figure 9.18. Sequential long-axis frames of a two-dimensional echocardiogram of a patient with flail posterior mitral leaflet, with matching drawings beneath each frame. *AML* = anterior mitral valve leaflet, *Ao* = aorta, *IVS* = interventricular septum, *LA* = left atrium, *PML* = posterior mitral valve leaflet, *PW* = posterior wall.

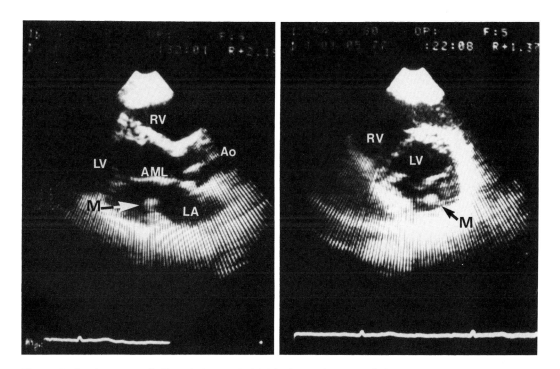

Figure 9.19. Long-axis (*left*) and short-axis (*right*) views of a mass (*M*) on the posterior mitral leaflet, which at surgery was a fibroadenoma. *AML* = anterior mitral valve leaflet, *Ao* = aorta, *LA* = left atrium, *LV* = left ventricle, *RV* = right ventricle.

tecting unusual flow directions that could be missed or underestimated by conventional Doppler techniques (18). Doppler echocardiography is the technique of choice for identifying and quantifying already known mitral insufficiency and monitoring the evolution of the disease. It is also the technique of choice for the differential diagnosis of other valvular pathology, including tricuspid regurgitation, aortic stenosis, and ventricular septal defect. These conditions and others like idiopathic hypertrophic subaortic stenosis (IHSS) may also be associated with mitral regurgitation. A Doppler study will be able to detect the presence or absence of these other conditions. Inaudible or atypical mitral regurgitation present in patients with low cardiac output after myocardial infarction or with congestive heart failure also may be detected by Doppler. These patients may benefit from vasodilators to reduce afterload if the correct diagnoses can be made.

FLAIL MITRAL LEAFLETS

Mintz et al. (19) demonstrated 2DE to be more sensitive than M-mode echocardiography for the diagnosis of flail mitral valve. Child et al. (20) described three criteria for a flail posterior mitral leaflet: (*a*) a systolic whipping arc-like motion into the left atrium; (*b*) a loss of the normal systolic coaptation of the anterior and posterior leaflets, and (*c*) a darting systolic mass of left atrial echoes representing flail mitral leaflets (Fig. 9.18).

A ruptured chordae tendineae is one of the more common causes for a flail mitral leaflet. Ballester et al. (21) studied a series of 32 patients

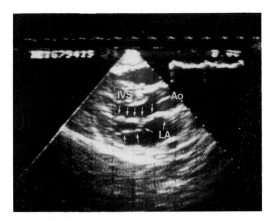

Figure 9.21. Long-axis view in a patient with anterior submitral and chordae tendineae calcification (*arrows*). *Ao* = aorta, *IVS* = interventricular septum, *LA* = left atrium.

with ruptured chordae tendineae and found that 65% had diastolic chaotic motion of the leaflets (seen best in the short-axis view), 55% had noncoaptation of anterior and posterior leaflets, and approximately 20% demonstrated systolic fluttering of the valve in the left atrium. A less common cause of flail mitral leaflet is ruptured papillary muscle, which sometimes can be diagnosed by 2DE.

OTHER MITRAL VALVE DISORDERS

Two-dimensional echocardiography has been used with great success to visualize masses on the mitral valve. Occasionally, nonendocarditic lesions of the mitral valve are encountered. Figure 9.19 shows a mitral leaflet mass in a patient who presented with an embolic cerebral vascular accident. At surgery this lesion was identified as a fibroma.

Patterns of mitral valve calcification have been studied by D'Cruz et al. (22). Figure 9.20 shows massive mitral annular and mitral apparatus calcification (anterior and posterior submitral calcification). In contrast, Figure 9.21 shows calcification of the chordae tendineae and anterior submitral calcification.

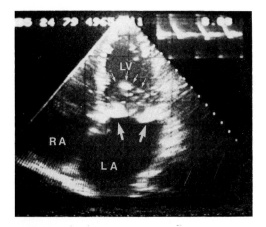

Figure 9.20. Apical four chamber view demonstrating massive mitral apparatus calcification (*arrows*). *LA* = left atrium, *RA* = right atrium.

REFERENCES

1. Levisman JA, Abassi AS, Pearce ML: Posterior mitral leaflet motion in mitral stenosis. *Circulation* 51:511, 1975.
2. Nichol PM, Gilbert BW, Kisslo JA: Two-dimensional echocardiographic assessment of mitral stenosis. *Circulation* 55:120, 1977.

3. Egeblad H, Berning J, Saunamaki K, Jacobensen JR, Wennevold A: Assessment of rheumatic mitral valve disease: Value of echocardiography in patients clinically suspected of predominant stenosis. *Br Heart J* 49:38, 1983.

4. Glover MU, Warren SE, Vieweg WVR, Ceretto WJ, Samtoy LM, Hagan AD: M-mode and two-dimensional echocardiographic correlation with findings at catheterization and surgery in patients with mitral stenosis. *Am Heart J* 105:98, 1983.

5. Henry WL, Griffith JM, Michaelis LL: Measurement of mitral valve orifice area in patients with mitral valve disease by real-time two-dimensional echocardiography. *Circulation* 51:827, 1975.

6. Wann LS, Weyman AE, Dillon JC, Feigenbaum H: Determination of mitral valve area by cross-sectional echocardiography. *Ann Intern Med* 88:337, 1978.

7. Gorlin R, Gorlin SG: Hydraulic formula for calculation of the area of stenotic mitral valve, other cardiac valves and central circulatory shunts. *Am Heart J* 41:1, 1951.

8. Martin RP, Rakowski H, Kleinman JH, Beaver W, London E, Popp RL: Reliability and reproducibility of two-dimensional echocardiographic measurement of the stenotic mitral valve orifice area. *Am J Cardiol* 43:560, 1979.

9. Sutton MJ St J, Oldershaw P, Sacchetti R, Paneth M, Lennox SC, Gibson RV, Gibson DG: Valve replacement without preoperative cardiac catheterization. *N Engl J Med* 305:1233, 1981.

10. Schweizer P, Bardos P, Erbel R, Meyer J, Merx W, Messmer BJ, Effert S: Detection of left atrial thrombi by echocardiography. *Br Heart J* 45:148, 1981.

11. Smith MD, Handshoe R, Handshoe S, Kwan OL, DeMaria AN: Comparative accuracy of two-dimensional echocardiography and Doppler pressure half-time methods in assessing severity of mitral stenosis in patients with and without prior commissurotomy. *Circulation* 73:100, 1986.

12. Shandheria BK, Tajik AJ, Reeder GS, Callahan MJ, Nishimura RA, Miller FA, Seward JB: Doppler color flow imaging: A new technique for visualization and characterization of the blood flow jet in mitral stenosis. *Mayo Clin Proc* 61:623, 1986.

13. Mintz GS, Kotler MN, Segal BL, Perry WR: Two-dimensional echocardiographic evaluation of a patient with mitral insufficiency. *Am J Cardiol* 44:670, 1979.

14. Mintz GS, Victor MF, Kotler MN, Parry WR, Segal BL: Two-dimensional echocardiographic identification of surgically correctable complications of acute myocardial infarction. *Circulation* 64:91, 1981.

15. Wann LS, Feigenbaum H, Weyman AE, Dillon JC: Cross-sectional echocardiographic detection of rheumatic mitral regurgitation. *Am J Cardiol* 51:1258, 1978.

16. Patel AK, Rowe GG, Thomsen JH, Dhanani SP, Kosolcharoen P, Lyle LEW: Detection and estimation of rheumatic mitral regurgitation in the presence of mitral stenosis by pulsed Doppler echocardiography. *Am J Cardiol* 51:986, 1983.

17. Ascah KJ, Stewart WJ, Jiang L, Guerrero JL, Newell JB, Gillam LD, Weyman AE: A Doppler two-dimensional echocardiographic method for quantitation of mitral regurgitation. *Circulation* 72:377, 1985.

18. Miyatake K, Izumi S, Okamoto M, Kinoshita N, Asonuma H, Nakagawa H, Yamamoto K, Takamiya M, Sakakibara H, Nimura Y: Semiquantitative grading of severity of mitral regurgitation by real-time two-dimensional Doppler flow imaging technique. *J Am Coll Cardiol* 7:82, 1986.

19. Mintz GS, Kotler MN, Seagel BL, Perry WR: Two-dimensional echocardiographic recognition of ruptured chordae tendineae. *Circulation* 57:244, 1978.

20. Child JS, Skorton DJ, Taylor RD, Krivokapich J, Abassi AS: M-mode and cross-sectional echocardiographic features of flail posterior mitral leaflets. *Am J Cardiol* 44:1383, 1979.

21. Ballester, M., Foale, R., Presbitrero, P., Yacoub, M., Richards, A., and McDonald, L.: Cross-sectional echocardiographic features of ruptured chordae tendineae. *Eur. Heart J.*, 4: 795, 1983.

22. D'Cruz I, Panetta F, Cohen H, Glick J: Submitral calcification or sclerosis in elderly patients. M-mode and two-dimensional echocardiography in "mitral annulus calcification." *Am J Cardiol* 44:31, 1979.

PART 2
Disorders of the Aortic Valve and Left Ventricular Outflow Tract

BISCUSPID AORTIC VALVE

Bicuspid aortic valve is the most common congenital deformity of the aortic valve and frequently is encountered in adults. Although this condition may have little clinical significance, its recognition may be important in determining the origin of a murmur and in recommending prophylaxis for bacterial endocarditis. M-mode echocardiographic criteria for diagnosis of bicuspid aortic valve have been developed, based on the degree of asymmetry of the closure line of the aortic valve leaflets within the aortic root during diastole (the eccentricity index) (1, 2). Although the eccentricity index is quite useful, it is not completely reliable, since it depends not only on the particular configuration of the leaflets but also on transducer angulation and placement. Therefore, some patients with bicuspid valves may have a normal eccentricity index and some patients may have a variable index, depending on transducer orientation (3) (Fig. 9.22).

Two dimensional echocardiography increases the accuracy of diagnosis of a bicuspid aortic valve by providing anatomic information in several planes. In the parasternal long-axis view, the aortic valve is seen in profile, and asymmetry of closure within the aortic root can be detected more consistently than with M-mode alone (Fig. 9.23A). However, the best view to assess the anatomy of the valve is the parasternal short-axis view, in which the aortic root is transected at the level of the aortic valve and all three leaflets of the normal aortic valve ordinarily can be seen (Figs. 5.24 and 5.25). If an acceptable parasternal short-axis view cannot be obtained, the aortic valve short axis usually can be visualized from the apex (by tilting the transducer slightly superiorly and medially from the four-chamber view (Fig. 5.30)) or from the subcostal approach. Using any of these approaches, it is usually possible to distinguish bicuspid from tricuspid aortic valves, regardless of whether the diastolic closure line is centered within the aortic root, by direct visualization of the two or three leaflets (Figs. 9.23B and 9.24). In either the parasternal short-axis view or the apical view, it is important to sweep the transducer in a superior-inferior plane so as to view the valve in its entirety throughout systole and diastole. In some cases of bicuspid aortic valve, especially when a left ventricular-aortic gradient is present, the valve during systole has a domed appearance in the long-axis view (Fig. 9.25) and appears to be a bull's eye in the short-axis view (Fig. 9.26).

AORTIC STENOSIS

Obstruction to left ventricular outflow can be due to valvular, subvalvular, or supravalvular aortic stenosis. It is often difficult to distinguish the site of obstruction by clinical means, and echocardiography can be of considerable diagnostic value. The spatial orientation and comprehensive anatomic information provided by 2DE is particularly valuable in this regard, with the parasternal long-axis and short-axis views generally being the most useful.

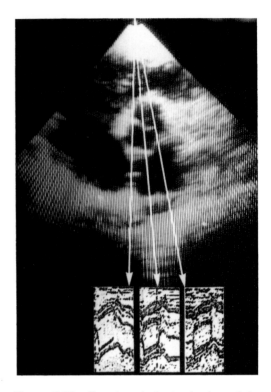

Figure 9.22. Parasternal short-axis view of the aortic root and valve during diastole of a patient with a bicuspid aortic valve, illustrating the appearance of the M-mode echocardiogram (*below*) with variation in the location of the diastolic aortic closure line within the root during diastole, according to the angulation of the M-mode beam.

VALVULAR AORTIC STENOSIS

Valvular aortic stenosis is by far the most common form of left ventricular outflow obstruction in adults. Characteristic echocardiographic features of aortic stenosis in adults include thickening, calcification, and limitation of opening of the valve leaflets (Figs. 9.27–9.31). Although these characteristics are typical of aortic stenosis, they are not specific enough for reliably differentiating valves with significant stenosis from valves with insignificant stenosis or no stenosis. This is because thickening, calcification, and limited opening also can be seen in patients with aortic sclerosis with multiple echoes in the aortic root and with insignificant aortic stenosis.

Ideally, it should be possible to determine the presence and severity of aortic stenosis by measuring the aortic valve area directly from a stop-

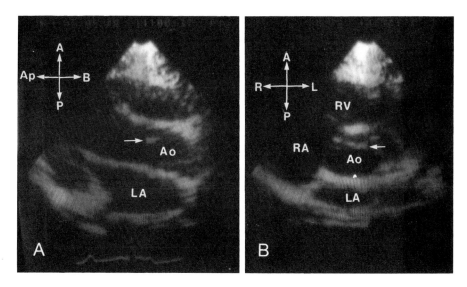

Figure 9.23. *A*, Parasternal long-axis view of aortic root in diastole, showing asymmetric coaptation point of aortic valve leaflets within the aortic root (*arrows*). *B*, Parasternal short-axis view corresponding to *A*, showing asymmetry of valve closure (*arrow*) and two leaflets of unequal size. *A* = anterior, *Ao* = aortic root, *Ap* = apex, *B* = base, *L* = left, *LA* = left atrium, *P* = posterior, *R* = right, *RA* right atrium, *RV* = right ventricle.

action systolic frame of the short-axis view of the aortic valve, as can be done with the mitral valve in mitral stenosis. Unfortunately, this has proved to be difficult in practice, mainly due to problems in accurately outlining the orifice area. In many cases there is incomplete visualization of the entire valve throughout systole, and frequently there is interference with visualization (with multiple

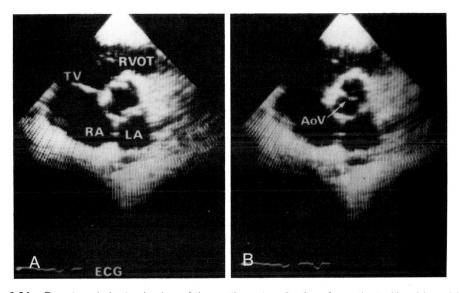

Figure 9.24. Parasternal short-axis view of the aortic root and valve of a patient with a bicuspid aortic valve in systole (*A*) and diastole (*B*), showing a normal leaflet separation in systole and a midline curvilinear valve closure line (*arrow*) in diastole with only two leaflets seen. *AoV* = aortic valve, *LA* = left atrium, *RA* = right atrium, *RVOT* = right ventricular outflow tract, *TV* = tricuspid valve.

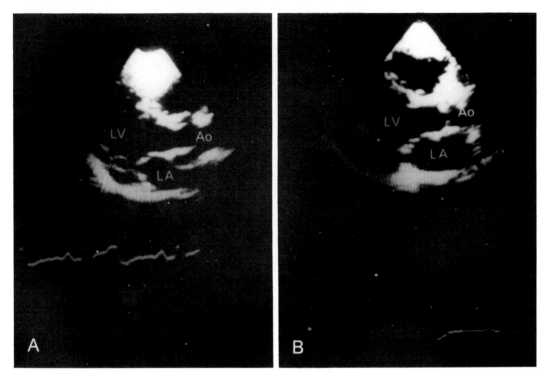

Figure 9.25. Parasternal long-axis views in systole of two patients with bicuspid aortic valves. *A,* Wide leaflet separation and the absence of doming in a patient without a left ventricular aortic gradient. *B,* Another patient with a 40 mm Hg gradient with both systolic doming and limited leaflet separation. *Ao* = aortic root, *LA* = left atrium, *LV* = left ventricle.

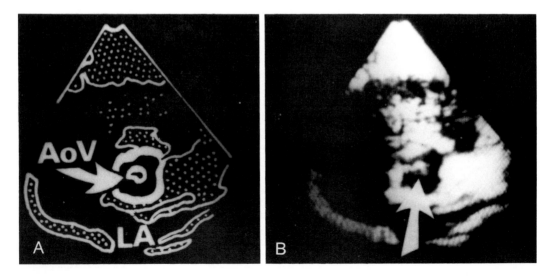

Figure 9.26. *A,* Drawing of parasternal short-axis view. *AoV* = aortic valve, *LA* = left atrium. *B,* Patient with a bicuspid aortic valve with doming, appearing as a bull's eye (circle within a circle).

echoes and reverberations-"blooming") because of extensive calcification of the leaflets and aortic root. In the cases where the valve orifice can be visualized and outlined adequately, transducer placement and angulation should be optimized and gain controls should be adjusted to provide the optimal settings, so that calcification does not result in blooming and thus present an apparent decrease in the actual orifice area. When these precautions are taken, it is possible to assess accurately the severity of aortic stenosis from the short-axis view in selected cases, especially in younger patients without severe calcification (4) (Fig. 9.27D).

to be more generally applicable in distinguishing between normal and stenotic valves, as well as between severely stenotic and mildly stenotic valves. This method does not require measurement of the orifice area, but instead measures maximum leaflet separation from a 2DE long- or short-axis view (Figs. 9.30 and 9.31). Although this is similar in principle to the technique used in M-mode echocardiography for assessing aortic stenosis, the 2DE technique has the advantage of utilizing multiple planes to select the view that best shows maximum leaflet separation.

Comparing this measure to hemodynamic data in adults with and without aortic stenosis, both Weyman et al. (5) and DeMaria et al. (4) found a significant correlation between maximum leaflet separation and the presence and degree of aortic stenosis (Fig. 9.32). A maximum leaflet separation of more than 20 mm was found only in normal subjects, and a leaflet separation of less than 14 mm was always associated with some degree of aortic stenosis. All patients with severe (critical) stenosis had a leaflet separation of between 1 and 12 mm.

In children with aortic stenosis, a much closer relationship exists between aortic leaflet separation, determined by 2DE, and aortic valve area, measured in the catheterization laboratory (6) (Fig. 9.33). The greater accuracy of 2DE in predicting the degree of aortic stenosis in children compared to adults is probably due to several factors. The predominant factor may be superior visualization of valve leaflets in children, generally due to the superiority of echoes in children and specifically due to the lack of calcification of the valve leaflets. The extensive calcification of aortic stenosis in adults tends to obscure the margins of the leaflets and makes accurate measurement of leaflet separation difficult, especially when the gain is too high and blooming occurs.

Another factor that may influence the accuracy of using maximum leaflet separation as an indicator of the severity of aortic stenosis is the effect of stroke volume (4). A diminished stroke volume can further reduce the maximum leaflet separation, resulting in overestimation of the severity of stenosis. This situation is more common in adults, as a result of left ventricular dysfunction secondary to long-standing systolic pressure overload from aortic stenosis or to coexisting ischemic heart disease. An additional common characteristic of aortic stenosis in adults, which may interfere with the extrapolation of measurement of leaflet separation to degree of stenosis, is the asymmetric involvement of the leaflets. There may be unequal separation between leaflets so that measurement of maximal leaflet separation between any two leaflets may not necessarily be representative of total orifice area (4). In contrast, congenital aortic stenosis is characterized by a symmetric, domed appearance (Figs. 9.25 and 9.26) in which the leaflets curve away convexly from the walls of the aortic root in the parasternal long-axis view and appear as a bull's eye in the parasternal short-axis view.

In summary, acquired aortic stenosis in adults is characterized by thickening and calcification of the leaflets, while in children systolic doming is typical. In both cases, leaflet separation during systole is diminished. The degree of limitation of leaflet separation is roughly proportional to the severity of stenosis, with a closer correlation being seen in children than in adults. Direct measurement of aortic valve orifice area from 2DE is potentially the most accurate method of quantitative assessment of aortic stenosis, but presently has limited applicability in adults due to difficulties in imaging.

Once again, Doppler echocardiography answers questions that 2DE and M-mode echocardiography cannot. A well-performed continuous wave Doppler study is not only able to differentiate aortic sclerosis from aortic stenosis, but can evaluate the severity of stenosis and measure the peak systolic gradient across the valve (7–10) (Fig. 9.34). Once the true peak systolic velocity is obtained by the proper orientation of the ultrasound beam inside the eccentric jet, it can be converted to a pressure gradient using the simplified Bernoulli equation:

$$\Delta P = 4 \times v^2$$

(peak systolic gradient across the aortic valve is

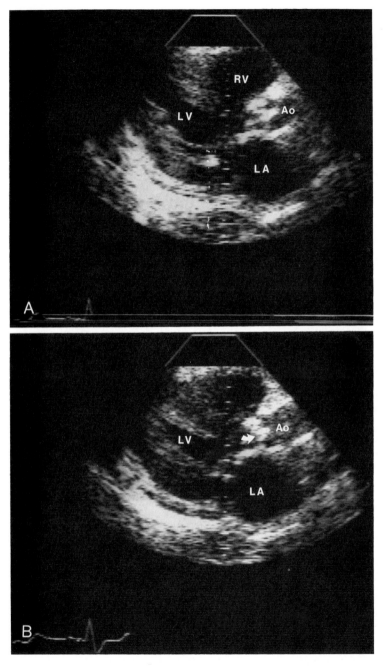

Figure 9.27. Parasternal long- (*A* and *B*) and short- (*C* and *D*) axis views of the aortic root (*Ao*) and valve of a patient with severe aortic stenosis. The bright and dense echoes of the aortic root and valve are consistent with calcification and thickening of these structures. *A* and *C* are diastole frames, and *B* and *D* are systolic frames. In *B*, the valve leaflets show little motion and separation (*arrow*) compared to *A*, consistent with severe stenosis. This is shown better in *C* and *D*, in which the valve orifice can be delineated (*arrows*). *LA* = left atrium, *LV* = left ventricle, *RVOT* = right ventricular outflow tract, *TV* = tricuspid valve.

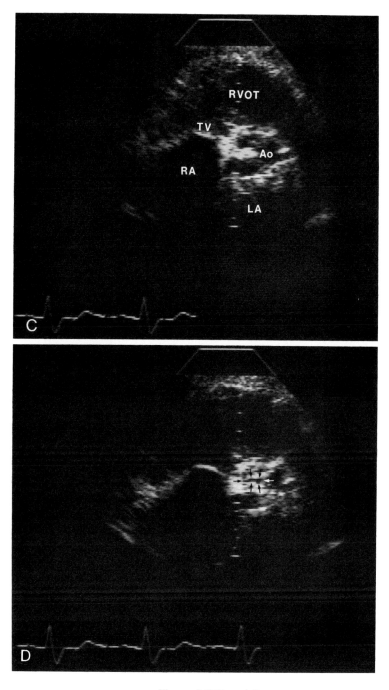

Figure 9.27C and D.

equal to four times the square of peak systolic velocity).

The key is to obtain true peak velocity. Any mistake (usually underestimation) will be squared. Consequently, small differences in velocities can produce large errors in estimating true pressure gradient. Pulsed Doppler is not usable for the diagnosis of aortic stenosis because the high velocities across the stenotic valve exceed the limits of this technique and aliasing occurs (Fig. 9.35).

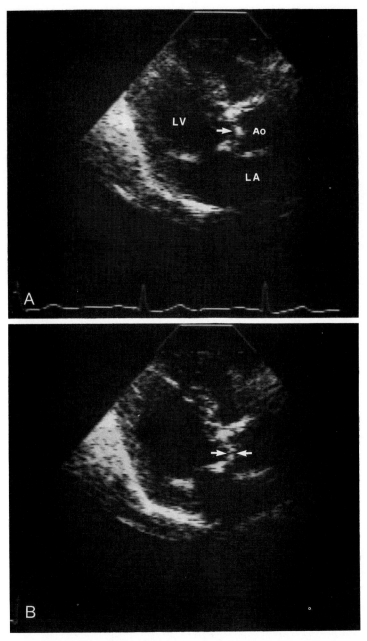

Figure 9.28. Parasternal long-axis view of the aortic root (*Ao*) and valve in diastole (*A*) and systole (*B*) of a patient with severe aortic stenosis, illustrating thickening, calcification, and limitation of valve opening. In *A*, *arrow* points to coapted aortic leaflets in diastole, and in *B*, *arrows* point to valve opening in systole. *LA* = left atrium, *LV* = left ventricle.

Even though improved equipment and transducers that provide simultaneous continuous wave Doppler and 2DE with better penetration and sensitivity are very helpful, the ability of the operator to find the direction of the eccentric jet is what ultimately determines the accuracy of a study. Although the location of the aortic valve and of the ascending aorta is easy to obtain with simultaneous Doppler and 2DE, the precise direction of a small high velocity jet is usually eccentric and

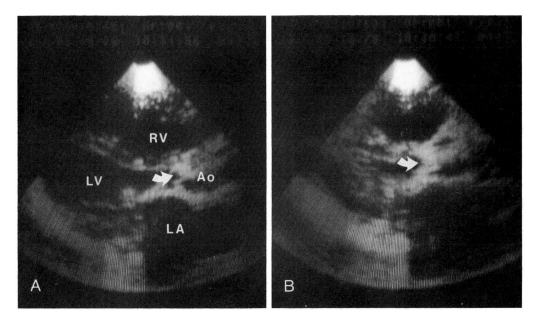

Figure 9.29. Parasternal long-axis views in diastole (*A*) and in systole (*B*) of a patient with severe aortic and mitral stenosis showing how heavy calcification of the aortic root and valve (*arrow*) would not allow measurement of leaflet separation. *Ao* = aortic root, *LA* = left atrium, *LV* = left ventricle, *RV* = right ventricle.

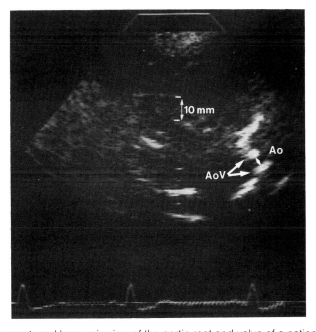

Figure 9.30. Partial parasternal long-axis view of the aortic root and valve of a patient with aortic stenosis (systolic frame). *Large arrows* point to two of the leaflets of the aortic valve, and the *double arrowhead* between the leaflets shows the maximum systolic leaf separation, which in this case measures 4mm. Ten mm size reference is shown. *Ao* = aorta, *AoV* = aortic valve.

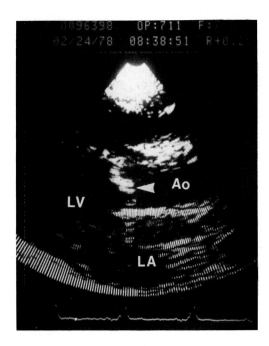

Figure 9.31. Parasternal long-axis view of the aortic root and valve of a systolic frame of a patient with severe aortic stenosis. The maximum leaflet separation is 2 mm. (This is probably underestimated because of the blooming due to calcification in the leaflets.) *Ao* = aortic root, *LA* = left atrium, *LV* = left ventricle.

cannot be predicted. Even when a high velocity jet is found, further search may reveal an even higher velocity jet and provide more accurate test results. This is one of the most challenging and time-consuming tests for a Doppler operator.

Since the direction of the jet is unpredictable, several acoustic windows must be used. The traditional windows are the suprasternal notch (Fig. 9.36) and the first or second right intercostal space with the patient turned to the right side. Less frequently, jet velocities are best obtained from the left sternal border, third right intercostal space, or subcostal view. The apical window has been considered useful. However, the general impression is that when good Doppler signals were recorded from both apical and high right parasternal windows or superstemal notches, the highest velocities more often were obtained from the latter positions than from the apex. The only advantage of the apical approach was that a good signal from the aortic jet could be obtained in practically every patient, especially older pa-

tients; however, a good signal from the aortic jet could not necessarily be obtained.

With the development of better equipment, the importance of the apical view has increased. In our own experience, using an Irex Meridien PCD4, the highest velocities are detected in the majority of cases from an apical view. But still other approaches are used routinely, even with the non-image transducer, which are usually better for the suprasternal notch and high right parasternal windows. The use of a cutaway mattress is essential for the apical view in order to study a patient adequately in the left lateral decubitus position.

The best location for the transducer in the apical area is usually lower and further to the left of the conventional five-chamber view. In this position, the apex is more to the left of the screen,

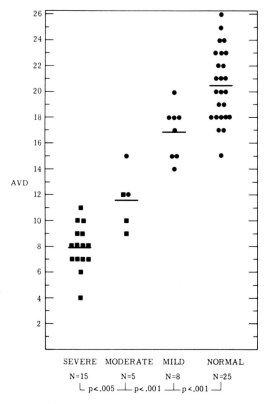

Figure 9.32. Relationship between aortic valve orifice diameter (*AVD*) measured from the two-dimensional echocardiogram and the severity of aortic stenosis in a group of patients studied by cardiac catheterization. (From Weyman AE, Feigenbaum H, Dillon JC, Chang S: Cross-sectional echocardiography in assessing the severity of valvular aortic stenosis. *Circulation* 52:828, 1975. With permission of the American Heart Association, Inc.)

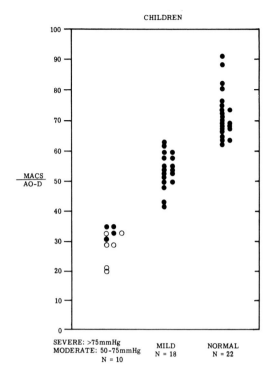

CHILDREN

Figure 9.33. The relationship between maximum aortic cusp separation (*MACS*) as a percentage of aortic diameter (*AO-D*) and degree of aortic stenosis determined by cardiac catheterization in a group of children studied by Weyman et al. (6). *Solid dots* indicate those children with moderate stenosis, and *open circles*, those with severe stenosis. (From Weyman AE, Feigenbaum H, Hurwitz RA, Girod DA, Dillon, JC: Cross-sectional echocardiographic assessment of the severity of aortic stenosis in children. *Circulation* 55:773, 1977. With permission of the American Heart Association, Inc.)

and the septum, instead of being oriented vertically, angles to the left. Using an online transducer, and with the patient in a left lateral decubitus position, access to the acoustic window is virtually impossible without a cutaway mattress.

Once this image is obtained, the continuous wave Doppler is placed simultaneously on the screen with the 2DE image. A search for the highest velocity jet is guided by the 2DE image and the audio signal. The audio signal is extremely important, because the direction of the jet is unpredictable. Next to the jet a harsh sound of high intensity is heard. As the beam moves closer to the jet, higher frequencies will be heard. When the continuous wave beam is fully inside

the jet, a clear, high frequency whistling sound is heard. To be able to record this high velocity it is necessary to scan with delicate, precise movements. The scan not only can move laterally, to the ascending aorta, but also more posteriorly and more anteriorly. Usually an exaggerated five-chamber view (more anteriorly) is better to locate the eccentric jet (Fig. 9.37). Once the highest velocity is found and the spectral analysis is recorded, the search for a higher velocity jet continues from other acoustic windows.

The technical skill of the operator is vitally important in estimating the pressure gradient across the aortic valve, since the severity of aortic stenosis is inferred from this gradient. However, one cannot forget that other factors also may interfere in this evaluation. Severe aortic stenosis may be underestimated in the presence of low cardiac output, even if the recording of the eccentric jet was recorded accurately, because reduced flow decreased the velocity. On the other hand, a mild or moderate stenosis may be overestimated if aortic insufficiency is present, since flow through the aortic valve is increased.

Time to peak systolic velocity can be helpful in estimating the severity of the aortic stenosis. An early peak with low velocity in late systole is found in mild aortic stenosis. As the severity of the aortic stenosis increases, the peak velocity occurs later in systole, and velocities stay high until end-systole.

Color flow mapping is especially useful in locating unusual and small eccentric jets and in

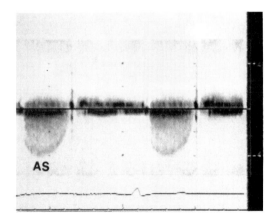

Figure 9.34. Continuous wave Doppler in a patient with aortic stenosis. The high velocity systolic jet (*AS*) moves away from the transducer in the apical view and is displayed below the baseline. The peak velocity is 4 m/sec.

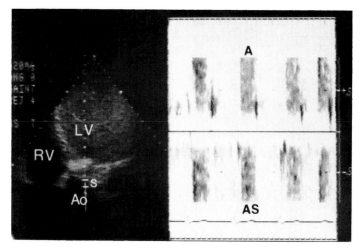

Figure 9.35. Pulsed Doppler in a patient with aortic stenosis. The sample volume (s) is placed in the ascending aorta (Ao) above the aortic valve. Because the velocity of the jet exceeds the limits of the pulsed Doppler, aliasing (A) occurs, and the peak velocity of the aortic stenosis jet (AS) cannot be obtained through standard pulsed Doppler techniques. LV = left ventricle, RV = right ventricle.

guiding the continuous wave beam to record an accurate spectral analysis (11). This technique is presented in the chapter on color flow echo Doppler.

SUBAORTIC STENOSIS

Subaortic stenosis is a relatively common form of congenital aortic stenosis which, on clinical grounds alone, can be difficult to distinguish from valvular aortic stenosis. Subaortic stenosis can oc-

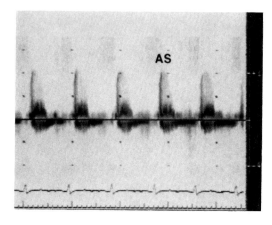

Figure 9.36. Continuous wave Doppler in a patient with aortic stenosis. From the suprasternal notch the high velocity systolic jet (AS) is toward the transducer and displayed above the baseline. The peak velocity is 4.2 m/sec.

cur in several forms, each of which is characterized by obstruction of the left ventricular outflow tract below the level of the aortic valve. The obstruction can be fixed or variable. In the fixed (discrete) form, the obstruction can be caused by the thin membranous ring that encircles the ventricle just below the base of the aortic valve, or it can be caused by a thicker fibromuscular ridge (collar). In a third form, there is a diffuse narrowing of the left ventricular outflow tract by a fibromuscular tunnel.

Although the diagnosis of subaortic stenosis may be suspected from M-mode echocardiography, recognition and characterization of this disorder definitely are facilitated by the enhanced spatial relationships of 2DE. In the parasternal long-axis view, the membranous form may be only partially visualized and appears as two linear echoes, adjacent to the outflow tract, which are in motion throughout the cardiac cycle (12) (Fig. 9.38). In some cases, it may be possible to visualize most or all of the membrane in this view (13) (Fig. 9.39), but the apical long-axis view may provide more consistent visualization of the membrane (14) (Fig. 9.40). The fibromuscular form of subaortic stenosis is characterized by a mass of echoes extending from the interventricular septum into the left ventricular outflow tract (13) (Fig. 9.41). The more diffuse form of subaortic fibromuscular hyperplasia forms a tunnel-like outflow tract.

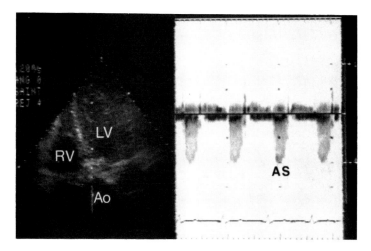

Figure 9.37. Continuous wave (CW) Doppler in a patient with aortic stenosis. The simultaneous two-dimensional image helps to guide the CW beam to find the true direction of the stenotic jet (*AS*) and the highest peak velocity. The peak velocity in this case was 4 m/sec. *Ao* = aorta, *LV* = left ventricle, *RV* = right ventricle.

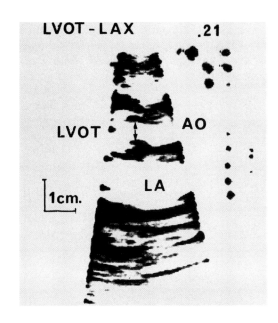

Figure 9.38. Appearance of membranous subaortic stenosis on a parasternal long-axis 30° sector scan. The membrane appears as a distinct linear structure adjacent to the walls of the aorta (*arrows*). *AO* = aorta, *LA* = left atrium, *LVOT* = left ventricular outflow tract. (From Weyman AE, Feigenbaum H, Hurwitz RA, Girod DA, Dillon JC, Chang S. Cross-sectional echocardiography in evaluating patients with discrete subaortic stenosis. *Am J Cardiol* 37:358, 1976, By permission of the *American Journal of Cardiology*).

The use of multiple transducer positions will provide the most diagnostic information and avoid missing subtle membranes or muscular ridges. This ability makes echocardiography superior to angiography for diagnosing this entity. However, at times it can be missed—especially in the presence of ventricular septal defect.

A full discussion of idiopathic hypertrophic subaortic stenosis (IHSS) with particular reference of the controversy of gradient as a cause or effect and "obstruction" is found in Chapter 18. In contrast to discrete subaortic stenosis, the outflow tract "obstruction" is present only (or to a greater extent) during systole rather than throughout the cardiac cycle, and can be increased in response to various maneuvers (e.g., valsalva, amylnitrate, isoproterenol, post-PVC beat). The other features of IHSS not seen in discrete subaortic stenosis include asymmetric septal hypertrophy (occasionally seen in discrete subaortic stenosis but more commonly seen in IHSS).

Doppler echocardiography is able to record flow velocity and has become an essential tool for the complete evaluation of the conditions mentioned above (15). While 2DE is able to image the pathologic anatomy, Doppler is able to identify the presence or absence of "obstruction" to flow through the left ventricular outflow tract, localize the level of the "obstruction," and quantify the degree of stenosis. The window of choice is the five-chamber apical view. Pulsed Doppler is capable of pinpointing the level of obstruction and

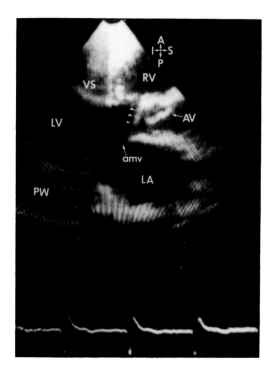

Figure 9.39. Parasternal long-axis view of a patient with discrete membranous subaortic stenosis, demonstrating a thin membrane (*arrowheads*) extending from the interventricular septum toward the anterior leaflet of the mitral valve. *A* = anterior, *amv* = anterior mitral valve leaflet, *AV* = aortic valve, *I* = inferior, *LA* = left atrium, *LV* = left ventricle, *P* = posterior, *PW* = posterior wall of the left ventricle, *RV* = right ventricle, *S* = superior, *VS* = ventricular septum. (From Wilcox WD, Seward JB, Hagler DJ, Mair DD, Tajik AJ: Discrete subaortic stenosis. Two-dimensional echocardiographic features with angiographic and surgical correlation. *Mayo Clin Proc* 55:425, 1980. By permission of the Mayo Clinic.)

mapping the pressure gradient through the left ventricular outflow tract (Fig. 9.42). Continuous wave Doppler is helpful in identifying the direction of flow and obtaining the peak systolic velocity (Fig. 9.43). The peak velocity usually exceeds the limits of the pulsed Doppler and aliasing is therefore recorded on the spectral analysis (Fig. 9.44). The use of other windows, such as the parasternal long axis, suprasternal notch, and subcostal, may help to identify better the direction of the jet and record the highest peak velocity. The use of multiple windows is mandatory for a thorough examination to assure that the highest

peak velocity has been detected. Further details of this technique can be found in the "Aortic Stenosis" section of this chapter.

SUPRAVALVULAR AORTIC STENOSIS

Supravalvular aortic stenosis is a congenital form of left ventricular outflow obstruction in which there is narrowing of the proximal ascending aorta. Its usual manifestation is an hourglass-shaped muscular narrowing, starting immediately distal to the coronary sinuses, but it can also be caused by a fibrous membrane (16). An example of the more common, muscular hyperplasia form is shown in Figure 9.45. The aortic root should be measured at the level of the aortic annulus for comparison to the area of suspected supravalvular stenosis in order to make the diagnosis. Normally the ascending aorta distal to the annulus is at least as wide as at the annular level, whereas in supravalvular stenosis the area of stenosis is narrower than at the annular level. In the four cases of hourglass-type of muscular supravalvular aortic stenosis described by Weyman, there was a 25–61% decrease in aortic diameter at the level of stenosis compared to the level of the aortic annulus (16).

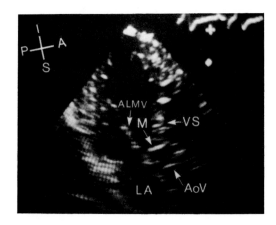

Figure 9.40. Apical long-axis view of a patient with discrete subaortic stenosis, illustrating the membrane (*M*) parallel to the aortic valve (*AoV*). *A* = anterior, *ALMV* = anterior leaflet of the mitral valve, *I* = inferior, *LA* = left atrium, *P* = posterior, *S* = superior, *VS* = ventricular septum. (From DiSessa TG, Hagen AD, Isabel-Jones, JB, Ti CC, Mercier JC, Friedman WF: Two-dimensional echocardiographic evaluation of discrete subaortic stenosis from the apical long axis view. *Am Heart J* 101:774, 1981. By permission of the CV Mosby Company.)

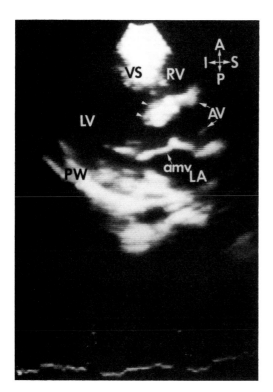

Figure 9.41. Parasternal long-axis view of a patient with a fibromuscular ridge (*arrowheads*) producing subaortic stenosis. The ridge has a broad attachment to the septal wall. (See legend to Figure 9.39 for abbreviations.) (From Wilcox WD, Seward JB, Hagler DJ, Mair DD, Tajik AJ: Discrete subaortic stenosis. Two-dimensional echocardiographic features with angiographic and surgical correlation. *Mayo Clin Proc* 55:425, 1980. By permission of the Mayo Clinic.)

As in subaortic stenosis, Doppler echocardiography has a very important role in the proper diagnosis of supravalvular aortic stenosis. Similarly, pulsed Doppler demonstrates the level of obstruction, and continuous wave Doppler quantifies the pressure gradient (17). The suprasternal notch and five-chamber apical views should be the principal approaches to localize the obstruction and identify the direction of the poststenotic jet.

AORTIC INSUFFICIENCY

Aortic insufficiency may be related to intrinsic disease of the cusp, to primary diseases of the aorta, or to a combination of both. As in any other valvular regurgitation, the main value of both 2DE and M-mode echocardiography is to characterize the etiology of the aortic insufficiency by recognizing the anatomy of the aortic cusps and of the ascending aorta (18). Therefore, when the diagnosis of aortic insufficiency is made by other techniques, the echocardiogram can reveal a bicuspid valve, prolapsed aortic cusp, calcifications or vegetations of the cusps, Valsalva sinus aneurysm, or dilatation and laceration of the ascending aorta—to name just a few. Thus, the diagnosis of aortic insufficiency usually is made only inferentially by 2DE and M-mode echocardiography, according to associated pathology. Direct evidence for aortic insufficiency must await Doppler inquiry.

The major reliable M-mode finding in aortic insufficiency is a high frequency diastolic fluttering of the anterior leaflet of the mitral valve that can be observed on both 2DE and M-mode echocardiography. However, if the regurgitant jet is not directed against the mitral leaflet, if the mitral valve is calcified or fibrotic, or if technical difficulties make the operator unable to direct the imaging beam to the portion of the leaflet affected by the jet, the fluttering of the mitral leaflet may be missed. On the other hand, a prosthetic mitral leaflet may not exhibit fluttering, and in the presence of atrial flutter or atrial fibrillation the fluttering may be obscured (Fig. 9.46C). Consequently, under these conditions aortic insufficiency can be missed. When present, the fluttering of the anterior leaflet of the mitral valve usually is

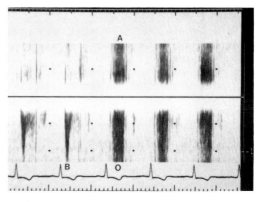

Figure 9.42. Pulsed Doppler in a patient with IHSS aortic stenosis. Pulsed Doppler is able to pinpoint the level of "obstruction" in the outflow tract. The first two systolic flows (*B*) represent the normal outflow velocities before the obstruction. Moving the sample volume one step ahead toward the aortic valve allows the "obstruction" (*O*) to be identified. Aliasing (*A*) occurs in the last three systolic flows.

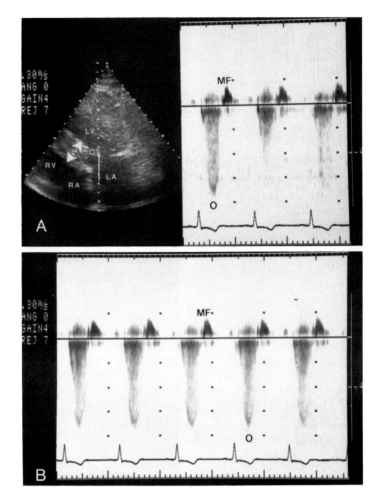

Figure 9.43. *A*, Continuous wave (CW) Doppler in a patient with IHSS. The simultaneous two-dimensional image is helpful to guide the CW beam to the outflow tract of the left ventricle (*OT*) and to obtain the peak systolic velocity. On a five-chamber apical view, the systolic jet after the "obstruction" of the outflow tract is away from the transducer, and velocities of approximately 7.5 m/sec were recorded (*O*). The *arrows* show the thickened interventricular septum (*IVS*). Some normal mitral forward flow (*MF*) is noted. *LA* = left atrium, *RA* = right atrium, *RV* = right ventricle. *B*, Full page of continuous wave Doppler in the same patient showing the high systolic velocities (*O*). Some normal mitral forward diastolic flow (*MF*) again is seen.

recognized better on the M-mode (Fig. 9.46*A* and *B*), which has a superior resolution and a higher sampling rate, than on the 2DE. However, if the resolution of the recording system is poor, the fluttering may resemble a thickened cusp, since the high frequency vibration will not be visible. More rarely, the fluttering may be observed on the interventricular septum if the insufficient jet is directed toward that structure.

Another important indirect finding in aortic insufficiency by echocardiography is left ventricular volume overload with left ventricular dilatation and increased left ventricular wall motion. However, these findings are not specific for aortic insufficiency and can be observed with any volume overload of the ventricle, such as in mitral regurgitation. Such findings may be absent when there is left ventricular dysfunction. The common association of aortic insufficiency with coronary heart disease may also confuse the proper evaluation of left ventricular wall motion and left ventricular internal dimensions. Nevertheless, the

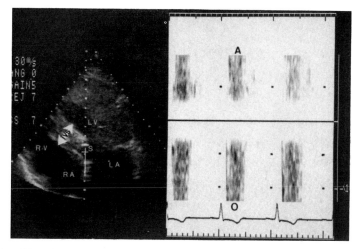

Figure 9.44. Pulsed Doppler in a patient with IHSS. Using a five-chamber apical view, the two-dimensional image guides the position of the sample volume (S) in the outflow tract of the left ventricle. When the level of "obstruction" is found, spectral analysis will show a high velocity systolic jet (O) with aliasing (A), but the actual peak systolic velocity cannot be recorded because it exceeds the limits of conventional pulsed Doppler techniques. *IVS* = interventricular septum, *LA* = left atrium, *LV* = left ventricle, *RA* = right atrium, *RV* = right ventricle.

study of ventricular size and function is important to follow the evolution of patients with aortic insufficiency (19).

Many studies have assessed efficiency of 2DE in establishing the proper time for aortic valve replacement in patients with aortic insufficiency (20–22). However, utilization of M-mode criteria alone has been extremely controversial (23). Stress echocardiography also has been studied with regard to the timing of aortic valve replacement

(24). It has now become clear that echocardiography cannot be the sole criterion used to judge the timing of surgical intervention and that clinical criteria and other studies must be used as well. Controversy notwithstanding, echocardiography is very precise for following deterioration of left ventricular function, and this is among the strongest criteria to influence consideration of surgery.

Doppler echocardiography has become the

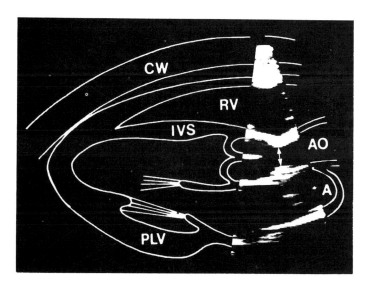

Figure 9.45. Parasternal long-axis view (30° sector scan) and diagram illustrating the appearance of muscular supravalvular aortic stenosis (*arrows*). *A* = atrium, *AO* = aorta, *CW* = chest wall, *IVS* = interventricular septum, *PLV* = posterior left ventricle, *RV* = right ventricle. (From Weyman AE, Caldwell RL, Hurwitz RA, Girod DA, Dillon JC, Feigenbaum H, Green D: Cross-sectional echocardiographic characterization of aortic obstruction. I. Supravalvular aortic stenosis and aortic hypoplasia. *Circulation* 57:491, 1978. With permission of the American Heart Association, Inc.).

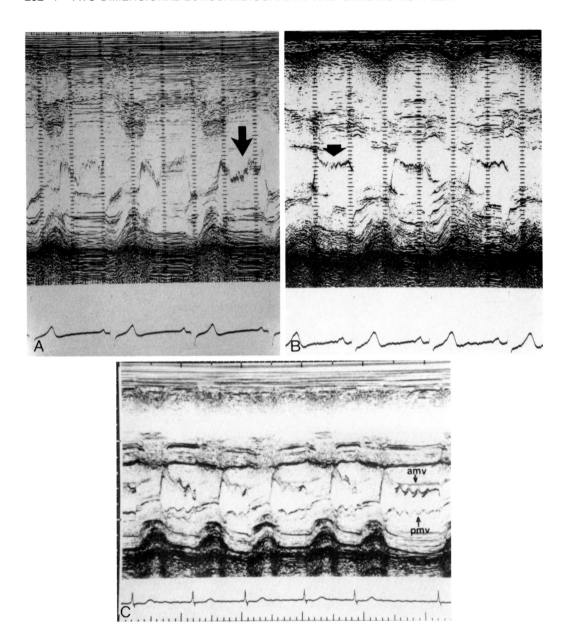

Figure 9.46. *A,* M-mode echocardiogram in a patient with aortic insufficiency. The *arrow* shows the high frequency diastolic fluttering of the anterior leaflet of the mitral valve associated with aortic insufficiency. *B,* M-mode echocardiogram in a patient with aortic insufficiency, showing the characteristic high frequency diastolic fluttering of the anterior mitral valve leaflet (*arrow*) (as seen in *A*). *C,* M-mode echocardiogram in a patient with atrial fibrillation. Diastolic fluttering of both anterior (*amv*) and posterior (*pmv*) leaflets of the mitral valve is noted. This coarse fluttering may obscure fine fluttering secondary to aortic insufficiency.

method of choice for the diagnosis of aortic insufficiency. It is able to identify directly the regurgitant jet and the severity of the disease in a semiquantitative fashion. Using simultaneous 2DE and Doppler echocardiographic equipment, the sample volume of the pulse Doppler is positioned in the left ventricular outflow tract behind the aortic valve in a five-chamber apical view. If aor-

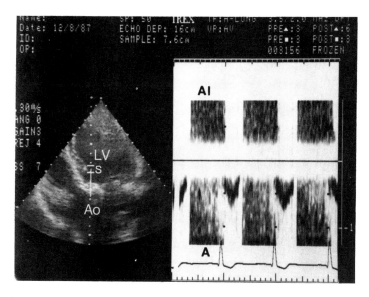

Figure 9.47. Pulsed Doppler in a patient with aortic insufficiency. The sample volume (s) is placed in the outflow tract of the left ventricle (LV) guided by the simultaneous two-dimensional image. The high velocity of the diastolic regurgitant jet toward the transducer (AI) exceeds the limits of the pulsed Doppler, and aliasing (A) occurs. Ao = aorta.

tic insufficiency is present, a harsh, high velocity, turbulent flow pattern will be recognized by the audio signal during diastole. Spectral analysis of the Doppler signal will show aliasing in the diastolic flow, with marked spectral broadening (Fig. 9.47). Aliasing occurs because the high velocity of the regurgitant jet exceeds the limits that the pulsed Doppler is able to record, and an ambiguous flow direction is observed on the spectral analysis. Once the jet is identified, pulsed Dopp-

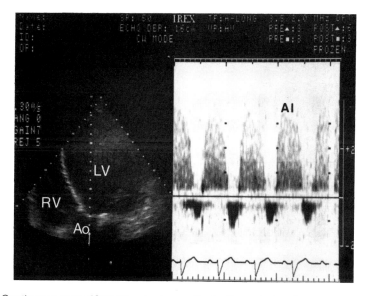

Figure 9.48. Continuous wave (CW) Doppler in a patient with aortic insufficiency. The simultaneous two-dimensional image is helpful to guide the CW beam parallel to the regurgitant jet. When the true direction is obtained, spectral analysis will display the full "envelope" of the diastolic flow toward the transducer (AI) through the incompetent aortic valve (Ao). LV = left ventricle, RV = right ventricle.

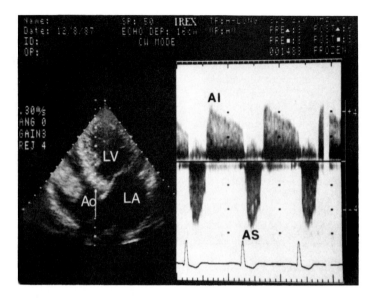

Figure 9.49. Continuous wave Doppler in a patient with severe aortic insufficiency and aortic stenosis. CW Doppler allows the analysis of the contour of the diastolic envelope of the regurgitant jet (*AI*). In severe cases, the maximal velocity decreased rapidly, and in mild cases, the decrease of the maximal velocity is less marked (see Fig. 9.48). This patient has significant aortic stenosis (*AS*) with a peak systolic velocity of approximately 5 m/sec. *Ao* = aorta, *LA* = left atrium, *LV* = left ventricle.

ler is used to determine the width and extension of the jet inside the left ventricle. The severity of aortic insufficiency can be estimated semiquantitatively by this mapping technique.

Even though pulsed Doppler is the principal method used to map a regurgitant jet, continuous wave Doppler is helpful to obtain the true ori-

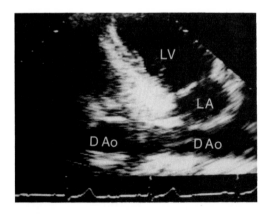

Figure 9.50. Two-chamber apical view visualization of the descending aorta (*D Ao*). The portion proximal to the aortic arch is located posteriorly to the left atrium (*LA*). *LV* = left ventricle.

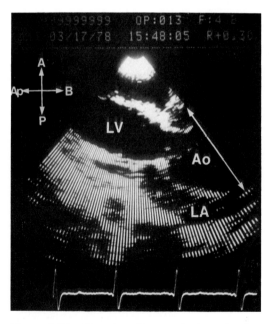

Figure 9.51. Parasternal long-axis view of a patient with Marfan's syndrome and a large aneurysm of the ascending aorta, measuring 9 cm in diameter (*arrow*). *Ao* = aorta, *LA* = left atrium, *LV* = left ventricle.

entation of the jet (25, 26). One cannot forget that the direction of the jet is unpredictable. Simultaneous 2DE and Doppler echocardiography are helpful, but are not enough to localize the Doppler beam or sample volume parallel to the regurgitant jet. The ideal 2DE image is the first step in localizing the aortic valve. From this point on, the search for the proper orientation of the jet starts by moving out of the two-dimensional plane with fine movements guided by the audio signal. Very often, based on a five-chamber apical view, the jet will cross the left ventricle horizontally instead of going vertically to the left ventricular apex. Even in severe cases the jet will reach the lateral wall proximal to the mitral valve.

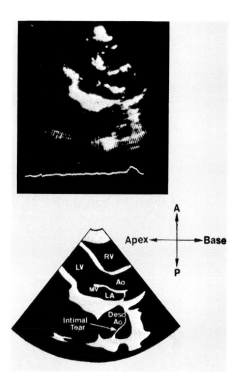

Figure 9.53. Parasternal long-axis view (*top*) and diagram (*bottom*) of a proven type III dissection of the thoracic aorta. *Arrow* denotes the intimal flap separating true from false lumen in an enlarged aorta (*Desc Ao*). *MV* = mitral valve. Other abbreviations are as in Figure 9.52. (From Mintz GA, Kotler, MN, Segal B, Parry WR: Two-dimensional echocardiographic recognition of the descending thoracic aorta. *Am J Cardiol* 44:232, 1979. By permission of the *American Journal of Cardiology*.)

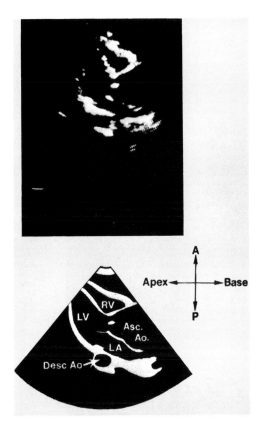

Figure 9.52. Parasternal long-axis views (*top*) and diagram (*bottom*) of a patient with a large aneurysm of the ascending aorta (*Asc. Ao.*) with a normal descending aorta (*Desc Ao*). *A* = anterior, *LA* = left atrium, *LV* = left ventricle, *P* = posterior, *RV* = right ventricle. (From Mintz GA, Kotler MN, Segal B, Parry WR: Two-dimensional echocardiographic recognition of the descending thoracic aorta. *Am J Cardiol* 44:232, 1979. By permission of the *American Journal of Cardiology*.)

Usually differentiation between the diastolic flow of aortic insufficiency and normal distolic flow through the mitral valve is easy because the quality of the Doppler signal is different. However, in the presence of associated mitral stenosis this differentiation may be difficult. In this case, positioning the sample volume of the pulsed Doppler in extreme positions permits characterization and allows the operator to compare and contrast the aortic insufficiency as well as mitral diastolic flow and avoid confusing these different entities. These extreme positions are exactly behind the aortic valve and in the midst of pure mitral flow. It should also be noted that the beam direction to obtain these two different flows is different.

Timing of the flows is also of great help. Aortic regurgitation starts at aortic valve closure before

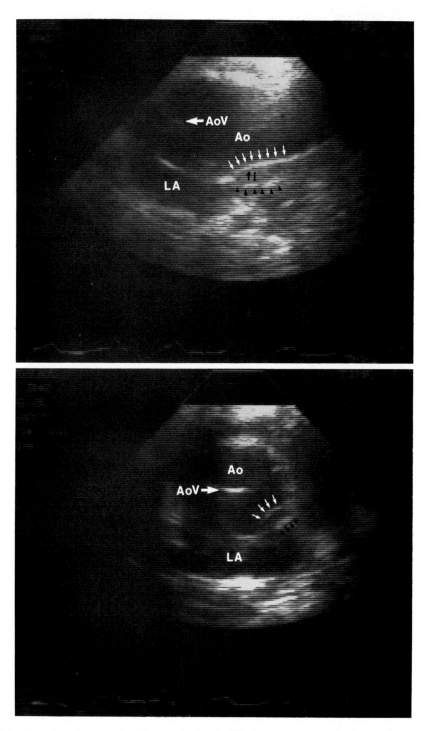

Figure 9.54. Parasternal long-axis (A) and short-axis (B) views of the proximal aorta in a patient with acute dissection along the posterior wall of the proximal aorta. In each view, *white arrows* indicate the dissected intimal flap, and *black arrowheads* indicate the true posterior aortic wall. *Ao* = aorta, *AoV* = aortic valve, *fl* = false lumen, *LA* = left atrium.

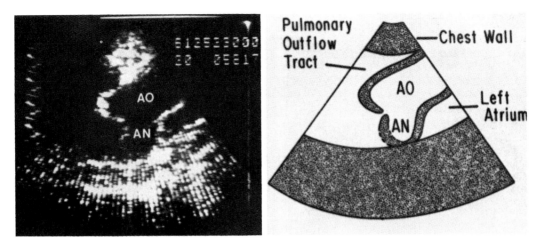

Figure 9.55. Parasternal long-axis view (*left*) and diagrammatic representation (*right*) of a Valsalva sinus aneurysm. *AN* = aneurysm, *AO* = aorta. (From DeMaria AN, Bommer W, Neuman A, Bogren H, Mason DT: Identification and localization of aneurysms of the ascending aorta by cross-sectional echocardiography. *Circulation* 59:755, 1979. With permission of the American Heart Association, Inc.)

the mitral valve opens. In severe mitral stenosis, with early mitral valve opening and aliasing occurring through most of diastole, it is more difficult to map the extension of the aortic insufficiency. Continuous wave Doppler may be useful in this differential diagnosis in that it is possible to record the full envelope of the diastolic flow without aliasing (Fig. 9.48). Also, the velocity pattern displayed on the spectral analysis from aortic insufficiency differs from the pattern of mitral stenosis. The severity of aortic insufficiency may be estimated also by the pattern of flow obtained by continuous wave Doppler. In severe aortic regurgitation, because the pressure gradient between the aorta and the left ventricle diminishes at end-diastole, the maximal velocity of the regurgitation on the spectral analysis decreased rapidly (Fig. 9.49).

The severity of aortic insufficiency also can be estimated by the increased velocity of forward aortic flow in systole. In the absence of aortic stenosis or high cardiac output, a higher peak systolic velocity will be present. This is related to the severity of aortic insufficiency due to increased flow volume across the aortic valve. Similarly, in aortic stenosis, the peak systolic velocity will overestimate the gradient across the aortic valve in the presence of significant aortic insufficiency (Fig. 9.49).

With modern equipment, the apical approach is most helpful in identifying the regurgitant jet and mapping its extension. The use of a parasternal long-axis view is necessary to complement the data. In technically difficult patients the subcostal view will sometimes be the one to assess aortic insufficiency best.

Using either continuous wave or pulsed Doppler, reverse flow velocity in diastole in both the ascending and descending aorta can be demonstrated from the suprasternal notch. This approach was more useful before the development of better transducers permitting simultaneous 2DE and Doppler visualization. Mild aortic insufficiency will not produce this reversed diastolic flow, and other conditions can mimic it. Therefore, it is most useful in moderate-to-severe and severe aortic insufficiency in assessing the severity of the insufficiency.

Color flow mapping is very useful, especially in detecting unusual flow directions that could be missed or underestimated by conventional Doppler (27). This technique is fully discussed in the chapter on color flow echocardiography.

ANEURYSMS OF THE THORACIC AORTA

The most proximal portion of the ascending aorta can be seen in the parasternal long-axis views, apical four- and two-chamber views, subcostal view, and sometimes the suprasternal view. The distal portion of the ascending aorta, as well as the arch and part of the descending aorta can be seen from the suprasternal view (Figs. 5.44 and 5.46). A portion of the descending aorta can be seen in the parasternal long- and short-axis views

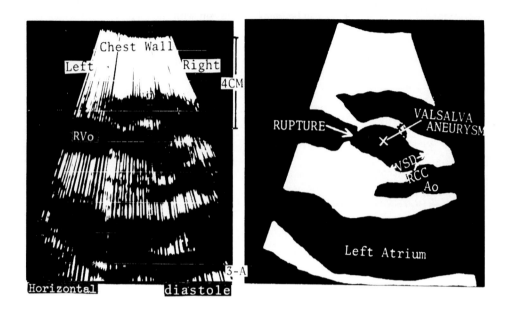

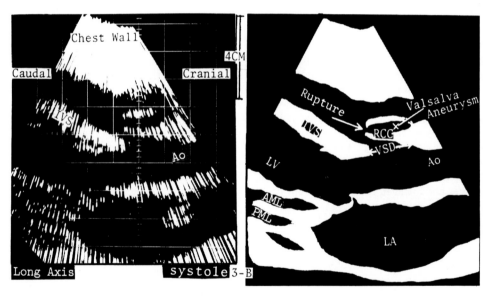

Figure 9.56. Parasternal short-axis view and diagrammatic representation (*top*) and long-axis view and diagrammatic representation (*bottom*) of a patient with a Valsalva sinus aneurysm that ruptured into the right ventricular outflow tract (*RVo*). A supracristal ventricular septal defect (*VSD*) was also present. The area of discontinuity between the right ventricular outflow tract and the aneurysm (*arrow*) was felt to be the site of rupture. *LV = left ventricle, PML = posterior mitral leaflet, RCC = right coronary cusp.* Other abbreviations are as in Figure 9.54. (From Matsumoto M, Matsuo H, Beppu S, Yoshioka Y, Kawashima Y, Nimura Y, Abe H: Echocardiographic diagnosis of ruptured aneurysm of sinus of Valsalva. *Circulation* 53:383, 1976. With permission of the American Heart Association, Inc.)

posterior to the left atrium (Fig. 5.17) as well as in the two-chamber apical view (Fig. 9.50).

Aneurysms of the ascending aorta can be identified in the parasternal long- and short-axis views by demonstration of progressive dilatation of the ascending aorta, starting from the level of Valsalva's sinuses (Figs. 9.51 and 9.52). Normally, the aortic root is widest at the level of the sinuses. A study by DeMaria et al. (28) demonstrated an excellent correlation between aortic dimension by 2DE and contrast angiography in 12 patients with aneurysms of the ascending aorta.

The suprasternal view of the aorta provides visualization of the aortic arch, the proximal portion of the descending aorta, and the origins of some of the arteries arising from the arch (Fig. 5.44). This view may be very useful in assessing the extent of an aneurysm. Likewise, other views of the descending aorta may help define the limits of the aneurysm (29) (Fig. 9.52).

DISSECTIONS

Dissections of the aorta are recognized best on 2DE by demonstration of a flap of intimal tissue within a dilated ascending or descending aorta (30, 31) (Figs. 9.53 and 9.54). This flap separates the true from the false lumen. The presence or absence of active blood flow in the false lumen has been shown to have both prognostic and therapeutic significance. It appears that patients who have no demonstrable flow in the false lumen are the best candidates for medical treatment. Patients with communication between the true lumen and the false channel may have a more favorable outlook if managed surgically. Doppler is also useful to detect aortic insufficiency, which occurs as a common complication of ascending aortic dissection.

VALSALVA SINUS ANEURYSMS

The right and noncoronary sinuses are seen in the parasternal long-axis view, while all three sinuses are visualized in the parasternal short-axis view. Although the diameter of the aorta at the level of the sinuses is normally slightly larger than at the level of the aortic annulus and at the proximal ascending aorta, asymmetric enlargement of one of the sinuses suggests the presence of a Valsalva sinus aneurysm (32) (Fig. 9.55).

An aneurysm of Valsalva's sinus can rupture into any of the cardiac chambers, depending on the location of the aneurysm (33). Diagnosis of a ruptured Valsalva sinus aneurysm depends upon demonstration of a discontinuity in the wall of

the sinus and, under the best circumstances, direct visualization of communication of the aneurysm with the chamber into which it has ruptured (Fig. 9.56). Doppler echocardiography plays an important role in identifying the precise area of the shunt.

REFERENCES

1. Nanda NC, Gramiak R, Manning J, Mahoney EB, Lipchik EO, DeWeese JA: Echocardiographic recognition of the congenital bicuspid aortic valve. *Circulation* 49:870, 1979.
2. Radford DJ, Bloom KR, Izwaka T, Moes CAF, Rowe RD: Echocardiographic assessment of bicuspid aortic valves. Angiographic and pathologic correlates. *Circulation* 53:80, 1976.
3. Fowles RE, Martin RP, Abrams TM, Schapira JN, French JW, Popp RL: Two-dimensional echocardiographic features of bicuspid aortic valve. *Chest* 75:434, 1979.
4. DeMaria AN, Bommer W, Joye J, Lee G, Bouteller J, Mason DT: Value and limitations of cross-sectional echocardiography of the aortic valve in the diagnosis and quantification of valvular aortic stenosis. *Circulation* 62:304, 1980.
5. Weyman AE, Feigenbaum H, Dillon JC, Chang S: Cross-sectional echocardiography in assessing the severity of valvular aortic stenosis. *Circulation* 52:828, 1975.
6. Weyman AE, Feigenbaum H, Hurwitz RA, Girod DA, Dillon JC: Cross sectional echocardiographic assessment of the severity of aortic stenosis in children. *Circulation* 55:773, 1977.
7. Otto CM, Pearlman AS, Comes KA, Reamer RP, Janko CL, Huntsman LL: Determination of the stenotic aortic valve area in adults using doppler echocardiography. *J Am Coll Cardiol* 7:509, 1986.
8. Skjaerpe T, Hegrenaes L, Hatle L: Noninvasive estimation of valve area in patients with aortic stenosis by Doppler ultrasound and two-dimensional echocardiography. *Circulation* 72:810, 1985.
9. Richards KL: Doppler echocardiographic quantification of stenotic valvular lesions. *Echocardiography* 4:289, 1987.
10. Currie PJ, Seward JB, Reeder GS, Vliestra RE, Bresnahan DR, Bresnahan JF, Smith HC, Hagler DJ, Tajik AJ: Continuous-wave Doppler echocardiographic assessment of severity of calcific aortic stenosis: A simultaneous Doppler-catheter correlative study in 100 adult patients. *Circulation* 71:1162, 1985.
11. Po-Hoey F, Kapur, KK, Nanda NC: Color-guided Doppler echocardiographic assessment of aortic valve stenosis. *J Am Coll Cardiol* 12:441, 1988.
12. Weyman AE, Feigenbaum H, Hurwitz RA, Girod DA, Dillon JC, Chang S: Cross-sectional echocardiography in evaluating patients with discrete subaortic stenosis. *Am J Cardiol* 37:358, 1976.
13. Wilcox WD, Seward JB, Hagler DJ, Mair KK, Tajik AJ: Discrete subaortic stenosis. Two-dimensional echocardiographic features with angiographic and surgical correlation. *Mayo Clin Proc* 55:425, 1980.

14. DiSessa TG, Hagan AD, Isabel-Jones JB, Ti CC, Mercier JC, Friedman WF: Two-dimensional echocardiographic evaluation of discrete subaortic stenosis from the apical long axis view. *Am Heart J* 101:774, 1981.

15. Kinney EL, Machado H, Cortada X, Galbut DL: Diagnosis of discrete subaortic stenosis by pulsed and continuous wave echocardiography. *Am Heart J* 110:1069, 1985.

16. Weyman AE, Caldwell RL, Hurwitz RA, Girod DA, Dillon JC, Feigenbaum H, Green D: Cross-sectional echocardiographic characterization of aortic obstruction. I. Supravalvular aortic stenosis and aortic hypoplasia. *Circulation* 57:491, 1978.

17. Lima CO, Sahn DJ, Valdes-Cruz LM, Allen HD, Goldberg SJ, Grenadier E, Barron JV: Prediction of the severity of left ventricular outflow tract obstruction by quantitative two-dimensional echocardiographic Doppler studies. *Circulation* 68:348, 1983.

18. Grayburn PA, Smith MD, Handshoe R, Friedman BJ, DeMaria AN: Detection of aortic insufficiency by standard echocardiography, pulsed Doppler echocardiography, and auscultation,. *Ann Intern Med* 104:599, 1986.

19. Kumpuris AG, Quinones MA, Waggoner AD, Kanon DJ, Nelson JG, Miller RR: Importance of preoperative hypertrophy, wall stress and end-systolic dimension as echocardiographic predictors of normalization of left ventricular dilatation after valve replacement in chronic aortic insufficiency. *Am J Cardiol* 49:1091, 1982.

20. Clark RD, Korcuska KL, Cohn K: Serial echocardiographic evaluation of left ventricular function in valvular disease including reproducibility guidelines for serial studies. *Circulation* 62:564, 1980.

21. Henry WL, Bonow RO, Rosing DR, Epstein SE: Observations on the optimum time for operative intervention for aortic regurgitation. II. Serial echocardiographic evaluation of asymptomatic patients. *Circulation* 61:484, 1980.

22. Bonow RO, Dodd JT, Maron BJ, O'Gara PT, White GG, McIntosh CL, Clark RE, Epstein SE: Long-term serial changes in left ventricular function and reversal of ventricular dilatation after valve replacement for chronic aortic regurgitation. *Circulation* 78:1108, 1988.

23. Fioretti P, Roelandt J, Bos RJ, Meltzer RS, van Hoogenhuijze D, Serruys PW, Nauta J, Hugenholtz PG: Echocardiography in chronic aortic insufficiency: Is valve replacement too late when left ventricular end-systolic dimension reaches 55 mm? *Circulation* 67:216, 1983.

24. Paulsen P: Aortic regurgitation. Detection of left ventricular dysfunction by exercise echocardiography. *Br Heart J* 46:380, 1981.

25. Labovitz AJ, Ferrara RP, Kern MJ, Bryg RJ, Mrosek DG, Williams GA: Quantitative evaluation of aortic insufficiency by continuous wave Doppler echocardiography. *J Am Coll Cardiol* 8:1341, 1986.

26. Masuyama T, Kodama K, Kitabatake A, Nanto S, Sato H, Uematsu M, Inoue M, Kamada T: Noninvasive evaluation of aortic regurgitation by continuous-wave Doppler echocardiography. *Circulation* 73: 460, 1986.

27. Perry GJ, Helmcke F, Nanda NC, Byard C, Soto B: Evaluation of aortic insufficiency by Doppler color flow mapping. *J Am Coll Cardiol* 9:952, 1987.

28. DeMaria AN, Bommer W, Neuman A, Weinert L, Bogren H, Mason DT: Identification and localization of aneurysms of the ascending aorta by cross-sectional echocardiography. *Circulation* 59:755, 1979.

29. Mintz GA, Kotler MN, Segal B, Parry WR: Two-dimensional echocardiographic recognition of the descending thoracic aorta. *Am J Cardiol* 44: 232, 1979.

30. Granato JE, Dee P, Gibson RS: Utility of two-dimensional echocardiography in suspected ascending aortic dissection. *Am J Cardiol* 56:123, 1985.

31. Dagli SV, Nanda NC, Roitman D, Moos S, Hsiung MC, Nath PH, Soto B: Evaluation of aortic dissection by Doppler color flow mapping. *Am J Cardiol* 56:497, 1985.

32. Matsumoto M, Matsuo H, Beppu S, Yoshioka Y, Kawashima Y, Nimura Y, Abe H: Echocardiographic diagnosis of ruptured aneurysm of sinus of Valsalva. *Circulation* 53:383, 1976.

33. Terdjman N, Bourdarias JP, Farcot JC, Gueret P, Dubourg O, Ferrier A, Hanania G: Aneurysms of sinus of Valsalva: Two-dimensional echocardiographic diagnosis and recognition of rupture into the right heart cavities. *J Am Coll Cardiol* 3:1227, 1984.

PART 3
The Tricuspid Valve

The ability to recognize tricuspid valve disease has been enhanced greatly by 2DE, which provides consistent visualization of the tricuspid valve in multiple views. Disorders involving the tricuspid valve are less common than disorders of the mitral or aortic valve. Consequently, it is important to examine carefully the tricuspid valve during a routine echocardiographic examination, as it is easy to overlook a problem that otherwise can be detected. The advent of Doppler echocardiography and color flow imaging has simplified the recognition of tricuspid value disease.

TRICUSPID STENOSIS

Tricuspid stenosis, which is almost always rheumatic in origin, is much less common than tricuspid regurgitation (1). Acquired tricuspid stenosis is due to chronic rheumatic valvulitis or fibrosis of the valve caused by foreign bodies, such as a transvenous permanent pacemaker (Fig. 9.57). Large right atrial tumors may produce a clinical picture suggestive of rapidly progressive tricuspid stenosis, but 2DE is able to differentiate between the two. Chronic rheumatic valvulitis virtually always is associated with rheumatic mitral valve disease.

Viewed by 2DE, the rheumatic tricuspid valve shows thickening and restricted anterior motion with diastolic doming, whereas the normal tricuspid valve opens widely (Fig. 9.58). In tricuspid stenosis, the valve remains in the echocardiographic plane throughout the cardiac cycle due to its restricted motion (2, 3). The M-mode echocardiogram usually shows thickening of the leaflets and reduction of the E-F slope (Fig. 9.59). Calcification of the tricuspid valve leaflets often produces multiple and disorganized echoes. Unfortunately, these M-mode findings are not diagnostic (4). Although 2DE has a high sensitivity and specificity in identifying tricuspid stenosis, it is a poor technique to evaluate its severity. The method of choice for evaluating the severity of tricuspid stenosis is Doppler echocardiography.

Doppler assessment of tricuspid stenosis uses similar techniques to those used in mitral stenosis. Continuous wave Doppler is able to record the spectral analysis of the high velocity diastolic flow through the tricuspid valve (Fig. 9.60). Both the parasternal and apical windows are used to find the highest velocity across the valve, guided mainly by the audio signal. Once the best spectral analysis is obtained, measurement of pressure halftime is used to quantitate tricuspid stenosis, as with mitral stenosis. Usually, pulsed Doppler is

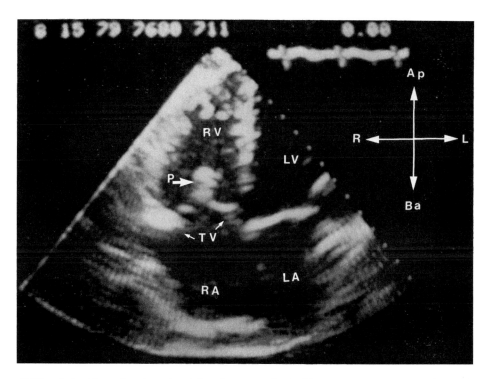

Figure 9.57. Apical four-chamber view taken from a patient with a transvenous pacemaker with manifestations of pure right heart failure. The pacing catheter (*P, large arrow*) is represented by heavy echoes. The tricuspid valve (*TV, small arrows*) appears thickened. No significant motion of the valve could be seen in real time. At surgery, both the pacing electrode and the *TV* showed a heavy buildup of fibrotic tissues. The fibrosis extended into the right atrial (*RA*) wall. *Ap* = apex, *Ba* = base, *L* = left, *LA* = left atrium, *LV* = left ventricle, *R* = right, *RV* = right ventricle.

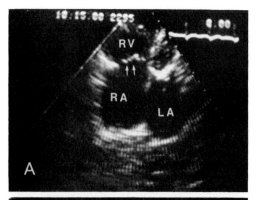

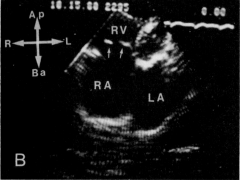

Figure 9.58. Apical four-chamber view of a patient with mitral and tricuspid stenosis, showing a dilated left atrium (*LA*), right ventricle (*RV*), and right atrium (*RA*) during systole (*A*) and diastole (*B*). The tricuspid valve (*arrows*) appears thickened. During diastole (*B*), opening of the valve is restricted. *Ap* = apex, *Ba* = base, *L* = left, *R* = right. (Courtesy of William Graettinger, M.D.)

not helpful, because the high velocity jet of tricuspid stenosis exceeds the limits of the technique and aliasing occurs.

TRICUSPID REGURGITATION

Tricuspid regurgitation is seen most commonly in conjunction with severe right ventricular failure, usually due to mitral valve dysfunction, cardiomyopathy, or coronary artery disease. Regurgitation also can be associated with pulmonary hypertension, tricuspid valve vegetations and tricuspid valve prolapse, and ruptured chordae tendineae (5). In most cases of tricuspid regurgitation the leaflets are intact anatomically, and the mechanism by which the valve becomes incompetent is dilatation of the tricuspid valve ring. Anatomic abnormalities that may be associated

with tricuspid regurgitation include dilatation of the right ventricle, right atrium, inferior vena cava, and hepatic veins (6). In severe cases of tricuspid regurgitation, systolic bowing of the interatrial septum may be seen.

The specific hemodynamic manifestation of tricuspid regurgitation is a systolic regurgitant wave from the right ventricle to the right atrium, extending into the inferior vena cava and hepatic veins. Contrast 2DE has been used in the past to document the systolic regurgitant wave. This technique uses a rapid peripheral venous bolus injection of 4–10 cc of contrast material, usually either agitated saline or indocyanine green dye. The contrast material appears on the video screen as a cloud of echoes, advancing from the right atrium to the right ventricle through the tricuspid valve. In the presence of tricuspid regurgitation, the microcavitations appear to move back and forth across the tricuspid valve (Fig. 9.61). Contrast material also may be seen regurgitating into the inferior vena cava and hepatic veins during systole (Figs. 9.62 and 9.63A and B). Color flow mapping is a useful imaging modality to assess tricuspid regurgitation (7).

The subcostal view is usually the best window to detect tricuspid regurgitation. This view provides the best plane for simultaneous visualization of the tricuspid valve, right atrium, inferior vena cava, and hepatic veins. In this view, systolic pulsation of the inferior vena cava and the hepatic veins can be appreciated. In patients with tricuspid regurgitation secondary to dilation of the tricuspid annulus, the right atrium, right ventricle, and tricuspid annulus usually are enlarged.

In some less common pathologic conditions, tricuspid regurgitation may be associated with anatomic abnormalities of the valve or subvalvular apparatus. These conditions include chronic rheumatic valvulitis, tricuspid endocarditis, Ebstein's anomaly, and tricuspid valve prolapse. Tricuspid regurgitation with tricuspid valve prolapse is more prevalent when associated with mitral valve prolapse (8). Diagnostic criteria for tricuspid valve prolapse by 2DE include the finding of a 2 mm posterior displacement during systole. The measurement is made from line, which connects the two points of attachment of the tricuspid valve to its ring. Tricuspid valve prolapse may occur independently but commonly is associated with prolapse of other valves. The best views to diagnose tricuspid valve prolapse are the parasternal long-axis view of the right ventricle (Figs. 9.64 and 9.65) or the apical four-chamber view.

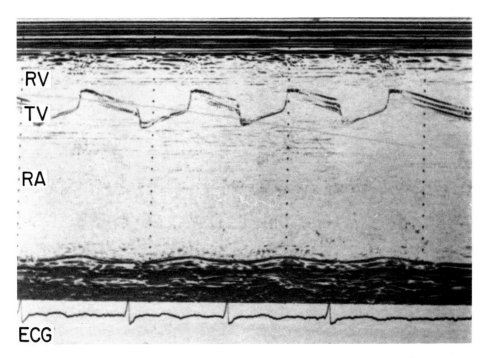

Figure 9.59. M-mode echocardiogram taken from a patient with tricuspid stenosis. The tricuspid valve (*TV*) is thickened, showing a diminished diastolic slope. The right atrium (*RA*) is significantly dilated. *RV* = right ventricle.

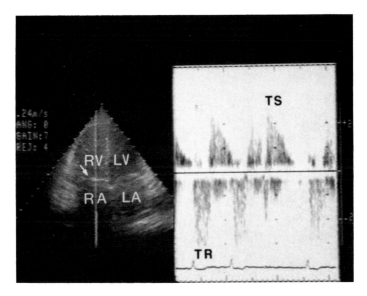

Figure 9.60. Continuous wave (CW) Doppler in a patient with tricuspid stenosis. The CW beam is guided by the simultaneous two-dimensional image through the thickened tricuspid valve (*arrow*). Spectral analysis shows the high velocity flow (over 2 m/sec) toward the transducer (*above the baseline*) during diastole, characteristic of tricuspid stenosis (*TS*). Some valvular regurgitation (*TR*) is also present and is represented by systolic flow away from the transducer (*below the baseline*). *LA* = left atrium, *LV* = left ventricle, *RA* = right atrium, *RV* = right ventricle.

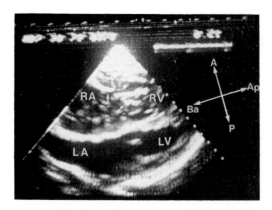

Figure 9.61. Subcostal view of a patient with tricuspid regurgitation following a peripheral injection with contrast material. The contrast material is represented by coarse echoes in the right ventricle (*RV*) and right atrium (*RA*). *A* = anterior, *Ap* = apex, *Ba* = base, *LA* = left atrium, *LV* = left ventricle, *P* = posterior.

The latter view allows a simultaneous assessment of mitral valve pathology (Fig. 9.66).

Carcinoid disease involving the tricuspid valve may produce stiff, immobile leaflets that are continuously open (9). Ebstein's anomaly of the tricuspid valve frequently is associated with tricuspid regurgitation. The principal abnormality in Ebstein's anomaly is downward displacement of the tricuspid valve into the right ventricle (10) (Figs. 9.67 and 9.68).

As in any other regurgitant valvular disease, both M-mode and 2DE are useful in demonstrating an anatomical defect that may cause tricuspid regurgitation. Also, these techniques can identify abnormalities secondary to tricuspid regurgitation, such as enlargement of right-sided chambers, inferior vena cava and hepatic vein dilatation, abnormal motion of the interventricular septum, or systolic pulsation of the interatrial septum or inferior vena cava. However, identifica-

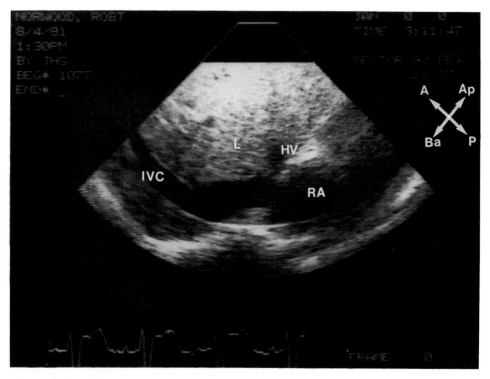

Figure 9.62. Subcostal view of a patient with resected tricuspid valve and severe tricuspid regurgitation. The inferior vena cava (*IVC*) and hepatic vein (*HV*) appear dilated. *A* = anterior, *Ap* = apex, *Ba* = base, *L* = liver, *P* = posterior, *RA* = right atrium.

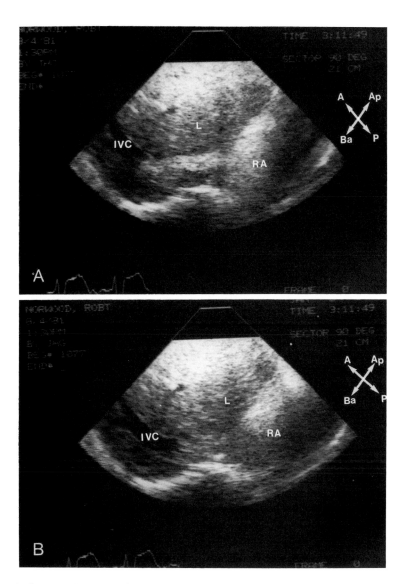

Figure 9.63. *A*, Same patient as in Figure 9.62 after the injection of echo contrast into the right atrium (*RA*). During systole a cloud of echoes fill up the *RA* as well as the inferior vena cava (*IVC*) and hepatic vein. *B*, Same patient as in *A*. During diastole the echo contrast is pushed back toward the *RA*. *A* = anterior, *Ap* = apex, *Ba* = base, *L* = liver, *P* = posterior.

tion and quantification of tricuspid regurgitation are made possible by Doppler echocardiography.

The parasternal, apical, and subcostal views are useful in evaluating tricuspid regurgitation. By placing the sample volume of the pulsed Doppler in the right atrium, immediately behind the tricuspid valve, tricuspid regurgitation's harsh sys-

tolic flow is recognized by the audio signal. The spectral analysis displays a systolic turbulent flow with marked spectral broadening on both sides of the baseline, because the high velocity of the jet exceeds the limits of pulsed Doppler. This phenomenon is called aliasing (Fig. 9.69). Once regurgitation is identified, the sample volume is

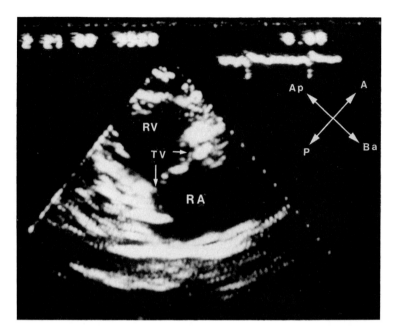

Figure 9.64. Parasternal long-axis view of the right ventricular (*RV*) inflow tract taken during systole. *Arrows* indicate the points of attachment of the tricuspid valve (*TV*) to its ring. The valve appears prolapsing into the right atrium (*RA*) beyond the level of the ring. *A* = anterior, *Ap* = apex, *Ba* = base, *P* = posterior.

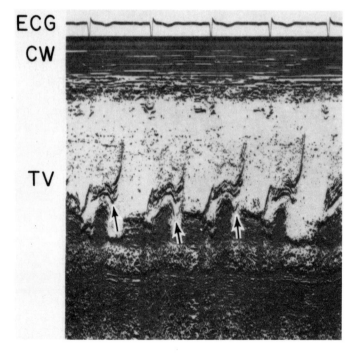

Figure 9.65. M-mode echogram of a tricuspid valve (*TV*). A late systolic posterior deflection (*arrows*) indicates prolapse of the valve. *CW* = chest wall.

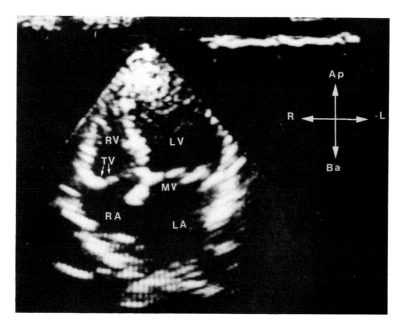

Figure 9.66. Apical four-chamber view taken from a patient with a flail mitral valve (*MV*) and mitral regurgitation. The tricuspid valve (*TV, arrows*) shows a distinct systolic prolapse into the right atrium (*RA*). *Ap* = apex, *Ba* = base, *L* = left, *LA* = left atrium, *LV* = left ventricle, *R* = right, *RV* = right ventricle.

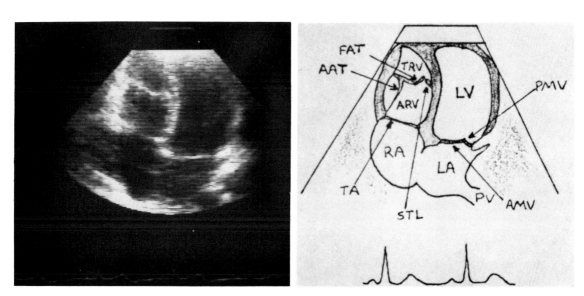

Figure 9.67. Apical four-chamber view (*left*) and schematic representation (*right*) in a patient with Ebstein's anomaly of the tricuspid valve (*TV*). The tricuspid anterior leaflet (*AAT*) can be seen originating from the tricuspid annulus (*TA*) and forming a notch, like a second attachment, where it becomes free of the wall of the "atrialized" right ventricle (*ARV*). Just the distal part of the leaflet, which begins after the notch, is free and represents the "true" anterior leaflet (*FAT*). The small septal leaflet of the tricuspid valve (*STL*) is well visualized. The true right ventricle (*TRV*) is represented by the area from the free portion of the anterior leaflet of the tricuspid valve to the right ventricular apex. The area between the tricuspid annulus and the attached portion of the anterior leaflet represents the atrialized right ventricle (ARV). The ratio of the mitral valve-to-apex distance: tricuspid valve-to-apex distance was found to be 2.5. *AMV* = anterior mitral leaflet, *LA* = left atrium, *LV* = left ventricle, *PMV* = posterior mitral leaflet, *PV* = pulmonary vein, *RA* = right atrium.

displaced for the purpose of mapping the jet in three dimensions (width, length, and depth), as in mitral regurgitation. The severity of the regurgitation can then be mapped (Fig. 9.70).

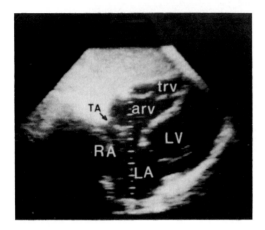

Figure 9.68. Subcostal view in a patient with Ebstein's anomaly. The tricuspid valve is clearly displaced toward the right ventricular apex, dividing this chamber into two portions: the atrialized right ventricle (*arv*) from the tricuspid annulus (*TA*) to the tricuspid valve and the true right ventricle (*trv*) form the tricuspid valve to the RV apex. *LA* = left atrium, *LV* = left ventricle, *RA* = right atrium.

Continuous wave Doppler complements the semiquantitative evaluation provided by pulsed Doppler. With higher limits of velocity, spectral analysis of the continuous wave Doppler is able to display the full envelope with marked spectral broadening of the regurgitant flow during systole (Fig. 9.71). The true direction of the flow can be appreciated without aliasing, displayed below the baseline, because the flow is directed away from the transducer during systole. The peak velocity and the rate of increase in velocity can also be evaluated. Using the simplified Bernoulli equation ($\Delta P = 4v^2$), the systolic pressure gradient between the right atrium and right ventricle can be obtained. If the right atrial systolic pressure is added to this result, the right ventricular systolic pressure is estimated noninvasively. The analysis of central venous pressure in the neck veins gives a good estimation of the right atrial pressure. With a normal right atrial pressure, 5 mm of Hg are added to the systolic pressure gradient. For example, for a tricuspid regurgitation envelope with a peak velocity of 3 m/sec, the estimated peak systolic gradient is 36 mm Hg (4×3^2), and the right ventricular systolic pressure is 41 mm Hg (36 + 5), assuming a normal right atrial systolic pressure of 5 mm Hg.

Studying the rate of increase of velocity of the regurgitant jet provides useful information. The

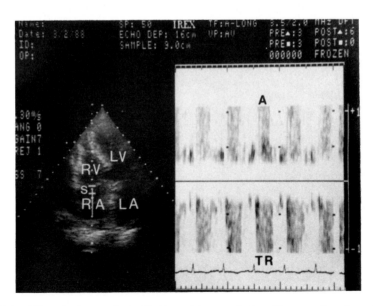

Figure 9.69. Pulsed Doppler in a patient with tricuspid regurgitation. The sample volume (*s*) is placed in the right atrium (*RA*) behind the tricuspid valve, guided by the simultaneous four-chamber apical view. The spectral analysis shows a high velocity systolic flow (*TR*) that exceeds the limits of the pulsed Doppler, and aliasing (*A*) occurs. *LA* = left atrium, *LV* = left ventricle, *RV* = right ventricle.

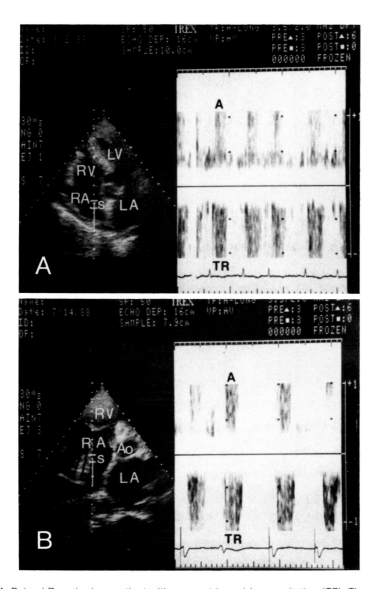

Figure 9.70. *A*, Pulsed Doppler in a patient with severe tricuspid regurgitation (*TR*). The sample volume (*s*) is placed in the right atrium (*RA*) far from the tricuspid valve, guided by simultaneous four-chamber two-dimensional apical view. Spectral analysis shows a strong signal of the *TR* with aliasing (*A*). *B*, A strong signal of tricuspid regurgitation (*TR*) with aliasing (*A*), using a parasternal short-axis view to place the sample volume (*s*) of the pulsed Doppler in the right atrium (*RA*), far from the tricuspid valve. *Ao* = aortic root, *LA* = left atrium, *LV* = left ventricle, *RV* = right ventricle.

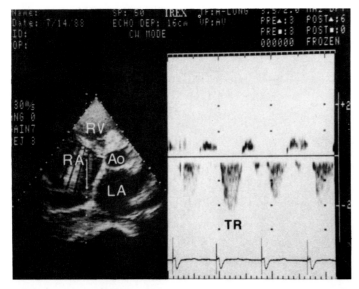

Figure 9.71. Continuous wave (CW) Doppler in a patient with tricuspid regurgitation (*TR*). A simultaneous parasternal short-axis view is used to guide the CW beam through the tricuspid valve. Spectral analysis is able to delineate the full envelope of the high velocity (over 2 m/sec) systolic flow of the *TR* away from the transducer (*below the baseline*). Ao = aortic root, *LA* = left atrium, *RA* = right atrium, *RV* = right ventricle.

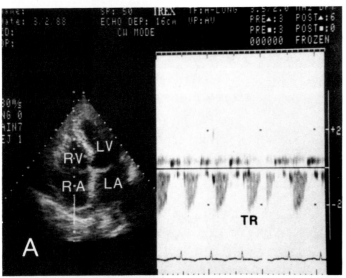

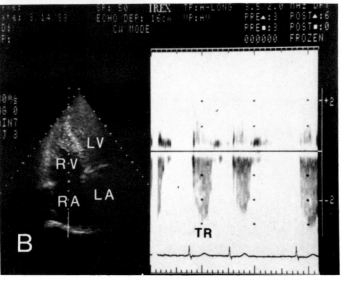

Figure 9.72. Continuous wave Doppler in tricuspid regurgitation (*TR*). Right ventricular function can be estimated by the analysis of the envelope of the *TR*. *A*, In patients with good right ventricular function the peak velocity is reached earlier in systole. *B*, In patients with right ventricular failure, the increase of the velocity is clearly slower. *LA* = left atrium, *LV* = left ventricle, *RA* = right atrium, *RV* = right ventricle.

peak velocity is reached earlier in systole in patients with good right ventricular function (Fig. 9.72*A*) than in patients with right ventricular failure (Fig. 9.72*B*), where the increase in velocity clearly is slower.

REFERENCES

1. Daniels SJ, Mintz GS, Kotler MN: Rheumatic tricuspid valve disease. Two-dimensional echocardiographic, hemodynamic, and angiographic correlations. *Am J Cardiol* 51:492, 1983.
2. Guyer DE, Gillam LD, Foale RA, Clark MC, Dinsmore R, Palacios I, Block P, King ME, Weyman AE: Comparison of the echocardiographic and hemodynamic diagnosis of rheumatic tricuspid stenosis. *J Am Coll Cardiol* 3:1135, 1984.
3. Nanna M, Chandaratna A, Reid C, Nimalasuriya A, Rahimtoola SH: Value of two-dimensional echocardiography in detecting tricuspid stenosis. *Circulation* 67:221, 1983.
4. Shimada R, Takeshita A, Nakamura M, Tokunaga K, Hirata T: Diagnosis of tricuspid stenosis by M-mode and two-dimensional echocardiography. *Am J Cardiol* 53:164, 1984.
5. Eckfeldt JH, Weir EK, Chesler E: Echocardiographic findings in ruptured chordae tendineae of the tricuspid valve. *Am Heart J* 105:1033, 1983.
6. Moreno FLL, Hagan AD, Holman, JR, Pryor, TA, Strickland RD, Castle CH: Evaluation of size and dynamics of the inferior vena cava as an index of right-sided cardiac function. *Am J Cardiol* 53:579, 1984.
7. Suzuki Y, Kambara H, Kadota K: Detection and evaluation of tricuspid regurgitation using a real-time, two-dimensional, color-coded, Doppler flow imaging system: Comparison with contrast two-dimensional echocardiography and right ventriculography. *Am J Cardiol* 57:811, 1986.
8. Ogawa S, Hayashi J, Sasaki H, Tani M, Handa S, Hakamura Y: Evaluation of combined valvular prolapse syndrome by two-dimensional echocardiography. *Circulation* 65:174, 1982.
9. Forman MB, Byrd BF, Oates JF, Robertson RM: Two-dimensional echocardiography in the diagnosis of carcinoid heart disease. *Am Heart J* 107:492, 1984.
10. Shiina A, Seward JB, Edwards WD, Hagler DJ, Tajik AJ: Two-dimensional echocardiographic spectrum of Ebstein's anomaly: Detailed anatomic assessment. *J Am Coll Cardiol* 3:356, 1984.

PART 4
The Pulmonic Valve

The pulmonic valve is a semilunar structure and comprises three cusps: anterior, right, and left. The right ventricular outflow tract and pulmonic valve can be visualized from the parasternal and subcostal views (Figs. 5.16, 5.24, and 5.41). The short-axis view at the level of the aortic valve will show the right ventricular outflow tract wrapping around the aorta, pulmonic valve, and pulmonary artery. In comparison to individuals without disease, these structures are imaged by M-mode echocardiography with less consistency and more difficulty. Whereas only a portion of the left pulmonic cusp is routinely seen with M-mode echocardiography, it is often possible to image two leaflets of the pulmonic valve with 2DE simultaneously and to assess directly the morphology of this valve.

PULMONIC STENOSIS

Pulmonic stenosis is one of the common congenital cardiac malformations seen in adult patients. Pulmonic stenosis may involve the pulmonic valve, the subvalvular region, or the pulmonary artery and its branches. However, approximately 80% of all cases of right ventricular outflow tract obstruction involve the pulmonic valve. The diagnosis of pulmonic stenosis by M-mode echocardiography is indirect, relying upon the demonstration of an exaggerated A wave in the tracing of the posterior leaflet motion resulting from a partial opening of the valve (Fig. 9.73). However, this is a nonspecific and insensitive sign of pulmonic stenosis. This pattern of early partial valve opening can be recognized readily from the 2DE (1).

Direct visualization of the anatomic features of the valve by 2DE is a much more specific method for diagnosis of pulmonic stenosis. The characteristic abnormality of congenital pulmonic stenosis is systolic doming of the valve, seen in both mild and severe stenosis (Fig. 9.74). The valve leaflets may be seen in the pulmonary artery lumen throughout systole and never assume a normal position parallel to the vessel wall. The leaf-

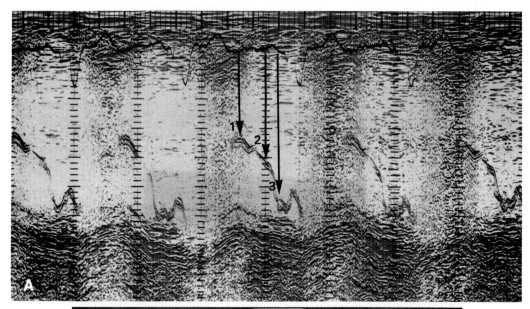

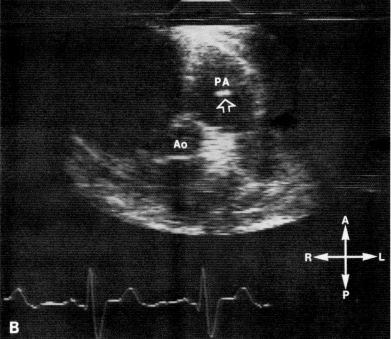

Figure 9.73. *A*, M-mode recording (*A*) and corresponding two-dimensional echocardiographic stop-frame photographs in the parasternal short-axis view of the pulmonary artery (*B, C,* and *D*) of a patient with pulmonic stenosis, demonstrating the early partial opening of the pulmonic valve (from position 1 (*A* and *B*) to position 2 (*A* and *C*) and the exaggerated A wave (position 3 (*A* and *D*). *Arrows* in *B, C,* and *D* point to the pulmonic valve position. *A* = anterior, *Ao* = aorta, *L* = left, *P* = posterior, *PA* = pulmonary artery, *R* = right.

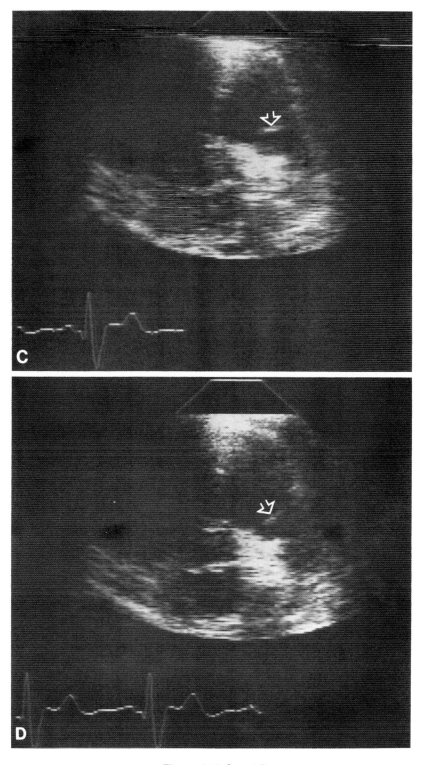

Figure 9.73.*C* and *D.*

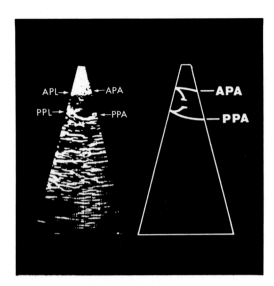

Figure 9.74. Parasternal long-axis view (*left*) and diagrammatic representation (*right*) of 30° sector scan of a patient with pulmonary stenosis, illustrating systolic doming of the valve leaflets. APL = anterior pulmonary leaflet, PPL = posterior pulmonary leaflet, APA = anterior wall of pulmonary artery, PPA = posterior wall of pulmonary artery. (From Weyman AE, Hurwitz RA, Girod DA, Dillon JC, Feigenbaum H, Green D: Cross-sectional echocardiographic visualization of the stenotic pulmonary valve. *Circulation* 56:769, 1977. With permission of the American Heart Association, Inc.)

lets may also appear thickened and exhibit extra echoes. The right ventricular pressure overload that occurs in pulmonic stenosis is associated with hypertrophy of the right ventricular free wall and with straightening of the ventricular septum that persists in diastole and systole. Pulmonic stenosis is a rare finding in adults, and the Doppler demonstration of an increased flow velocity in the pulmonary artery should prompt a search for other etiologies that result in an increased flow volume through the right heart.

Doppler echocardiography can demonstrate increased flow velocity across the pulmonic valve and is used to generate estimates of the pressure gradient across it (2). The parasternal short-axis view is the window of choice to guide the Doppler beam parallel to the flow from the right ventricular outflow tract to the pulmonary artery. Continuous wave Doppler is the method of choice to detect the peak systolic velocity across the pulmonic valve and to evaluate the severity of the stenosis (Fig. 9.75). Pulsed Doppler may not be helpful in recording the peak systolic velocity because of aliasing. However, it is very helpful in finding the level of obstruction, i.e., infundibular, valvular, or supravalvular (3). Once the level of obstruction is found by pulsed Doppler, the highest peak systolic velocity is obtained by further orientation of the transducer, guided by the audio signal. The peak systolic pressure gradient is again estimated by use of the modified Bernoulli equa-

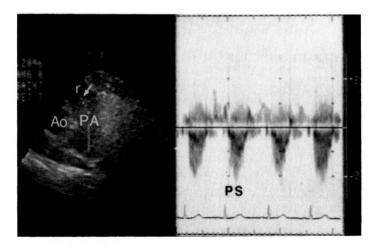

Figure 9.75. Continuous wave (CW) Doppler in a patient with pulmonic stenosis. A simultaneous short-axis parasternal view is used to guide the CW beam through the pulmonic valve (*arrow*). Spectral analysis shows the high velocity (over 2 m/sec) systolic flow of pulmonic stenosis (*PS*) away from the transducer (*below the baseline*). Ao = aorta, PA = pulmonary artery, r = right ventricular outflow tract.

tion ($\Delta P = 4v^2$), where the peak systolic pressure gradient across the pulmonic valve is equal to four times the peak systolic velocity squared. Color flow mapping also has been used to detect eccentric flow jets (see Chapter 7, Color Flow Mapping). When tricuspid regurgitation is present, the velocity of the regurgitant blood can be used to estimate right ventricular systolic pressure.

PULMONIC INSUFFICIENCY

Pulmonic insufficiency is usually the consequence of pulmonary hypertension or bacterial endocarditis. Although in this situation there are no morphologic abnormalities of the valve, echocardiography may suggest this diagnosis by demonstrating diastolic fluttering of the tricuspid valve. Contrast 2DE studies have been used in the assessment of pulmonic insufficiency (4). An agitated saline solution containing microbubbles is injected into a peripheral vein while the right ventricular outflow tract is being imaged. Pulmonic insufficiency would result in passage of contrast from the pulmonary artery, across the pulmonic valve, and into the right ventricular outflow tract during diastole (Fig. 9.76).

Doppler echocardiography is the method of choice to diagnose pulmonic insufficiency. From the parasternal window, the Doppler beam is parallel to the flow from the right ventricular outflow tract to the pulmonary artery. The sample volume of the pulsed Doppler is placed in the right ventricular outflow tract behind the pulmonic valve, guided by the simultaneous 2DE image. If pulmonic insufficiency is present, a harsh, high velocity, turbulent flow will be heard in the audio signal during diastole. Spectral analysis of the Doppler signal will show aliasing in the diastolic flow (Fig. 9.77). Aliasing occurs because the high velocity of the regurgitant jet exceeds the limits that pulsed Doppler is able to record and an ambiguous direction of the flow is observed. The width and extension of the jet inside the right ventricle is mapped by moving the sample volume of the pulsed Doppler inside the right ventricular outflow tract.

Continuous wave Doppler is helpful in recording the peak velocity and the full envelope of diastolic flow without aliasing (Fig. 9.78). Mild pulmonic insufficiency is a frequent finding in "normal" patients having Doppler examinations. The pressure gradient across the pulmonic valve can be estimated if pulmonic insufficiency is demonstrated by Doppler echocardiography (5). Since

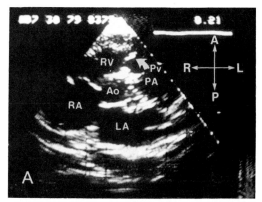

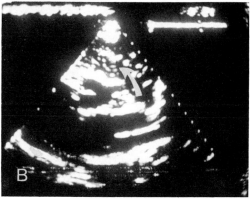

Figure 9.76. Parasternal short-axis views of the pulmonary outflow tract before (*A*) and after (*B*) the peripheral injection of agitated saline. In *A*, *arrow* indicates the position of the pulmonic valve (*PV*). In *B*, *arrow* indicates the contrast effect of the agitated saline within the right ventricular outflow tract during diastole. *A* = anterior, *AO* = aorta, *L* = left, *LA* = left atrium, *P* = posterior, *PA* = pulmonary artery, *R* = right, *RA* = right atrium, *RV* = right ventricle.

right ventricular and right atrial pressure are equal at end-diastole, the pulmonary artery diastolic pressure can be estimated by adding the end-diastolic pressure gradient calculated across the pulmonic valve to the right atrial pressure (6).

PULMONARY HYPERTENSION

Both M-mode and 2DE have a low sensitivity and specificity for the diagnosis of pulmonary hypertension. Neither method can quantitate pulmonary artery pressure. The diagnosis of pulmonary hypertension by M-mode echocardiography depends upon the demonstration of a decrease in A wave magnitude with flat diastolic slope, midsystolic notching, and an increase in

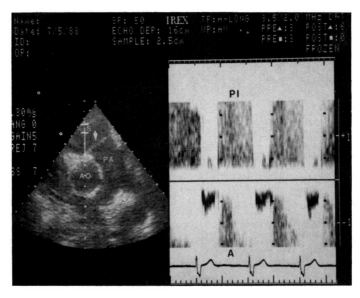

Figure 9.77. Pulsed Doppler in a patient with pulmonic insufficiency (*PI*). The sample volume (*s*) is placed in the right ventricular outflow tract behind the pulmonic valve (*arrow*) guided by a simultaneous short-axis parasternal two-dimensional view. Spectral analysis shows the high velocity diastolic flow of pulmonic insufficiency (*PI*) with aliasing (*A*). *AO* = aorta, *PA* = pulmonary artery.

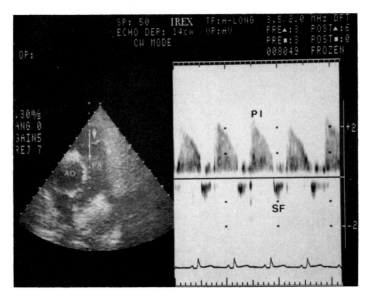

Figure 9.78. Continuous wave (CW) Doppler in a patient with pulmonic insufficiency (*PI*). A simultaneous parasternal short-axis two-dimensional view is used to guide the CW beam through the pulmonic valve (*arrow*). The full envelope of the high velocity diastolic flow of *PI* is represented in the spectral analysis above the baseline (flow toward the transducer). The normal forward systolic flow (*SF*) is represented below the baseline, following the QRS complex of the ECG (flow away from the transducer). *AO* = aorta, *PA* = pulmonary artery.

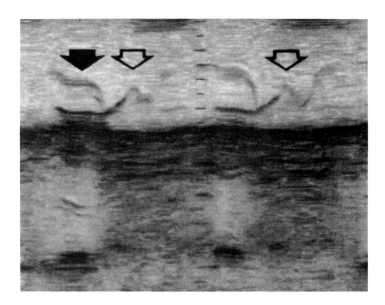

Figure 9.79. M-mode echocardiogram of the pulmonary valve in a patient with pulmonary hypertension. Absence of the *A* wave on a flat diastolic slope (*closed arrow*) and a systolic notch (*open arrow*) are the M-mode findings suggestive of pulmonary hypertension.

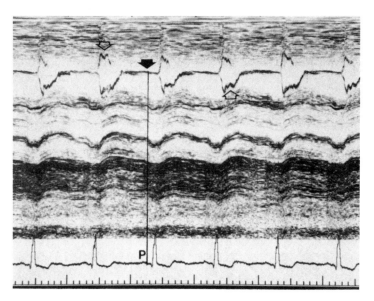

Figure 9.80. M-mode echocardiogram of the pulmonary valve in a patient with pulmonary hypertension. In such patients, the pulmonary valve is better seen, and often two of the cusps can be recorded. The *closed arrow* shows the absence of the *a* wave on a flat diastolic slope, following the P wave of the ECG. The *open arrow* shows the systolic notch in the anterior leaflet and in one of the posterior leaflets of the pulmonary valve.

right ventricular presystolic ejection time (de-layed opening) and decrease in ejection time (Figs. 9.79 and 9.80). Since there is no structural ab-normality of the pulmonic valve, 2DE adds little to the diagnosis other than the nonspecific dem-

onstration of a dilated pulmonary artery, which usually is present in chronic pulmonary hyper-tension. Figure 9.81 shows the abnormal closed position of the pulmonic valve in early systole, with bowing of the leaflets into the right ventric-

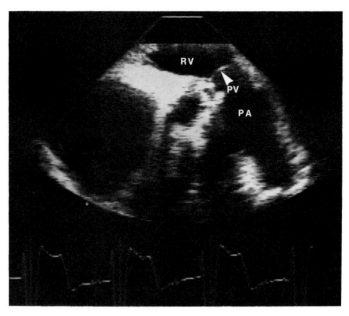

Figure 9.81. Parasternal short-axis view of the right ventricular outflow tract illustrating the closed position and bowing of the pulmonic valve (*arrow, PV*) in a patient with pulmonary hypertension. *PA* = pulmonary artery, *RV* = right ventricle.

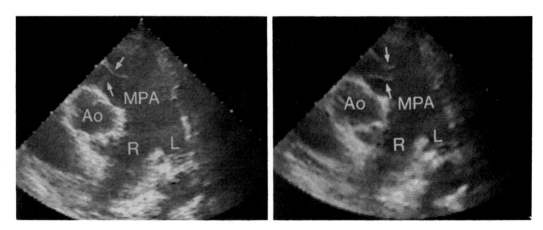

Figure 9.82. Parasternal short-axis views in a patient with idiopathic dilatation of the pulmonary artery. The dramatic dilatation of the main pulmonary artery (*MPA*) can be appreciated when compared to the diameter of the aorta (*Ao*). Both right (*R*) and left (*L*) branches of the pulmonary artery also are dilated and visualized much further than usual. *Left*, Two of the leaflets of the pulmonary valve (*arrows*) are identified clearly, closed in diastole. *Right*, The same patient showing the pulmonary leaflets (*arrows*) opening in systole.

ular outflow tract in a patient with pulmonary hypertension.

Idiopathic dilatation of the pulmonary artery is suspected when a dilated pulmonary artery is seen in the absence of signs of pulmonary hypertension, pulmonic stenosis, or left-to-right shunt. In such cases, it will be noted that the pulmonic valve is seen more readily than in normal individuals because of the prominence of the pulmonary artery (Fig. 82*A* and *B*). Doppler echocardiography is able to demonstrate the presence of pulmonic insufficiency and tricuspid regurgitation, usual findings in pulmonary hypertension. The study of the spectral analysis of the systolic flow through the pulmonary artery and of the preejection time is also very important for the diagnosis of pulmonary hypertension. This pathology will increase the preejection interval (from the beginning of the QRS to the onset of systolic flow), and peak systolic velocity is reached earlier in systole (shortening of the acceleration time). Also, the pulmonary systolic flow may present a midsystolic notch, as seen in M-mode tracings.

Another pulmonary artery abnormality that can be recognized by 2DE and Doppler echocardiography is branch stenosis of this vessel. The suprasternal and parasternal approaches have been utilized to identify both left and right pulmonary artery stenosis.

REFERENCES

1. Weyman AE, Hurwitz RA, Girod DA, Dillon JC, Feigenbaum H, Green D: Cross-sectional echocardiographic visualization of the stenotic pulmonary valve. *Circulation* 56:769, 1977.
2. Johnson GL, Kwan OL, Handshoe S, Noonan JA, DeMaria AN: Accuracy of two combined two-dimensional echocardiography and continuous wave Doppler recordings in the estimation of pressure gradient in right ventricular outlet obstruction. *J Am Coll Cardiol* 3:1013, 1984.
3. Hagler DJ, Tajik AJ, Seward JB, Ritter DG: Noninvasive assessment of pulmonary valve stenosis, aortic valve stenosis, and coarctation of the aorta in critically ill neonates. *Am J Cardiol* 57:369, 1986.
4. Meltzer RS, Vered Z, Hegesh T, Benjamin P, Visser CA, Shem-Tov AA, Neufeld HN: Diagnosis of pulmonic regurgitation by contrast echocardiography. *Am Heart J* 107:102, 1984.
5. Masuyama T, Kodama K, Kitabatake A: Continuous-wave Doppler echocardiographic detection of pulmonary regurgitation and its application to noninvasive estimation of pulmonary artery pressure. *Circulation* 74:484, 1986.
6. Chan KL, Currie PJ, Seward JB, Hagler DJ, Mair DD, Tajik AJ: Comparison of three Doppler ultrasound methods in the prediction of pulmonary artery pressure. *J Am Coll Cardiol* 9:549, 1987.

10

Echocardiography of Mitral Valve Prolapse

Robert M. Davidson, M.D.

Since the first descriptions of the echocardiographic findings of mitral valve prolapse (MVP) in 1970–1971 (1–3), echocardiography has become the standard technique to diagnose or to confirm the clinical diagnosis of this disorder. At the present time, echocardiography probably is utilized more often in the average outpatient echocardiography laboratory for this purpose than for the evaluation of any other condition. In one such representative laboratory, almost one-half of all patients referred for echocardiographic examination in an average year were referred for evaluation of known or suspected MVP (R. M. Davidson, unpublished observations).

Despite the widespread utilization of echocardiography for this purpose and the general acceptance of this technique as the "gold standard" for the diagnosis of MVP, there has been increasing concern and debate over the validity of previously accepted criteria for the echocardiographic diagnosis of MVP, as well as over the role of echocardiography in the diagnosis of this syndrome.

ANATOMIC-PATHOLOGIC BASIS OF MITRAL VALVE PROLAPSE

Before discussing the specific echocardiographic findings of MVP, it would be worthwhile to review the basic anatomic abnormalities characteristic of this disorder. These have been described by various investigators to consist of: (*a*) displacement of part or all of one or both leaflets into the left atrium during systole, resulting in "billowing" or "ballooning" of the valve into the atrium, (*b*) redundancy (increased size) of the valve leaflets, (*c*) increased thickness of the valve leaflets, (*d*) mitral annular dilatation (and "disjunction"), (*e*) failure of leaflet apposition, and

(*f*) elongation, thickening, and abnormal insertion of the chordae tendineae, sometimes with rupture (4–14). Histologically, the basis of idiopathic (primary) MVP generally is believed to be myxomatous degeneration (6, 8, 13), although it recently has been demonstrated that in a significant proportion of patients with MVP the etiology is postinflammatory (following acute rheumatic carditis) (15–17).

ECHOCARDIOGRAPHY OF MITRAL VALVE PROLAPSE

Echocardiographic characteristics of normal mitral valve motion during systole have been well established by two-dimensional and M-mode echocardiographic techniques. As ventricular diastole ends and systole begins (between the *A* and *C* points on the M-mode echo [Fig. 10.1*A*]), the edges of the anterior and posterior leaflets of the mitral valve move toward each other and make contact (coaptation), resulting in closure of the valve (Fig. 10.1*B* in the two-dimensional parasternal long-axis view). The leaflets remain together until the beginning of diastole (point *D* on the M-mode echo). During this time (the *C* to *D* interval on the M-mode echo), there is normally an anterior (upward) motion of the valve structure as the ventricle contracts. There is also an inferior (caudal) motion of the mitral annulus and valve, toward the left ventricular apex (18, 19), which can best be appreciated on the parasternal long-axis view of the two-dimensional image.

In contrast to normal mitral valve motion, the most consistent echocardiographic abnormality of MVP, both by M-mode and by two-dimensional techniques, is posterior and superior displacement of all or part of one or both leaflets into the left atrium during systole (1–3). Figure

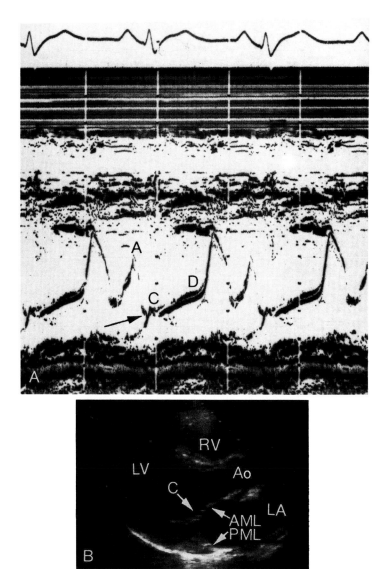

Figure 10.1. *A*, M-mode echocardiogram of normal mitral valve, illustrating normal coaptation of the anterior and posterior leaflets at point *C* (*arrow*), with gradual anterior motion of the closed valve during systole (between points *C* and *D*). *B*, Two-dimensional parasternal long-axis view of a normal mitral valve during systole, illustrating the normal appearance of the closed valve and the coaptation point of the anterior and posterior leaflets (*C*). *RV* = right ventricle, *LV* = left ventricle, *Ao* = aorta, *LA* = left atrium, *AML* = anterior mitral leaflet, *PML* = posterior mitral leaflet.

10.2 illustrates typical M-mode tracings showing this characteristic feature. This posterior displacement can involve one or both leaflets and can occur either in mid-to-late systole only (Fig. 10.2*A*) or throughout systole (holosystolic "hammocking") (Fig. 10.2*B*). The type of prolapse pattern (mid-to-late systolic versus holosystolic) can vary not only among patients, but even within an individual patient. Several studies have shown that conditions that decrease left ventricular size, such as standing, administration of amyl nitrite, performance of Valsalva's maneuver, or the devel-

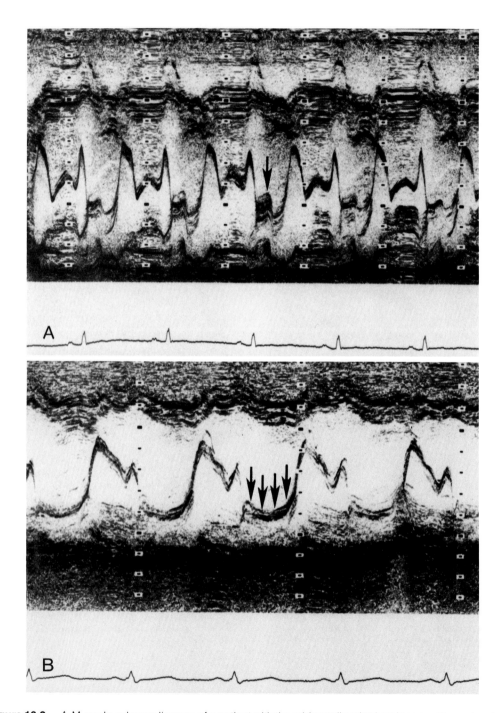

Figure 10.2. *A*, M-mode echocardiogram of a patient with the midsystolic mitral prolapse pattern, showing the abrupt and marked posterior motion of both leaflets (*arrow*) into the left atrium at midsystole. *B*, M-mode echo of a patient with the holosystolic mitral prolapse pattern, showing the "hammock"-type motion (*arrows*).

NORMAL

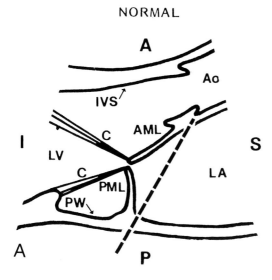

ANTERIOR AND POSTERIOR
LEAFLET PROLAPSE

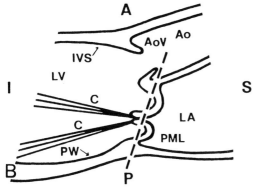

late systolic prolapse pattern to the holosystolic pattern (1–3, 20–23).

The anatomic basis of MVP can be appreciated best utilizing the two-dimensional echo technique, where systolic displacement of the mitral valve leaflet(s) into the left atrium can be seen best in either the parasternal long-axis view or the apical four-chamber view. In these views, one or both leaflets can be seen to "bow" or "arch" superiorly (cephalad) and posteriorly through the plane of the mitral valve annulus into the left atrium. (19, 24–27) (Figs. 10.3–10.6).

Although the above-described abnormalities of MVP are the major echocardiographic findings, a number of other abnormalities also have been

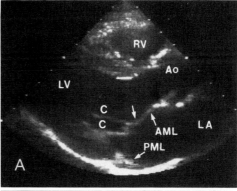

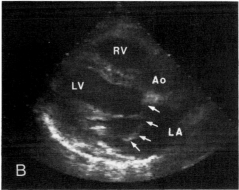

Figure 10.3. *A,* Diagrammatic representation of a parasternal long-axis view of the heart during systole, illustrating the normal closed position of the mitral leaflets and their relationship to the plane of the mitral annulus (*dashed line*). *B,* The same view, illustrating a patient with mitral prolapse, showing the superior displacement of both leaflets beyond the plane of the mitral annulus, into the left atrium. *I* = inferior, *A* = anterior, *S* = superior, *P* = posterior, *LV* = left ventricle, *C* = chordae tendineae, *IVS* = interventricular septum, *AML* = anterior mitral leaflet, *PML* = posterior mitral leaflet, *Ao* = aorta, *AOV* = aortic valve, *LA* = left atrium, *PW* = posterior left ventricular wall. (From Feigenbaum H: *Echocardiography,* ed 4. Philadelphia, Lea & Febiger, 1986, p. 272.)

opment of tachycardia or ectopic beats can lead to earlier systolic posterior displacement of the mitral leaflets or the conversion of the mid-to-

Figure 10.4. Parasternal long-axis views of systolic frames of two-dimensional echoes. *A,* A patient with mild MVP. The *arrow* points to the point of superior bowing of the anterior mitral leaflet toward the left atrium. *B,* A patient with marked MVP, showing a very large and thick anterior mitral leaflet (*arrows*) bowed superiorly beyond the plane of the mitral annulus. *RV* = right ventricle, *LV* = left ventricle, *C* = chordae tendineae, *Ao* = aorta, *LA* = left atrium, *AML* = anterior mitral leaflet, *PML* = posterior mitral leaflet.

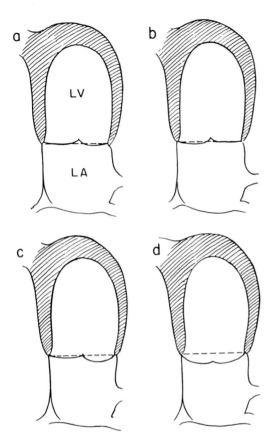

Figure 10.5. Diagrammatic representation of the left ventricle (*LV*) and left atrium (*LA*) in the apical four-chamber view illustrating mild prolapse of the posterior leaflet (*a*), anterior leaflet (*b*), moderate prolapse of both leaflets (*c*), and severe prolapse of both leaflets (*d*). In *a* and *b* the coaptation point is above the plane of the mitral annulus (*dashed line*), whereas in *c* it is at the plane, and in *d* it is below the plane. (From Perloff JK, Child JS, Edwards JE: New guidelines for the clinical diagnosis of mitral valve prolapse. *Am J Cardiol* 57:1127, 1986. Reproduced by permission of Technical Publishing.)

described in both M-mode and two-dimensional echocardiograms in patients with this disorder, and are of interest and useful to varying degrees. Haikal and associates (28) summarized and reviewed 12 different types of abnormalities on M-mode echo alone which have been described in patients with MVP. One such abnormality, which had been described a number of years ago on the M-mode echo, is the presence of multiple echoes during systole (Fig. 10.7). This finding, subsequently analyzed by two-dimensional echo-

cardiography, is believed to represent the superimposition of echoes as the M-mode beam transects a redundant valve (and/or chordae tendineae) at various points, as well as due to artifact of beam width (20, 24, 26, 29) (Figs. 10.8 and 10.9). It should be noted that the presence of multiple parallel systolic echoes sometimes can be seen in normal individuals (28–31) and does not by itself constitute a diagnostic sign of MVP (Fig. 10.10).

Another echocardiographic feature noted in some patients with MVP is increased thickness of the mitral valve (30–34) (Fig. 10.11). Although this finding occasionally is seen in normal subjects, Nishimura and associates (31) found that patients with MVP frequently had a valve thickness of 5 mm or more (measured during diastole on the M-mode tracing), whereas normal subjects had a thickness of less than 5 mm (Fig. 10.12).

An increased diastolic excursion and rate of opening of the anterior leaflet of the mitral valve also are noted sometimes in echocardiograms of patients with MVP. This has been referred to as a "whip-like" motion (19, 24) sometimes resulting in the anterior leaflet contacting the interventricular septum (31, 32, 35) (Figs. 10.9*B*, 10.11*B*, and 10.13). Again, this is an inconsistent finding and one commonly seen in normal subjects, and thus not a useful sign for diagnosing MVP (28).

Among other M-mode abnormalities occasionally noted in patients with MVP is one that usually is associated with idiopathic subaortic stenosis rather than MVP: systolic anterior motion of the mitral valve (SAM). This finding, when seen in patients with MVP, is probably secondary to redundancy of the chordae tendineae (25, 36, 37).

Two other echocardiographic findings sometimes noted in MVP include excessive posterior coaptation of the mitral leaflets and an abnormal "curling" motion of the mitral valve annulus (19, 20, 38). The point of leaflet coaptation has been found to be abnormally posterior (closer to the posterior wall of the left atrium) on the parasternal long-axis view in patients with MVP compared to normal subjects, probably secondary to excessively large anterior leaflets (Fig. 10.14). This abnormality, along with the abnormal "curling" motion of the mitral annulus, in which the annulus moves in a normal caudal direction, but not simultaneously in the normal anterior motion, probably accounts for at least some of the posterior motion of the mitral leaflets seen in the M-mode echo (19, 20, 38).

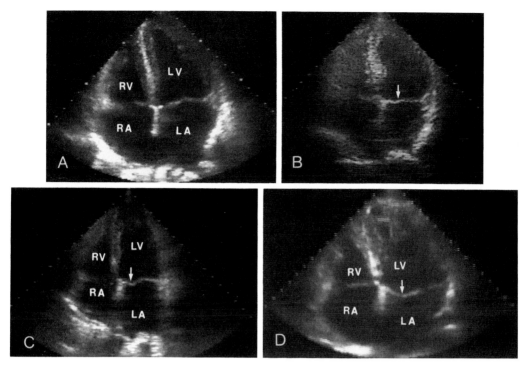

Figure 10.6. Two-dimensional apical four-chamber views of a normal patient (*A*), a patient with mild prolapse of the anterior leaflet (*B*), a patient with moderate prolapse of the anterior leaflet (*C*), and a patient with severe prolapse of the anterior leaflet (*D*). The *arrows* indicate the point of maximal prolapse. *RV* = right ventricle, *RA* = right atrium, *LV* = left ventricle, *LA* = left atrium.

Failure of leaflet coaptation (apposition) is believed by some authors to be a characteristic functional abnormality of MVP, accounting for the presence of mitral regurgitation, when present (6). This abnormality is actually synonymous with a flail leaflet, which can be seen on the echocardiograms of some patients with MVP (Fig. 10.15), but is neither characteristic nor unique for MVP patients (28).

The most recently recognized echocardiographic sign of MVP is mitral annular dilatation. In studies utilizing the two-dimensional technique, linear measurement of mitral annular size and calculated estimates of annular circumference and area corresponded with the presence and severity of MVP. Patients with MVP, especially if severe, had a larger annular size than normal subjects (39–41). (The techniques for calculating mitral annular size are beyond the scope of this chapter and are detailed in the referenced articles).

It recently has been suggested that there are two distinct phenotypic types of patients with MVP:

one characterized by mitral leaflet billowing and normal anulus size, and the other characterized by a dynamic expansion of the mitral anulus during systole and absence of leaflet billowing (42).

Although all of these echocardiographic signs are helpful in recognizing patients with MVP, it has become increasingly apparent that many normal subjects also have findings on M-mode and/or two-dimensional echocardiography that suggest MVP and that there is obvious overlap between the appearance of normal and prolapsed mitral valves in regard to echocardiographic findings. Current thinking is that rather than being two completely distinct entities, a continuum probably exists between normal and prolapsed mitral valves, and thus there may be an area of uncertainty in diagnosis based on echo findings alone (14, 23, 28, 43–52). Although the ultimate clinical definition of mitral valve prolapse remains to be defined and there is no true "gold standard" for establishing the diagnosis, guidelines have been drawn to distinguish between "normal" and "prolapse" patterns on both M-mode and two-dimen-

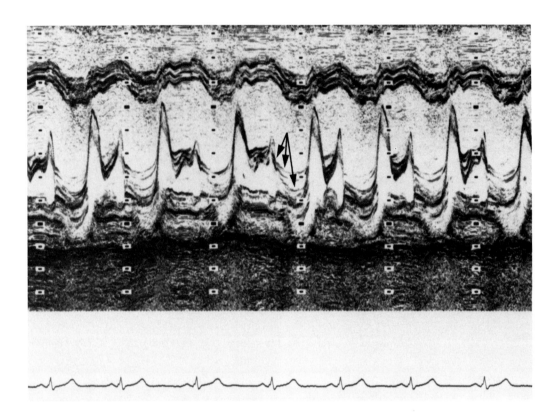

Figure 10.7. M-mode echocardiogram of a patient with pansystolic mitral prolapse, illustrating multiple echoes during systole (*arrows*).

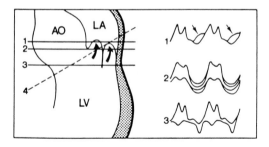

Figure 10.8. Diagrammatic illustration of a two-dimensional parasternal long-axis view (the orientation is vertical rather than horizontal, as is current custom), of a patient with mitral prolapse, showing the various M-mode patterns of mitral valve motion obtained by different transducer positions (sectors), resulting in multiple systolic echoes and a pansystolic prolapse pattern only in position 3. *Ao* = aorta, *LA* = left atrium, *LV* = left ventricle. (From Sahn DS, Allen HD, Goldberg SJ, Friedman WF: Mitral valve prolapse in children. A problem defined by real-time cross-sectional echocardiography. *Circulation:* 53, 656, 1976. Reproduced by permission of the American Heart Association, Inc.)

sional echoes, based on the extent of posterior and superior displacement of the mitral leaflets. Since mild degrees of systolic displacement of one or both leaflets can be seen in normal subjects, criteria have been recommended for the minimum amount of displacement to qualify as prolapse. On the M-mode tracing, the degree of displacement is determined by drawing a line from the C point to the D point (Fig. 10.16). There is some disagreement in the literature as to how much a leaflet must be displaced below this line to be considered diagnostic of prolapse. Haikal and associates (28) found that *any late* systolic posterior motion was highly specific for MVP. Other echocardiographers have used as a diagnostic criterion a minimum displacement of 2.0 mm (43, 45), while still others have suggested 3.0 mm (28, 31, 53), and as much as 5 mm has also been suggested (54). Obviously, using the 3 mm (or 5 mm) measurement as a minimum criterion increases the specificity of diagnosis, while the 2 mm criterion increases the sensitivity. In a study of 343 patients with MVP who had at least 3 mm

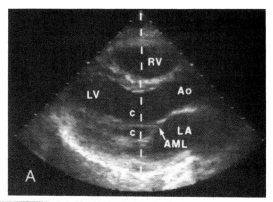

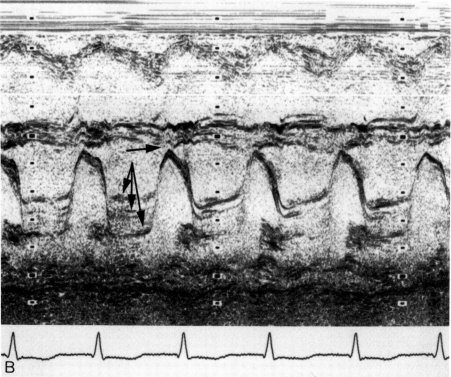

Figure 10.9. Long-axis parasternal two-dimensional echocardiogram (*A*) and M-mode echocardiogram (*B*) of a patient with mitral valve prolapse indicating intersection of an M-mode beam (*dashed line*) with several (thickened) chordae and the mitral valve leaflet, resulting in multiple systolic echoes on the M-mode echo of the mitral valve during systole (*vertical arrows*). Also illustrated is the increased excursion of the mitral leaflet in diastole, with a very small *E* point-septal separation (*horizontal arrow*). *RV* = right ventricle, *LV* = left ventricle, *Ao* = aorta, *LA* = left atrium, *C* = chordae tendinae, *AML* = anterior mitral leaflet.

of displacement below the *C–D* line, the range of displacement was 3 to 22 mm, and the mean was 7 mm (31), suggesting that 3 mm is not an unrealistic lower limit for diagnosis. In a recent review, Devereux and coauthors (14) suggested using 2 mm of posterior displacement as a minimum criterion for MVP if a pattern of late systolic displacement is seen, but using 3 mm as a

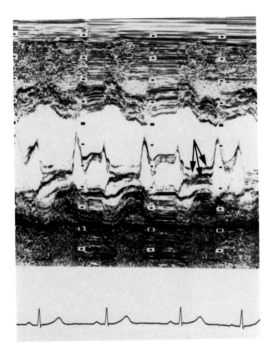

Figure 10.10. M-mode echocardiogram of a normal patient, showing multiple echoes during systole (*arrows*).

minimum when a holosystolic pattern is seen, and *then* only in conjunction with confirmation by two-dimensional echocardiography.

Similarly, utilizing two-dimensional echo, attempts have been made to determine which view is most useful in the diagnosis of MVP and to define the limit of normal leaflet displacement superior or posterior to the plane of the mitral valve annulus (Figs. 10.3 and 10.5). Morganroth and coworkers (55) suggested in 1981 that the apical four-chamber view should be the "standard for the diagnosis of idiopathic mitral valve prolapse syndrome," based on the increased sensitivity of detecting mild-to-moderate prolapse compared to the parasternal long-axis view. Since then, others have confirmed the increased sensitivity of the apical view, but have also observed a decreased specificity, such that an unacceptably high frequency of probably normal individuals are found to have some degree of superior displacement of one or both leaflets on the apical four-chamber view (40, 46, 47, 53, 56–59). A number of studies have shown a correlation between the extent of displacement and the severity of prolapse as determined by various criteria (27, 40, 45, 47, 48, 51, 53, 56, 60–62). Several techniques have been described to estimate the extent of prolapse. Figure 10.5 illustrates one method to differentiate mild, moderate, and severe MVP on the apical four-chamber view. Based on clinical grounds, it has been suggested that mild superior displacement of only the anterior mitral leaflet or of both mitral leaflets seen on the apical four-chamber view alone is probably not an adequate basis for the diagnosis of MVP, since this is frequently seen in normal subjects. Severe displacement in this view or any degree of superior displacement of either or both leaflets in the parasternal long-axis view is, however, sufficient

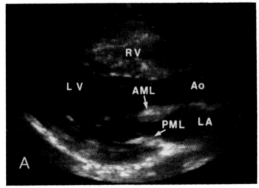
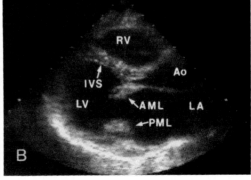

Figure 10.11. Parasternal long-axis views of two patients with mitral valve prolapse and markedly thickened leaflets. *A*, An early diastolic frame. *B*, A diastolic frame taken at the maximum leaflet excursion (in a different patient), illustrating the near-contact of the anterior mitral leaflet and the interventricular septum. *RV* = right ventricle, *LV* = left ventricle, *Ao* = aorta, *LA* = left atrium, *AML* = anterior mitral leaflet, *PML* = posterior mitral leaflet, *IVS* = interventricular septum.

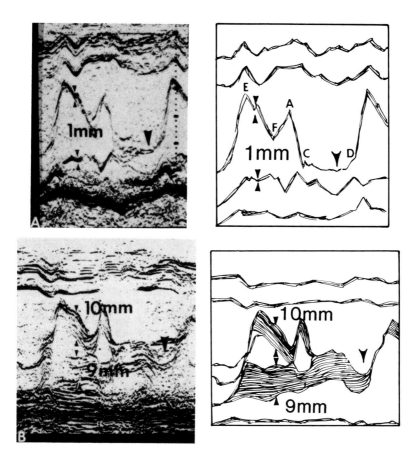

Figure 10.12. M-mode echocardiograms (*left* and diagrammatic representations (*right*) of two patients with mitral valve prolapse. The patient shown in *A*, has normal leaflet thickness. *B*, the patient has an abnormally thick leaflet. The large *arrowheads* show the point of prolapse and the *small arrowheads* show the thickness of the anterior and posterior leaflets at the midpoint of the E-F slope. (From Nishimura RA, McGoon MD, Shub C, Miller FA Jr., Ilstrup DM, Tajik AJ: Echocardiographically documented mitral-valve prolapse. Long term follow-up of 237 patients. *New Engl J Med* 313: 1306, 1985. Reproduced by permission of the Massachusetts Medical Society).

basis for the echocardiographic diagnosis of MVP (14, 46–48, 57). (It should be noted that severe prolapse, when present, is likely to be seen on both views (46)). The etiology of apparent, but "false positive" prolapse on the apical four-chamber view has been postulated recently by Levine and coworkers to be due to the nonplanar ("saddle") shape of the normal mitral annulus. This results in the *appearance* of leaflet displacement superior to the annulus in the apical four-chamber view without *actual* leaflet displacement (63, 64). Bearing this in mind, it is most appropriate to utilize both the apical four-chamber view and the parasternal long-axis view in the diagnosis of MVP. Thus, this diagnosis is relatively certain when leaflet

displacement of any degree is seen in both views or when leaflet displacement is moderate to severe if seen in the apical four-chamber only.

Since the advent of two-dimensional echocardiography, there has also been considerable discussion over the merits of this technique versus M-mode echocardiography in the diagnosis of MVP. Since both techniques are now used routinely in conjunction with each other, this question would appear somewhat irrelevant today; however, it is still of some importance, since in some instances there appears to be prolapse by one technique and not by the other and thus some uncertainty as to which technique is of more diagnostic importance. The sensitivity of M-mode

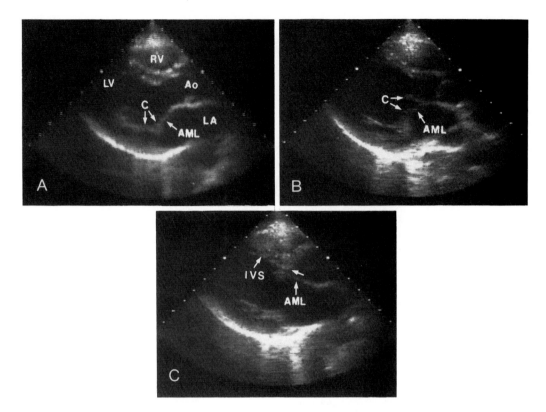

Figure 10.13. Sequential diastolic frames of a parasternal long-axis view of a patient with mitral valve prolapse, illustrating the "whip-like" motion of the anterior mitral leaflet and chordae tendineae and contact with the interventricular septum (*arrow*). RV = right ventricle, LV = left ventricle, Ao = aorta, LA = left atrium, AML = anterior mitral leaflet, C = chordae tendineae, IVS = interventricular septum.

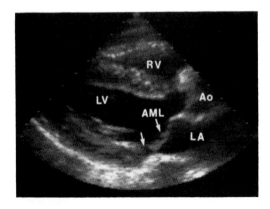

Figure 10.14. Parasternal long-axis view of a diastolic frame of a patient with mitral valve prolapse, illustrating a large anterior leaflet and an excessively posterior coaptation point (*arrow*). RV = right ventricle, LV = left ventricle, AO = aorta, LA = left atrium, AML = anterior mitral leaflet.

echocardiography in the diagnosis of MVP has been found to be anywhere from 50% to 82%, using auscultatory and/or angiographic standards for comparison (15, 32, 53, 56, 65), while the sensitivity of the two-dimensional technique has been found to range from 60% to 100% (46, 56, 65), according to the particular criteria used for diagnosis. In two studies directly comparing the two techniques, two-dimensional echocardiography was more sensitive than M-mode echocardiography in the same patient population, although not more specific (56, 65). In several studies there was a tendency for a higher correlation between the techniques (increased sensitivity of M-mode) when the degree of prolapse was more severe (55, 65), and one study showed a correlation between the amount of posterior leaflet displacement on the M-mode echo and the amount of superior leaflet displacement on the apical four-

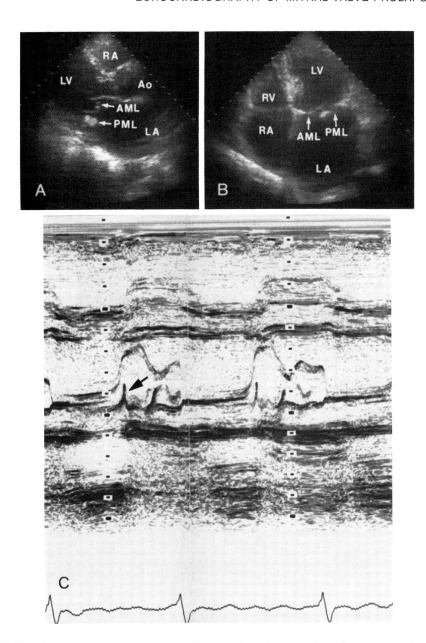

Figure 10.15. *A*, Parasternal long-axis view. *B*, Apical four-chamber view. *C*, M-mode echocardiogram from a patient with mitral valve prolapse and a flail leaflet. In the two-dimensional echo views (*A* and *B*), taken during systole, a markedly thickened posterior mitral leaflet is seen which does not coapt with the anterior leaflet. In the M-mode tracing (*C*), early diastolic motion of the posterior leaflet is seen (*arrow*), a common sign of a flail mitral leaflet. *RV* = right ventricle, *LV* = left ventricle, *RA* = right atrium, *Ao* = aorta, *LA* = left atrium, *AML* = anterior mitral leaflet, *PML* = posterior mitral leaflet.

chamber view (51). Although an occasional patient may display the diagnostic criteria for prolapse as seen in the M-mode tracing and not in the two-dimensional portion of the study (56), the opposite situation is much more likely to be the case, primarily as a result of technical limitations of the M-mode technique (65).

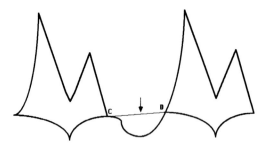

Figure 10.16. Diagrammatic representation of an M-mode echocardiographic tracing of mitral valve motion in a patient with mitral valve prolapse, illustrating the method of drawing a line (*arrow*) from the *C* point to the *D* point in order to measure the maximum posterior displacement of the mitral valve during systole.

TECHNICAL CONSIDERATIONS AND SOURCES OF ERROR

There are a number of factors in both the performance and interpretation of echocardiograms that can lead to misdiagnosis of MVP, resulting in either a false-positive or false-negative diagnosis. The multiplicity of diagnostic criteria of MVP by M-mode and two-dimensional echocardiography is obviously a source of under- and overdiagnosis. However, even when these criteria are clearly defined and the echocardiographers are experienced, there is still a significant inter- and intraobserver variability in interpretation for both M-mode and two-dimensional echocardiograms (60). As would be expected, the greatest discrepancies involve patients with mild MVP. It is unlikely that this problem will be resolved, since there is necessarily some degree of subjectivity in reading, even when applying standard criteria. As might be expected, less variability in interpretation is seen when the echocardiogram is of high technical quality (14, 66).

One other consideration in interpretation is that MVP can be diagnosed mistakenly in the presence of two commonly encountered conditions: pericardial effusion and mitral stenosis. In pericardial effusion, either late systolic or pansystolic posterior motion of the mitral valve can be recorded on the M-mode echocardiogram, presumably as a result of exaggerated ("swinging") motion of the entire heart during systole. This phenomenon of "pseudoprolapse" can be recognized by the simultaneous posterior motion of the right ventricular wall, interventricular septum

and posterior left ventricular wall, along with the mitral valve (Fig. 10.17). This finding characteristically disappears after resolution of the effusion (67–69).

Another condition that can result in a "pseudoprolapse" pattern is mitral stenosis, in which there is frequently systolic bowing of one or both leaflets into the left atrium (70) (Fig. 10.18). Because of the characteristic appearance of mitral stenosis on echocardiography, ordinarily there should be no difficulty in recognizing its presence and not mistaking it for MVP.

In regard to the technical aspects of obtaining an echocardiogram, it has been shown repeatedly that both patient position and transducer position can influence the appearance of the mitral valve on the echocardiogram, especially in the case of the M-mode. Both false-positive and false-negative prolapse patterns can be obtained on M-mode echocardiograms by improper positioning of the transducer on the chest wall. By placing the transducer high on the chest wall and angling caudally, posterior systolic valve motion can be seen in the absence of MVP as a result of movement of the heart and mitral valvular apparatus away from the transducer during systole. For the same reason, a false-negative pattern can be seen in patients with MVP by placing the transducer too low on the chest wall and angling in a cephalad direction. The optimal transducer position is perpendicular to the chest wall and heart, with resultant simultaneous recording of the mitral leaflets anterior to the left atrial wall (32, 43, 45, 71). Unfortunately, optimal transducer positioning is not always possible due to chest wall configuration, and false-positive and false-negative M-mode echoes may not be totally avoidable. Fortunately, two-dimensional echocardiography largely eliminates this problem. However, it has been shown that medial and tangential angling of the two-dimensional echo beam across the plane of the mitral valve can give the appearance of excessive posterior coaptation and superior arching of the anterior leaflets in normal subjects, resulting in a false-positive diagnosis of MVP (18).

Patient position can also influence the appearance of the mitral valve in systole. Yoon and Han (72) demonstrated that the M-mode echocardiogram can be negative for MVP in the left lateral decubitus position, but positive in the supine position, presumably as a result of a slight increase in left ventricular size in the decubitus position. Similarly, an M-mode echo may be negative for

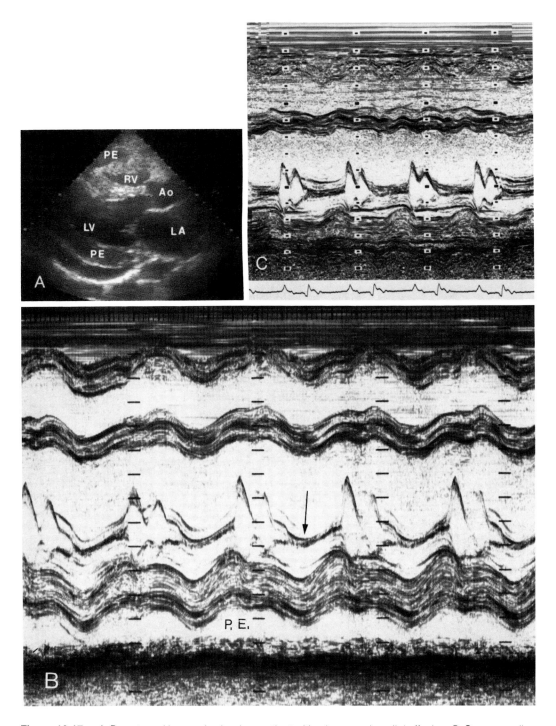

Figure 10.17. *A*, Parasternal long-axis view in a patient with a large pericardial effusion. *B*, Corresponding M-mode echocardiogram. *C*, M-mode echocardiogram in the same patient after pericardiocentesis. *B* and *C* illustrate the "pseudoprolapse" pattern on the M-mode tracing (*B*, *arrow*). There is still a small effusion present in *C*, but the "pseudoprolapse" pattern is much less marked. *PE* = posterior pericardial effusion. *RV* = right ventricle, *LV* = left ventricle, *Ao* = aorta, *LA* = left atrium.

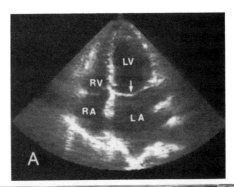

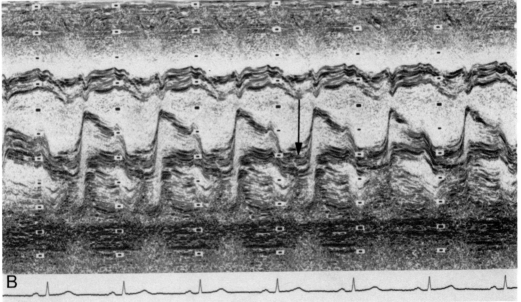

Figure 10.18. *A* and *B*, Apical four-chamber view and M-mode echocardiogram, respectively, of a patient with rheumatic mitral stenosis, illustrating a "pseudoprolapse" pattern (*arrows*). *RV* = right ventricle, *RA* = right atrium, *LV* = left ventricle, *LA* = left atrium.

MVP in the supine position, but positive in the standing position in some patients with MVP, as well as in some normal subjects (23, 43), also presumably reflecting a change in ventricular size and perhaps other factors. Therefore, although the sensitivity of (M-mode) echocardiography in the diagnosis of MVP may be increased by performing the study with the patient in the upright position, there is a tendency for false-positive results, and (supine) two-dimensional echocardiography remains a more reliable technique (23).

CLINICAL-ECHOCARDIOGRAPHIC CORRELATES IN MVP

When M-mode echocardiography was first introduced for the detection of MVP, it was already apparent that it was capable of providing additional clinical insight into this syndrome. For example, it was noted that there was a correlation between the timing of the mid-to-late systolic posterior motion of the mitral valve with the timing of the midsystolic click on phonocardiography. It was also observed that there tended to be a correlation of the type of murmur with the type of prolapse seen on the M-mode echo. Patients with mid-to-late systolic murmurs tended to have a mid-to-late systolic prolapse pattern, and patients with holosystolic murmurs tended to have a holosystolic prolapse pattern (1, 2, 20, 31). (However, other investigators, found a poor correlation between the auscultatory findings and the type of prolapse seen on echocardiography (24, 29, 32, 57)).

More recently, a great deal of attention has focused on the question of the clinical significance of echocardiographically detected MVP, especially in subjects with minimal or no auscultatory findings. In a recent review using auscultation and/or phonocardiography as the standard for diagnosis, the prevalence of MVP in the general population ranged from 0.4% to 17.0%, while the prevalence detected by M-mode echocardiography ranged from 2.5% to 21%, and the prevalence by two-dimensional echocardiography ranged from 1.2% to 34.5%. In each case the prevalence varied according to age and sex, with the lowest incidence in males, the very young, and the elderly (49). Several studies have also shown a correlation of the presence of MVP on either M-mode or two-dimensional echo with body dimensions, in that subjects who were tall and thin had a significantly higher prevalence of MVP than those who were short and obese, with 59% of female ballet dancers having echocardiographic evidence of MVP (44, 50, 51). The increased prevalence of MVP in females may be explained in part by the increased ratio of mitral annulus size and leaflet dimensions to body surface area in normal females (42).

With MVP being such a frequently found abnormality on echocardiography, using even more stringent criteria, the clinical significance of this finding has been repeatedly questioned, and the whole issue of "silent" MVP (i.e., an abnormal echo in the absence of signs or symptoms suggesting MVP) remains controversial. Although the vast majority of subjects found to have MVP by echo have a benign clinical history and probably have a normal life span (14, 31), other persons with MVP have significant complications of this disorder, including severe mitral regurgitation, arrhythmias, bacterial endocarditis, or cerebral emboli. Attempts therefore have been made to distinguish these two seemingly disparate groups by their echocardiographic findings.

Approximately 70% of subjects suspected by history and/or examination to have MVP are also found by Doppler echocardiographic study to have mitral regurgitation (53, 56). Moreover, there is a significant correlation between the presence and degree of regurgitation with the degree of prolapse, as well as with the size of the mitral annulus, the presence and degree of leaflet deformity, and the presence of abnormal leaflet coaptation (34, 40, 41, 73). Perhaps of even greater clinical significance, there is a higher incidence of high grade arrhythmias, symptoms of congestive heart failure, and endocarditis in patients with severe prolapse (40) and in MVP patients with thicker and more redundant valves (34, 73, 74). Also, rupture of the chordae tendineae was found to be much more common among MVP patients with thickened mitral valves than in those with normal valve thickness (30). Similarly, a very significant association has been demonstrated between the presence of leaflet redundancy by M-mode echo (middiastolic valve thickness of 5 mm or greater) and the occurrence of sudden death, infective endocarditis, or cerebral embolic events (10.3% incidence of any of these events in the group with a redundant valve versus 0.7% incidence in the group without redundancy) (31).

MVP thus appears to be a spectrum of diseases rather than a single entity, ranging from subjects with "silent" prolapse, equivocal findings on echocardiography, and a benign clinical course to those with obvious clinical and echocardiographic findings and a tendency for complications. Consequently, various schemes have been proposed to classify this syndrome according to the clinical and echocardiographic presentation. To this end, Devereux and associates (14) recently proposed a series of clinical and echocardiographic criteria for the diagnosis of MVP, which appear very reasonable based on all available information (see Table 10.1). It should be noted that these criteria do not include the apical four-chamber view, because of the problem of poor specificity. In a somewhat similar approach to the same goal of the reliable diagnosis of MVP, Perloff and associates (9, 48) proposed a series of major and minor clinical and echocardiographic criteria similar to the Jones criteria for rheumatic fever (9, 48). Table 10.2 summarizes their echocardiographic criteria in which the apical four-chamber view is utilized, but are felt only to be diagnostic in themselves when the degree of leaflet displacement is marked.

The debate over the absolute criteria for the diagnosis of MVP is likely to continue for awhile, especially over the question of "silent" prolapse. But the echocardiographic criteria given in these two tables should serve as a practical guide to a clinically useful echocardiographic diagnosis of this syndrome. Still unresolved, but discussed in detail in the recent literature, is the question of what is the absolute "gold standard" for the diagnosis of MVP—auscultation, echocardiography, or a combination of the two. At present, it would seem most appropriate to describe the echocardiographic findings in a given patient as

Table 10.1. Echocardiographic Criteria for the Clinical Diagnosis of MVP

Criterion	Technical Considerations	Accuracy
A. M-Mode Echo Criteria (2-D Targeted)		
Late systolic prolapse equal to or greater than 2 mm	Continual visualization of mitral leaflet interfaces from C to D points on multiple cycles; longitudinal and transverse sweeps should be obtained	High if "pseudoprolapse" due to overall heart motion in presence of pericardial effusion is excluded
Holosystolic prolapse equal to or greater than 3 mm	Must avoid high parasternal interspace; should have systolic billowing of mitral leaflets documented by two-dimensional echocardiography in parasternal long-axis view	High only if documented by two-dimensional echocardiography; otherwise relatively poor
B. Two-Dimensional Echo Criteria		
Systolic leaflet billowing into left atrium in parasternal long-axis view	Review is necessary in stop-frame mode to document leaflet protrusion across annular plane	Sensitivity moderate, specificity very high

Table 10.2. Major and Minor Echocardiographic Criteria for the Diagnosis of MVP

A. Major Criteria (Which Establish the Diagnosis of MVP)

I. Two-Dimensional/Doppler Echocardiography
Marked systolic displacement of mitral leaflets with coaptation point at or on the left atrial side of the anulus
Moderate systolic displacement of the leaflets with at least moderate mitral regurgitation, chordal rupture, and annular dilatation

II. Two-Dimensionally Targeted M-Mode Echocardiography
Marked (equal to or greater than 3 mm) late systolic buckling posterior to the C–D line

B. Minor Criteria (Which Arouse Suspicion but Do Not Establish the Diagnosis of MVP)

I. Two-Dimensional/Doppler Echocardiography
Moderate superior systolic displacement of mitral leaflets with Doppler mitral regurgitation

II. Two-Dimensionally Targeted M-Mode Echocardiography
Moderate (2 mm) late systolic buckling posterior to the C–D line
Holosystolic displacement (3 mm) posterior to the C–D line

C. Nonspecific Findings (Which Do Not Bear on the Diagnosis of MVP)

Two-Dimensional Echocardiography
Isolated mild-to-moderate superior systolic displacement of mitral leaflets, especially in the apical four-chamber view

"consistent with," "suggestive of," or "no evidence of" mitral valve prolapse, according to the findings. Thus the final clinical diagnosis should be determined by the clinician, based on the entire presentation. It would also seem appropriate, based on the data discussed earlier, no longer to state merely whether or not prolapse is seen on the echocardiogram, but to describe in some detail the appearance of the valve and the extent of prolapse, since clinical characterization of the patient is dependent on this information, and diagnostic and therapeutic decisions may be made based on the severity of prolapse.

REFERENCES

1. Shah PM, Gramiak R: Echocardiographic recognition of mitral valve prolapse (abstr). *Circulation* 45:III–45, 1970.
2. Dillon JC, Haine CL, Chang S, Feigenbaum H: Use of echocardiography in patients with prolapsed mitral valve. *Circulation* 43:503–507, 1971.
3. Kerber RE, Isaeff DM, Hancock EW: Echocardiographic patterns in patients with the syndrome of systolic click and late systolic murmur. *N Engl J Med* 284:691–693, 1971.
4. Barlow JB, Bosman CK: Aneurysmal protrusion of the posterior leaflet of the mitral valve. An auscultatory-electrocardiographic syndrome. *Am Heart J* 71:166–178, 1966.
5. Criley JM, Lewis KB, Humphries JO, Ross RS: Prolapse of the mitral valve: Clinical and cine-angiographic findings. *Br Heart J* 28:488–496, 1966.
6. Barlow JB, Pocock WA: The mitral valve prolapse enigma-two decades later. *Mod Concepts Cardiovasc Dis* 53:13–17, 1984.

7. Isner JM, Roberts WC: Morphologic observations on the mitral valve at necropsy in patients with systolic clicks with or without systolic murmurs and/or echocardiographic evidence of mitral valve prolapse (Abstr). *Am J Cardiol* 43:368, 1979.

8. Rippe J, Fishbein MC, Carabello B, Angoff G, Sloss L, Collins JJ Jr, Alpert JS: Primary myxomatous degeneration of cardiac valves. Clinical, pathological, haemodynamic, and echocardiographic profile. *Br Heart J* 44:621–629, 1980.

9. Perloff JK, Child JA: Clinical and epidemiologic issues in mitral valve prolapse: Overview and perspective. *Am Heart J* 113:1324–1332, 1987.

10. Siegel RJ, Fishbein MC, Criley JM: Functional anatomy of the mitral valve in health and disease: Emphasis on rheumatologic disorders: Part II. *Cardiovasc Rev Rep* 7:431–455, 1986.

11. Hutchins GM, Moore GW, Skoog DK: The association of floppy mitral valve with disjunction of the mitral annulus fibrosis. *N Engl J Med* 314:535–540, 1986.

12. Roberts WC, McIntosh CL, Wallace RB: Mechanisms of severe mitral regurgitation in mitral valve prolapse determined from analysis of operatively excised valves. *Am Heart J* 113:1316–1323, 1987.

13. Virmani R, Atkinson JB, Byrd BF III, Robinowitz M, Forman MB: Abnormal chordal insertion: A cause of mitral valve prolapse. *Am Heart J* 113:851–858, 1987.

14. Devereux RB, Kramer-Fox R, Shear MK, Kligfield P, Pini R, Savage DD: Diagnosis and classification of severity of mitral valve prolapse: Methodologic, biologic, and prognostic considerations. *Am Heart J* 113:1265–1280, 1987.

15. Marcus R, Sareli P, Antunes M, Magalhaes M, Meyer T, Grieve T, Barlow J: Functional pathology of mitral regurgitation in active rheumatic carditis—Surgical and echocardiographic observations (Abstr). *J Am Coll Cardiol* 7:8A, 1986.

16. Tomaru T, Uchida Y, Mohri N, Mori W, Furuse A, Asano K: Postinflammatory mitral and aortic valve prolapse: A clinical and pathological study. *Circulation* 76:68–76, 1987.

17. Lembo NJ, Dell'Italia LJ, Crawford MH, Miller JF, Richards KL, O'Rourke RA: Mitral valve prolapse in patients with prior rheumatic fever. *Circulation* 77:830–836, 1988.

18. Gilbert BW, Schatz RA, VonRamm OT, Behar VS, Kisslo JA: Mitral valve prolapse: two-dimensional echocardiographic and angiographic correlation. *Circulation* 54:716–723, 1976.

19. Fraker TD Jr, Johnson ML, Kisslo JA: Echocardiographic diagnosis of mitral valve disease. In Kisslo JA (Ed): *Two-Dimensional Echocardiography*. New York, Churchill Livingstone, 1980, pp 52–53.

20. Popp RL, Brown OR, Silverman JF, Harrison DC: Echocardiographic abnormalities in the mitral valve prolapse syndrome. *Circulation* 49:428–433, 1974.

21. Winkle RA, Goodman DJ, Popp RL: Simultaneous echocardiographic-phonocardiographic recordings at rest and during amyl nitrite administration in patients with mitral valve prolapse. *Circulation* 51:522–529, 1975.

22. Devereux RB, Perloff JK, Reichek N, Joseph-son ME: Mitral valve prolapse. *Circulation* 54:3–14, 1976.

23. Noble LM, Dabestani A, Child JA, Krivokapich J: Mitral valve prolapse. Cross sectional and provocative M-mode echocardiography. *Chest* 82:158–163, 1982.

24. Sahn DJ, Allen HD, Goldberg SJ, Friedman WF: Mitral valve prolapse in children. A problem defined by real-time cross-sectional echocardiography. *Circulation* 53:651–657, 1976.

25. Rakowski H, Martin RP, Popp RL: Two-dimensional echocardiographic findings in mitral valve prolapse (Abstr). *Circulation* 55 and 56 (Suppl III):III–154, 1977.

26. Cohen MV: Real-time sector scan study of the mitral valve prolapse syndrome. *Br Heart J* 40:964–971, 1978.

27. Morganroth J, Jones RH, Chen CC, Naito M: Two dimensional echocardiography in mitral, aortic and tricuspid valve prolapse. *Am J Cardiol* 46:1164–1177, 1980.

28. Haikal M, Alpert MA, Whiting RB, Ahmad M, Kelly D: Sensitivity and specificity of M mode echocardiographic signs of mitral valve prolapse. *Am J Cardiol* 50:185–190, 1982.

29. DeMaria An, King JF, Bogren HG, Lies JE, Mason DT: The variable spectrum of echocardiographic manifestations of the mitral valve prolapse syndrome. *Circulation* 50:33–41, 1974.

30. Naggar CZ, Pearson WN, Seljan MP, Maddock LK, Masrof S, Elwood DJ: Frequency of complications of mitral valve prolapse in subjects aged 60 years and older. *Am J Cardiol* 58:1209–1212, 1986.

31. Nishimura RA, McGoon MD, Shub C, Miller FA Jr, Ilstrup DM, Tajik AJ: Echocardiographically documented mitral valve prolapse. Long-term follow-up of 237 patients. *N Engl J Med* 313:1305–1309, 1985.

32. DeMaria AN, Neuman A, Lee G, Mason DT: Echocardiographic identification of the mitral valve prolapse syndrome. *Am J Med* 62:819–829, 1977.

33. Chandraratna PAN, Nimalasuriya A, Kawanishi D, Duncan P, Rosin B, Rahimtoola SH: Identification of the increased frequency of cardiovascular abnormalities associated with mitral valve prolapse by two-dimensional echocardiography. *Am J Cardiol* 54:1283–1285, 1984.

34. Marks AR, Choong CY, Sanfilippo AJ, Ferré M, Weyman AE: Identification of high-risk and low-risk subgroups of patients with mitral valve prolapse. *N Engl J Med* 320:1031–1036, 1989.

35. Higgins CB, Reinke RT, Gosink B, Leopold GR: The significance of mitral valve prolapse in middle-aged and elderly men. *Am Heart J* 91:292–296, 1976.

36. Gardin JM, Talano JV, Stepanides L, Fizzano J, Lesch M: Systolic anterior motion in the absence of asymmetric septal hypertrophy. A buckling phenomenon of the chordae tendineae. *Circulation* 63:181–188, 1981.

37. Kessler KM, Anzola E, Sequeira R, Serafini AN, Myerberg RJ: Mitral valve prolapse and systolic anterior motion: A dynamic spectrum. *Am Heart J* 105:685–688, 1983.

38. Matthews E, Henry WL, Ronan JA, Griffith JM: Two dimensional echo evaluation of mitral valve prolapse—An explanation of the patterns seen with M-mode echocardiograms (Abstr). *Circulation* 54 (Suppl II):II–235, 1976.
39. Ormiston JA, Shah PM, Tei C, Wong M: Size and motion of the mitral valve annulus in man. II. Abnormalities in mitral valve prolapse. *Circulation* 65:713–719, 1982.
40. Cohen IS: Two-dimensional echocardiographic mitral valve prolapse: Evidence for a relationship of echocardiographic morphology to clinical findings and to mitral annular size. Am Heart J 113:859–868, 1987.
41. Pini R, Devereux RB, Greppi B, Roman MJ, Hochreiter C, Kramer-Fox R, Niles NW, Kligfield, P, Erlebacher JA, Borer JS: Comparison of mitral valve dimensions and motion in mitral valve prolapse with severe mitral regurgitation to uncomplicated mitral valve prolapse and to mitral regurgitation without mitral valve prolapse. *Am J Cardiol* 62:257–263, 1988.
42. Pini R, Greppi B, Kramer-Fox R, Roman MJ, Devereux RB. Mitral valve dimensions and motion and familial transmission of mitral valve prolapse with and without mitral leaflet billowing. *J Am Coll Cardiol* 12:1423–1431, 1988.
43. Markiewicz W, Stoner J, London E, Hunt SA, Popp RL: Mitral valve prolapse in one hundred presumably healthy young females. *Circulation* 53:464–473, 1976.
44. Savage DD, Garrison RJ, Devereux RB, Castelli WP, Anderson SJ, Levy D, McNamara PM, Stokes J III, Kannel WB, Feinleib M: Mitral valve prolapse in the general population. I. Epidemiologic features: The Framingham Study. *Am Heart J* 106:571–576, 1983.
45. Wann LS, Grove JR, Hess TR, Glisch L, Ptacin MJ, Hughes CV, Gross CM: Prevalence of mitral prolapse by two dimensional echocardiography in healthy young women. *Br Heart J* 49:334–340, 1983.
46. Akpert MA, Carney RJ, Flaker GC, Sanfelippo JF, Webel RR, Kelly DL: Sensitivity and specificity of two-dimensional echocardiographic signs of mitral valve prolapse. *Am J Cardiol* 54:792–796, 1984.
47. Warth DC, King ME, Cohen JM, Tesoriero VL, Marcus E, Weyman AE: Prevalence of mitral valve prolapse in normal children. *J Am Coll Cardiol* 5:1173–1177, 1985.
48. Perloff JK, Child JS, Edwards JE: New guidelines for the clinical diagnosis of mitral valve prolapse. *Am J Cardiol* 57:1124–1129, 1986.
49. Levy D, Savage D: Prevalence and clinical features of mitral valve prolapse. *Am Heart J* 113:1281–1290, 1987.
50. Cohen JL, Austin SM, Segal KR, Millman AE, Kim CS: Echocardiographic mitral valve prolapse in ballet dancers: A function of leanness. *Am Heart J* 113:341–344, 1987.
51. Kriwisky M, Froom P, Gross M, Ribak J, Lewis BS: Usefulness of echocardiographically determined mitral leaflet motion for diagnosis of mitral valve prolapse in 17- and 18-year old men. *Am J Cardiol* 59:1149–1151, 1987.

52. Devereux RB: Diagnosis and prognosis of mitral valve prolapse. *N Engl J Med* 320:1077–1078, 1989.
53. Panidis IP, McAllister M, Ross J, Mintz GS: Prevalence and severity of mitral regurgitation in the mitral valve prolapse syndrome: A Doppler echocardiographic study of 80 patients. *J Am Coll Cardiol* 7:975–981, 1986.
54. Blich A, Vignola PA, Walker H, Kaplan AD, Chiotellis PN, Lees RS, Myers GS: Echocardiographic spectrum of posterior systolic motion of the mitral valve in the general population. *J Clin Ultrasound* 5:243–247, 1977.
55. Morganroth J, Mardelli TJ, Naito M, Chen CC: Apical cross-sectional echocardiography. Standard for the diagnosis of idiopathic mitral valve prolapse syndrome. *Chest* 79:23–28, 1981.
56. Abbasi AS, DeCristofaro D, Anabtawi J, Irwin L: Mitral valve prolapse: Comparative study of M-mode, two-dimensional and Doppler echocardiography. *J Am Coll Cardiol* 2:1219–1223, 1983.
57. Krivokapich J, Child JS, Dadourian BJ, Perloff JK: Reassessment of echocardiographic criteria for diagnosis of mitral valve prolapse. *Am J Cardiol* 61:131–135, 1988.
58. Hagege AA, Abascal VM, Novick SS, Weyman AE, Levine RA: Prospective study of mitral valve prolapse: Further evidence for "normality" of displacement in the apical 4-chamber view only (Abstr). *J Am Coll Cardiol* 11:125A, 1988.
59. Sanfilippo AJ, Popovic AD, Harrigan P, Handschumacher MD, Weyman AE, Levine RA: Two to five year echocardiographic follow-up of patients with mitral valve prolapse: Is apical four-chamber view displacement a precursor of abnormality (Abstr)? *J Am Coll Cardiol* 13:226A, 1989.
60. Wann LS, Gross CM, Wakefield RJ, Kalbfleisch JH: Diagnostic precision of echocardiography in mitral valve prolapse. *Am Heart J* 109:803–808, 1985.
61. Schreiber TL, Feigenbaum H, Weyman AE: Effect of atrial septal defect repair on left ventricular geometry and degree of mitral valve prolapse. *Circulation* 61:888–896, 1980.
62. Weyman AE: *Cross-Sectional Echocardiography.* Philadelphia, Lea & Febiger, 1982, pp 174–175.
63. Levine RA, Triulzi MO, Harrigan P, Weyman AE: The relationship of mitral annular shape to the diagnosis of mitral valve prolapse. *Circulation* 75:756–767, 1987.
64. Handschumacher MD, Hagege AA, Harrigan P, Sanfilippo AJ, Weyman AE, Levine RA: Direct demonstration of mitral leaflet annular relationships by three-dimensional echocardiography: Implications for the diagnosis of mitral valve prolapse (Abstr). *J Am Coll Cardiol* 11:126A, 1988.
65. Alpert MA, Haikal M, Carney RJ: Factors predisposing to false negative M-mode echocardiograms in patients with two-dimensional echocardiographic criteria for mitral valve prolapse. *Am Heart J* 113:1250–1252, 1987.
66. Meltzer RS, Devereux RB, Goldman ME, Kronzon I, Meller J, Teichholz LE, Thornton JC: Observer variability in M-mode echocardiographic diagnosis of mitral valve prolapse: Effect of tracing quality and depth of prolapse. *J Cardiovasc Ultrasonogr* 6:39–48, 1987.

67. Levisman JA, Abbasi AS: Abnormal motion of the mitral valve with pericardial effusion: Pseudo-prolapse of the mitral valve. *Am Heart J* 91:18–20, 1976.
68. Vignola PA, Pohost GM, Curfman GD, Myers GS: Correlation of echocardiographic and clinical findings in patients with pericardial effusion. *Am J Cardiol* 37:701–707, 1976.
69. Nanda NC, Gramiak R, Gross CM: Echocardiography of cardiac valves in pericardial effusion. *Circulation* 54:500–504, 1976.
70. Nichol PM, Gilbert BW, Kisslo JA: Two-dimensional echocardiographic assessment of mitral stenosis. *Circulation* 55:120–128, 1977.
71. Weiss AN, Mimbs JW, Ludbrook PA, Sobel BE: Echocardiographic detection of mitral valve prolapse. Exclusion of false positive diagnosis and determination of inheritance. *Circulation* 52:1091–1096, 1975.
72. Yoon MS, Han J: Comparison of supine and left lateral decubitus positions in M-mode echocardiographic findings in mitral valve prolapse by auscultation. *Am J Cardiol* 57:350–352, 1986.
73. Grayburn PA, Berk MR, Kwan OL, Spain MG, Harrison MR, Smith MD, DeMaria AN: Relation of valvular anatomy and coaptation to mitral regurgitation in mitral valve prolapse: Assessment by color flow Doppler imaging (Abstr). *J Am Coll Cardiol* 11:126A, 1988.
74. Darcy TP, Virmani R, Cohen IS, Robinowitz M: Mitral valve prolapse associated with sudden death: Morphologic spectrum and distinguishing features (Abstr). *J Am Coll Cardiol* 11:125A, 1988.

11

Evaluation of Prosthetic Heart Valves by Echocardiography

James R. Katz, M.D.
Lawrence S. C. Czer, M.D.

INTRODUCTION

Cardiac valvular prostheses are generally categorized as mechanical or biologic according to the material utilized in the construction of the mobile occluder element. Mechanical prosthetic valves can be classified further according to the design of the occluder element, which may be a caged ball, caged disc, tilting disc, or bileaflet structure (Table 11.1). Bioprostheses are constructed from a variety of biologic materials and are classified by the type of material used (Table 11.2). Echocardiographic findings are generally similar within each class of mechanical or biologic prostheses. This chapter focuses on five commonly used prostheses: the Starr-Edwards caged ball, Bjork-Shiley tilting disc, St. Jude bileaflet, and the Hancock and Carpentier-Edwards bioprosthetic valves.

M-MODE AND TWO-DIMENSIONAL ECHOCARDIOGRAPHY

Starr-Edwards Valve

Earlier Starr-Edwards Silastic prosthetic valves, such as the aortic 1260 Starr-Edwards valve, can be distinguished echocardiographically in that both anterior and posterior surfaces of the ball can be recorded readily (Fig. 11.1A). As the velocity of sound transmission through Silastic is slow relative to that of soft tissue, an apparent increase in ball diameter measured by M-mode technique is found. Additionally, the posterior surface of the ball is recorded posterior to the suture ring (4, 94).

Later Starr-Edwards prosthetic valves such as the mitral model 6400 with constituent hollow titanium metal ball allows only visualization of the anterior surface of the ball by echocardiogra-

phy. On occasion, the posterior echo of the ball may be obtained when the valve is examined off-axis. The opening and closing motion of the Starr-Edwards prosthesis is recorded readily in the aortic or mitral position. In the mitral position the valve remains open throughout diastole; a slope resembling that of mitral stenosis is encountered. Measurement of ball excursion and opening and closing velocities have not been shown to be of value in the evaluation of suspected prosthetic valve malfunction; position of the patient and gravitational effects may affect the opening velocity of the mitral valve (4). In the aortic position during systole, bouncing motion of the poppet occurs with an opening and reclosure motion. Combined echophonocardiography is of lesser importance in evaluation of A_2-mitral valve opening (MVO) interval, as loud prosthetic sounds are commonly encountered with Starr-Edwards prostheses.

Abnormal findings: Inability to demonstrate multiple clicks on echophonocardiography in association with the absence of poppet bouncing may suggest a thrombosed poppet (80).

Patients reported by Brodie et al. (5) with paravalvular regurgitation had A_2-MVO intervals (0.04–0.07 sec) that were considerably shorter than normal. One patient each with left ventricular dysfunction and prosthetic obstruction had respective A_2-MVO intervals of 0.06 and 0.08 sec. By comparison, the normal interval was 0.10 ± 0.02 sec. All patients with mitral Starr-Edwards paraprosthetic regurgitation also had normal to vigorous septal motion on two-dimensional echocardiography. Despite the presence of normal cage and suture ring echoes, a thrombosed mitral Starr-Edwards valve has been recognized by the absence of independent anterior poppet motion (87).

Table 11.1. Mechanical Prosthetic Valves

Caged ball
  Harken
  Starr-Edwards[a] Models 1000, 1200[a], 1260[a], 2300,
        2310, 2320, 2400, 6000, 6120[a],
        6300, 6310, 6320, 6400
  Magovern-Cromie[a]
  Smeloff-Sutter[a] (formerly Smeloff-Cutter)
  Braunwald-Cutter
  DeBakey-Surgitool

Caged disc
  Harken
  Kay-Suzuki
  Kay-Shiley
  Cross-Jones
  Beall[a] model 106[a]
  Starr-Edwards models 6500, 6520
  Cooley-Cutter

Tilting disc
  Wada-Cutter
  Lillihei-Kaster[a]
  Bjork-Shiley[a] (Delrin disc, *spherical disc*[a],
        60° convexo-concave, *monostrut*[a,b])
  Medtronic-Hall[a] (formerly Hall-Kaster)
  Omniscience[a]

Bileaflet
  Gott-Daggett
  St. Jude[a]
  Duromedics

[a]Currently available.
[b]Investigational use only (in United States).

Bjork-Shiley Valve

In the aortic position the opening of the disc valve is not readily appreciated, but may be recorded by echophonocardiography as a soft sound occurring 0.04 sec after the first sound, followed by a soft early-to-midsystolic ejection murmur. In the mitral position, the Bjork-Shiley valve generally does not produce an opening sound. However, phonocardiography occasionally may record a soft prosthetic opening sound at the left sternal border or apex (99).

The opening motion of the disc is readily recorded by M-mode echo (48), whereas two-dimensional echocardiography is of lesser utility because of side lobe and reverberating echoes. A Bjork-Shiley valve in the aortic position produces reverberating echoes behind the aortic root in the left atrium. In the mitral position, with the onset of diastole, there is a brisk opening movement, sharp E point and prolonged E–F slope. Abrupt closure of the prosthetic valve with ventricular systole produces a loud closure sound at the apex,

unless first degree atrioventricular block or left ventricular dysfunction are associated abnormalities. Because tilting disc mitral valve opening sounds cannot be heard, echophonocardiography should be done to record the A_2-MVO interval. Typically 0.05–0.09 sec, the A_2-MVO interval is generally shorter than other prosthetic valves and similar to intervals recorded with other tilting disc valves (58).

Abnormal findings: Of seven patients described by Chandraratna et al. (56), four had a marked reduction or absence of the closing click, and three had significant aortic incompetence with clearly audible valve clicks. Cardiac catheterization was performed for clinical evidence of prosthetic dysfunction. Three patients were noted to have periprosthetic leaks, three had extensive clot formation in and around the valve, and the seventh patient, who clinically had reduction of the intensity of the closing click, had normal disc motion with marked left ventricular dysfunction. Normal echocardiographic disk movement and paradoxic septal motion were demonstrated in this latter patient. Echocardiographic findings suggestive of aortic prosthetic dysfunction included complete absence of disc motion, reduction of velocity of opening and closing, dense echoes in the aortic root with loss of clear delineation of the posterior aortic root, or diastolic fluttering of the anterior mitral valve leaflet. Ben-Zvi et al. (57) recorded echocardiographic find-

Table 11.2. Bioprostheses

Porcine aortic valve heterograft
  Hancock[a]
  Carpentier-Edwards[a]
  Angell-Shiley
  Hancock II[a,b]
  Tascon[a,b]
  BioImplant[a,b] (St. Jude; formerly Liotta)
  Intact[a,b] (Medtronic)

Bovine pericardium
  Ionescu-Shiley
  Hancock pericardial
  Mitroflow (Mitral Medical)
  Carpentier-Edwards pericardial

Homograft
  Human aortic valve[a]
  Dura mater[a]

Autograft
  Fascia lata

[a]Currently available.
[b]Investigational use only (in United States).

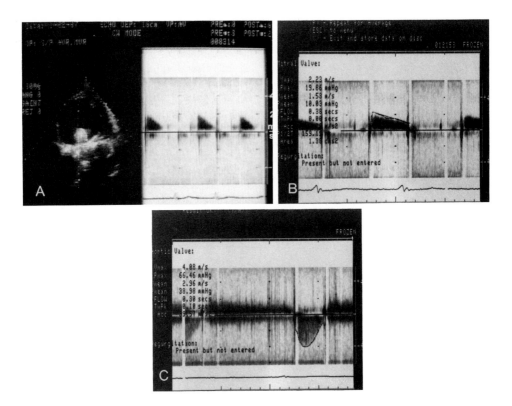

Figure 11.1. Normal mitral and aortic Starr-Edwards prostheses. Forty-seven-year-old male, 16 years after aortic and mitral valve replacements with Starr-Edwards prostheses, had a 1-year history of congestive heart failure and ascites. *Panels A* and *B* are apical four-chamber simultaneous two-dimensional/continuous wave and continuous wave only images, respectively, demonstrating a 2.2 m/sec V_{max} and pressure half-time of 159 msec for the mitral prosthesis. *Panel C* shows a V_{max} of 4.0 m/sec for the aortic prosthesis. Cinefluoroscopy of the valves was unremarkable, and marked left ventricular dysfunction was present on two-dimensional echocardiographic evaluation.

ings in two patients with thrombosis of an aortic Bjork-Shiley prosthesis to include absence of prosthetic disc motion, associated with dense aortic root echoes, and no clear delineation of anterior and posterior walls. Repeat echocardiograms obtained after thrombectomy and debridement of the thrombosed Bjork-Shiley prostheses revealed a normal pattern of disc motion and clear separation of the aortic walls.

Following prosthetic mitral valve replacement, 27 patients with Lillehei-Kaster valves were reported by Brodie et al. (5). A_2-MVO intervals as recorded by echophonocardiography or phonocardiography alone were reported to range from 0.07 to 0.12 sec in 29 patients with normally functioning Lillehei-Kaster mitral prostheses. Intervals in this case were similar to those reported by Gibson et al. (58). The intervals were significantly

shorter than this in patients with obstructed prostheses (0.03–0.06 sec) and in patients with paravalvular regurgitation (0.05 and 0.06 sec). Intervals in patients with left ventricular dysfunction were either short or normal (0.06–0.10 sec). Prolongation of the A_2-MVO interval and marked variation in this interval from beat to beat as reported in mitral ball valve prostheses (82–84, 86, 88, 98, 103, 104) were not noted in the study of Brodie et al. (5). Their study suggested that echocardiography of the left ventricle was useful in distinguishing between paravalvular regurgitation, prosthetic valve obstruction, and left ventricular dysfunction. Brodie et al. (5), Bernal-Ramirez and Phillips (50), and others (81) have found normal or vigorous septal motion in patients with paravalvular regurgitation, whereas hypokinetic or paradoxic septal motion was more likely with prosthetic obstruction or left ventricular dysfunction. Additional echocardiographic findings suggestive of a thrombosed mitral tilting disc valve include a rounded and slowed pattern of opening and closure with loss of distinct E-point associated with diminution in the respective opening and closing rates to less than 180 mm/sec and 300 mm/sec, flattened diastolic slope, and diminished amplitude of disc excursion (50, 52). Dense echos in the region of the suture ring accompanied by reduced or absent disc excursion were reported by Copans (52) in patients with thrombosed Bjork-Shiley mitral prostheses undergoing echocardiography. A second echocardiographic pattern reported by Bernal-Ramirez and Phillips (50) was an unusual hump during the opening phase associated with normal or hyperkinetic septal motion and correlating with significant paravalvular leak.

Abnormal echoes in the region of the disc with limitation of disc excursion have been reported in thrombotic jamming of the tricuspid Bjork-Shiley prosthesis (51).

St. Jude Valve

Leaflet motion of the St. Jude aortic prosthesis may be recorded by M-mode echocardiography (60, 79, 96). During systole, separation of the anterior and posterior leaflets is present, and in some patients two distinct leaflets may be visualized in the aortic root. However, the pattern is usually indistinguishable from that obtained in patients with an aortic eccentric monocuspid valve. During systole, the two leaflets of the St. Jude prosthesis seat against and are difficult to separate from the suture ring. In the aortic position, leaflet motion with opposing leaflets separated by an echo-free space is demonstrable in only 24% of patients, whereas leaflet separation is observed in 85% of patients with the St. Jude valve in the mitral position (79). Reverberating echoes resulting in left atrial echo artifacts are encountered with both eccentric monocuspid and bileaflet aortic prostheses. In the mitral position, an echo-free space separating the two leaflets of the St. Jude prosthesis is recorded commonly during diastole by M-mode techniques. Occasionally, asynchronous early diastolic closure of the posterior leaflet is observed in patients with atrial fibrillation and long cycle lengths (60). Direct visualization of leaflet motion by two-dimensional echocardiography is occasionally possible if the leaflets open in a direction perpendicular to the echo-

cardiographic plane of the long axis of the left ventricle, as with the parasternal short-axis window (60, 64). A mitral valve opening sound is not audible; therefore the A_2-MVO interval as recorded by combined echophonocardiography is useful. In normally functioning St. Jude mitral valves characterized in two studies, measured A_2-MVO intervals were 0.08 ± 0.02 sec (79) and 0.10 ± 0.02 sec (60).

Abnormal findings: In patients with a clotted St. Jude mitral prosthesis, the A_2-MVO opening interval may be shortened markedly (96). Abnormal rounding of the opening motion compared to a baseline study has been reported by these same investigators.

Hancock and Carpentier-Edwards Bioprostheses

In the mitral position, an opening sound may be detected by auscultation in approximately one-half of the patients (99). The sound occurs 0.07–0.11 sec after the second heart sound and is best heard at the apex; visualization of the individual leaflet opening during diastole and merging together during systole is possible and allows derivation of A_2-MVO intervals for Hancock prostheses by M-mode echocardiography.

The echocardiographic features of bioprosthetic valves include two strong distinct parallel bands of echoes from the near and far portions of the circular stent (42). The outer surfaces of the anterior and posterior bands correspond to the actual stent diameter. The stent moves anteriorly with systole and posteriorly with diastole. Two-dimensional echocardiography allows assessment of valve alignment, as well as leaflet and ring motion (2, 4). Differentiation of valvular problems from left ventricular dysfunction has also been possible by two-dimensional echocardiography.

The diagnostic accuracy (97%) of two-dimensional echocardiography is superior to M-mode echocardiography (67%) in assessing bioprosthetic valves (37, 43). Variables analyzed in the two-dimensional studies included: (*a*) contour of the sewing ring and prosthetic stents and occurrence of adjacent extraneous echoes; (*b*) sewing ring motion not excluding and consonant with surrounding cardiac tissues; and (*c*) normal porcine leaflet thickness less than 3 mm.

Abnormal findings: Schapira et al. (37) found that of 33 patients with suspected bioprosthetic valve or left ventricular dysfunction, 16 had an abnormal bioprosthetic valve confirmed by surgery or autopsy, with normal left ventricular function. Fifteen of these patients had abnormal two-dimensional echocardiographic studies, demonstrating valve masses in 6, thickening of leaflets in 6, mass with valve dehiscence in 2, and valve dehiscence in 1 patient. In comparison, M-mode echocardiography missed valve masses, leaflet thickening, and leaflet dehiscence with alarming frequency. M-mode and two-dimensional echocardiography were also useful in distinguishing prosthetic valvular from left ventricular dysfunction.

With mitral insufficiency due to valve ring dehiscence or paravalvular leaks, alterations of stent position and mobility have been described (35). The major M-mode features of prosthetic regurgitation in the mitral position diagnostic of a torn and flail porcine cusp were localized fuzzy cusp echoes with fluttering of the cusp in both systole and diastole (36). In 4 of 5 patients with ruptured and flail porcine mitral cusps, the two-dimensional echocardiogram demonstrated rapid systolic motion of the involved leaflet into the atrium beyond the line of valve closure (Figs. 11.2–11.5). With native aortic valve regurgitation, diastolic flutter may occur in a normal porcine mitral valve (44). Excessive anterior stent movement and systolic slope of a porcine prosthesis should arouse suspicion of paravalvular leak (44).

The presence of reduced initial diastolic slope of the porcine valve as reported with stenosis of other tissue valves (35, 85, 105) was not a particularly diagnostic feature in the patients studied

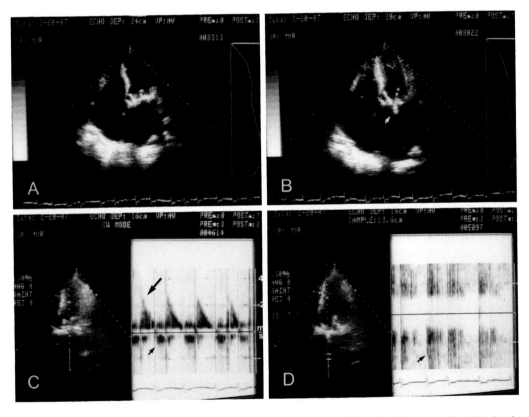

Figure 11.2. Mitral bioprosthetic leaflet tear. Seventy-four-year-old female, 10 years after mitral valve replacement for rheumatic mitral disease, presented with progressive heart failure and an apical systolic murmur. *Panels A and B* are atrial four-chamber diastolic and systolic two-dimensional images, respectively. The latter depicts prolapse of the torn leaflet into the left atrium (*arrow, panel B*). Continuous wave Doppler (*panel C*) shows a 3.0 m/sec peak diastolic velocity without obvious prolongation of $P_{1/2}t$ (*large arrow*) and systolic atrial disturbance (*small arrow*). The pulsed mode Doppler (*panel D*) confirms a significant regurgitant jet near the back wall of the left atrium (*small arrow*).

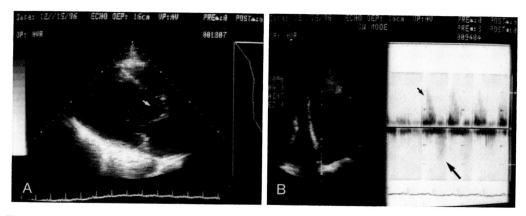

Figure 11.3. Aortic bioprosthetic leaflet tear. Twenty-nine-year-old male, 10 years after porcine aortic valve replacement for rheumatic aortic insufficiency; presented with a loud regurgitant murmur and recurrent superventricular tachycardia. Parasternal long-axis view demonstrates diastolic prolapse of the ruptured leaflet into the left ventricular outflow tract (*arrow, panel A*). Simultaneous two-dimensional/continuous wave image displays a diastolic disturbance (*small arrow, panel B*) subsequently mapped in pulsed mode as significant aortic regurgitation. Note the V_{max} is increased at 4.0 m/sec (*large arrow*), reflecting the enhanced stroke volume and not stenosis.

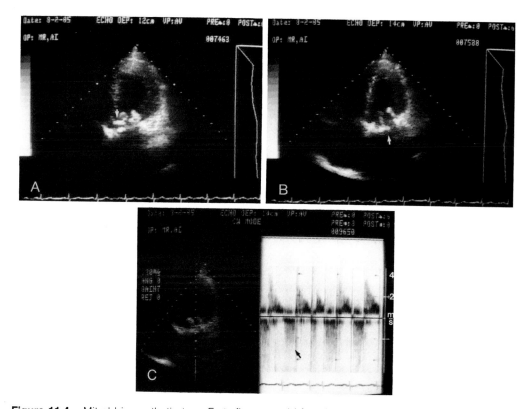

Figure 11.4. Mitral bioprosthetic tear. Forty-five-year-old female, 9 years after #29 porcine mitral valve replacement for rheumatic mitral stenosis; presented with an apical murmur and suspected subacute bacterial endocarditis. *Panels A* and *B* are apical four-chamber views, showing suspect vegetation prolapsing through the stent into LV inflow tract with diastole and systole, respectively (*arrows*). *Panel C* shows V_{max} is increased at greater than 3.0 m/sec with a rapid dropoff representing a normal $P_{1/2}t$; prosthetic mitral regurgitation is also present (*arrow*). At surgery, a torn and mildly calcified leaflet attached via a small pedicle was observed. There was no active infection.

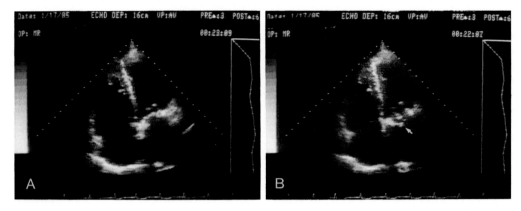

Figure 11.5. Mitral bioprosthetic tear. Sixty-three-year-old female, 8 years after porcine mitral valve replacement and coronary artery bypass surgery, presented with progressive dyspnea and fatigue. Diastolic and systolic two-dimensional images (*panels A and B*, respectively) depict prolapse of the torn leaflet into the left atrium (*arrow, B*). Leaflet calcification and tear with prolapse into the left atrium were demonstrated at surgery.

by Alam et al. (36). Reduced porcine bioprosthetic leaflet or closely corresponding anterior stent E–F slope appears to be of limited value in diagnosing porcine valve stenosis. This finding is common and in accord with reports of a mild diastolic hemodynamic gradient, even when these valves are functioning normally (44). Although leaflet motion in vitro and in vivo (41) has been related to stroke volume with partial opening of one leaflet in low flow states, i.e., less than 20 cc stroke volume (41), the M-mode and two-dimensional echocardiographic findings of dense leaflet echoes associated with low rate of diastolic movement of leaflet or stent should arouse suspicion of mitral bioprosthetic stenosis (35). Alam et al. (36) found thickening of the porcine cusp in the mitral position with loss of cusp detail to be more specific than reduced diastolic slope in diagnosing porcine valve stenosis. Other investigators have noticed a reduced ratio of internal stent diameter relative to a normal external stent diameter (35). Normal ultrasonic internal and external stent diameters have been reported with ranges of 0.56–0.74 by Horowitz et al. (42) and 0.7–0.9 by Chandraratna and San Pedro (45). Reduction in stent ratio, diminution in the space between the posterior stent echo and the posterior aortic root, no demonstrable systolic posterior space between leaflet, and stent with or without apparent diminution of aortic bioprosthetic leaflet excursion may indicate valve thrombosis (45).

Effect of Cardiac Arrhythmias and Conduction Disturbances on Prosthetic Valve Motion

The echocardiographic motion of normally functioning prosthetic valves can be influenced by various rhythm and conduction disturbances (66). These altered motion patterns may be mistaken for the echocardiographic appearance of malfunction in prosthetic valves and are clinically important. Panidis et al. (66) noted that echocardiographic findings during different arrthymias were similar for the various types of valve prostheses.

Prosthetic mitral valve closure occurs 60–80 msec following the Q wave (Q–C interval) in patients with normal P-R intervals in sinus rhythm (66) and in patients with complete atrioventricular block and implanted dual chamber pacemakers with programmable P-Q intervals (67). Earlier end-diastolic prosthetic mitral valve closure occurs when there is P-R interval prolongation: the Q-C interval is typically less than 60 msec. Premature closure of mitral valve prostheses in diastole has been reported to occur in patients with first degree atrioventricular block, atrial fibrillation with ventricular rates of fewer than 60 beats/min, atrial flutter, complete heart block, and VVI pacemakers (66). In general, the longer the P-R interval, the earlier the prosthetic mitral valve closes during end-diastole.

The proposed mechanisms of mitral valve closure have been categorized as "atriogenic" (where by closure results from termination of atrial systole) and "ventriculogenic" (whereby closure results from the onset of ventricular systole). These mechanisms were reviewed recently by Little et al. (100). Native atrioventricular valves were studied echocardiographically in atrioventricularly sequentially paced patients. The ventricular A point bore a constant temporal relation to the P wave over the range of P-Q intervals from 75 to 175 msec, suggesting "atriogenic" valve closure over this range. However, the interval from the P wave to completion of valve closure progressively shortened as the P-Q interval was decreased, suggesting progressive increasing ventricular contribution to completion of atrioventricular valve closure with shortening of the P-Q interval. During complete heart block, a rounded closing motion of the prosthetic mitral valve was observed during atrial systole-induced closure of the valve, while the closing motion of the valve was sharp when ventricular systole completed the prosthetic closure.

A late diastolic, anteriorly directed "bump" or "notch" on the prosthetic mitral valve echocardiogram can be observed corresponding to the P wave on the electrocardiogram and representing the effect of atrial contraction. This late diastolic bump induced by atrial contraction should be distinguished from an early diastolic bump on a Bjork-Shiley valve, which may indicate a paravalvular leak (50) or clot formation (49). It must also be distinguished from an early diastolic notch on a Beall valve or Starr-Edwards valve, suggesting variance of the prosthetic valve (95). Diastolic closure and reopening of a native or prosthetic mitral valve is well reported with atrial fibrillation, atrial flutter, atrial tachycardia, and complete heart block (66, 89, 106).

Panidis et al. (66) suggested an inverse relation between the preceding QRS cycle length (R to R interval of QRS on the electrocardiogram) and the Q-C interval of the prosthetic mitral valve in patients with atrial fibrillation. With R-R intervals of more than 1000 msec (ventricular rates of fewer than 60 beats/min), the Q-C interval was always less than 70 msec. This is in contrast to R-R intervals of less than 1000 msec (ventricular rates greater than 60 beats/min), where the Q-C interval was always greater than 70 msec. They proposed that in atrial fibrillation with ventricular rates of fewer 60 beats/min, closure of the prosthetic mitral valve is not accomplished by ventricular contraction. The mechanism of this early closure of the prosthetic mitral valve during atrial

fibrillation with prolonged filling periods may be associated with an increment in left ventricular pressure, resulting in a ventriculoatrial gradient across the mitral valve or development of a critical left ventricular "locking" volume (66, 97).

Patients with long R-R cycles may demonstrate premature diastolic closure of the prosthetic mitral valve (4). Premature closure of central disk or ball occluder-type mitral prosthetic valves in atrial fibrillation with long R-R intervals may be gravity-dependent and favored by factors contributing to diminution of transmitral flows, such as low cardiac output or large valvular orifice size. Premature closure of a prosthetic mitral valve was noted only when the atrial side of the prosthesis was below or level with the left ventricle and with occluders of a specific gravity greater than that of blood (65). Premature gravity-dependent closure of the posterior leaflet or bileaflet mitral prostheses has also been reported in patients with atrial fibrillation and long R-R intervals (60). The same investigators also reported gravitationally dependent diastolic fluttering of both leaflets during atrial fibrillation and long R-R cycles in the absence of aortic insufficiency.

Early diastolic closure of the prosthetic mitral valve with a reopening in late diastole has been reported in atrial flutter with a more than 2:1 atrial ventricular block and in atrial tachycardia with varying atrioventricular block. In contrast to atrial flutter, where the opening and closing of the Bjork-Shiley prosthetic mitral valve was sharp, Panidis et al. (66) noted a unique echocardiographic feature of atrial tachycardia with variable block. This was a rounded opening and closing motion of the prosthesis following the P waves and seemingly independent of ventricular contraction. Rounded late diastolic reopening of a Bjork-Shiley mitral valve prosthesis was also noted in a patient with atrioventricular sequentially paced dissociative rhythm, where the P-R interval was in the 400–440 msec range (66). Thus, the appearance of late diastolic rounded opening and closing motion of the prosthetic mitral valve in a patient with atrial tachycardia and variable block or dissociative rhythm may be mistaken for the opening bump of a dysfunctional monocuspid prosthetic mitral valve.

DOPPLER ECHOCARDIOGRAPHY
General Considerations

In vivo assessment of valve prostheses has previously been obtained in normal or dysfunctional prosthetic valves only by invasive investigation (15, 18, 38, 39, 53, 62, 107, 108). Doppler echocardiography has the potential to provide similar information by noninvasive means.

Evaluation of forward flow

Velocity profiles across the prosthetic valve are obtained by placing the transducer in the apical position in patients with a mitral or tricuspid prosthesis; and in the apical, suprasternal, or right parasternal positions in patients with aortic prostheses. The Doppler beam should be placed as perpendicular as possible to the plane of the valve ring in patients with a central flow valve; some angulation is required to obtain the maximal flow velocity in patients with a tilting disc valve, as flow through such valves is best demonstrated at the major orifice with weaker signals at the minor orifice (22). For caged-ball or caged-disc valves, velocities will be maximal around the periphery of the occluder. Bileaflet valves such as the St. Jude have three flow orifices with nearly equal maximal velocities. Bioprosthetic valves exhibit central flow characteristics. The audio signal of the Doppler spectrum is useful as a guide in the scanning procedure and may aid in identifying the optimum probe position.

Deviations of the Doppler probe from the ideal position (i.e., where the incident sound beam coincides with the direction and position of the vectors of V_{max}; cosine $0° = 1$) can result in a significant underestimation of the actual gradient. However, if the deviation is less than $15°–20°$, the errors will be relatively small because the values of the cosine function remain close to unity in this range (cosine $15° = 0.966$, cosine $20° = 0.939$). Holen et al. (53) showed that the tilting disc structure in the mitral position does not prevent the attainment of a satisfactory probe position. Thus, Doppler assessment of pressure gradient in nine adult patients with Bjork-Shiley mitral prostheses accurately and reliably predicted the mean transprosthetic diastolic gradient determined by catheterization to within 0.5 mm Hg.

Overestimation of Doppler-derived gradients may occur, especially with aortic prostheses. The proximal velocity term of the Bernouli equation may be substantial, and ignoring this term may lead to significant overestimation of the transprosthetic gradient. Moreover, pressure recovery may occur downstream from the valve, where the distal pressure is measured by catheter techniques; immediately adjacent to the occluder, higher velocities occur and thus a greater pressure drop is calculated. Recovery of downstream pressure is possible when flow is laminar and loss of energy by turbulence is minimal. The St. Jude valve has hemodynamic features which may allow this phenomenon to occur (113, 114).

It has been noted that prosthetic mitral valve Doppler profiles resemble mitral stenosis (16, 19, 74). There are three ways of expressing the magnitude of the obstruction to the mitral prosthesis: mean transprosthetic gradient, effective prosthetic mitral area, and pressure half-time. Holen et al. (18, 19, 39) characterized the obstructive features of normally functioning Hancock, Bjork-Shiley, and Lillihei-Kaster mitral valves. The ultrasound-derived mean transprosthetic mitral gradient and effective valve area corresponded well with catheterization-derived values in their study and values reported by others (47). Hatle and others (12, 74) have used the mean transprosthetic gradient and pressure half-time for porcine (Hancock) and tilting disc mitral (Bjork-Shiley) prostheses. Tabulated data from many investigators for mean transprosthetic gradients, effective prosthetic mitral area, and pressure half-time are listed in Tables 11.3 and 11.4.

A wide range of effective mitral orifice areas for each type and size of prosthesis has been reported (22). This variation has also been reported at catheterization and has been attributed to valve orientation and inertia of the prosthetic leaflets (90). In vitro, effective orifice area increases with prosthesis size (7). In vitro and in vivo, the effective valve area changes with flow across the valve (6, 40, 41, 61, 62) and can vary throughout diastole, usually being largest in the first third of diastole (91). The Doppler pressure half-time method utilizes the deceleration of velocities early in diastole and should measure the largest effective orifice at any cardiac output. Although the maximum detected flow is dependent on the cardiac output and on the presence of valvular regurgitation, the mitral pressure half-time is less subject to these variables. The evaluation of prosthetic pressure half-time may allow clear separation of the patient with prosthetic mitral stenosis from that with a paraprosthetic leak and regurgitation (Figs. 11.6 and 11.7).

Serial increases in calculated prosthetic valve area and diminution in pressure half-time associated with a systolic atrial disturbance have been recorded by Ferrara et al. (54), suggesting that Doppler echocardiography can adequately differentiate between (a) enhanced transprosthetic flow secondary to regurgitation with attendant increase in mitral valve area due to diastolic flow around a dehisced stent and (b) stenosis or enhanced flow due to increase in cardiac output (as with A-V pacing or isoproterenol). The former would be expected to demonstrate a systolic flow disturbance in the left atrium associated with an increased peak velocity and diminished pressure half-time, whereas the latter would demonstrate increased peak diastolic velocity and increased pressure half-time in the absence of a systolic left atrial disturbance (stenosis) or decrease in pressure half-time in the absence of a systolic left atrial disturbance (enhanced output).

Evaluation of regurgitant flow

In general, most normally functioning mechanical valve designs produce mild amounts of orifice regurgitation. The largest regurgitant volumes have been observed with the St. Jude (7.6–10.6 ml/beat) and Bjork-Shiley valves (5.5–8.5 ml/beat), as documented from in vitro laser Doppler studies by Yoganathan et al. (7). By comparison, bioprosthetic valve designs such as the Carpentier-Edwards valve produce much less orifice regurgitation (0.8–1.2 ml/beat) (7). Knowledge of the prosthetic design, therefore, is a necessary prerequisite for differentiating between abnormal and normal orifice regurgitation.

Paravalvular regurgitation may be difficult to distinguish from orifice regurgitation. Some authors found the orientation of the regurgitant jet to be helpful, with very eccentric jets indicating paravalvular leak (23); others, however, discerned no distinguishing feature of paravalvular regurgitation (21, 22, 54, 110). Transesophageal color Doppler may allow differentiation of paravalvular from valvular regurgitation, because it is possible to determine the origin of regurgitatant jets, especially for mitral prostheses, by this approach.

Doppler ultrasound may fail to penetrate prosthetic valves, and therefore regurgitant flow may be "masked" when the prosthesis is interposed between the ultrasound source and the chamber being interrogated (111). In this situation, significant regurgitant may be missed. Transesophageal Doppler echocardiography may be very helpful in the evaluation of mitral prostheses (112), since the left atrium can be interrogated without attenuation or distortion of the ultrasound signal by the prosthesis.

Starr-Edwards Valve

The Doppler assessment of a caged ball valve such as the Starr-Edwards in the mitral position is the most difficult of all mitral prostheses (1, 22). The sample volume or continuous wave beam must be placed beside the ball at the sewing ring to obtain adequate tracings (Table 11.3, Fig. 11.8). Williams and Labovitz (22) reported mean prosthetic mitral valve area in 10 patients with Starr-Edwards valve to be 2.0 ± 0.3 cm^2. Smaller effective orifice areas of the Starr-Edwards mitral prosthesis were associated with a higher peak diastolic gradient, ranging from 4 to 19 mm Hg (mean: 10 mm Hg) in the five patients with Starr-Edwards prostheses in whom this parameter was measured. Panidis et al. (1) found similar calculated effective orifice areas and peak diastolic gradients in three patients with clinically normal Starr-Edwards mitral prostheses. Peak velocity was 1.8 ± 0.4 m/sec, and the mean diastolic gradient was 5 ± 2 mm Hg. The results of Doppler measurements of effective mitral valve area parallel measurements obtained in vitro and in vivo from catheterization (8, 70).

In the aortic position, normal Starr-Edwards prosthetic function may be associated with peak gradients of up to 64 mm Hg (1, 22, 106) (Table 11.5). Williams and Labovitz (22) studied six normally functioning Starr-Edwards aortic prostheses, with mean transvalvular gradients ranging from 12 to 50 mg Hg (mean: 29.3 ± 13.3 mm Hg). Panidis et al. (1) studied four normally functioning prostheses, finding normal peak transvalvular gradients ranging from 36 to 43 mm Hg (mean: 40 ± 3 mm Hg). Peak velocities of 3.2 ± 0.2 m/sec were noted. Of the 12 normal aortic Starr-Edwards recipients described by Ramirez et al. (73), two patients with 22 mm valves had gradients of 64 mm Hg. The strong negative correlation ($r = 0.99$) between peak systolic flow velocity and valve size reported by these investigators amplifies the importance of obtaining prosthesis size in aortic caged ball recipients. Thus, higher Doppler gradients across normally functioning Starr-Edwards aortic prostheses were encountered and agree with values reported in vitro and at catheterization (8, 71, 72).

In vitro regurgitant volumes of Starr-Edwards prostheses are among the lowest of all prosthetic designs because of complete occlusion of the primary flow orifice when closed (8). Williams and Labovitz (22) and Panidis et al. (1) reported "insignificant" regurgitation in Starr-Edwards prostheses in both mitral and aortic positions.

Abnormal function: Williams et al. (22) described one patient with an aortic Starr-Edwards valve whose peak gradient was 64 mm Hg. Valve size and surgical findings were not reported, although valve stenosis was stated to be confirmed at operation. The potential for subvalvular left

Table 11.3. Normal Function of Mitral Valve Prostheses by Doppler Echocardiography

Valve	Author	N	Peak Velocity	Peak Gradient	Mean Gradient	$P_{1/2}t$	Orifice (cm²)	Regurgitation	Comments
Starr-Edwards	Panidis IP et al. (1)	3	1.8 ± 0.4	13 ± 5	5 ± 2		2.1 ± 0.5	1/3	Insignificant
	Williams GA and Labovitz AJ (22)	10		10 (five pts range 4–19 mm Hg)			2.0 ± 0.3	3/10	No correlation between stent size and calculated valve area
Bjork-Shiley	Holen J et al. (19)	9					2.13 ± 0.72		Immediate postoperative period
	Williams GA and Labovitz AJ (22)	36		10 (19 patients)			2.5 ± 0.8	4/36	Mild regurgitation; no correlation between Doppler-derived effective orifice area to stent size
	Sagar KB et al. (21) #29	7		7.0 ± 3.7	2.0 ± 0.08		2.1 ± 0.2	4/17	Mild regurgitation
	Panidis IP et al. (1) #31	10		6.0 ± 3.0	2.0 ± 1.9		2.2 ± 0.3	3/8	Insignificant regurgitation
							2.2 ± 0.4		
	Holen J et al. (53)	9			5.2 ± 2.6				Simultaneous manometric (transseptal left atrial and retrograde left ventricular catheterization) and continuous wave Doppler data-confirmed accuracy of instantaneous or mean pressure gradient to within ± 0.5 mm Hg
St. Jude	Weinstein IR et al. (63)	13	1.38 ± 0.33		2.3 ± 0.9	61.2 ± 16.9		1/13	No difference between 29 and 31 mm valves.
	Panidis IP et al. (1)	44	1.6 ± 0.3	11 ± 4	5 ± 2		3.0 ± 0.6	14/44	No significant difference in peak velocity, peak and mean gradients when patients with 27, 29, or 31 St. Jude valves compared

Bioprostheses								
Panidis IP et al. (1)	6	1.9 ± 0.3	15 ± 5	7 ± 1	(100)	2.2 ± 0.7	0	
Gibbs JL et al. (34)	38	1.64 ± 0.2			90		4/38	Weak correlation between $P_{1/2}t$ and time since implantation; mitral regurgitation detected in patients 3 yr postimplant
Holen J et al. (39)	8			5.4			1/8	
Simpson IA et al. (20)	90	0.9–2.0		3.5	81		3/47	Mild regurgitation; trend toward longer $P_{1/2}t$ with 29 versus 31 or 33 valves
Ryan T et al. (38)	29	1.36 ± .24			136 ± 18		1/29	Mitral regurgitation clinically undetected in patients 97 months postoperative with V_{max} 1.75 m/sec; poor correlation of $P_{1/2}t$ with prosthetic mitral valve size; $^{25}/_{28}$ implants 31–35 mm range; possible relationship between $P_{1/2}t$ and age of implant
Sagar KB et al. (21) #27	3		10.0 ± 4	5.0 ± 2.0		1.3 ± 0.8		
#29	9		7.0 ± 3	2.0 ± 0.7		1.5 ± 0.2		
#31	8		4.0 ± 0.7	2.0 ± 0.9		1.6 ± 0.2		
#33	3		3.0 ± 2.0	2.0 ± 2.0		1.9 ± 0.2		Normal function defined as mean gradient 8 mm Hg and absence of clinical and hemodynamically significant obstruction and regurgitation across the prosthesis
Williams GA and Labovitz AJ (22)	16		15 (3 patients)			2.1 ± 0.7 (1.1 to 4 cm²)	3/16	No correlation between valve area and stent size. Minimal mitral regurgitation in 3 patients
Holen J et al. (19)	8					1.40 ± 0.68 Ae		Effective valve area (Ae) obtained in the immediate postoperative period (see text)

Table 11.4. Abnormal Function of Mitral Valve Prostheses by Doppler Echocardiography

Valve	Author	N	Peak Velocity	Peak Gradient	Mean Gradient	$P_{1/2}t$	Orifice (cm²)	Regurgitation	Comments
Starr-Edwards	Veyrat C et al. (23)	6							Two patients with perivalvular leak; preoperative estimate of circumference of paravalvular leak
Bjork-Shiley Lillehei-Kaster	Williams GA and Labovitz AJ (22)	4					0.65 0.5 2.2	0 0 3+	Tissue ingrowth Tissue ingrowth Severe regurgitation and dehiscence confirmed by catheterization
							2.0	1+	Mild regurgitation on Doppler 2 + on catheterization
	Sagar KB et al. (21)	1 4			22 mm Hg 10 mm Hg		0.5–0.6 2.0 (2 patients)	0	Tissue ingrowth and thrombus Mitral valve area by catheterization. Close correlation between Doppler and catheterization mean gradient; and between Doppler and catheterization mitral valve area
	Panidis IP et al. (1)	1	No demonstrable flow						Autopsy-proven thrombosis and fibrosis of prosthesis
	Nitter-Hauge (17)	3	2.25 m/sec 1.72 1.34					+ – +	One patient each with Bjork-Shiley, Lillihei-Kaster and Hall-Kaster prostheses; all had thrombus. Peak V_{max} > "normal", prolonged $P_{1/2}t$ (unspecified)
	Ferrara RP et al. (54)	1	1.0 2.8				2.0 2.2 2.7	– + +	Immediately postsurgery. New systolic murmur, heart failure with endocarditis 2 weeks following mitral valve replacement; Doppler demonstrated regurgitation and progressive decrease in $P_{1/2}t$; catheterization and surgery confirmed dehiscence.
	Veyrat C et al. (23)	3							Mapping of paravalvular leak

	Reference	n						Paravalvular regurgitation	
St. Jude	Weinstein IR et al. (63)	1						1/1	Significant regurgitation by Doppler 1-month postop
	Panidis IP et al. (1)	1			31			+	Endocarditis with death; no catheterization data
Bioprostheses	Panidis IP et al. (1) H27	1			25	17		Significant	Degeneration; 3+ mitral regurgitation at catheterization
	H27	1			36	18		Present	Degeneration; 3+ mitral regurgitation at catheterization
	C-E29	1			11	4		Significant	Degeneration; 3+ mitral regurgitation at catheterization
	C-E31	1			15	5		Significant	Degeneration; 3+ mitral regurgitation at catheterization
	C-E31	1			23	8		Significant	Degeneration; 3+ mitral regurgitation at catheterization
	Wilkins GT (15)	7		3.5–10.4			1.5–2.6		All 6–7 yrs postimplant. All presented with signs of atrioventricular valve dysfunction
	Sagar KR (21)	12		15–25 (six patients with MS, six with MR)			(est. 0.7–1.3)	6/12	Six patients with stenosis (1/6 with 1+ mitral regurgitation at catheterization). Six patients with mitral regurgitation and mean regurgitation unreported; Doppler unable to distinguish valvular from paravalvular regurgitation
	Williams GA and Labovitz AJ (22)	1					1.8	3+	Degeneration; 3+ mitral regurgitation at catheterization
	Veyrat C et al. (23)	3						3/3	One third incorrectly identified as having paravalvular regurgitation
	Ryan T et al. (38)	11	2.11 ± 0.49 (MS) 2.06 ± 0.53 (MR + MS)	12–24 (MS)			220 ± 63	10/11 (2+)	$P_{1/2}t > 180$ cms in seven of eight patients with prosthetic stenosis; patients with prosthetic dysfunction younger than those with normally functioning prostheses (51 ± 12 yrs versus 61 ± 10 yrs)

Table 11.5. Normal Function of Aortic Valve Prostheses by Doppler Echocardiography

Valve	Author	N	Peak Velocity	Peak Gradient	Mean Gradient	Regurgitation	Comments
Starr-Edwards	Williams GA and Labovitz AJ (22)	6		29 ± 13		2/6	Insignificant
	Panidis IP et al. (1)	4	3.2 ± 0.2	40 ± 3	24 ± 4	3/4	Insignificant
	Ramirez ML #22	2	4.0 ± 0.0			6/12	Strong negative correlation (r = 0.99) between peak systolic flow velocity and volume size
	et al. (73) #24	5	3.45 ± 0.6				
	#26	5	3.0 ± 0.23				
Bjork-Shiley	Sagar KB #23	6		33 ± 4	14 ± 7	4/20	Insignificant
	et al. (21) #25	9		19 ± 5	13 ± 5		
	#27	5		16 ± 5	10 ± 2		
	Williams GA and Labovitz AJ (22)	33		22 ± 10.0		14/33	Insignificant
	Panidis IP et al. (1)	8	2.6 ± 0.5	27 ± 9	14 ± 6	5/8	Insignificant
	Ramirez ML #21	4	2.76 ± 0.9			2/21	Negative correlation (r = 0.80) between peak systolic flow velocity and valve size
	et al. (73) #23	5	2.76 ± 0.42				
	#25	4	2.06 ± 0.31				
	#27	5	1.81 ± 0.20				
	#29	2	1.87 ± 0.17				
St. Jude	Weinstein IR et al. (63)	7	1.97 ± 0.52				
	Panidis IP et al. (1)	38	2.3 ± 0.6	22 ± 12	12 ± 7	22/38	Insignificant aortic regurgitation
Bioprostheses	Panidis IP et al. (1)	9	2.6 ± 0.6	30 ± 12	17 ± 10	4/9	Mild aortic insufficiency (AI)
	Sagar KB #23	7		18 ± 4	12 ± 2	5/22	Mild AI
	et al. (21) #25	10		16 ± 2	11 ± 3		
	#27	5		15 ± 3	10 ± 3		

Study	N	Velocity	Age	Fraction	Comments
Williams GA and Labovitz AJ (22)	27		23 ± 10	8/31	AI in clinically normal patients
Simpson IA et al. (20)	19		18 ± 9	5/19	Mild AI
Ramirez ML and Wong M (27)	20	2.52 ± 0.10			Defines intra- and interobserver variability
Gibbs JL et al. (34)	24	2.44 ± 0.48		2/24	Peak velocity correlated weakly with time since implantation; AR detected in patients 3.5 ± 5.5 years postoperatively; the latter with peak velocity of 3.2 m/sec (clinically normal)
Ramirez ML et al. (73)	106	Carpentier-Edwards #21 3.25 ± 1.42 #23 2.95 ± 0.07 #25 2.76 ± 0.55 #27 2.45 ± 0.39 #29 2.41 ± 0.44 #31 2.36 ± 0.43 Hancock #21 3.50 #23 2.94 ± 0.24 #25 2.48 ± 0.32 #27 2.38 ± 0.39 #29 2.23 ± 0.04 #31 2.00		9/41	Both valve types showed significant negative correlation between valve size and peak aortic flow velocity (see text)

Table 11.6. Abnormal Function of Aortic Valve Prostheses by Doppler Echocardiography

Valve	Author	Size	N	Peak Velocity	Peak Gradient	Mean Gradient	Regurgitation	Comments
Starr-Edwards	Williams IR et al. (22)		1		64			50 mm gradient at catheterization; dysfunction confirmed at operation, but surgical finding not reported
	Veyrat C et al. (23)		7				4/7	Four patients with paravalvular leak; preoperative estimate of circumference of paravalvular leak accurate in 3/4
Bjork-Shiley	Williams GA and Labovitz AJ (22)		4		55		0	48 mm Hg peak to peak gradient to surgery
					100		0	3+ AI at catheterization
					0		2+	2+ AI at catheterization
					0		2+	2+ AI at catheterization
	Sagar KB et al. (21)		8				6/8	Severe AI in two; Doppler unable to distinguish valvular from paravalvular regurgitation; 2/8 stenosis
	Panidis JP et al. (1)		1		26	14	yes	Significant AI on Doppler; 2+ AI at catheterization
	Veyrat C et al. (23)		3					
St. Jude	Weinstein IR et al. (63)		3				3/3	2/3 AI unsuspected clinically; severity unreported
	Panidis JP et al. (1)	19	1		44	18	3+	Significant AI at catheterization
		19	1		45	18	3+	1/3 had increased flow velocity and gradient by Doppler compared to normals
		23	1		55	37	2–3+	
	Veyrat C et al. (23)		1				1/1	Preoperative estimate of circumference of paravalvular tear
Bioprostheses	Sagar KA et al. (21)		14			30–68	11/14	Good correlation (r = 0.94) between Doppler and catheterization-derived mean gradients (Hancock and Bjork-Shiley prostheses) for stenotic or normal prostheses
	Williams GA and Labovitz AJ (22)		2	4.0	64 (stenosis) / 0 (regurgitation)		3+	Calcified bioprosthesis (stenosis); pathology of incompetent valve unreported, 3+ AI on catheterization

ventricular outflow tract obstruction should be recognized and necessitates interrogation of the outflow tract using pulsed or high pulse repetition frequency modes. Veyrat et al. (23) identified four paraprosthetic leaks among seven abnormal Starr-Edwards aortic prostheses (Table 11.6); and by Doppler echocardiography, preoperative estimation of the circumferential extent of the paravalvular leak was accurately obtained in all.

Bjork-Shiley Valve

Doppler echocardiographic evaluation of flow characteristics of tilting disc valves, like the Bjork-Shiley, is easier than the Doppler assessment of peripheral flow valves such as the Starr-Edwards and Beall valves (1, 22) (Fig. 11.9, *panel D*). Holen et al. (53) evaluated nine patients with clinically normal Bjork-Shiley mitral prostheses using simultaneous manometric (transseptal, left atrial, and retrograde left ventricular catheterization) and continuous wave Doppler, confirming the accuracy of Doppler-derived instantaneous or mean pressure gradient to within 0.5 mm Hg of that determined by manometry (Table 11.3). They found a mean transprosthetic mitral gradient of 5.2 ± 2.6 mm Hg (range: 2.0–11.0 mm Hg) and found that a satisfactory Doppler probe position was possible with posteriorly directed flow of the disc's major orifice.

In the immediate postoperative period, Holen

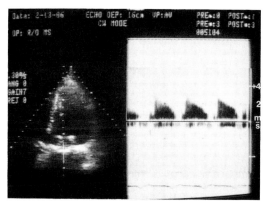

Figure 11.6. Mitral bioprosthetic stenosis. Seventy-year-old male, 10 years after #31 porcine mitral valve replacement; presented with progressive dyspnea. Two-dimensional/continuous wave image demonstrates a 2.9 m/sec V_{max} and prolonged $P_{1/2}t$ of 275 msec consistent with porcine mitral stenosis. At surgery the porcine bioprosthesis demonstrated multiple nodular calcifications within the cusps and along the commissures. Mild strut creep was present.

et al. (19) calculated effective valve areas (A_e) as a measure of flow obstruction in the prosthetic mitral valve implants. Along with other investigators (13, 14, 18), Holen found A_e to be independent of cardiac output and heart rate at rest. The A_e of 2.13 ± 0.72 as determined by Doppler closely approximated those calculations (by the Gorlin formula) performed simultaneously by manometry. This was also true in the study of Bjork et al. (47), in which Gorlin-based manometric determinations of prosthetic valve area were corrected by a factor of 0.6. This correction reflects the in vivo dependency of the ratio of ultrasound-to-catheterization gradient on orifice size, where increasing ratios (and the necessity for correction factor) were encountered with smaller orifices. For the 27, 29, and 31 Bjork-Shiley mitral prostheses, the effective valve areas were 1.65, 2.24, and 2.07 cm², respectively. For the 20 and 25 Lillehei-Kaster mitral prostheses, the effective valve areas were 1.41 and 2.33, respectively (19).

Williams et al. (22) reported mitral valve orifice calculations using the pressure half-time method as reported by Hatle (12) in 36 patients with normally functioning mitral Bjork-Shiley prostheses (Table 11.3). These 36 clinically normal patients had a mean valve area of 2.5 ± 0.8 cm², ranging from 1.8 to 3.7 cm². Average peak diastolic gradient when reported in 19 of the 36 patients was 10 mm Hg. Sagar et al. (21) and Panidis et al. (1) reported mitral valve orifice calculations by the pressure half-time method in a range similar to that reported by Williams (22). Also, Sagar et al. (21) and Panidis et al. (1) reported an average peak diastolic gradient of 6–10 mm Hg and mean diastolic transvalvular gradients of 2–5 mm Hg (Table 10.3). These values of mean transprosthetic diastolic gradient are in agreement with others obtained by a simultaneous manometric and Doppler ultrasonic study reported by Holen et al. (53) and confirmed the mild obstructive nature of a normally functioning tilting disc valve in the mitral position. Minimal regurgitation is a normal finding and is demonstrable in as many as one of three patients by pulsed Doppler as a systolic disturbance adjacent to the mitral prosthesis in the left atrium (1, 21, 22).

Williams and Labovitz (22) reported peak transvalvular gradients measured in 33 patients with Bjork-Shiley aortic prosthesis to range from 5 to 38 mm Hg (mean: 21.5 ± 10.0) (Table 10.5). Seventy percent of normal patients had peak gradients of 22 mm Hg or less. Where Doppler-derived systolic transvalvular gradients were plotted for Bjork-Shiley and porcine aortic prostheses, a

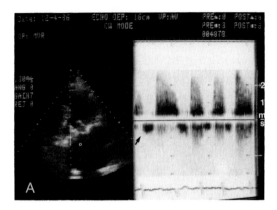

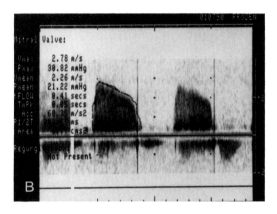

Figure 11.7. Mitral bioprosthetic stenosis. Sixty-three-year-old female, 3 years after #29 Hancock mitral valve replacement for rheumatic mitral stenosis; presented with recurrent congestive heart failure and atrial fibrillation. Note a 2.8 m/sec V_{max} and suggestion of a regurgitant (systolic) atrial disturbance on simultaneous two-dimensional/continuous wave imaging (*arrow, panel A*). Continuous wave (*panel B*) shows pressure half-time of 281 msec, consistent with prosthetic stenosis. Only trace of mitral regurgitation was present.

weak correlation was found ($r = -0.35$), the gradients increasing with decreasing valve size. The only gradients over 32 mm Hg were seen in valves of size 23 mm or less. Sagar et al. (21) also noted that the six patients with a 23 mm Bjork-Shiley prosthesis had the highest peak gradients (33 ± 4 mm Hg) and mean gradients (14 ± 7 mm Hg). The ranges of mean peak gradient and mean systolic gradient were 16–33 mm Hg and 10–14 mm Hg, respectively, in the study of normal aortic Bjork-Shiley prostheses (sizes 23, 25, and 27) reported by Sagar et al. (21) (Table 11.5).

The range of peak systolic and mean systolic transvalvular gradients for normal Bjork-Shiley aortic prostheses of unspecified size were also reported by Panidis et al. (1) to be 13–36 mm Hg (mean: 27 ± 9 mm Hg) and 6–23 mm Hg (mean: 14 ± 6 mm Hg). The range of peak velocity was 1.8–3.0 m/sec (mean: 2.6 ± 0.5 m/sec). Thus, it appears that a normally functioning Bjork-Shiley prosthesis in the aortic position is associated with a peak gradient of < 40 mm Hg by Doppler ultrasonography.

Regurgitation across the aortic Bjork-Shiley

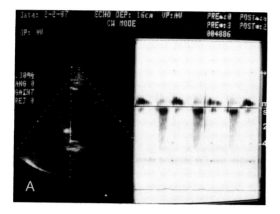

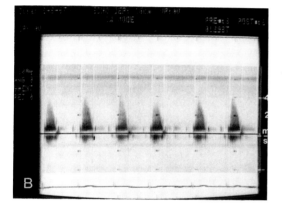

Figure 11.8. Aortic caged ball valve stenosis. Seventy-three-year-old male, 16 years after Smeloff-Sutter (medium size) aortic valve replacement for rheumatic aortic stenosis, presented with typical exertional angina. Cardiac catheterization revealed triple vessel disease: Retrograde or transseptal left heart catheterization was not performed. Simultaneous two-dimensional/continuous wave Doppler (*panel A*) shows 4.4 m/sec V_{max}. Nonimaging Pedof continuous wave (*panel B*) from the right parasternal position, in comparison, underestimates the V_{max} recorded with the imaging transducer.

prosthesis of an insignificant nature (i.e., confined to the valvular or immediate subvalvular outflow area) was demonstrable in up to 42% of normal patients (Table 11.5). The insufficiency was holodiastolic, and localization of the origin of insufficiency to the valve or paravalvular area was not possible using the apical window (1).

Abnormal function: Sagar et al. (21) and Williams and Labovitz (22) collectively evaluated nine patients with dysfunctional Bjork-Shiley mitral prostheses by Doppler echocardiography, cath-

eterization, or subsequent surgery (Table 11.4). Patients with tissue ingrowth or thrombus of the Bjork-Shiley prosthesis typically had prosthetic mitral valve areas (by the pressure half-time method) of 0.5–0.7 cm² with close correlation between Doppler-derived and catheterization-derived values for mitral valve area (21, 22) and mean transprosthetic gradient (21). A mean mitral transprosthetic gradient of 22 mm Hg was reported by Sagar et al. (21) in their patient with a thrombosed Bjork-Shiley mitral prosthesis. Ex-

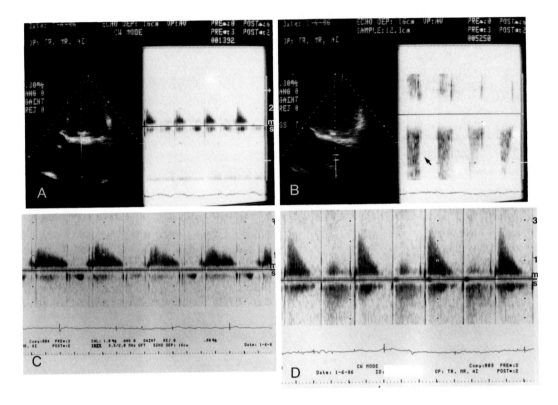

Figure 11.9. Mitral Harken disc perivalvular regurgitation, tricuspid Harken disc stenosis, and normal aortic Bjork-Shiley prosthesis. Sixty-nine-year-old female, 13 years after Harken mitral and tricuspid #21 Bjork-Shiley aortic valve replacements, and VVI pacemaker implant presented with predominantly right-sided congestive heart failure, hemolytic anemia, and syncope.

An apical four-chamber, two-dimensional/continuous wave image with continuous wave cursor on axis to the mitral central occluder disc (*panel A*) does not reveal the presence of 3+ mitral regurgitation as does the off-axis pulsed-mode image (*panel B, arrow*). Cinefluoroscopy revealed an excessive degree of valve rocking, suggesting the possibility of perivalvular disruption. Surgery revealed a 4 to 5 mm hole in the posterior mitral anulus, the site of the perivalvular leak.

Panel C demonstrates a prosthetic tricuspid V_{max} of 1.8 m/sec and $P_{1/2}t$ of 190 msec, suspicious for prosthetic stenosis. Cinefluoroscopy revealed severe restriction of disc movement within its cage. At surgery the tricuspid prosthesis was entirely normal but was unable to open completely, because the cage was partially embedded in the interventricular septum.

The nonimaging Pedof continuous wave transducer (*panel D*) demonstrates an aortic prosthetic V_{max} of 3.0 m/sec, within the range of normal.

amination of normal Doppler-derived mean transprosthetic gradients as listed in Table 11.3 would substantiate this as an abnormal value.

Panidis et al. (1) described a patient with no demonstrable transmitral flow on Doppler interrogation. At autopsy, thrombosis and fibrosis of the prosthesis were encountered. Nitter-Hauge (17) reported three patients with Bjork-Shiley mitral prosthetic dysfunction due to thrombus formation. The patient with fixation of the valve in the open position by thrombus formation at the minor orifice showed maximal velocity and fall in peak pressure greater than normal (though unspecified), whereas a second patient with thrombus of the minor orifice resulting in pure prosthetic stenosis (confirmed at operation) showed a high normal maximal diastolic velocity associated with a prolonged pressure half-time.

Sagar et al. (21) and Williams and Labovitz (22) reported catheterization-confirmed prosthetic regurgitation to be associated with calculated mitral valve areas of > 2.0 cm^2 associated with significant systolic atrial disturbance. In the two patients with prosthetic regurgitation reported by Sagar et al. (21), mean transprosthetic gradient was less than 10 mm Hg. Ferrara et al. (54) have convincingly demonstrated the utility of Doppler echocardiography in diagnosing dysfunctional and progressive prosthetic regurgitation in a patient who developed bacterial endocarditis 2 weeks following Bjork-Shiley mitral valve replacement. Dehiscence confirmed by catheterization and surgery was associated with a progressive increase in maximal diastolic velocity, diminution in pressure half-time, and thus increase in calculated mitral valve area by the pressure half-time method.

Most investigators report the inability to differentiate prosthetic from paraprosthetic regurgitation in a Bjork-Shiley mitral valve by Doppler interrogation alone (21, 22, 54). However, Veyrat et al. (23) described a group of 19 patients with dysfunctional mitral prostheses (3 with Bjork-Shiley) and were able to identify the site and magnitude of dysfunction in bioprostheses and mechanical prostheses. They found pulsed Doppler and surgical results correlated well for both the site of dysfunction (80% of patients) and the size of the leak (81% of patients). Two of three patients with paraprosthetic leaks around a Bjork-Shiley mitral valve were identified, and estimates of leak circumference by pulse Doppler approximated the surgical findings.

Malfunction of the Bjork-Shiley prosthesis in the aortic position has been reported (1, 21–23)

(Table 10.6). Good correlation between Doppler echocardiography and cardiac catheterization for the mean gradient of normally functioning and stenotic aortic prostheses was reported by Sagar et al. (21). However, alteration of mechanical prosthetic function during retrograde catheterization across a tilting disc valve may negate the accuracy of catheterization in diagnosing prosthetic dysfunction. This is in part because of catheter-induced regurgitation (21). The maximal instantaneous pressure gradient or mean transprosthetic gradient across a suspect dysfunctional Bjork-Shiley aortic prosthesis should be compared to baseline postoperative studies. Significant prosthetic dysfunction may be present with little transprosthetic gradient when there is left ventricular dysfunction (22) or aortic insufficiency (1, 22). As there appears to be a significant learning curve when dysfunctional native aortic valves are examined (26, 29), the serial evaluation of tilting disc valves in the aortic position should be performed by experienced operators so as to avoid potential underestimation of maximal instantaneous pressure gradient.

St. Jude Valve

The hemodynamic advantages of the mitral St. Jude valve, including a lower transvalvular gradient and a larger effective orifice area, especially in smaller annular sizes, have been demonstrated by angiographic (109) and early postoperative hemodynamic studies (61). Mean mitral valve gradient was measured from direct postoperative (to 48 hr) left atrial and left ventricular pressures by Chaux et al. (62). This gradient ranged from 1.4 ± 0.2 to 1.9 ± 0.6 mm Hg in 26 patients with St. Jude mitral prostheses, sizes 25, 27, 29, and 31 mm. This range of postoperative transprosthetic gradients parallels that reported by Weinstein (63) using Doppler echocardiography and averaging 2.3 ± 0.9 mm Hg for 29 and 31 mm prostheses (Table 11.3).

A larger mean transprosthetic Doppler mitral gradient of 5 ± 2 mm Hg was reported by Panidis et al. (1) in 44 patients with St. Jude prostheses. No significant difference in peak velocity or peak and mean gradients was evident when patients with 27, 29, or 31 mm St. Jude valves were compared by Panidis et al. (1) or by Weinstein et al. (63) in patients with a 29 or 31 mm St. Jude valve in the mitral position. The two studies listed in Table 11.3 suggest that a mean transprosthetic mitral gradient of > 7 mm Hg should raise suspicion of possible prosthetic malfunction.

Weinstein et al. (63) reported pressure half-time to be 61 ± 16.9 msec in their 13 normal mitral St. Jude recipients (Table 11.3). The range of pressure half-time of 44 to 122 msec would be expected for normal mitral St. Jude valves based on the pressure half-time-derived calculations of mitral valve area (1.8–5.0 cm^2) in the 44 normal patients described by Panidis et al. (1). Mitral orifice area calculated by the pressure half-time method (1) was 3.0 ± 0.6 cm^2. Mitral valve areas derived from the Gorlin formula were reported by Chaux et al. (62) to range from 2.1 ± 0.5 to 3.1 ± 0.9 cm in the 26 patients with a 25, 27, 29, or 31 mm St. Jude prosthesis in the immediate postoperative period. Under conditions of maximal orifice utilization (flow) during isoproterenol infusion, calculated orifice areas ranged from 3.5 ± 1.6 to 4.4 ± 2.2 cm^2 for 27, 29, and 31 mm prostheses. Similar in vivo determinations of Doppler-derived estimates of effective valve orifice areas for St. Jude prostheses in response to exercise or isoproterenol infusion have not been published.

Weinstein et al. (63) found Doppler echocardiography provided data suitable for analysis in 7 of 10 patients with clinically normal aortic St. Jude prostheses (Table 11.5). Respective mean and maximal velocities were 1.23 ± 0.25 and 1.97 ± 0.52 for normal St. Jude aortic prostheses, in comparison with 0.89 ± 0.14 and 1.22 ± 0.19 m/sec for normal aortic valves. Larger prosthetic valves tended to generate smaller mean and peak flow velocities, although the number of patients with each size valve was too small to allow a meaningful comparison. Panidis et al. (1), in a study including 38 patients with normal St. Jude aortic prostheses, found a peak velocity of 2.3 ± 0.6 m/sec and mean systolic transvalvular gradient of 12 ± 7 mm Hg (Table 11.5). The peak velocity and the peak and mean gradients of the St. Jude valve in the aortic position were lower than in those of the Bjork-Shiley (eight patients), Starr-Edwards (four patients), or tissue valve (nine patients). These differences reached statistical significance only when compared with the Starr-Edwards valve. When patients with size 19, 21, 23, or 25 mm St. Jude valve in the aortic position were compared by Panidis et al. (1), peak velocity and peak and mean gradients tended to be higher in patients with a smaller valve size. As in the study of Weinstein et al. (63), these differences did not reach statistical significance.

Insignificant aortic regurgitation, suggested by the detection of a diastolic regurgitant jet in the left ventricular outflow tract immediately below the prosthetic aortic valve, was detected by Doppler technique in 58% of patients with an aortic St. Jude valve.

Abnormal function: Panidis et al. (1) and Weinstein et al. (63) reported one patient each with dysfunction of the mitral St. Jude prosthesis. Significant regurgitation by Doppler echocardiography associated with peak and mean diastolic gradients of 31 and 8 mm Hg, respectively, 1 month postoperatively resulted in reoperation (without catheterization) in the patient described by Panidis et al. (1). The patient described by Weinstein et al. (63) had a paravalvular leak suspected by physical examination and confirmed by Doppler echocardiography, although the magnitude of regurgitation and diastolic gradients were unreported.

Utilization of pressure half-time may be invaluable in the serial assessment of St. Jude mitral valve function. Pressure half-time of a normally functioning St. Jude mitral prosthesis is not significantly different from that of a normal native mitral valve and approximates 60 msec (63). An increase in transmitral maximal velocity above the normal range for the St. Jude mitral prosthesis (Table 11.3) associated with a normal or near normal pressure half-time would suggest enhanced transmitral flow due to increased cardiac output or valvular/paravalvular regurgitation. The latter is associated with a significant and systolic disturbance in the left atrium as mapped by pulsed Doppler technique. However, the regurgitation may be masked by reverberations from the prosthesis, especially in the apical four-chamber view. A prolonged pressure half-time is expected to be a more reliable indicator of prosthetic stenosis than peak or mean transprosthetic gradient, as it is independent of cardiac output. In addition, peak or mean transmitral gradient across dysfunctional St. Jude mitral prostheses may be normal or near normal in the presence of severe left ventricular dysfunction or low cardiac output.

Panidis et al. (1) described three patients with significant regurgitation of an aortic St. Jude prosthesis. One of the three had an increased mean gradient and flow velocity, whereas the other two had an increased flow velocity at mildly elevated mean gradients (valvular sizes unspecified). Regurgitation was clinically unsuspected in two of the three patients. Veyrat et al. (23) identified one patient with a paraprosthetic leak around a St. Jude aortic device and estimated (preoperatively) the extent of the circumferential tear.

Prosthetic aortic regurgitation is confirmed by finding a diastolic flow disturbance > 2 cm below the prosthetic ring in the outflow tract. The presence of a diastolic disturbance associated with an increase in maximal velocity should aid in the differentiation of prosthetic regurgitation from stenosis. Additionally, the peak instantaneous pressure estimated on spectral display of Doppler velocities occurs earlier in insufficient valves as compared with stenotic prostheses. However, these findings are not unique to the St. Jude aortic prosthesis.

Hancock and Carpentier-Edwards Valves

Normal mitral porcine xenograft function assessed by Doppler echocardiography has been reported by many investigators (1, 19–22, 34, 38, 39) and is tabulated in Table 11.3. Holen et al. (39) compared mean manometric pressure gradient via simultaneous left atrial and left ventricular catheterization (P_c) with mean diastolic pressure gradient determined from noninvasive ultrasound data (P_u) in eight clinically normal Hancock mitral valve recipients. In these patients, P_c was 5.4 mm, and the difference between P_c and P_u was 0.3 ± 0.9 mm Hg. Wilkins et al. (15) also reported a close relationship ($r = 0.96$) between simultaneous P_c and P_u with simultaneous transseptal left atrial and left ventricular catheterization in seven patients with clinically abnormal porcine mitral valves.

Normally functioning prosthetic mitral xenografts (29 patients) were reported by Ryan et al. (38) to be associated with $V_{max} \le 1.8$ m/sec, pressure half-time ≤ 160 msec, and absence of a systolic left atrial disturbance. Ryan et al. (38) were unable to correlate pressure half-time with the size of the mitral porcine xenograft: 25 of 28 prostheses fell within the narrow range of 31–35 mm. Simpson et al. (20) reported 44 normal recipients of Wessex porcine mitral prostheses to have a P_u of 3.5 ± 0.9 mm Hg, typical pressure half-time of 81 ± 21 msec, and a range of peak diastolic velocities for 29 and 31 mm valves only ($n = 31$) of 1.41–1.66 m/sec. In 38 normal recipients of a mitral Carpentier-Edwards prosthesis, Gibbs et al. (34) reported a weak correlation ($r = 0.44$) between the time since mitral valve implantation and the pressure half-time. Mean pressure half-time was 90 ± 23 msec for 27, 29, and 31 mm valves (range unreported), and mean peak velocity for the same valve sizes was 1.64 ± 0.24 m/sec. Similar pressure half-time val-

ues are expected, although unreported, in the data of Panidis et al. (1) and Williams and Labovitz (22), with respective calculated prosthetic mitral valve areas (by the pressure half-time method) of 2.2 ± 0.7 cm² (six patients) and 2.1 ± 0.7 cm² (16 patients).

It appears that normal mitral porcine xenograft function is associated with a peak diastolic velocity < 2.0 m/sec, pressure half-time typically ≤ 160–180 msec, and no demonstrable systolic left atrial disturbance. Some investigators, however, have described "minimal" regurgitation of a normal mitral porcine xenograft as a systolic disturbance at the valve level unassociated with an increase in peak diastolic velocity in up to 20% of patients studied (20, 22, 34, 38, 39).

In the aortic position, normal porcine xenograft function has been characterized by numerous investigators (1, 20–22, 27, 34), and the findings are tabulated in Table 11.5. Peak systolic gradients recorded in nine patients with normal porcine aortic xenografts by Panidis et al. (1) ranged from 12 to 53 mm Hg (mean: 30 ± 12 mm Hg). Mean systolic gradients ranged from 5 to 36 mm Hg (mean: 17 ± 10 mm Hg). They reported that peak velocities ranged from 1.8 to 3.6 m/sec. Mean peak velocity was 2.6 ± 0.6 ($n = 9$), similar to the mean peak velocities of 2.44 ± 0.48 ($n = 24$) and of 2.52 ± 0.10 ($n = 20$) reported respectively by Gibbs et al. (34) and Ramirez and Wong (27). Ramirez and Wong were also able to demonstrate a 0.8% intraobserver and 2.7% interobserver coefficient of variation when their 20 patients underwent three serial Doppler echocardiographic studies over a 1-month period.

Sagar et al. (21) and Ramirez et al. (73) showed a negative correlation between peak aortic flow velocities and valve size for both Carpentier-Edwards and Hancock porcine xenografts. Ramirez et al. (73) showed a significant negative correlation of $r = -0.96$ and $r = -0.95$, respectively, in 41 Carpentier-Edwards and 32 Hancock valves, when valve size was compared with peak aortic flow velocity. A poorer negative correlation ($r = -0.35$) was obtained by Williams and Labovitz (22) when peak systolic gradient was plotted as a function of valve size for 36 patients with Hancock or Bjork-Shiley aortic prostheses. Of these 36 patients, only 11 were recipients of porcine aortic xenografts, and the only peak systolic gradients over 32 mm Hg were seen in valves of size 23 mm or less. Gibbs et al. (34) found no significant difference in peak velocities between 24 Carpentier-Edwards aortic xenografts of dif-

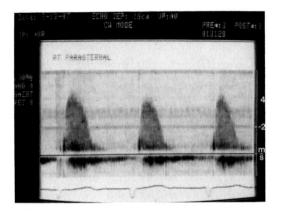

Figure 11.10. Aortic bioprosthetic/patient mismatch. Seventy-nine-year-old female after #23 Carpentier-Edwards aortic valve replacement for calcific aortic stenosis; underwent routine early postoperative evaluation here using the nonimaging continuous wave Pedof transducer in the right parasternal position. Note the V_{max} of 4.5 m/sec, predicting a peak gradient of 80 mm Hg. The patient was asymptomatic, the gradient representing a smaller stent diameter and relative stenosis due to patient/prosthesis mismatch.

ferent sizes, although peak velocity correlated weakly with time since implantation.

Unusually high velocities may be found across normally functioning aortic bioprostheses of smaller anulus size, especially early postoperatively (Fig. 11.10), when cardiac output is increased due to anemia and high catecholamine levels.

Mild regurgitation undetected clinically in 20–25% of patients has been reported by many investigators (1, 20–22, 27, 34, 73), and Doppler echocardiography did not distinguish between valvular and paravalvular regurgitation (21, 22). Gibbs et al. (34) reported aortic bioprosthetic insufficiency in two clinically normal patients 3.5 and 5.5 yr postoperatively. As a clear diastolic murmur is not usually audible in these patients, its definite presence should indicate closer follow-up of the patient (4).

Abnormal function (Figs. 11.2–11.7): Panidis et al. (1) reported 5 patients with dysfunction of either Hancock or Carpentier-Edwards mitral bioprostheses 6–7 yr following mitral valve replacement (Table 11.4). Overall, Doppler echocardiography correctly identified the presence (although in one case underestimated the severity) of regurgitation in all 5 patients and showed higher-than-normal values for peak velocity and

mean gradients across the prostheses in 3 patients.

Using a simultaneous Doppler catheter study in 12 patients with clinically suspected atrioventricular prosthetic valve dysfunction, Wilkins et al. (15) validated continuous wave Doppler echocardiographic measurements of mitral (and tricuspid) valve gradients. The group included 7 patients with Hancock or Carpentier-Edwards prostheses. Mean gradients ranging from 3.5 to 10.4 mm Hg and valve areas (by the half-time method) ranging from 1.5 to 2.6 cm² were reported. Only 2 of 7 patients presented by Wilkins et al. (15) had demonstrable mitral regurgitation on Doppler interrogation: None had severe stenosis.

Twelve patients with dysfunction of a Hancock mitral prosthesis were segregated successfully by Doppler echocardiography into groups with stenosis or regurgitation. The 6 patients with stenosis had mean diastolic transprosthetic gradients ranging from 15 to 25 mm Hg. Pressure half-times were unreported, and from illustration, it appears stenotic prostheses were characterized by half-time-derived mitral valve areas of 0.7–1.3 cm². All patients with stenosis and 3 of 6 patients with regurgitation were subjected to catheterization. A good correlation between Doppler mean gradient and catheterization mean gradient was obtained ($r = 0.93$, including some patients with Bjork-Shiley prostheses), as was good correlation between catheterization mitral valve area and Doppler-derived mitral valve area ($r = 0.98$, including some patients with Bjork-Shiley prostheses).

Of the 11 patients with dysfunctional porcine mitral prostheses evaluated by Ryan et al. (38), 8 had bioprosthetic stenosis with pressure half-time ranging from 150 to 350 msec (mean: 220 ± 63 msec), and 7 of 8 had one of ≥ 180 msec. Normal patients and patients with purely regurgitant prostheses had, in comparison, a mean pressure half-time of 136 ± 18 msec. The range of pressure half-time reported by Ryan et al. (38) for stenotic bioprostheses would result in pressure half-time-derived mitral valve areas of 0.6 to 1.5 cm². Mean transprosthetic gradient was reported to range from 12 to 24 mm Hg in patients with bioprosthetic stenosis. Of interest, patients with dysfunction of a prosthetic mitral valve were younger than those with normally functioning prostheses (51 ± 12 years versus 61 ± 10 years).

Fourteen patients with dysfunction of a Hancock aortic prosthesis were studied by Doppler echocardiography and cardiac catheterization and reported by Sagar et al. (21) (Table 11.6). Three of 14 had bioprosthetic stenosis with a range of mean gradients of 30–68 mm Hg. Eleven of 14 had aortic regurgitation on Doppler echocardiography, which was severe in 6. Doppler- and catheterization-derived mean gradients (Hancock and Bjork-Shiley prostheses in the aortic position) correlated well ($r = 0.94$) for stenotic and normal prostheses. Williams and Labovitz (22) described two patients with bioprosthetic aortic dysfunction. One patient with a calcified prosthesis had a V_{max} of 4.0 m/sec and no demonstrable aortic insufficiency; the other had no demonstrable gradient with 3+ aortic insufficiency on Doppler echocardiography and catheterization. Pathology was unreported on this latter case. Distinction between aortic bioprosthetic incompetence due to degeneration or paraprosthetic leak (Fig. 11.3) has not yet been reported by Doppler echocardiography. However, color Doppler may yet prove revealing in this area.

TRICUSPID VALVE

The Doppler echocardiographic findings for normal tricuspid valve prostheses are described by Gibbs et al. (34). Nine clinically normal recipients of Carpentier-Edwards tricuspid prostheses had a mean peak velocity of 1.49 ± 0.12 m/sec. This group included small numbers of valves of different sizes (25, 27, 29, 31, and 35 mm) with a mean $P_{1/2}t$ of 163 ± 50 msec. No correlation between peak velocity or $P_{1/2}t$ and either patient age or time since implantation was found. Gibbs et al. found considerable beat-to-beat variation in pressure half-time across tricuspid xenografts ranging from 10 to 140 msec (mean: 54 msec). They speculated that the variation probably represented changes in valve orifice area due to the effects of respiration and varying cycle length. In contrast, only slight beat-to-beat variation in native (12) or prosthetic mitral xenograft (0–40 msec; mean: 16 msec) (34) pressure half-time has been observed, even in atrial fibrillation.

Continuous wave Doppler echocardiographic measurement of tricuspid prosthetic valve gradients has been reported by Wilkins et al. (15) and Perez (76). In three collective patients with dysfunctional Starr-Edwards, Bjork-Shiley, and Hancock tricuspid prostheses, Doppler echocardiographically derived mean transprosthetic gradients ranged from 3.8 to 15 mm Hg. This closely approximated mean transprosthetic gradients obtained at catheterization. However, mean trans-

valvular gradients may not be detectable by Doppler echocardiography, when a reduced cardiac output is imposed by other valvular disease. Apparent false-positive M-mode and two-dimensional echocardiographic findings of (native) tricuspid stenosis have been reported in the absence of demonstrable tricuspid valve gradient at catheterization (77, 78) due to the presence of low output syndromes associated with mitral valve disease.

Veyrat et al. (75), in 41 abnormal native tricuspid valve patients evaluated by Doppler echocardiography, found high diagnostic accuracy in segregation of patients with predominant tricuspid stenosis from predominant regurgitation. This differentiation was based on the presence of alterations in the early diastolic flow velocity (diastolic "D" summit or significant increase in duration of the D wave corrected for heart rate) in patients with stenosis. Deceleration half-time, the time interval between peak flow velocity and half-peak velocity, has been reported to be prolonged in patients with native tricuspid valve stenosis (mean: 350 ± 25 msec) versus normal subjects (120 ± 15 msec). The pressure gradient recorded from catheterization appeared to correlate better with deceleration half-time ($r = 0.92$) than with Doppler echocardiography-derived mean transvalvular gradient calculated from Bernoulli's law in the 18 patients with tricuspid stenosis reported by Nakamura et al. (78).

Patients with abnormal tricuspid prosthetic function by Doppler echocardiographic assessment are reported by Wilkins et al. (15) and Perez et al. (76). As is the case with mitral prostheses, tricuspid prosthetic dysfunction may be characterized by increased diastolic velocities with paravalvular/valvular regurgitation or stenosis. However, prolonged pressure or deceleration half-times may be more indicative of relative or absolute stenosis (Fig. 11.9C).

REFERENCES

1. Panidis IP, Ross J, Mintz GS: Normal and abnormal prosthetic valve function as assessed by Doppler echocardiography. *J Am Coll Cardiol* 8:317–326, 1986.
2. Kotler MN, Mintz GS, Segal BL, Parry WR: Clinical uses of two dimensional echocardiography. *Am J Cardiol* 45:1061–1082, 1980.
3. Kotler MN, Goldman A, Parry WR: Noninvasive evaluation of cardiac valve prostheses. Cardiac imaging: New technologies and clinical applications. In Brest AN (ed): *Cardiovascular Clinics.* Philadelphia, FA Davis, 1986, pp 201–241.

4. Kotler MN, Mintz GS, Panidis I, Morganroth J, Segal BL, Ross J: Noninvasive evaluation of normal and abnormal prosthetic valve function. *J Am Coll Cardiol* 2:151–173, 1983.

5. Brodie BR, Grossman W, McLaurin L, Starek PJK, Craige E: Diagnosis of prosthetic mitral valve malfunction with combined echo-phonocardiography. *Circulation* 53:93–100, 1976.

6. Gray RJ, Chaux A, Matloff JM, DeRobertis M, Raymond M, Stewart M, Yoganathan A: Bileaflet, tilting disc and porcine aortic valve substitutes: In vivo hydrodynamic characteristics. *J Am Coll Cardiol* 3:321–327, 1984.

7. Yoganathan AP, Chaux A, Gray RJ, Woo YR, DeRobertis M, Williams FP, Matloff JM: Bileaflet, tilting disc and porcine aortic valve substitutes: In vitro hydrodynamic characteristics. *J Am Coll Cardiol* 3:313–320, 1984.

8. Rashtian MY, Stevenson DM, Allen DT, Yoganathan AP, Harrison EC, Edmiston WA, Faughan P, Rahimtoola SH: Flow characteristics of four commonly used mechanical heart valves. *Am J Cardiol* 58:743–752, 1986.

9. Gabbay S, McQueen DM, Yellin EL, Becker RM, Frater RWM: In vitro hydrodynamic comparison of mitral valve prostheses at high flow rates. *J Thorac Cardiovasc Surg* 76:771–787, 1978.

10. Gillam LD, Choong CY, Wilkins GT, Marshall JE: The effect of aortic insufficiency on Doppler pressure half-time calculations of mitral valve area in mitral stenosis. *Circulation* 74 (Suppl II):II-217, 1986.

11. Fujii K, Kitabatake A, Tanouchi J, Ishihara K, Uematsu M, Yoshida Y, Ito H, Tominaga N, Inoue M: Stenotic orifice area determined by Doppler echocardiography is independent of hemodynamic conditions. *Circulation* 74 (Suppl II):II-216, 1986.

12. Hatle L, Angelsen B, Tromsdal A: Noninvasive assessment of atrioventricular pressure half-time by Doppler ultrasound. *Circulation* 60:1096–1104, 1979.

13. Holen J, Aaslid R, Landmark K, Simonsen S: Determination of pressure gradient in mitral stenosis with a noninvasive ultrasound Doppler technique. *Acta Med Scand* 199:455–460, 1976.

14. Holen J, Aaslid R, Landmark K, Simonsen S, Ostrem T: Determination of effective orifice area in mitral stenosis from noninvasive ultrasound Doppler data and mitral flow rate. *Acta Med Scand* 201:83–88, 1977.

15. Wilkins GT, Gillam LD, Kritzer GL, Levine RA, Palacios IF, Weyman AE: Validation of continuous-wave Doppler echocardiographic measurements of mitral and tricuspid prosthetic valve gradients: A simultaneous Doppler-catheter study. *Circulation* 74:786–795, 1986.

16. Raizada V, Hoyt TW, Corlew S, Abrams J: A study of the diastolic flow velocity profile of the clinically uncomplicated mitral porcine bioprosthesis using an echo-Doppler technique. *Jap Heart J* 24:59–66, 1983.

17. Nitter-Hauge S: Doppler echocardiography in the study of patients with mitral disc valve prostheses. *Br Heart J* 51:61–69, 1984.

18. Holen J, Nitter-Hauge S: Evaluation of obstructive characteristics of mitral disc valve implants with ultrasound Doppler techniques. *Acta Med Scand* 201:429–434, 1977.

19. Holen I, Hoie J, Semb B: Obstructive characteristics of Bjork-Shiley, Hancock, and Lillehei-Kaster prosthetic mitral valve in the immediate postoperative period. *Acta Med Scand* 204:5–10, 1978.

20. Simpson IA, Reece IJ, Houston AB, Hutton I, Wheatley DJ, Cobbe SM: Noninvasive assessment by Doppler ultrasound of 155 patients with bioprosthetic valves: A comparison of the Wessex porcine, low profile Ionescu-Shiley, and Hancock pericardial bioprostheses. *Br Heart J* 56:83–88, 1986.

21. Sagar KB, Wann S, Paulsen WHJ, Romhilt DW: Doppler echocardiographic evaluation of Hancock and Bjork-Shiley prosthetic valves. *J Am Coll Cardiol* 7:681–687, 1986.

22. Williams GA, Labovitz AJ: Doppler hemodynamic evaluation of prosthetic (Starr-Edwards and Bjork-Shiley) and bioprosthetic (Hancock and Carpentier-Edwards) cardiac valves. *Am J Cardiol* 56:325–332, 1985.

23. Veyrat C, Witchitz S, Lessana A, Ameur A, Abitbol G, Kalmanson D: Valvar prosthetic dysfunction. Localization and evaluation of the dysfunction using the Doppler technique. *Br Heart J* 54:273–284, 1985.

24. Veyrat C, Abitbol G, Bas S, Manin JP, Kalmanson D: Quantitative assessment of valvular regurgitations using the pulsed Doppler technique. Approach to the regurgitant lesion. *Ultrasound Med Biol* 10:201–213, 1984.

25. Blumlein S, Bouchard A, Schiller NB, Dae M, Byrd BF III, Ports T, Botvinick EH: Quantitation of mitral regurgitation by Doppler echocardiography. *Circulation* 74:306–314, 1986.

26. Currie PJ, Hagler DJ, Seward JM, Reeder GS, Fyfe DA, Bove AA, Tajik AJ: Instantaneous pressure gradient: A simultaneous Doppler and dual catheter correlative study. *J Am Coll Cardiol* 7:800–806, 1986.

27. Ramirez ML, Wong M: Reproducibility of standalone continuous-wave Doppler recording of aortic flow velocity across bioprosthetic valves. *Am J Cardiol* 55:1197–1199, 1985.

28. Smith MD, Kwan OL, DeMaria AN: Value and limitations of continuous-wave Doppler echocardiography in estimating severity of valvular stenosis. *JAMA* 25:3145–3151, 1986.

29. Panidis IP, Mintz GS, Ross J: Value and limitations of Doppler ultrasound in the evaluation of aortic stenosis: A statistical analysis of 70 consecutive patients. *Am Heart J* 112:150–158, 1986.

30. Zhang Y, Nitter-Hauge S, Ihlen H, Rootwelt K, Myhre E: Measurement of aortic regurgitation by Doppler echocardiography. *Br Heart J* 55:32–38, 1986.

31. Hoffmann A, Pfisterer M, Stulz P, Schmitt HE, Burkart F, Burckhardt D: Noninvasive grading of aortic regurgitation by Doppler ultrasonography. *Br Heart J* 55:283–285, 1986.

32. Goldberg SJ, Allen HD: Quantitative assessment by Doppler echocardiography of pulmonary or

aortic regurgitation. *Am J Cardiol* 56:131–135, 1985.

33. Gross CM, Wann LS: Doppler echocardiographic diagnosis of porcine bioprosthetic cardiac valve malfunction. *Am J Cardiol* 53:1203–1205, 1984.
34. Gibbs JL, Wharton GA, Williams GJ: Doppler echocardiographic characteristics of the Carpentier-Edwards xenograft. *Eur Heart J* 7:353–356, 1986.
35. Horowitz MS, Goodman DJ, Hancock EW, Popp RL: Noninvasive diagnosis of complications of the mitral bioprosthesis. *J Thorac Cardiovasc Surg* 71:450–457, 1976.
36. Alam M, Madrazo AC, Magilligan DJ, Goldstein S: M mode and two dimensional echocardiographic features of porcine valve dysfunction. *Am J Cardiol* 43:502–509, 1979.
37. Schapira JN, Martin RP, Fowles RE, Rakowski H, Stinson EB, French JW, Shumway NE, Popp RL: Two dimensional echocardiographic assessment of patients with bioprosthetic valves. *Am J Cardiol* 43:510–519, 1979.
38. Ryan, T, Armstrong, WF, Dillon JC, Feigenbaum H: Doppler echocardiographic evaluation of patients with porcine mitral valves. *Am Heart J* 111:237–244, 1986.
39. Holen J, Simonsen, S, Froysaker T: Determination of pressure gradient in the Hancock mitral valve from noninvasive ultrasound Doppler data. *Scand J Clin Lab Invest* 41:177–183, 1981.
40. Czer LSC, Gray RJ, Bateman TM, DeRobertis MA, Resser K, Chaux A, Matloff JM: Hemodynamic differentiation of pathologic and physiologic stenosis in mitral porcine bioprostheses. *J Am Coll Cardiol* 7:284–294, 1986.
41. Bommer W, Yoon D, Grehl TM, Mason DT, Neumann A, DeMaria AN: In vitro and in vivo evaluation of porcine bioprostheses by cross-sectional echocardiography. *Am J Cardiol* 41:405, 1978.
42. Horowitz MS, Tecklenberg PL, Goodman DJ, Harrison DC, Popp RL: Echocardiographic evaluation of the stent mounted aortic bioprosthetic valve in the mitral position. In vitro and in vivo studies. *Circulation* 54:91–96, 1976.
43. Martin RP, French JW, Popp RL: Clinical utility of two-dimensional echocardiography in patients with bioprosthetic valves. *Adv Cardiol* 27:294–304, 1980.
44. Bloch WN Jr, Felner JM, Wickliffe C, Symbas PN, Schlant RC: Echocardiogram of the porcine aortic bioprosthesis in the mitral position. *Am J Cardiol* 38:293–298, 1976.
45. Chandraratna PAN, San Pedro SB: Echocardiographic features of the normal and malfunctioning porcine xenograft valve. *Am Heart J* 95:548–554, 1978.
46. Bjork VO, Henze A: Ten years' experience with the Bjork-Shiley tilting disc valve. *J Thorac Cardiovasc Surg* 78:331–342, 1979.
47. Bjork VO, Book K, Cernigliaro C, Holmgren A: The Bjork-Shiley tilting disc valve in isolated mitral lesions. *Scand J Thorac Cardiovasc Surg* 7:131–148, 1973.
48. Douglas JE, Williams GD: Echocardiographic

evaluation of the Bjork-Shiley prosthetic valve. *Circulation* 50:52–57, 1974.
49. Clements SD Jr, Perkins JV: Malfunction of a Bjork-Shiley prosthetic heart valve in the mitral position producing an abnormal echocardiographic pattern. *J Clin Ultrasound* 6:334, 1978.
50. Bernal-Ramirez JA, Phillips JH: Echocardiographic study of malfunction of the Bjork-Shiley prosthetic heart valve in the mitral position. *Am J Cardiol* 40:449–453, 1977.
51. Raj MVJ, Srinivas V, Evans DW: Thrombotic jamming of a tricuspid prosthesis. *Br Heart J* 38:1355–1358, 1976.
52. Copans H, Lakier JB, Kinsley RH, Colsen PR, Fritz VU, Barlow JM: Thrombosed Bjork-Shiley mitral prostheses. *Circulation* 61:169–174, 1980.
53. Holen J, Simonsen S, Froysaker T: An ultrasound Doppler technique for the noninvasive determination of the pressure gradient in the Bjork-Shiley mitral valve. *Circulation* 59:436–442, 1979.
54. Ferrara RP, Labovitz AJ, Wiens RD, Kennedy HL, Williams GA: Prosthetic mitral regurgitation detected by Doppler echocardiography. *Am J Cardiol* 55:229–230, 1985.
55. Bjork VO, Holmgren A, Olin C, Ovenfors CA: Clinical and haemodynamic results of aortic valve replacement with the Bjork-Shiley tilting disc valve prosthesis. *Scand J Thor Cardiovasc Surg* 5:177–191, 1971.
56. Chandraratna PAN, Lopez JM, Hildner FJ, Samet P, Ben-Zvi J, Gindlesperger D: Diagnosis of Bjork-Shiley aortic valve dysfunction by echocardiography. *Am Heart J* 91:318–324, 1976.
57. Ben-Zvi J, Hildner FJ, Chandraratna PA, Samet P: Thrombosis on Bjork-Shiley aortic valve prosthesis. Clinical, arteriographic, echocardiographic and therapeutic observations in seven cases. *Am J Cardiol* 34:538–544, 1974.
58. Gibson TC, Starek PJK, Moos S, Craige E: Echocardiographic and phonocardiographic characteristics of the Lillehei-Kaster mitral valve prosthesis. *Circulation* 49:434–440, 1974.
59. Forman R, Gersh BJ, Fraser R, Beck W: Hemodynamic assessment of Lillehei-Kaster tilting disc aortic and mitral prostheses. *J Thorac Cardiovasc Surg* 75:595–598, 1978.
60. Feldman HJ, Gray RJ, Chaux A, Halpern SW, Kraus R, Allen HN, Matloff JM: Noninvasive in vivo and in vitro study of the St. Jude mitral valve prosthesis. Evaluation using two dimensional and M mode echocardiography, phonocardiography and cinefluoroscopy. *Am J Cardiol* 49:1101–1109, 1982.
61. Gray R, Chaux A, Matloff J, Raymond M: Early postoperative hemodynamic comparison of St. Jude cardiac prostheses and porcine xenografts, at rest and with stress. *Circulation* 59–60 (Suppl II):II-222, 1979.
62. Chaux A, Gray RJ, Matloff JM, Feldman H, Sustaita H: An appreciation of the new St. Jude valvular prosthesis. *J Thorac Cardiovasc Surg* 81:202–211, 1981.
63. Weinstein IR, Marbarger JP, Perez JE: Ultrasonic assessment of the St. Jude prosthetic valve: M mode,

two-dimensional, and Doppler echocardiography. *Circulation* 68:897–905, 1983.

64. Tri TB, Schatz RA, Watson TD, Bowen TE, Schiller NB: Echocardiographic evaluation of the St. Jude medical prosthetic valve. *Chest* 80:278–284, 1981.

65. Busch UW, Pechacek LW, Garcia E, Mathus VS, Hall RJ: Premature closure of prosthetic mitral valves as a consequence of gravity. *Cath Cardiovasc Diag* 8:131–136, 1982.

66. Panidis IP, Morganroth J, David D, Chen CC, Kotler MN: Prosthetic mitral valve motion during cardiac dysrhythmias as determined by echocardiography. *Am J Cardiol* 51:996–1004, 1983.

67. Freedman RA, Yock PG, Echt DS, Popp RL: Effect of variation in PQ interval on patterns of atrioventricular valve motion and flow in patients with normal ventricular functions. *J Am Coll Cardiol* 7:595–602, 1986.

68. Williams JCP, Vandenberg RA, Sturm RE, Wood EF: Presystolic atriogenic mitral reflux developed at abnormally long PR intervals. *Cardiovasc Res* 3:271–277, 1968.

69. Panidis IP, Ross J, Munley B, Nestico P, Mintz GS: Diastolic mitral regurgitation in patients with atrioventricular conduction abnormalities: A common finding by Doppler echocardiography. *J Am Coll Cardiol* 7:768–774, 1986.

70. McAnulty JH, Morton M, Rahimtoola SH, Kloster FE, Ahuja N, Starr AE: Hemodynamic characteristics of the composite strut ball valve prostheses (Starr-Edwards track valves) in patients on anticoagulants. *Circulation* 58 (Suppl I): I-159–I-161, 1978.

71. Russell T II, Kremkau EL, Kloster F, Starr A: Late hemodynamic function of cloth-covered Starr-Edwards valve prostheses. *Circulation* 45–46 (Suppl I):I-8–I-13, 1972.

72. Kloster FE, Farrehi C, Mourdjinis A, Hodan RP, Starr A, Griswold HE: Hemodynamic studies in patients with cloth-covered composite-seat Starr-Edwards valve prostheses. *J Thorac Cardiovasc Surg* 60:879–888, 1970.

73. Ramirez ML, Wong M, Sadler N, Shah PM: Doppler evaluation of 106 bioprosthetic and mechanical aortic valves. *J Am Coll Cardiol* 5:527, 1985.

74. Hatle L, Angelsen B: Pulsed and continuous wave Doppler in diagnosis and assessment of various heart lesions: Prosthetic valves. In: *Doppler Ultrasound in Cardiology*, ed 2. Philadelphia, Lea & Febiger, 1985, pp 188–205.

75. Veyrat C, Kalmanson D, Farjon M, Manin JP, Abitbol G: Noninvasive diagnosis and assessment of tricuspid regurgitation and stenosis using one and two dimensional echo-pulsed Doppler. *Br Heart J* 47:596–605, 1982.

76. Perez JE, Ludbrook PA, Ahumada GG: Usefulness of Doppler echocardiography in detecting tricuspid valve stenosis. *Am J Cardiol* 55:601–603, 1985.

77. Guyer DE, Gillam LD, Foale RA, Clark MC, Dinsmore R, Palacios I, Block P, King ME, Weyman AE: Comparison of the echocardiographic and hemodynamic diagnosis of rheumatic tricuspid stenosis. *J Am Coll Cardiol* 3:1135–1144, 1984.

78. Nakamura K, Satomi G, Ogasawara S, Oteki H, Hirosawa K: Noninvasive evaluation of tricuspid stenosis with Doppler echocardiography. *Circulation* 70 (Suppl II):II-394, 1984.

79. Panidis IP, Ren JF, Kotler MN, Mintz GS, Mundth ED, Goel IP, Ross J: Clinical and echocardiographic evaluation of the St. Jude cardiac valve prosthesis: Follow-up of 126 patients. *J Am Coll Cardiol* 4:454–462, 1984.

80. Simon EB, Kotler MN, Segal BL, Parry W: Clinical significance of multiple systolic clicks from Starr-Edwards prosthetic aortic valves. *Br Heart J* 39:645–650, 1977.

81. Miller HC, Gibson DG, Stephen SJD: Role of echocardiography and phonocardiography in diagnosis of mitral paraprosthetic regurgitation with Starr-Edwards prostheses. *Br Heart J* 35:1217–1225, 1973.

82. Pfeifer J, Goldschlager N, Sweatman T, Gerbode F, Selzer A: Malfunction of mitral ball valve prosthesis due to thrombus. *Am J Cardiol* 29:95–99, 1972.

83. Belenkie I, Carr M, Schlant RC, Nutter DO, Symbas PN: Malfunction of a Cutter-Smeloff mitral ball valve prothesis: Diagnosis by phonocardiography and echocardiography. *Am Heart J* 86:399–403, 1973.

84. Schlager J, Mannix EP Jr, Wolf RE: Auscultatory and phonocardiographic sign of ball variance in a mitral prosthetic valve. *Am Heart J* 81:809–816, 1971.

85. Mary DAS, Pakrashi BC, Catchpole RW, Ionescu MI: Echocardiographic studies of stented fascia lata grafts in the mitral position. *Circulation* 49:237–245, 1974.

86. Lee SJK, Zaragoza AJ, Callaghan JC, Couves CM, Sterns LP: Malfunction of the mitral valve prosthesis (Cutter-Smeloff). *Circulation* 41:479–484, 1970.

87. Berndt TB, Goodman DJ, Popp RL: Echocardiographic and phonocardiographic confirmation of suspected caged mitral valve malfunction. *Chest* 70:221, 1976.

88. Craige E, Hutchin P, Sutton R: Impaired function of cloth-covered Starr-Edwards mitral valve prosthesis. *Circulation* 41:141–148, 1970.

89. Hultgren HN, Hubis H: A phonocardiographic study of patients with the Starr-Edwards mitral valve prosthesis. *Am Heart J* 69:306–319, 1965.

90. Chaitman BR, Bonan R, Lepage G, Tubau JF, David PR, Dydra I, Grondin CM: Hemodynamic evaluation of the Carpentier-Edwards porcine xenograft. *Circulation* 60:1170–1182, 1979.

91. Ubago JL, Figueroa A, Colman T, Ochoteco A, Duran CG: Hemodynamic factors that affect calculated orifice areas in the mitral Hancock xenograft valve. *Circulation* 61:388–394, 1980.

92. Becker RM, Strom J, Frishman W, Oka Y, Lin YT, Yellin EL, Frater RWM: Hemodynamic performance of the Ionescu-Shiley valve prosthesis. *J Thorac Cardiovasc Surg* 80:613–620, 1980.

93. Cosgrove DM, Lytle BW, Gill CC, Golding LAR, Stewart RW, Loop FD, Williams GW: In vivo hemodynamic comparison of porcine and pericardial valves. *J Thorac Cardiovasc Surg* 89:358–368, 1985.

94. Johnson ML, Paton BC, Holmes JH: Ultrasonic evaluation of prosthetic valve motion. *Circulation* 41–42 (Suppl II):II-3–9, 1970.

95. Busch UW, Mathur VS, Garcia E, Hall RJ: Echocardiography and prosthetic valve malfunction (letter to editor). *Am J Cardiol* 42:690, 1978.

96. DePace NL, Kotler MN, Mintz GS, Lichtenberg R, Goel IP, Segal BL: Echocardiographic and phonocardiographic assessment of the St. Jude cardiac valve prosthesis. *Chest* 80:272–280, 1981.

97. David D, Michelson EL, Naito M, Chen CC, Schaffenburg M, Dreifus LS: Diastolic "locking" of the mitral valve: The importance of atrial systole and intraventricular volume. *Circulation* 67:640, 1983.

98. McHenry MM, Smeloff EA, Fong WY, Miller GE, Ryan PM: Critical obstruction of prosthetic heart valves due to lipid absorption by Silastic. *J Thorac Cardiovasc Surg* 59:413–425, 1970.

99. Smith ND, Raizada V, Abrams J: Auscultation of the normally functioning prosthetic valve. *Ann Int Med* 95:594–598, 1981.

100. Little RC: The mechanism of closure of the mitral valve: A continuing controversy. *Circulation* 59:615–618, 1979.

101. Kyllonen K, Mattila T, Hartikainen M, Tala P: Mitral valve replacement with ball and tilting disc valve prosthesis. *Scand J Thor Cardiovasc Surg* 10:15–20, 1976.

102. Rostad H, Fjeld NB, Hall KV: Experiences with various types of mitral valve prostheses. *Scand J Thor Cardiovasc Surg* 10:113–116, 1976.

103. Leatherman LL, Leachman RD, McConn RG, Hallman GL, Cooley DA: Malfunction of mitral ball-valve prostheses due to swollen poppet. *J Thorac Cardiovasc Surg* 57:160–163, 1969.

104. Sanderson RG, Hall AD, Thomas AN: The clinical diagnosis of ball variance in a mitral valve prosthesis. *Ann Thorac Surg* 6:473–475, 1968.

105. Horowitz MS, Goodman DJ, Popp RL: Echocardiographic diagnosis of calcific stenosis of a stented aortic homograft in the mitral position. *J Clin Ultrasound* 2:179–183, 1974.

106. Burggraf GW, Craige E: The first heart sound in complete heart block. *Circulation* 50:17–24, 1974.

107. Nitter-Hauge S, Froysaker T, Hall KV: Clinical and haemodynamic results following mitral valve replacement with the new Lillehei-Kaster pivoting disc valve prosthesis. *Scand J Thor Cardiovasc Surg* 11:15–24, 1977.

108. Nitter-Hauge S, Hall KV, Froysaker T: Mitral valve replacement. A comparative clinical and haemodynamic study of the new Lillehei-Kaster and Bjork-Shiley prostheses. *Scand J Thor Cardiovasc Surg* 11:111–117, 1977.

109. Lillehei CW: Worldwide experience with the St. Jude medical valve prosthesis: Clinical and hemodynamic results. *Contemp Surg* 20:17–32, 1982.

110. Alam M, Rosman H, Lakier JB, Kemp S, Khaja F, Hautamaki K, Magilligan DJ, Stein PD: Doppler and echocardiographic features of normal and dysfunctioning bioprosthetic valves. *J Am Coll Cardiol* 10:851–858, 1987.

111. Sprecher DL, Adamick R, Adams D, Kisslo J: In vitro color flow, pulsed and continuous wave Doppler ultrasound masking of flow by prosthetic valves. *J Am Coll Cardiol* 9:1306–1310, 1987.

112. Bolger A, Czer L, Freidman A, Kleinman J, DeRobertis M, Chaux A, Maurer G: Intraoperative transesophageal color Doppler imaging: Advantages and limitations. *J Am Coll Cardiol* 11:217A, 1988.

113. Czer LSC, Matloff J, Chaux A, DeRobertis M, Yoganathan A, Gray R: A 6 year experience with the St. Jude Medical valve: hemodynamic performance, surgical results, biocompatibility and followup. J Am Coll Cardiol 6: 904–12, 1985.

114. Czer LSC: Dopper assessment of prosthetic valves. International J of Cardiac Imaging 4: 9–10, 1989.

12

Doppler Echocardiographic Correlation with Cardiac Catheterization in Valvular Heart Disease

Philip J. Currie

INTRODUCTION

Doppler echocardiography represents a major advance in noninvasive hemodynamic evaluation of patients with valvular heart disease. Clinical applications include estimation of pressure gradients across stenotic lesions (1–11), determination of valve areas (12–20), determination of cardiac output (21, 22), estimation of right heart and pulmonary artery pressures (23–32), detection and quantitation of valvular regurgitation (33–41), and cardiac shunting (42).

These assessments can be made with the patient at rest or in hemodynamic states altered by exercise, hand grip, Valsalva's maneuver, or pharmacologic intervention (Fig. 12.1). In addition, Doppler echocardiography can provide valuable information for serial follow-up of patients with valvular heart disease.

With any technical advance, validation studies are necessary to establish accuracy. In the case of Doppler echocardiography, the clinical gold standard for hemodynamic assessment is cardiac catheterization. However, there are prerequisites for accurate comparison of these techniques:

1. Measurements must be performed in the same or comparable physiologic states.
2. Results should be directly comparable to those obtained by the time-tested standard.
3. Meticulous care should be taken to optimize both techniques (for example, use of a dual catheter technique for pressure gradient measurement instead of catheter withdrawal across a stenosis).

4. Doppler-catheter hemodynamics should be assessed as both instantaneous and beat-to-beat relationships.
5. The validity and accuracy of the standard should be examined critically. All too frequently, discrepancies are attributed to inaccuracies of the new technique without considering how "golden" the gold standard is.
6. Comparisons should not be made without control over the gold standards and patient safety. Human experimentation should be preceded by careful animal or in vitro studies.
7. Catheterization or Doppler techniques should not be oversimplified, as new errors can be introduced.
8. Validation studies should also include comparison against other available methods, rather than just against a gold standard. This allows a better perspective on the usefulness of the new technique, either alone or in combination.

PRESSURE GRADIENT ESTIMATION

Most Doppler-derived hemodynamics are based on the Bernoulli equation. This equation is applied to Doppler-derived velocity data to determine gradient, pressure, flow, and valve area. The Bernoulli equation can be simplified markedly for ease of use. Modifications have been described in detail by Hatle and Angelsen (43). Numerous in vitro (44), canine (10, 11), and human studies (7–9, 24) have confirmed the validity of the modified formula in determining pressure gradient and derived hemodynamics. The modi-

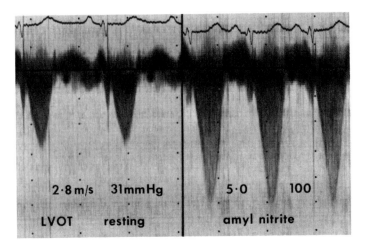

Figure 12.1. Left ventricular outflow tract (*LVOT*) Doppler spectral tracings of a patient with hypertrophic obstructive cardiomyopathy. Tracings recorded from the apical transducer position with the patient at rest and following inhalation of amyl nitrite. The resting gradient of 31 mm Hg more than tripled (100 mm Hg) with amyl nitrite. Doppler calibration markers are 1 m/sec apart.

fications consist of eliminating the flow acceleration and viscosity terms, leading to the equation:

$$P_1 - P_2 = 1/2p\,(v_2^2 - v_1^2) \qquad 12.1$$

Flow acceleration refers to the force necessary to overcome fluid inertia—negligible in blood. Viscosity or frictional forces of blood can be negated. The constant ($\frac{1}{2}p$) is reduced to the number 4.0. The correct value, allowing for the conversion of units, is actually 3.94. Therefore, there is a slight tendency to overestimate the gradient. This is balanced by the tendency to underestimate velocity with Doppler, due to the inability to have a zero angle between the ultrasound beam and the maximum velocity jet. The third modification is elimination of initial velocity (v_1) from the Bernoulli equation. With a significant stenosis, the square of the velocity proximal to the stenosis (v_1) is much smaller than the square of the distal velocity (v_2). Consequently, the (v_1) term can be ignored, leaving the modified Bernoulli equation (1):

$$\text{Pressure gradient} = 4v_2^2 \qquad 12.2$$

In patients at either extreme of blood viscosity, exclusion of the viscosity term from the Bernoulli equation may not be valid. These situations include severe anemia or hyperviscosity (patients with cyanotic congenital heart disease). Also, the velocity (v_1) proximal to the stenosis may not always be negligible. The most commonly encountered situations where v_1 is increased and should be included in the equation are high output states, aortic regurgitation, coarctation of the aorta (45), and prosthetic aortic valves (46). When in doubt, it is always best to measure the proximal velocity (v_1) and, if significant, to include it in the equation:

$$\text{Pressure gradient} = 4(v_2^2 - v_1^2)$$

Doppler examination is generally performed without correcting for the presumed angle between the ultrasound beam and the maximum systolic jet. This practice is supported by studies showing accurate correlation between Doppler-derived and catheter-measured gradients using a nonimaging Doppler transducer without angle correction (7, 8, 24). This is in contrast to reports where angle correction has been advocated, based on estimates of blood flow direction using either two-dimensional echo (47) or color flow Doppler imaging of the systolic jet (48). Angle correction is fraught with potential error and should not be used.

Color flow Doppler imaging can better display jet direction. However, no comparisons have been made between comprehensive interrogation with the nonimaging continuous wave Doppler transducer and color flow Doppler-guided jet direction for angle correction. Also, transducer positions used to optimize color flow imaging may lead to a large angle between the continuous wave Dopp-

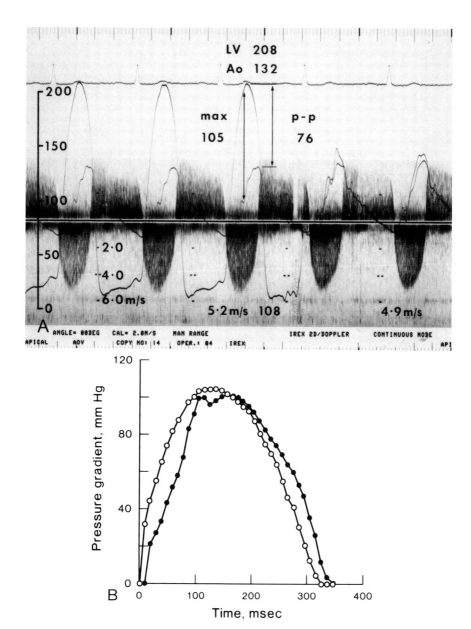

Figure 12.2. *A*, Simultaneous Doppler and dual catheter pressure recordings in a patient with severe aortic stenosis. The maximal catheter gradient (*max*) of 105 mm Hg corresponded closely to the maximal instantaneous Doppler gradient of 108 mm Hg. The peak-to-peak catheter pressure gradient (*p-p*) is 76 mm Hg. The peak left ventricular (*LV*) pressure and the peak aortic (*Ao*) pressures are nonsynchronous. Note the effect of a catheter across the stenotic aortic valve: A rise in the ascending aortic pressure and a fall in Doppler maximum velocity from 5.2 m/s to 4.9 m/s. *B*, Instantaneous Doppler and catheter pressure gradients in the same patient as *A*. Gradients are derived from the digitized Doppler spectral velocity envelope and simultaneous left ventricular and ascending aortic pressure waveforms of the third beat from *A*. The instantaneous catheter gradient (*closed circles*) is comparable with the Doppler-derived gradient (*open circles*). Note the slight phase delay related to the fluid-filled catheter system. The mean catheter gradient is 70 mm Hg, and the mean Doppler-derived gradient is 75 mm Hg.

ler beam and maximum blood flow jet. This obligates angle correction in patients where the smaller nonimaging transducer would be less likely to require angle correction. The arbitrary addition of angle correction may result in random overestimation of velocity. On the other hand, not using angle correction can never result in overestimation and, at most, may lead to only a small systematic underestimation.

A consideration in estimating pressure gradients is the Doppler technique used—pulsed wave, high pulse repetition frequency (HPRF) Doppler, or continuous wave. Pulsed wave Doppler is unable to quantitate velocities higher than normal due to aliasing. Therefore, it has no place in the quantitation of pressure gradients across stenotic lesions. Results of a study by Stewart et al. (49) demonstrated HPRF Doppler to be less accurate than continuous wave Doppler in estimation of high velocity jets.

The Doppler signal is a continuum of instantaneous events related to instantaneous changes in the direction and velocity of the reflecting object. In the heart, instantaneous blood flow velocity and pressure gradient can be determined throughout the cardiac cycle. The maximum instantaneous velocity—which yields the maximum instantaneous gradient—is most commonly determined. A common mistake is comparing this Doppler-derived maximum instantaneous gradient with the catheter-measured peak-to-peak gradient. In stenotic outflow cardiac lesions, the catheter-measured peak-to-peak gradient represents the difference between the peak ventricular and peak arterial pressures. However, these pressures are nonsynchronous. All comparisons should be between instantaneous pressure gradients.

The peak-to-peak catheter gradient is a convenient and established measurement. However, it does not follow hydraulic principles, as it is the difference of two nonsynchronous peak pressures. Therefore, it has no relationship to an instantaneous gradient (Fig. 12.2). The application of continuous wave Doppler in the assessment of stenotic pressure gradients has been shown to be correct in aortic stenosis over a wide range of severity (8, 9) (Figs. 12.3 and 12.4), in other left ventricular outflow obstructive lesions (5, 7) (Figs.

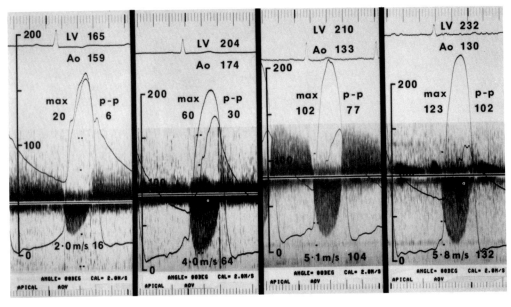

Figure 12.3. A composite of simultaneous Doppler-catheter pressure measurements in four patients with varying degrees of aortic stenosis and dual catheter left ventricular (*LV*) and ascending aortic (*Ao*) pressure measurements. The maximum catheter (*max*) gradient is greater than the peak-to-peak (*p-p*) catheter gradient at each level of stenosis. The maximum Doppler-derived gradients accurately measure the simultaneously recorded maximum catheter gradient, but overestimate the peak-to-peak gradient. Doppler calibration markers are 2 m/sec apart. (From Currie PJ, et al. Continuous-wave Doppler echocardiographic assessment of severity of calcific aortic stenosis: A simultaneous Doppler-catheter correlation study in 100 adult patients. *Circulation* 71:1162–1169, 1985. By permission of the American Heart Association, Inc.)

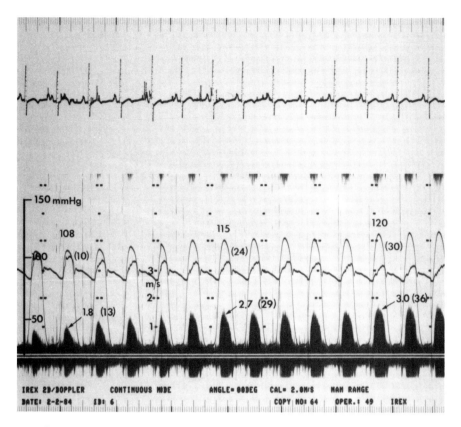

Figure 12.4. Simultaneous Doppler and dual catheter pressure recordings in an open-chest dog model of aortic stenosis (10). Tightening of an ascending aortic snare has produced concurrent beat-to-beat increase in maximum catheter pressure gradient and a corresponding increase in the maximum Doppler gradient. Doppler calibration markers are 2 m/sec, and the Doppler transducer is directly on the ascending aorta above the aortic snare. At the beginning of the tracing, there is no gradient. As tightening increases, there is a maximum catheter gradient of 30 mm Hg with a corresponding maximum Doppler gradient of 30 mm Hg. Note that catheter pressures were measured with transducer-tipped catheters. (Courtesy of Dr. Mark Callahan, Mayo Clinic.)

12.5 and 12.6), and in various types of right ventricular outflow obstructive lesions (7) (Figs. 12.6 and 12.7).

A Doppler-derived maximum pressure gradient is not equivalent to a catheter-measured peak-to-peak pressure gradient (7, 8, 10) (Figs. 12.2, 12.5, 12.7, and 12.8). Unfortunately, reports have equated the two (1, 2, 6), leading to some clinical confusion. When reporting pressure gradients, it is crucial to convey to the clinician that a Doppler measurement is a maximum instantaneous gradient. Estimating the peak-to-peak catheter gradient from the maximum Doppler gradient may be less reliable, even when regression equations are used (8).

The mean Doppler-determined gradient may

be the most useful clinical expression of pressure gradient, as it is directly comparable to the mean gradient measured by catheter. Also, both mean gradients represent an average over systole rather than instantaneous (Fig. 12.9). Disadvantages include the need for software to calculate the maximum velocities, mean velocities, and gradients, and it is more time-consuming to trace the Doppler spectral envelope on line. However, when an incomplete spectral envelope is obtained, the maximum gradient obtained may be more accurate than the derived mean gradient.

In the presence of cardiac arrhythmias, the maximum Doppler gradient should not be determined from a single beat. An average gradient needs to be derived from consecutive beats and

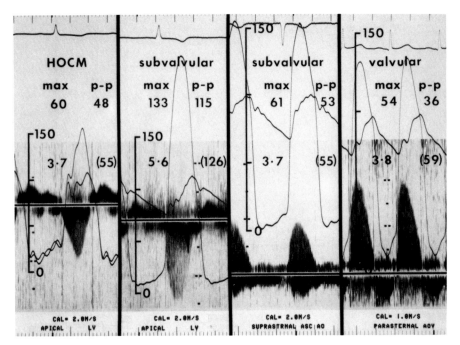

Figure 12.5. A composite of simultaneous Doppler-catheter pressure measurements in four patients with varying left ventricular outflow tract obstructive lesions and dual catheter left ventricular and ascending aortic pressure measurements. The lesions (from the *left*) are: hypertrophic obstructive cardiomyopathy (*HOCM*), fibromuscular subvalvular aortic stenosis, discrete membranous subvalvular aortic stenosis, and congenital valvular aortic stenosis. The maximum catheter (*max*) gradient is greater than the peak-to-peak (*p-p*) catheter gradient at each level of stenosis. Maximum Doppler-derived gradients accurately reflect the simultaneous recorded maximum catheter gradient, but overestimate the peak-to-peak gradient. Calibration markers and the Doppler transducer sites are shown at the *bottom* of each tracing.

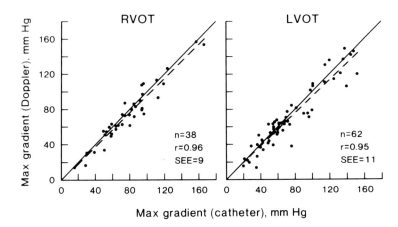

Figure 12.6. Correlation between simultaneous maximal (*Max*) Doppler-derived and catheter pressure gradients in 100 patients with stenotic cardiac lesions. Thirty-eight patients have right ventricular outflow obstructive (*RVOT*) lesions, and 62 have left ventricular outflow obstructive lesions (*LVOT*) (7). This demonstrates the close Doppler/catheter pressure gradient correlation for both LVOT and RVOT stenotic lesions. The *dotted line* represents the regression line, and the *solid line*, the line of identity. (Reprinted with permission from the American College of Cardiology and Currie PJ, et al: Instantaneous pressure gradient: A simultaneous Doppler and dual catheter correlative study. *J Am Coll Cardiol* 7:800–806, 1986.)

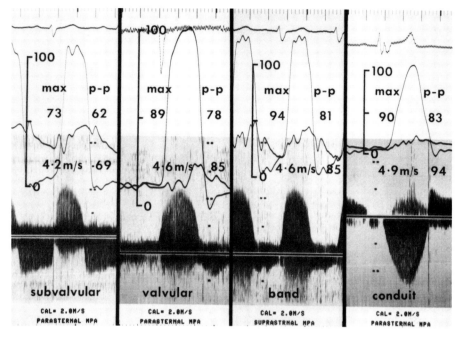

Figure 12.7. A composite of simultaneous Doppler-catheter pressure measurements in four patients with a variety of right ventricular outflow tract obstructive lesions in whom dual catheter right ventricular and pulmonary artery pressure measurements were obtained. The lesions (from the *left*) are: fibromuscular subvalvular pulmonary stenosis, congenital valvular pulmonary stenosis, pulmonary artery band, and a stenotic right ventricular-to-pulmonary artery conduit. The maximum catheter (*max*) gradient is greater than the peak-to-peak (*p-p*) catheter gradient at each level of stenosis. The maximum Doppler-derived gradients accurately measure the simultaneously recorded maximum catheter gradient, but overestimate the peak-to-peak gradient. Doppler calibration markers are 2 m/sec apart, and the Doppler transducer sites are shown at the *bottom* of each tracing.

reported as such (Fig. 12.8). Beats that are not optimal, due to change in transducer position or other technical factors, should not be included in the averaging, as they may not reflect real beat-to-beat variation in hemodynamics.

Comparisons of Doppler- and catheter-determined gradients have shown a much closer correlation between simultaneous measurements (7, 8) (Fig. 12.10). Disparities between nonsimultaneous measurements should not be written off as Doppler inaccuracies, since variations in hemodynamic state must be considered. The technique of catheter gradient measurement should be evaluated, since the catheter across the stenosis potentially further compromises the orifice (Fig. 12.2).

Doppler echocardiography provides an important noninvasive technique for serial noninvasive evaluation of patients. Transducer position, heart rate, and blood pressure measurements at the time of Doppler examination are essential for accurate serial follow-up.

A number of potential sources of error exist for cardiac catheterization. The catheter pullback technique of pressure gradient measurement has more potential for error than a dual catheter technique, where instantaneous and mean pressure gradients can be measured accurately. Other important considerations are the fidelity of the catheter pressure measurement system and the inherent presence of catheter-induced artifact. An underdamped system or catheter artifact may lead to errors in estimation of maximum and mean pressure gradients, which may be interpreted incorrectly as inaccuracies in the Doppler-derived gradient.

Transseptal catheterization is being increasingly used to estimate pressure gradients in aortic stenosis. This supersedes catheter withdrawal of a retrograde aortic catheter or the less accurate

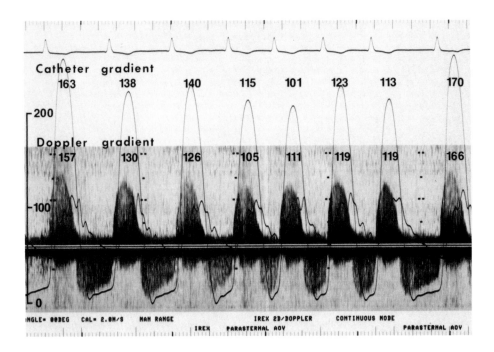

Figure 12.8. Simultaneous Doppler-catheter pressure measurements with a dual left ventricular and ascending aortic catheter technique, showing the beat-to-beat comparison in a patient with atrial fibrillation and severe aortic stenosis. The catheter and Doppler-derived gradients are maximum systolic gradients. The Doppler echo was recorded with the transducer in the right parasternal position. Note that aortic regurgitation was also detected. (From Currie PJ, et al: Continuous-wave Doppler echocardiographic assessment of severity of calcific aortic stenosis: A simultaneous Doppler-catheter correlation study in 100 adult patients. *Circulation* 71:1162–1169, 1985. By permission of the American Heart Association, Inc.)

method of simultaneous left ventricular and peripheral artery pressure recordings (50). Mean gradients rather than maximum instantaneous Doppler gradient or peak-to-peak catheter gradient are now reported. Valve area calculations are used by both echocardiographic and cathe-

terization laboratories to minimize the problems of nonsimultaneous measurements.

VALVE AREA DETERMINATION

Pressure gradient alone may not be sufficient to determine the severity of stenosis. In patients

Figure 12.9. Correlation of simultaneous mean Doppler-derived and catheter pressure gradients in 100 adult patients with aortic stenosis (8). The regression equation is: Catheter gradient = 5.2 + 0.98 × Doppler-determined gradient. The *dotted line* represents the regression line, and the *solid line* the line of identity. (From Currie PJ, et al: Continuous-wave Doppler echocardiographic assessment of severity of calcific aortic stenosis: A simultaneous Doppler-catheter correlation study in 100 adult patients. *Circulation* 71:1162–1169, 1985. By permission of the American Heart Association, Inc.)

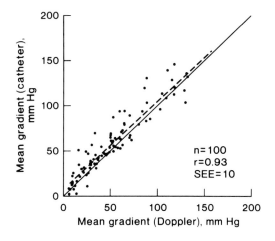

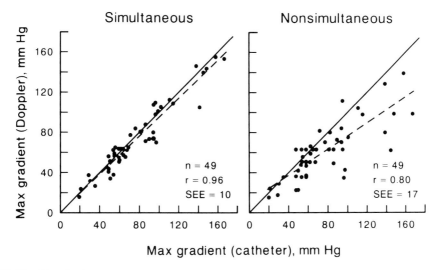

Figure 12.10. Nonsimultaneous versus simultaneous Doppler catheter correlation in the study of 100 stenotic outflow tract lesions of Currie et al. (7), shown in Fig. 12.6. There is a closer correlation of simultaneous than nonsimultaneous maximal Doppler and catheter pressure gradients. The regression equations are: Doppler gradient = 0.98 × catheter gradient − 1.4; and Doppler gradient = 0.78 × catheter gradient + 5.2. The *dotted line* represents the regression line, and the *solid line* the line of identity. (Reprinted with permission from the American College of Cardiology and Currie PJ, et al: Instantaneous pressure gradient: A simultaneous Doppler and dual catheter correlative study. *J Am Coll Cardiol* 7:800–806, 1986.)

with low cardiac output, suspected aortic stenosis, and left ventricular dysfunction, aortic valve area determination may be necessary for clinical decision making.

Cardiac catheterization using the Gorlin formula remains the gold standard for determining valve area (51). This formula was derived from hydraulic equations describing steady-state flow through an orifice and relates flow to mean velocity and cross-sectional area of the orifice. As standard cardiac catheterization cannot measure velocity, mean velocity with the square root of the mean pressure difference is substituted. In addition, various other modifications were made to derive the Gorlin formula (52):

$$\text{Valve area} = \frac{[CO/(DFP \text{ or } SEP) \times HR]}{(44.5 \times c \times \sqrt{\text{mean } \Delta P})} \quad (12.4)$$

where DFP = diastolic filling period, HR = heart rate, c = empiric constant, and ΔP = mean pressure difference across the aortic valve.

Several studies have shown errors in valve area calculations made using the Gorlin formula. This is particularly true with extremes of pressure gradient or flow (20). As pressure difference approaches zero, calculated valve area approaches infinity. The catheterization methods to estimate flow across the stenotic valve are less than optimal in the presence of valvular regurgitation, low output states, and cardiac arrhythmias. All catheterization techniques estimating cardiac output (thermodilution, dye dilution, angiographic, and Fick) have significant limitations and potential errors (53).

Initial studies evaluating Doppler methods of estimating mitral and aortic valve areas used the Gorlin equation (15, 19). The mean pressure gradient was determined from the maximum Doppler spectral envelope, and the cardiac output was obtained by thermodilution. These studies established the method's validity for estimating valve area. However, the studies also showed an inaccuracy in determining flow across the stenotic valve in the presence of regurgitation.

Studies in patients with aortic valve stenosis have shown that Doppler-derived aortic valve area correlates closely with catheterization data (12–19) (Figs. 12.11 and 12.12). Aortic valve area (area_{AV}) can be determined by two-dimensional/Doppler echo based on the continuity equation (13) according to the formula:

$$\text{area}_{AV} = \text{mean velocity}_{LVOT} \times \pi/4 \\ \times [\text{diameter}_{LVOT}]^2 / \text{mean velocity}_{AV} \quad 12.5$$

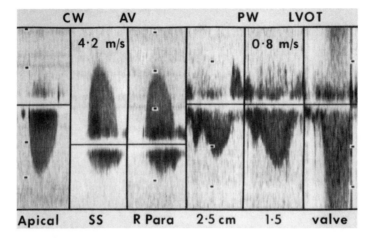

Figure 12.11. Composite Doppler tracings in a patient with severe aortic stenosis (*SS*), illustrating the Doppler data needed for aortic valve area calculation (13). It is essential to use multiple transducer positions to obtain the best continuous wave (*CW*) Doppler signal across the aortic valve. In this patient, the best signal was from the right parasternal (*R para*) position with a maximum velocity of 4.2 m/sec and a mean velocity of 3.2 m/sec. Careful examination by pulsed wave (*PW*) Doppler is needed from the apical five-chamber view to obtain the best left ventricular outflow tract (*LVOT*) signal. This signal was obtained at a depth of 1.5 cm into the LVOT with the maximum LVOT velocity of 0.8 m/sec and the mean velocity of 0.5 m/sec. With the LVOT diameter of 2.5 cm measured by two-dimensional echo parasternal long-axis view, the estimated aortic valve (*AV*) area is 0.77 cm², using the Doppler formula: valve area$_{AV}$ = mean velocity$_{LVOT}$ × $\pi/4$ [diameter$_{LVOT}$]²/mean velocity$_{AV}$.

where mean velocity$_{LVOT}$ = mean velocity of the left ventricular outflow tract obtained by pulse wave Doppler interrogation of the LVOT in the apical five-chamber view; diameter LVOT = diameter of the left ventricular outflow tract obtained by measuring immediately beneath the aortic annulus in the parasternal long-axis two-

dimensional echo view; mean velocity$_{AV}$ = mean velocity of the aortic valve obtained by continuous wave Doppler interrogation of multiple transducer positions to obtain the highest signal (Fig. 12.11).

Understanding potential errors is critical in the correct application of this method. The left ventricular outflow tract (LVOT) diameter, LVOT

Figure 12.12. Correlation of Doppler estimated aortic valve area (*AVA*) calculated totally noninvasively versus aortic valve area determined at cardiac catheterization (*CATH*) by the Gorlin formula in a study of 48 adults with aortic stenosis. (Reprinted with permission from the American College of Cardiology and Otto CM, et al: Determination of the stenotic aortic valve area in adults using Doppler echocardiography. *J Am Coll Cardiol* 7:509–517, 1986.)

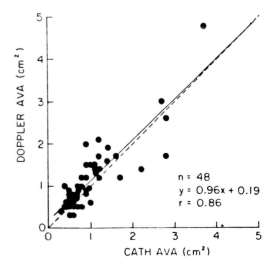

Doppler velocity, and aortic valve velocity may be measured inaccurately. This method assumes the left ventricular outflow tract is circular. Although there is good reproducibility of subvalvular diameter measurements in patients with normal aortic valves, it has not been established in patients with calcific aortic stenosis and associated left ventricular hypertrophy. Subvalvular velocity must be measured carefully by pulsed wave Doppler mapping of the LVOT. The velocity in the LVOT significantly increases immediately beneath the valve, compared to the most appropriate sampling site, 1.0–2.0 cm beneath the valve (13) (Fig. 12.11). It is most appropriate to measure flow across the LVOT rather than mitral diastolic flow. This is because, according to the continuity equation, the flow measured $LVOT = flow_{AV}$. Therefore, aortic or mitral regurgitation or intracardiac shunts will not lead to inaccuracies with catheterization techniques of blood flow determination (13).

Hatle et al. (54) validated a simple method to estimate mitral valve area, based on the Doppler-derived mitral diastolic pressure half-time. This is the time elapsed between the maximum early diastolic pressure gradient to half this diastolic pressure gradient (55) (Fig. 12.13). The diastolic half-time represents a measure of the rate of left atrial emptying, which is independent of the severity of associated mitral regurgitation. Diastolic half-time measured by either catheterization or Doppler techniques are directly comparable.

Potential pitfalls of Doppler include:

1. With rapid heart rates or prominent A waves, the slope of early diastolic flow—and therefore the diastolic half-time—is difficult to measure.
2. In the presence of aortic regurgitation, it can be difficult to record a clear mitral diastolic Doppler spectral envelope.
3. A significant angle error may occur (Fig. 12.14).

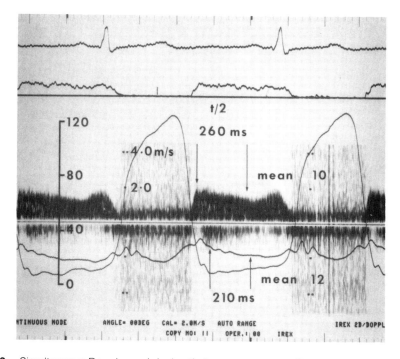

Figure 12.13. Simultaneous Doppler and dual catheter pressure recordings in a patient with severe pure mitral stenosis. One catheter is in the left ventricle across the aortic valve, and the other catheter is in a pulmonary artery wedge position. The Doppler-derived diastolic half-time of 260 msec (*ms*) corresponds to the catheter-measured diastolic half-time of 210 msec (*ms*). The Doppler-derived mean gradient of 10 mm Hg corresponds to the catheter-measured mean gradient of 12 mm Hg. The Doppler-derived mitral valve area using the formula (54) (mitral valve area = 220/Doppler diastolic half-time) is 0.8 cm², which correlates with the catheter-derived mitral valve area using the Gorlin formula of 0.9 cm².

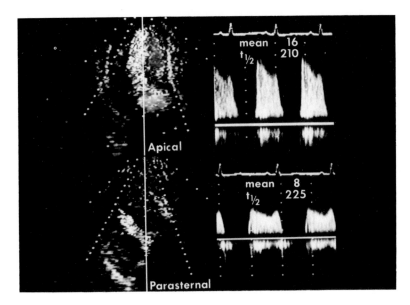

Figure 12.14. Composite color flow Doppler and continuous wave Doppler of the mitral valve in the apical and low parasternal views in a patient with moderately severe mitral stenosis. This ilustrates the effect on mean diastolic mitral gradient of a significant angle between the diastolic jet and ultrasound beam. In the apical view, the mean gradient was 16 mm Hg, but dropped to 8 mm Hg when there was a significant angle error. This demonstrates the use of color flow imaging in minimizing angle error. There was little difference in Doppler diastolic half-time ($t_{1/2}$) between the two views. See this figure in Color Atlas.

The potential pitfalls of catheterization include:

1. Disparity between the pulmonary capillary wedge pressure and true left atrial pressure may cause a major error in mean gradient measurement (56).
2. Associated tricuspid regurgitation may cause cardiac output estimation to be inaccurate.
3. Mitral regurgitation may cause underestimation of mitral valve area as calculated by the Gorlin formula.

Estimating prosthetic valve area by cardiac catheterization has seen limited study (57). Applying the Gorlin formula to prosthetic valves may not be satisfactory, since inlet geometries and flow rates differ from those of stenotic native valves. Theoretical hydraulic considerations suggest that Doppler methods of assessing prosthetic valve area with the continuity equation may be satisfactory, despite poor correlation with the Gorlin-estimated valve area (57).

CARDIAC OUTPUT ESTIMATION

Blood flow through a vessel is related to cross-sectional area (CSA) and mean velocity (V). De-termining stroke volume (SV) requires measurement of the cross-sectional area of the vessel or valve—usually by two-dimensional echocardiography—and the time velocity integral (TVI). The TVI corresponds to the area under the Doppler spectral envelope measured by either computer or planimetry.

$$SV = CSA \times TVI \qquad 12.6$$

Many studies have validated Doppler for non-invasive determination of intracardiac blood flow and cardiac output (21, 22, 58). The limitations of the technique involve determination of the appropriate cross-sectional area and Doppler velocity signals (58–61). Multiple sites have been used to measure blood flow. These include the ascending aorta, left ventricular outflow tract, mitral valve, pulmonary valve, and tricuspid valve. Various methods have been advocated to measure cross-sectional area, especially of the atrioventricular valves (22).

Accurate determination of cardiac output assumes that cross-sectional area, and blood flow velocity measurements are made at the same level. The cross-sectional area often is assumed to be circular and without any significant dynamic change during systole. The other assumption is that sample volume represents the characteristics of flow across the entire cross-section measured (laminar flow).

The gold standard for determining cardiac output is catheterization using Fick, indicator dilution, or thermodilution methods. These techniques have inherent inaccuracies (53). Also, they represent an averaged cardiac output over many cardiac cycles and represent effective blood flow. Doppler techniques represent beat-to-beat measurements at various sites and represent absolute blood flow (including regurgitant or shunt flow) at that measurement site. The clinical usefulness of noninvasive cardiac output determination deserves further study. The most common uses of Doppler-determined blood flow are in shunt quantitation, regurgitant ratio determination, and area$_{AV}$ estimation.

VALVULAR REGURGITATION QUANTITATION

The major difficulty in assessing valvular regurgitation in patients with valvular heart disease is that no technique can accurately quantitate the severity of the regurgitant lesion. All clinically used techniques are, at best, semiquantitative. Therefore, validation studies of newer Doppler techniques must take into account the insensitivity of standard angiographic techniques.

Adequacy of an angiographic study depends on balancing many factors (62, 63). These are

1. Positioning the catheter to avoid interference with the valve;
2. Adjusting the volume and rate of contrast delivery to obtain the best chamber opacification while avoiding catheter recoil, inducing cardiac arrhythmias and toxic effects of contrast volume;
3. Making sure that increased cardiac chamber size does not prevent optimal opacification and that there is entire simultaneous visualization of the chambers in the field of view.

Both semiquantitative (flow mapping) and quantitative (regurgitant fraction) Doppler methods have been used to assess valvular regurgitation (33–35, 38–41).

Flow mapping determines spatial distribution of the regurgitant jet (length and area) into the regurgitant chamber. This is performed by spatial mapping with either pulsed wave or color flow Doppler and provides a semiquantitative index of severity of regurgitation. However, the measurement made by Doppler flow mapping is quite different from the qualitative densitometric assessment of contrast opacification of the regurgitant chamber compared to the chamber of contrast injection. Doppler data are interpreted using a scale of 0 to 4+ (64). Both Doppler and an-

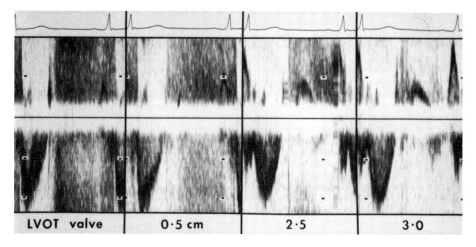

Figure 12.15. Composite pulsed wave Doppler spectral tracings recorded from the apical transducer position in a patient with moderate aortic regurgitation. The sample volume was initially immediately beneath the aortic valve level, demonstrating the typical aliased diastolic signal of aortic regurgitation. As the sample volume is moved further into the left ventricular outflow tract (*LVOT*), so the aortic regurgitation is less obvious to 3.0 cm below the valve; the aortic regurgitation is essentially gone.

giographic techniques have limited quantitative value and provide only a semiquantitative estimate of severity of valvular regurgitation.

Pulsed wave Doppler spatial mapping plots the distribution of regurgitant flow determined by the area of aliased Doppler signal in a tomographic two-dimensional image. Since regurgitant blood jets are high velocity, they are detected by pulsed wave Doppler as aliased Doppler signals (Fig. 12.15). Consequently, typical pulsed wave Doppler regurgitant signals are easy to differentiate. Careful examination is needed, using multiple sample sites in multiple tomographic planes, to produce accurately a three-dimensional impression of "volume" for the regurgitant jet of blood.

Color flow Doppler has demonstrated that regurgitant jets can travel in unusual directions. For example, an anteriorly directed mitral regurgitant jet is produced by ruptured chordae tendineae of the posterior mitral leaflet (Fig. 12.16). Color flow Doppler has helped us understand the limitations of pulsed wave Doppler mapping in only a single tomographic plane. Thus meticulous pulsed wave Doppler technique is necessary, which is also time-consuming.

Color flow Doppler imaging is the newest among Doppler echocardiographic techniques. Initial studies show that color flow Doppler is useful in the noninvasive semiquantitation of valvular regurgitation (34, 38–40, 64, 65) (Fig. 12.16 and 12.17). Direct visualization of the blood flow jet by color flow Doppler allows faster estimation of valvular regurgitation than standard pulsed wave Doppler spatial mapping. With color flow im-

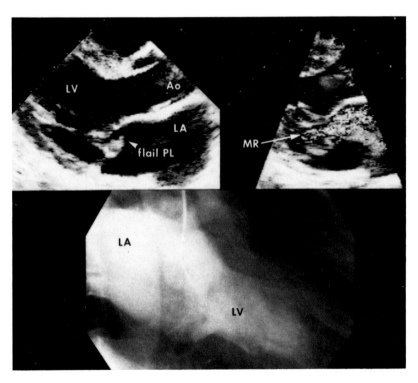

Figure 12.16. Composite of two-dimensional/Doppler echocardiograms and cineangiogram in a patient with severe mitral regurgitation. *Upper left panel,* Parasternal long-axis, two-dimensional echo view in systole, showing the left ventricle (*LV*), left atrium (*LA*), ascending aorta (*Ao*), and flail posterior leaflet (*PL*) of the mitral valve. *Upper right panel,* Color flow Doppler mapping in the same view as in *A,* demonstrating an anteriorly directed mitral regurgitant jet (*MR*) indicative of posterior leaflet pathology. The mitral regurgitation, by imaging in multiple tomographic views, was graded as severe. *Lower panel,* A systolic still frame left ventricular cineangiogram in the same patient in the right anterior oblique projection. The left ventricle (*LV*) and left atrium (*LA*) are shown. There is greater opacification of the left atrium than the left ventricle with retrograde filling of the pulmonary veins, indicating severe mitral regurgitation by Sellers' criteria (70). See this figure in Color Atlas.

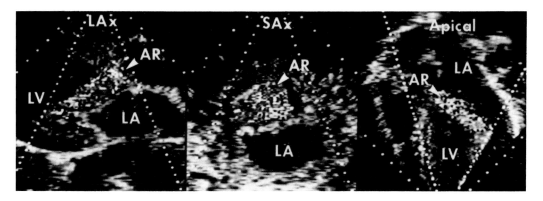

Figure 12.17. Composite two-dimensional echo views with color flow Doppler mapping in a patient with severe aortic regurgitation (*AR*). This illustrates the use of multiple tomographic views to define the volume of a regurgitant jet and semiquantitate the severity of aortic regurgitation. The *left panel* is a parasternal long-axis view (*LAx*) demonstrating the aortic regurgitant jet directed along the anterior leaflet of the mitral valve into the left ventricle (*LV*). In the *middle panel*, a parasternal short-axis view (*SAx*), the aortic regurgitant jet opacifies most of the left ventricular outflow tract. The *right panel*, an apical five-chamber view (apex down), shows the aortic regurgitant jet in the left ventricle. *LA*, Left atrium. See this figure in Color Atlas.

aging, the entire depth and width of the regurgitant jet can be measured. Severity is then estimated by developing a three-dimensional impression of the size of the regurgitant jet of blood relative to the regurgitant chamber. Attempts have been made to quantitate the spatial distribution of the regurgitant jet (i.e., length, area, width) and relate it to catheter-derived parameters (34, 40).

An important consideration in the optimal use of color flow Doppler echocardiography is the appropriate selection of patients. Generally, a patient with an adequate two-dimensional echo image will have a satisfactory color flow Doppler image. Obtaining the best color flow image is aided by:

1. Obtaining the best two-dimensional image possible;
2. Making certain that the lesion to be imaged by color flow is as close to the transducer as possible; all current commercially available two-dimensional Doppler systems suffer from far field insensitivity of color flow Doppler mapping of regurgitant jets;
3. Orienting the color flow jet so that it is as parallel to the ultrasound beam as possible, to optimize directional information; balancing these seemingly contradictory considerations usually results in the optimal transducer position for color flow imaging being between the parasternal and apical positions;

4. Attempting to develop a three-dimensional impression of the volume of the regurgitant jet by imaging in multiple views (parasternal long- and short-axis views as well as the apical view) (Fig. 12.17);
5. Understanding the effect on the spatial distribution of the regurgitant jet by changing the instrument used, the transducer's carrier frequency, the color flow map algorithm, the pulse repetition frequency, the scanning sector angle, the color frame rate, the color flow filter, or the color gain settings (64) (Fig. 12.18);
6. Converging jets, such as those caused by aortic regurgitation and mitral inflow, especially with higher velocity mitral stenosis, can be difficult to interpret.
7. Taking into consideration aliasing, wall motion ghosting, artifacts produced by valves, and shadowing produced by prosthetic valves (66).

The following methods have been proposed to quantitate valvular regurgitation better.

1. Differential Doppler flow measurements can be used to calculate the regurgitant ratio by applying techniques similar to those used to quantitate shunt flow (67).
   Aortic regurgitant fraction (RF):

$$RF\ (\%) = \frac{LVOT\ flow - systemic\ flow}{LVOT\ flow} \times 100$$

12.7

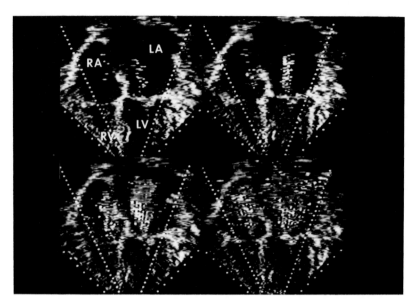

Figure 12.18. Composite of an apical four-chamber echo view (apex down) with color flow Doppler mapping in a patient with severe mitral and tricuspid regurgitation, with increasing color flow settings. This illustrates the major influence of these settings in assessing jet distribution. The left atrium (*LA*), left ventricle (*LV*), right atrium (*RA*), and right ventricle (*RV*) are labeled. *Upper panels* have too low color gain. *Lower left panel* is optimal, and *lower right panel* has too high a gain setting. See this figure in Color Atlas.

where systemic flow = tricuspid valve, mitral valve, or pulmonary flow, and LVOT = left ventricular outflow tract flow

Mitral regurgitant fraction (RF):

$$\text{RF } (\%) = \frac{\text{Mitral flow} - \text{systemic flow}}{\text{Mitral flow}} \times 100 \quad (12.8)$$

where systemic flow = tricuspid valve, pulmonary valve, or LVOT flow.

2. Regurgitation can be assessed by a pulsed wave Doppler technique measuring the amount of diastolic flow reversal in the descending arch of the aorta (35). The area under the diastolic portion of this Doppler spectral profile is divided by the area under the systolic portion, yielding a regurgitant fraction.
3. By using continuous wave Doppler spectral recordings of aortic regurgitation, the pressure decay in the aortic to left ventricular diastolic pressure gradient can be estimated. This is calculated by estimating the Doppler diastolic half-time and the Doppler pressure decay slope (36, 67).

Of all the techniques listed above, color flow Doppler mapping appears to have the most clinical utility. There are a number of potential pitfalls and artifacts that should be considered before valid assessment can be made with color flow Doppler. Unfortunately, a major limitation in the assessment of valvular regurgitation is that all clinically used techniques are only semiquantitative.

INTRACARDIAC PRESSURE ESTIMATION

Calculations of intracardiac pressures by Doppler are indirect. These involve using a Doppler-derived pressure gradient (ΔP) and a second known (or assumed) pressure according to the formula:

$$\Delta P = P_1 - P_2 = 4v^2 \quad\quad 12.9$$

where P_1 and P_2 = pressures on either side of a stenosis.

When the distal pressure (P_2) is known,

$$P_1 = P_2 + 4v^2 \quad\quad 12.10$$

and when the proximal pressure (P_1) is known,

$$P_2 = P_1 + 4v^2 \quad\quad 12.11$$

Right ventricular systolic pressure (RVSP) can be estimated using the formula:

$$RVSP = \Delta P + RA \qquad 12.12$$

where ΔP is derived from the Doppler-determined maximum systolic velocity of tricuspid regurgitation, and the RA pressure is derived from any number of methods. These methods include clinical estimation of jugular venous pressure, a derived regression equation, or an assumed constant (24). Correlative studies confirm this to be an accurate Doppler technique for estimation of right ventricular systolic pressure (23, 24) (Figs. 12.19 and 12.20).

This method is widely applicable due to the large percentage of patients with Doppler-detected tricuspid regurgitation even if not clinically apparent or hemodynamically significant (24). If the right atrial pressure is estimated or assumed, the right ventricular systolic pressure can be cal-

culated indirectly (23, 24). However, it has been shown that the most significant error in this technique is not because of the Doppler-derived pressure gradient measurement, but is due to the inaccuracy of *RA* pressure estimation (24) (Figs. 12.21 and 12.22).

There are a number of methods to determine the pulmonary artery systolic pressure, including:

1. *Measuring duration of the right ventricular isovolumetric relaxation interval.* This interval between pulmonary valve closure and tricuspid valve opening ($P_c - T_o$ interval) is measured by recording valve closure and tricuspid valve opening (27). Then a nomogram, based on the $P_c - T_o$ interval and heart rate, is used to estimate pulmonary artery pressure (68). There is a proportional increase in this interval with increasing pulmonary artery pressure and an inverse relationship to heart rate. The technique requires accurate recording to the

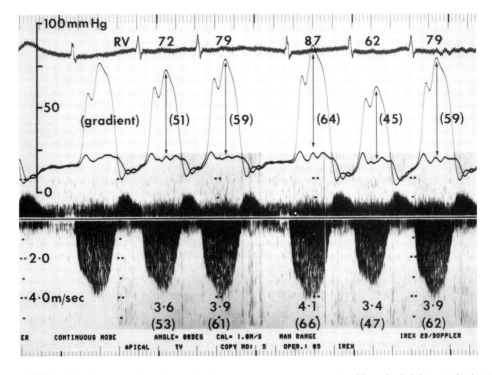

Figure 12.19. Simultaneous Doppler-catheter pressure measurements with a dual right ventricular and right atrial catheter technique, showing the beat-to-beat comparison in a patient with atrial fibrillation and tricuspid regurgitation. The maximum catheter and Doppler-derived gradients correlate closely despite an irregular heart rate. The Doppler transducer was in the apical position. (Reprinted with permission from the American College of Cardiology and Currie PJ, et al: Continuous wave Doppler determination of right ventricular pressure: A simultaneous Doppler-catheterization study in 127 patients. *J Am Coll Cardiol* 6: 750–756, 1985.)

Figure 12.20. Correlation of simultaneous Doppler-derived and catheter-measured right ventricular-right atrial maximal (*Max*) pressure gradients in 111 patients with analyzable Doppler-detected tricuspid regurgitation from a study by Currie et al. (24). The regression equation is:
Doppler gradient
$$= 2.2 + 0.88 \times \text{catheter gradient}$$
The *dotted line* represents the regression line, and the *solid line*, the line of identity. (Reprinted with permission from the American College of Cardiology and Currie PJ, et al: Continuous wave Doppler determination of right ventricular pressure: A simultaneous Doppler-catheterization study in 127 patients. *J Am Coll Cardiol* 6:750–756, 1985.)

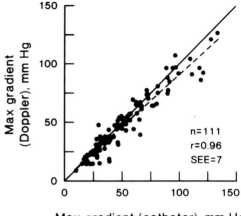

$P_c - T_o$ interval and is limited to patients without cardiac arrhythmias. However, this measurement may be useful when valve motion of the tricuspid and pulmonary valves can be recorded but complete spectral envelopes are unobtainable.

2. *Pulsed wave Doppler recordings of the pulmonary artery flow velocity.* Quantitative analysis of the pulmonary artery spectral envelope determines the preejection period, acceleration time, right ventricular ejection time, and the acceleration time corrected for heart rate

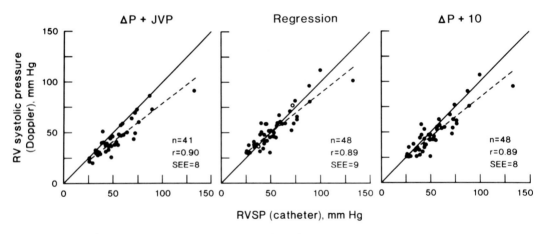

Figure 12.21. Composite graphs showing correlation of three methods of Doppler estimation of right ventricular systolic pressure with the catheter-measured pressures in the simultaneous Doppler-catheter study in 127 patients by Currie et al. (24). This shows a good correlation between Doppler-estimated and catheter-measured right ventricular systolic pressure, but the most accurate pressure used the derived regression equation. *Left panel,* Estimated right ventricular (*RV*) systolic pressure (Doppler gradient (*FP*) and jugular venous pressure (*JVP*)) versus catheter right ventricular systolic pressure (*RVSP*). The *dotted line* is the regression line, and the *solid line* is the line of identity. *Center panel,* Estimated RVSP using previously derived regression equations versus catheter-measured right ventricular systolic pressure. *Closed circles* are estimates using the low regression (*RVSP = FP + 14*) in patients with a jugular venous pressure of 2–20 cm H$_2$O, and the *open circles* are the other two patients with a jugular venous pressure of 3–20 cm H$_2$O in whom the high regression equation was used (*RVSP = 1.1 × FP + 20*). *Right panel,* Estimated *RVSP* (Doppler gradient (*FP*) + 10 mm Hg) versus the catheter *RVSP*. (Reprinted with permission from the American College of Cardiology and Currie PJ, et al: Continuous wave Doppler determination of right ventricular pressure: A simultaneous Doppler-catheterization study in 127 patients. *J Am Coll Cardiol* 6:750–756, 1985.)

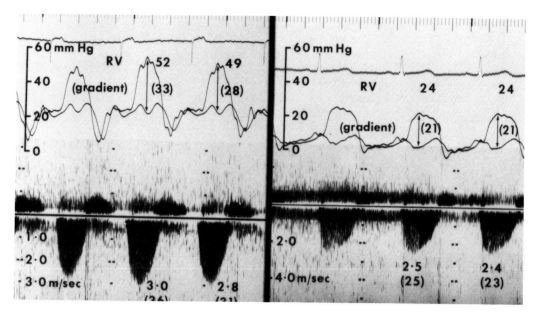

Figure 12.22. The effect of right atrial pressure estimation on the prediction of right ventricular (*RV*) systolic pressure is demonstrated by simultaneous Doppler and catheter pressure recordings in patients with similar maximal systolic pressure gradients. *Left panel,* Patient with constrictive pericarditis and a markedly increased right atrial pressure. *Right panel,* Patient with an atrial septal defect and a maximal gradient of 21 mm Hg. However, the right atrial pressure is low, resulting in a lower right ventricular systolic pressure despite a maximal Doppler gradient comparable to that in the *left panel.* (Reprinted with permission from the American College of Cardiology and Currie PJ, et al: Continuous wave Doppler determination of right ventricular pressure: A simultaneous Doppler-catheterization study in 127 patients. *J Am Coll Cardiol* 6:750–756, 1985).

(25, 26, 30, 32). A number of studies have shown these indices correlate well with catheter-measured pulmonary artery pressure (25, 26, 30) and total pulmonary resistance (30, 32).

Pulmonary artery diastolic pressure (PADP) can be estimated according to the formula:

$$PADP = \Delta P + RVEDP$$

where ΔP = end-diastolic pressure gradient between the pulmonary artery and the right ventricle. This is estimated from the end-diastolic regurgitant velocity determined from Doppler recording of the pulmonary regurgitation (28) (Fig. 12.23). The right ventricular end-diastolic pressure (RVEDP) is assumed to be small (approximately 5 mm Hg). The major error with this technique is the potential inability to obtain the maximum diastolic signal of pulmonary regurgitation and the assumption that RVEDP is small. As Doppler-detected pulmonary regurgitation is

very commonly obtained even in normal subjects, PADP is very frequently obtainable. This greatest value of the technique is the confirmation of the severity of pulmonary hypertension obtained by the tricuspid regurgitation technique.

It has been proposed that the left ventricular end-diastolic pressure (LVEDP) can be derived from Doppler-detected aortic regurgitation according to the formula:

$$LVEDP = DBP - \Delta P \qquad 12.14$$

where ΔP = end-diastolic pressure gradient between the aorta and the left ventricle. This is estimated from the end-diastolic regurgitant velocity determined by Doppler recording of the aortic regurgitation. The DBP is the diastolic aortic blood pressure measured by sphygmomanometric arm cuff pressure (69).

There are serious limitations to this technique. The degree of error for estimating both diastolic blood pressure and the pressure gradient is as

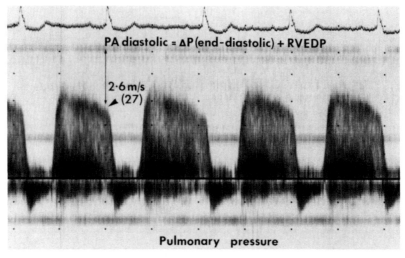

PA diastolic = ΔP(end-diastolic) + RVEDP

2·6 m/s
(27)

Pulmonary pressure

Figure 12.23. Doppler tracing showing calculation of diastolic PA pressure. Continuous wave Doppler spectral tracing through the pulmonary valve, with the transducer in the high left parasternal position, demonstrates normal pulmonary systolic velocity and pulmonary regurgitation. Pressure is calculated using the equation (28), PA diastolic = ΔP (end-diastolic) + RVEDP, where PA diastolic = pulmonary artery diastolic pressure, P = Doppler-derived end-diastolic pressure gradient from the pulmonary regurgitant spectral tracing, and RVEDP = right ventricular end-diastolic pressure.

great as the difference between normal and significantly abnormal LVEDP.

Doppler-detected mitral regurgitation can be used to estimate left atrial pressure according to the formula:

$$LA = SBP - \Delta P \qquad 12.15$$

where SBP is the systolic aortic blood pressure measured by sphygmomanometry. ΔP is the systolic pressure gradient between the left ventricle and the left atrium, derived from the maximum systolic velocity of Doppler-detected mitral regurgitation. This technique has only limited application because errors in the estimation of systolic blood pressure and in determination of pressure gradient are similar to the difference between normal and significantly abnormal left atrial pressures. In addition, determination of maximum velocity of mitral regurgitation may be difficult to obtain in patients with mitral valve prolapse or flail leaflets, where mitral regurgitation jets may be directed eccentrically. The resultant left atrial pressure does not represent either A or V wave pressures, but rather the left atrial pressure at the maximum instantaneous pressure difference between left ventricle and left atrium.

SUMMARY

Doppler echocardiography represents an exciting technique that has added a major and expanding dimension in the noninvasive evaluation of patients with congenital and acquired heart disease. However, increased technical and interpretive skills are required by echocardiographer to apply these techniques accurately.

The future role of Doppler echocardiography depends on validation against catheterization. However, these studies require careful interpretation. Measurements should be performed in the same or comparable physiologic state. Meticulous care should be taken to optimize both techniques. Accuracy of the gold standard should be examined critically. If accurate validation studies cannot be performed with patients due to inaccurate or inappropriate gold standards or inability to control parameters accurately, then careful animal studies or in vitro studies should be done. Oversimplification of either catheterization or Doppler techniques may lead to additional error. When there are many different Doppler methods developed to determine the same cathetherization parameter, validation studies should include not only the comparison with catheterization, but also with the other Doppler methods.

These correlative studies permit recognition of the limitations and pitfalls of both Doppler and catheterization. This leads to their better use in patients with heart disease.

REFERENCES

1. Lima CO, Sahn DJ, Valdes-Cruz LM, Allen HD, Goldberg SJ, Grenadier E, Vargas-Barron J: Prediction of the severity of left ventricular outflow tract obstruction by quantitative two-dimensional echocardiographic Doppler studies. *Circulation* 68:348–354, 1983.
2. Stamm RB, Martin RP: Quantification of pressure gradients across stenotic valves by Doppler ultrasound. *J Am Coll Cardiol* 2:707–718, 1983.
3. Johnson GL, Kwan OL, Handshoe S, Noonan JA, DeMaria AN: Accuracy of combined two-dimensional echocardiography and continuous-wave Doppler recordings in the estimation of pressure gradient in right ventricular outlet obstruction. *J Am Coll Cardiol* 3:1013–1018, 1984.
4. Hatle L, Angelsen BA, Tromsdal A: Non-invasive assessment of aortic stenosis by Doppler ultrasound. *Br Heart J* 43:284–292, 1980.
5. Hatle L: Noninvasive assessment and differentiation of left ventricular outflow obstruction with Doppler ultrasound. *Circulation* 64:381–387, 1981.
6. Berger M, Berdoff RL, Gallerstein PE, Goldberg E: Evaluation of aortic stenosis by continuous-wave Doppler ultrasound. *J Am Coll Cardiol* 3:150–156, 1984.
7. Currie PJ, Hagler DJ, Seward JB, Reeder GS, Fyfe DA, Bove AA, Tajik AJ: Instantaneous pressure gradient: a simultaneous Doppler and dual catheter correlative study. *J Am Coll Cardiol* 7:800–806, 1986.
8. Currie PJ, Seward JB, Reeder GS, Vlietstra RE, Bresnahan DR, Bresnahan JF, Smith HC, Hagler DJ, Tajik AJ: Continuous-wave Doppler echocardiographic assessment of severity of calcific aortic stenosis: A simultaneous Doppler-catheter correlation study in 100 adult patients. *Circulation* 71:1162–1169, 1985.
9. Smith MD, Dawson PL, Elion JL, Wisenbaugh T, Kwan OL, Handshoe S, DeMaria AN: Systematic correlation of continuous-wave Doppler and hemodynamic measurements in patients with aortic stenosis. *Am Heart J* 111:245–252, 1986.
10. Callahan M, Tajik AJ, Su-Fan Q, Bove AA: Validation of instantaneous pressure gradients measured by continuous wave Doppler in experimentally induced aortic stenosis. *Am J Cardiol* 56:989–993, 1985.
11. Valdes-Cruz LM, Horowitz S, Sahn DJ, Larson D, Lima CO, Mesel E: Validation of a Doppler echocardiographic method for calculating severity of discrete stenotic obstructions in a canine preparation with a pulmonary artery band. *Circulation* 69:1177–1181, 1984.
12. Kosturakis D, Allen HD, Goldberg SJ, Sahn DJ, Valdes-Cruz LM: Noninvasive quantification of stenotic semilunar valve areas by Doppler echocardiography. *J Am Coll Cardiol* 3:1256–1262, 1984.
13. Skjaerpe T, Hegrenaes L, Hatle L: Noninvasive estimation of valve area in patients with aortic stenosis by Doppler ultrasound and two-dimensional echocardiography. *Circulation* 72:810–818, 1985.
14. Teirstein P, Yeager M, Yock PG, Popp RL. Doppler echocardiographic measurement of aortic valve area in aortic stenosis: A noninvasive application of the Gorlin formula. *J Am Coll Cardiol* 8:1059–1065, 1986.
15. Ohlsson J, Wranne B. Noninvasive assessment of valve area in patients with aortic stenosis. *J Am Coll Cardiol* 7:501–508, 1986.
16. Otto CM, Pearlman AS, Comess KA, Reamer RP, Janko CL, Huntsman LL. Determination of the stenotic aortic valve area in adults using Doppler echocardiography. *J Am Coll Cardiol* 7:509–517, 1986.
17. Come PC, Riley MF, McKay RG, Safian R: Echocardiographic assessment of aortic valve area in elderly patients with aortic stenosis and of changes in valve area after percutaneous balloon valvuloplasty. *J Am Coll Cardiol* 10:115–124, 1987.
18. Richards KL, Cannon SR, Miller JF, Crawford MH. Calculation of aortic valve area by Doppler echocardiography: A direct application of the continuity equation. *Circulation* 73:964–969, 1986.
19. Warth DC, Stewart WJ, Block PC, Weyman AE: A new method to calculate aortic valve area without left heart catheterization. *Circulation* 80:978–983, 1984.
20. Cannon SR, Richards KL, Crawford M: Hydraulic estimation of stenotic orifice area: A correction of the Gorlin formula. *Circulation* 71:1170–1178, 1985.
21. Huntsman LL, Stewart DK, Barnes SR, Franklin SB, Colocousis JS, Hessel EA: Noninvasive Doppler determination of cardiac output in man: Clinical validation. *Circulation* 67:593–602, 1983.
22. Fisher DC, Sahn DJ, Friedman MJ, Larson D, Valdes-Cruz LM, Horowitz S, Goldberg SJ, Allen HD: The mitral valve orifice method for noninvasive two-dimensional echo Doppler determinations of cardiac output. *Circulation* 67:872–877, 1983.
23. Yock PG, Popp RL: Noninvasive estimation of right ventricular systolic pressure by Doppler ultrasound in patients with tricuspid regurgitation. *Circulation* 70:657–62, 1984.
24. Currie PJ, Seward JB, Chan K, Fyfe DA, Hagler DJ, Mair DD, Reeder GS, Nishimura RA, Tajik AJ: Continuous wave Doppler determination of right ventricular pressure: A simultaneous Doppler-catheterization study in 127 patients. *J Am Coll Cardiol* 6:750–756, 1985.
25. Kitabatake A, Inoue M, Asao M, Masuyama T, Tanouchi J, Morita T, Mishima M, Uemastu M, Shimazu T, Hori M, Abe H: Noninvasive evaluation of pulmonary hypertension by a pulsed Doppler technique. *Circulation* 68:302–309, 1983.
26. Chan KL, Currie PJ, Seward JB, Hagler DJ, Mair DD, Tajik AJ. Comparison of three Doppler ultrasound methods in the prediction of pulmonary artery pressure. *J Am Coll Cardiol* 9:549–554, 1987.
27. Hatle L, Angelsen BAJ, Tromsdal A: Non-invasive estimation of pulmonary artery systolic pressure with Doppler ultrasound. *Br Heart J* 45:157–165, 1981.
28. Masuyama T, Kodama K, Kitabatake A, Sato H,

Nanto S, Inoue M: Continuous-wave Doppler echocardiographic detection of pulmonary regurgitation and its application to noninvasive estimation of pulmonary artery pressure. *Circulation* 74:484–492, 1986.

29. Matsuda M, Sekiguchi T, Sugishita Y, Kuwako K, Iida K, Ito I: Reliability of non-invasive estimates of pulmonary hypertension by pulsed Doppler echocardiography. *Br Heart J* 56:158–164, 1986.

30. Martin Duran R, Larman M, Trugeda A, Vazquez De Prada JA, Ruano J, Torres A, Figueroa A, Pajaron A, Nistal F: Comparison of Doppler-determined elevated pulmonary arterial pressure with pressure measured at cardiac catheterization. *Am J Cardiol* 57:859–863, 1986.

31. Isobe M, Yazaki Y, Yakaku F, Koizumi K, Hara K, Tsuneyoshi H, Yamaguchi T, Machii K: Prediction of pulmonary arterial pressure in adults by pulsed Doppler echocardiography. *Am J Cardiol* 57: 316–321, 1986.

32. Dabestani A, Mahan G, Gardin JM, Takenaka K, Burn C, Allfie A, Henry WL. Evaluation of pulmonary artery pressure and resistance by pulsed Doppler echocardiography. *Am J Cardiol* 59:662–668, 1987.

33. Quinones MA, Young JB, Waggoner AD, Ostojic MC, Ribeiro LGT, Miller RR: Assessment of pulsed Doppler echocardiography in detection of quantitation of aortic and mitral regurgitation. *Br Heart J* 44:612–620, 1980.

34. Perry GJ, Helmcke R, Nan da N, Byard C, Soto B.: Evaluation of aortic insufficiency by Doppler color flow mapping. *J Am Coll Cardiol* 9:952–959, 1987.

35. Kitabatake A, Ito H, Inoue M, Tanouchi J, Ishihara K, Morita T, Fujii, Yoshida Y, Masuyama T, Yoshima H, Hori M, Kamada T: A new approach to noninvasive evaluation of aortic regurgitant fraction by two-dimensional Doppler echocardiography. *Circulation* 72:523–529, 1985.

36. Teague SM, Heinsmer JA, Anderson JL, Anderson JL, Sublett K, Olson EG, Voyles WF, Thadani U: Quantification of aortic regurgitation utilizing continuous wave Doppler ultrasound. *J Am Coll Cardiol* 8:592–599, 1986.

37. Labovitz AJ, Ferrara RP, Kern MJ, Bryg RJ, Mrosek DG, Williams GA: Quantitative evaluation of aortic insufficiency by continuous wave Doppler echocardiography. *J Am Coll Cardiol* 8:1341–1347, 1986.

38. Touche T, Prasquier R, Nitenberg N, De Zuttere D, Gourgon R: Assessment and follow-up of patients with aortic regurgitation by an updated Doppler echocardiography measurement of the regurgitant fraction in the aortic arch. *Circulation* 72:819–824, 1985.

39. Suzuki Y, Kambara H, Kadota K, Tamaki S, Yamazato A, Nohara R, Osakda G, Kawai C: Detection and evaluation of tricuspid regurgitation using a real time, two dimensional, color-coded Doppler flow imaging system: comparison with contrast two dimensional echocardiography and right ventriculography. *Am J Cardiol* 57:811–815, 1986.

40. Helmcke F, Nanda NC, Hsiung MC, Soto B, Adey CK, Goyal RG, Gatewood RP: Color Doppler assessment of mitral regurgitation with orthogonal planes. *Circulation* 75:175–183, 1987.

41. Blumlein S, Bouchard, A, Schiller NB, Dae M, Byrd BF III, Ports T, Botvinick EH: Quantitation of mitral regurgitation by Doppler echocardiography. *Circulation* 74:306–314, 1986.

42. Sanders SP, Yeager S, Williams RG: Measurement of systemic and pulmonary blood flow and QP/QS ratio using Doppler and two-dimensional echocardiography. *Am J Cardiol* 51:952–956, 1983.

43. Hatle L, Angelsen B: *Doppler Ultrasound in Cardiology: Physical Principles and Clinical Applications*, ed 2. Philadelphia, Lea & Febiger, 1985, p 8.

44. Teirstein PS, Yock PG, Popp RL: The accuracy of Doppler ultrasound measurement of pressure gradients across irregular, dual, and tunnellike obstructions to blood flow. *Circulation* 72:577–584, 1985.

45. Hatle L, Angelsen B: *Doppler Ultrasound in Cardiology: Physical Principles and Clinical Applications*, ed 2. Philadelphia, Lea & Febiger, 1985, p 217.

46. Hatle L, Angelsen B: *Doppler Ultrasound in Cardiology: Physical Principles and Clinical Applications*, ed 2. Philadelphia, Lea & Febiger, 1985, p 196.

47. Valdez-Cruz LM, Sahn DJ, Scagnelli S, Lima CO: Accuracy of continuous wave 2D echo Doppler studies for prediction of gradients across pulmonary artery bands: Clinical studies (Abstr). *J Am Coll Cardiol* 3:603, 1984.

48. Sahn DJ, Valdes-Cruz LM, Swensson RE, Scagnelli S, Dalton N: Potential for angular errors in Doppler gradient estimates: a study of spatial orientation of jet lesions using real-time color flow Doppler imaging (Abstr). *Circulation* (Suppl II):II-115, 1984.

49. Stewart WJ, Galvin KA, Gillam LD, Guyer DE, Weyman AE: Comparison of high pulse repetition frequency and continuous wave Doppler echocardiography in the assessment of high flow velocity in patients with valvular stenosis and regurgitation. *J Am Coll Cardiol* 6:565–571, 1985.

50. Folland ED, Parisi AF, Carbone C: Is peripheral arterial pressure a satisfactory substitute for ascending aortic pressure when measuring aortic valve gradients? *J Am Coll Cardiol* 4:1207–1212, 1984.

51. Gorlin R, Gorlin SG: Hydraulic formula for calculation of the area of the stenotic mitral valve, other cardiac valves and central circulatory shunts. I. *Am Heart J* 41:1–29, 1951.

52. Carabello BA, Grossman W: Calculation of stenotic valve orifice area. In Grossman W (ed): *Cardiac Catheterization and Angiography*, ed 3. Philadelphia, Lea & Febiger, 1986, p 143.

53. Reddy PS, Curtiss EI, Bell B, O'Toole JD, Salerni R, Leon DF, Shaver JA: Determinants of variation between Fick and indicator dilution estimates of cardiac output during diagnostic catheterization. Fick vs. dye cardiac outputs. *J Lab Clin Med* 87:568–576, 1976.

54. Hatle L, Angelsen B, Tromsdal A: Noninvasive assessment of pressure half-time by Doppler ultrasound. *Circulation* 60:1096–1104, 1979.

55. Libanoff AJ, Rodbard S: Atrioventricular pressure half-time. Measure of mitral valve orifice area. *Circulation* 38:144–150, 1968.

56. Kane PB, Askanazi J, Neville JF, Mon RL, Hanson EL, Webb WR: Artifacts in the measurement of pulmonary artery wedge pressure. *Crit Care Med* 6:36–38, 1978.

57. Wilkins GT, Gillam LD, Kritzer GL, Levine RA, Palacios IF, Weyman AE: Validation of continuous-wave Doppler echocardiographic measurements of mitral and tricuspid prosthetic valve gradients: A simultaneous Doppler-catheter study. *Circulation* 74:786–795, 1986.

58. Sahn DJ: Determination of cardiac output by echocardiographic Doppler methods: Relative accuracy of various sites for measurement. *J Am Coll Cardiol* 6:663–664, 1985.

59. Stewart WJ, Jiang L, Mich R, Pandian N, Guerrero JL, Weyman AE: Variable effects of changes in flow rate through the aortic, pulmonary and mitral valves on valve area and flow velocity: Impact on quantitative Doppler flow calculations. *J Am Coll Cardiol* 6:653–662, 1985.

60. Panidis IP, Ross J, Mintz GS: Effect of sampling site on assessment of pulmonary artery blood flow by Doppler echocardiography. *Am J Cardiol* 58:1145–1147, 1986.

61. Lighty GW Jr, Gargiulo A, Kronzon I, Politzer F: Comparison of multiple views for the evaluation of pulmonary arterial blood flow by Doppler echocardiography. *Circulation* 74:1002–1006, 1986.

62. Croft CH, Lipsomb K, Mathis K, Firth BG, Nicod P, Tilton G, Winniford MD, Hillis LD: Limitations of qualitative angiographic grading in aortic or mitral regurgitation. *Am J Cardiol* 53:1593–1598, 1984.

63. Hillis LD, Grossman W: Cardiac ventriculography. In Grossman W (ed): *Cardiac Catheterization and Angiography*, ed 3. Philadelphia, Lea & Febiger, 1986, p 200.

64. Omoto R, Matsumura M: Acquired valvular disease. In Omoto R (ed): *Color Atlas of Real-Time Two-Dimensional Doppler Echocardiography*, ed 2. Tokyo, Shindan-To-Chiryo, 1984, p 69.

65. Miyatake K, Okamoto M, Kinoshita N, Izumi S, Owa M, Takao S, Sakakibara H, Nimura Y: Clinical applications of a new type of real-time two-dimensional Doppler flow imaging system. *Am J Cardiol* 54:857–868, 1984.

66. Takamoto S: Pitfalls and artifacts. In Omoto R (ed): *Color Atlas of Real-Time Two-Dimensional Doppler Echocardiography*, ed 2. Tokyo, Shindan-To-Chiryo, 1984, p 41.

67. Goldberg SJ, Allen HD: Quantitative assessment by Doppler echocardiography of pulmonary or aortic regurgitation. *Am J Cardiol* 56:131–135, 1985.

68. Burstin L: Determination of pressure in the pulmonary artery by external graphic recordings. *Br Heart J* 29:396–404, 1967.

69. Grayburn PA, Handshoe R, Smith MD, Harrison MR, DeMaria AN: Quantitative assessment of the hemodynamic consequences of aortic regurgitation by means of continuous wave Doppler recordings. *J Am Coll Cardiol* 10:135–141, 1987.

70. Sellers RD, Levy MF, Amplatz K, Lillehei CW: Left retrograde cardioangiography in acquired cardiac disease: Technique, indications, and interpretations in 700 cases. *Am J Cardiol* 14:437–447, 1964.

13

Assessment of Ischemic Heart Disease and Left Ventricular Function by Stress Echocardiography

Randall G. Wilson, M.D.
Mee-Nin Kan, M.D.
Navin C. Nanda, M.D.

INTRODUCTION

The early detection of coronary artery disease (CAD) is a major clinical challenge for which many diagnostic techniques have been developed. Common to all current noninvasive tests is the principle of stress-induced augmentation of myocardial oxygen demand. In patients with CAD, stress-induced myocardial ischemia allows measurement of some parameter that reflects the amount and location of the ischemic myocardium.

For more than 50 years the standard test for CAD has been the exercise electrocardiogram (ECG). However, the S-T segment changes used to diagnose CAD can be altered or masked by ventricular hypertrophy, bundle branch block, and drug effects. This decreases the sensitivity and specificity of the test, lowering the predictive value of an exercise ECG.

A potentially more sensitive index of myocardial ischemia involves observation of changes in cardiac wall motion. Occlusion of a main coronary branch has been shown to produce an immediate and progressive decrease in the amplitude of systolic contraction (1). This is rapidly followed (within 1 min) by systolic expansion. These changes are reversible if interruption of coronary blood flow is not prolonged.

Of principal importance is the observation that regional myocardial dysfunction can occur before any S-T segment changes develop (2). Since echocardiography is sensitive to these abnormalities of regional wall motion, the exercise echocardiogram was the next logical step in the quest for improved diagnostic accuracy.

Before examining exercise echocardiography in detail, however, it is necessary to understand the heart's response to exercise.

CARDIAC RESPONSE TO EXERCISE

The effect of exercise on the heart is complex and depends on the type of exercise, the position of the subject during exercise, and the work load achieved. The two types of exercise, isometric and isotonic, differ substantially in their diagnostic usefulness.

Isometric exercise is sustained muscular contraction against a fixed resistance and usually is performed clinically with the aid of a hand-grip dynamometer. In normal subjects, this type of exercise produces a modest increase in cardiac output. The increase is mainly secondary to a reflex-mediated increase in heart rate. Blood pressure also rises, but there is little effect on left ventricular end-systolic volume (LVESV), left ventricular end-diastolic volume (LVEDV), stroke volume, or ejection fraction (EF)

In patients with CAD, the increased heart rate and blood pressure can induce myocardial ischemia, regional wall motion abnormalities (WMA), and decreased EF. Changes in the LVESV and LVEDV can be variable; however, both usually decrease slightly.

Ischemia is a less frequent response to isometric exercise than to isotonic exercise. This lower sensitivity limits the clinical and investigational value of isometric exercise.

Isotonic exercise, also called dynamic exercise, produces a graded increase in myocardial oxygen consumption and cardiac output through increases in heart rate and stroke volume. The data on changes in ventricular volumes are conflicting because of the different exercise methodologies used (e.g., upright versus supine, treadmill versus bicycle ergometer). When exercise is performed on a bicycle ergometer with the subject in the upright position, the heart rate and rate-pressure product are usually slightly higher, whereas with the subject in the supine position, LVEDV and stroke volume are slightly higher. However, when absolute changes from rest to exercise are compared, the increase in heart rate, blood pressure, stroke index, and cardiac index are similar in both supine and upright bicycle ergometry.

Multistage maximal treadmill exercise is the most common protocol in use today. This produces increases in cardiac output, stroke volume, and EF in normal subjects, but produces less significant changes in EF in patients with CAD. Treadmill exercise yields a higher maximum myocardial oxygen consumption at maximal exercise than does either supine or upright bicycle ergometer exercise. However, heart rate, rate-pressure product, and cardiac output are similar. At submaximal levels of exercise to similar levels of myocardial oxygen consumption, the heart rate and blood pressure are higher on the bicycle ergometer.

Many patients prefer treadmill exercise to the bicycle ergometer. Patients are more familiar with walking than cycling, and the bicycle ergometer tends to produce leg fatigue at only moderate levels of exercise. This tends to lower the sensitivity of the test, since the patient's exercise on the bicycle ergometer is often limited to submaximal levels.

M-MODE AND TWO-DIMENSIONAL ECHOCARDIOGRAPHY

The first echocardiographic technique to be used in conjunction with exercise testing was M-mode echocardiography. This established the usefulness of echocardiography as an adjunct to stress testing, but the limitations imposed by its "ice pick" view led to its replacement by two-dimensional echocardiography.

The superiority of two-dimensional echocardiography lies in its ability to produce real-time comprehensive images of cardiac structures in multiple tomographic planes. This allows assessment of left and right ventricular regional wall motion and quantification of left ventricular EF. When used in conjunction with a graded exercise test, it can identify patients with significant CAD

and test for multivessel disease in patients with previous myocardial infarction or stable angina.

The exercise protocol used in combination with echocardiography depends to a large extent on the equipment available and on the examiner's experience. However, there are two basic protocols. The first uses supine or semisupine bicycle ergometer exercise, with the echocardiogram recorded before and during exercise. The second uses a treadmill exercise protocol, with the echocardiograms performed before and immediately after exercise.

In the early days of exercise echocardiography, most believed that exercise-induced WMA disappeared quickly when exercise ceased. For that reason, supine and semisupine bicycle ergometry were the most popular methods of exercise. This approach produced studies of adequate quality 71–78% of the time (3–5). The sensitivity of exercise echocardiography was between 68% and 76%, and the specificity was between 92% and 100%.

Results of several bicycle ergometer studies showed that exercise-induced WMA lasted from 1 to 3 min after exercise ceased (3). One report found persistence of WMA up to 30 min postexercise (6). As a result, Maurer and Nanda (7) investigated treadmill exercise with echocardiograms obtained before and after exercise.

Approximately 85% of these echocardiographic studies were adequate for interpretation. Other investigators have published similar results of between 87% and 92% adequate studies (6, 8, 9). Maurer and Nanda (7) also demonstrated a sensitivity of 83% and a specificity of 92% for detecting CAD by echocardiography. The sensitivity of echocardiography to CAD was highest in patients with three-vessel disease (92%) and two-vessel disease (100%). In patients with single-vessel disease, on the other hand, the sensitivity was only 50%. Subsequent investigations by Heng et al. (8) and Jaarsma et al. (9) have produced similar sensitivity and specificity data.

Assessment of exercise two-dimensional echocardiograms for WMA is accomplished by dividing each view into segments and analyzing each for the presence and extent of asynergy (hypokinesis, akinesis, or dyskinesis). Since distinguishing between types of asynergy can be difficult at times, especially in the vigorously contracting heart, a highly trained observer is required. However, the ability to make these distinctions is improved by computer techniques such as closed loop analysis of a single cardiac cycle and by side-by-side comparison of rest and exercise echocardiograms.

Left ventricular wall thickening or thinning during systole is defined more easily in the vigorously contracting heart, although poor endocardial images are a major limitation of the technique. In the apical window, large areas of the endocardium are parallel to the sound beam and produce poor images. Similarly, the parasternal view is limited because interposed lung tissue makes this view difficult to obtain during or immediately after exercise.

The subcostal window has been suggested as an alternative to the traditional apical and parasternal examination (10). Endocardial echoes are identified more readily in subcostal four-chamber and short-axis views, since the endocardium tends to be perpendicular to the ultrasound beam.

Measuring left ventricular EF before and after exercise may improve the recognition of exercise-induced ischemia. Using two-dimensional echocardiography, Zwehl et al. (11) studied 10 normal subjects in the supine position at rest and during peak bicycle exercise. Apical and parasternal images were used to calculate left ventricular (LV) volumes according to the formula:

$$\text{Volume} = \tfrac{5}{6}\,(\text{area of cross-section})\,(\text{LV long axis}) \quad 13.1$$

Left ventricular EF increased significantly from 63.4% at rest to 72.1% at peak exercise, LVESV decreased, and LVEDV remained unchanged. Estimation of left ventricular EF was reproducible, demonstrating a mean error of less than 10%.

Crawford et al. (12) exercised normal subjects and patients with ischemic heart disease in an upright bicycle ergometer. Two-dimensional echocardiography was performed, and apical (four-chamber, long-axis) views were used to calculate left ventricular volumes using Simpson's rule. The EF was calculated at rest, during peak exercise, and after nitroglycerin had been administered. Normal subjects demonstrated significant increases in peak exercise LVEDV and EF compared with those for the resting state. In contrast, patients with heart disease showed no differences, except that roughly one-third showed a significant increase in EF during exercise when nitroglycerin was given.

Limacher et al. (13) performed two-dimensional echocardiography with the subject at rest and immediately after maximal treadmill exercise. In normal subjects, EF went from 66% at rest to 73% after exercise. In patients with ischemic heart disease, the mean EF went from 56% at rest to 53% after exercise. Two patients demonstrated a decrease in EF without an abnormal change in wall motion. Limacher et al. concluded that the sensitivity of exercise echocardiography was increased slightly by considering the EF along with assessment of wall motion.

In a study by Heng et al. (8), exercise two-dimensional echocardiography was performed in conjunction with thallium imaging. In patients with normal perfusion, EF increased from 52% to 67% during exercise. In patients with reversible thallium defects, EF went from 53% to 43%. No significant change in EF was noted in patients with irreversible thallium defects. These three patient groups were not differentiated by changes in other parameters, such as heart rate and rate-pressure product.

Since left ventricular EF is more a measure of global than regional function, a decrease in EF is not specific for myocardial ischemia. Still, calculating the EF may be of some value in patients with heart disease. In this group, changes in EF help determine the extent of ventricular dysfunction induced by exercise and can help assess the effects of therapeutic intervention.

TWO-DIMENSIONAL ECHOCARDIOGRAPHY: COMPARISON WITH OTHER TECHNIQUES

Exercise electrocardiography and two-dimensional echocardiography have similar specificity in detecting exercise-induced ischemia. However, in most studies the sensitivity of exercise echocardiography is higher in patients with more extensive heart disease. This is even more pronounced in patients with extensive heart disease and no prior myocardial infarction. Combining the two techniques may improve the sensitivity of exercise electrocardiography, especially in patients with multivessel disease.

Wann et al. (3) compared exercise two-dimensional echocardiography against thallium scintigraphy. Areas of exercise-induced WMA identified by two-dimensional echocardiography correlated well with defects identified via reversible thallium perfusion. Maurer and Nanda (7) demonstrated similar results and also showed that two-dimensional echocardiography could identify exercise-induced right ventricular asynergy, but thallium scintigraphy could not. When right ventricular asynergy was considered, echocardiography demonstrated a higher sensitivity to ischemic heart disease than did thallium scintigraphy.

Radionuclide angiography (RNA) is a well-validated and popular noninvastive technique used to evaluate ventricular wall motion and EF, both at rest and during exercise. Ginzton et al. (10) studied segmental wall motion by exercise echocardiography using subcostal views. In both normal and postmyocardial infarction patients, echocardiographic wall motion analysis correlated well with RNA.

In other studies, the two techniques for detecting ischemic heart disease have been compared. Visser et al. (5) compared two-dimensional echocardiography and RNA in the same patients, using the same supine bicycle exercise protocol. Although two-dimensional echocardiography provided a better view of the interventricular septum and inferior wall of the LV, RNA had a better sensitivity for ischemic heart disease (91% versus 76%). Limacher et al. (13) compared RNA during bicycle exercise with two-dimensional echocardiography done after treadmill exercise. Exercise echocardiography demonstrated a superior sensitivity (92% versus 75%), but the work load for the treadmill exercise was higher than for the bicycle exercise. The improved sensitivity of echocardiography could well have been influenced by this increased opportunity to induce ischemia.

Crawford et al. (14) compared left ventricular EF determined by two-dimensional echocardiography and RNA, using upright bicycle ergometry in patients with coronary artery disease. The EF determined by RNA at maximum exercise was higher than that calculated by two-dimensional echocardiography. However, the RNA value corresponded to the value determined by echocardiography at 1 min before maximum exercise. When angina occurred during exercise, echocardiography detected the rapid increase in EF on a beat-to-beat basis. The sampling time for RNA is much longer (2 min), which may account for the apparently high EF at maximum symptom-limited exercise.

STANDARD DOPPLER ECHOCARDIOGRAPHY

Combined two-dimensional and Doppler echocardiography can be used to advantage during exercise stress testing. Indices derived from aortic blood flow velocity have been shown to decrease immediately after occlusion of a coronary artery. These indices include aortic peak flow velocity, maximum acceleration of flow, and stroke volume (15, 16). Aortic blood flow measurements made at the time of cardiac catheterization have correlated well with these same indices (17). Stroke volume can be determined noninvasively by taking the product of the aortic flow velocity integral, obtained by Doppler, and the aortic valve area, determined by two-dimensional echocardiography. Cardiac output derived from these measurements has been shown to correlate well with results obtained by thermodilution or the Fick method.

Results of recent studies have shown that, using the suprasternal notch approach, pulsed or continuous wave Doppler can be used to assess changes in aortic peak flow velocity and acceleration. These studies were performed during and immediately after supine or upright exercise in normal subjects and in patients with coronary artery disease (18–20). In these normal volunteers, satisfactory studies were obtained 100% of the time.

Daley et al. (21) found that peak flow velocity and stroke volume at rest are lower with the subject in the upright position than in the supine position. However, at peak exercise there is no significant positional difference in peak flow velocity, stroke volume, and maximum acceleration. This suggests that combined two-dimensional and Doppler exercise studies should be done with the subject in the upright position, since the degree of increase in these indices with exercise is much greater in this position.

Results of various studies have shown that the increase in aortic peak velocity at peak exercise was between 60% and 120%, using treadmill exercise. Using supine bicycle exercise, the increase was only between 45% and 50%. The increase in stroke volume index at peak exercise was between 50% and 66% using treadmill exercise. The same measurement taken during supine bicycle exercise showed only an 18% increase. In one study, the aortic flow velocity integral actually decreased by 12% during peak exercise on a supine bicycle. Increase in maximum acceleration is more than 100% in treadmill exercise, but is only 76% in supine bicycle exercise.

Older normal individuals have been shown to have lower peak flow velocity and acceleration at rest, but the degree of change at peak exercise was similar to the younger age group (< 40 years old). Bryg et al. (22) performed Doppler studies in normal subjects and patients with CAD. During exercise, CAD patients demonstrated a lower percent increase in peak flow velocity, maximal flow acceleration, stroke volume index, and cardiac index than did normal subjects. The stroke volume index increased in normal subjects during submaximal treadmill exercise and remained unchanged or decreased slightly at maximum exercise. Cardiac index increased progressively at each exercise work level.

In CAD patients, three patterns of peak velocity response were defined. A type I response was an increase in peak flow velocity during maximum treadmill exercise to nearly double the resting value. This response was similar to that seen in normal subjects. Among patients with CAD, this reponse usually was seen in those with one-vessel disease and normal LV function at rest. A type II response was an increase in peak flow velocity of lesser magnitude with no decrease in velocity at maximum exercise. The type III response was a decrease in peak flow velocity at maximum exercise.

The type II and III responses were seen in patients with more severe CAD and left ventricular dysfunction at rest. The greatest differences between normal subjects and CAD patients in exercise Doppler-derived measurement of aortic flow are in CAD patients with multivessel disease and left ventricular dysfunction at rest. Thus Doppler echocardiography may be a useful adjunct to routine exercise testing to weed out false-positive tests.

The major problem encountered during exercise Doppler was the inability to acquire peak flow velocities continuously during the exercise period. This was especially true with pulsed Doppler systems and in older patients who may not have had laminar flow in the ascending aorta. Respiration and body movement made it difficult to maintain the same transducer angulation and sample volume position throughout exercise, resulting in flow spectral variations. Therefore, measurements should be made from beats that show the highest peak velocity.

There is also the problem of aliasing during exercise when pulsed Doppler is used, but in most normal subjects the highest peak velocity during exercise does not significantly exceed the Nyquist limit. This problem can be alleviated by lowering the baseline, using a Doppler transducer with a lower transmitted frequency, or switching to a continuous wave Doppler system.

COLOR DOPPLER ECHOCARDIOGRAPHY

Conventional Doppler studies have difficulty in maintaining transducer angulation and sample volume position during exercise. This increases the difficulty of evaluating valvular function in a vigorously contracting heart. The suprasternal notch approach also prevents left ventricular wall motion from being demonstrated simultaneously with changes in aortic flow. Using Doppler color flow mapping (color Doppler) allows simultaneous assessment of these indices as well as evaluation of exercise-induced valvular dysfunction and EF.

The apical window is best suited for exercise testing, as the mitral and tricuspid valves are evaluated most easily from this position. Some patients with CAD may develop mitral regurgitation during exercise, due to ischemic dysfunction involving the papillary muscle. In this case, traditional two-dimensional echocardiography and conventional pulsed Doppler are of little help. Mitral regurgitation cannot be evaluated by two-dimensional echocardiography, and mapping by conventional pulsed Doppler is not practical in an exercising patient. Doppler color flow mapping can reliably detect mitral regurgitation and assess its severity and can be used during and immediately after supine bicycle exercise.

A recent investigation found mitral regurgitation in 59% of the CAD patients studied, 69% of whom had three-vessel disease (23). Exercise-induced mitral regurgitation often developed before any new asynergy of the left ventricular walls. In a few patients, exercise-induced mitral regurgitation existed without coexisting new WMA.

The drawback to color Doppler involves motion artifact, which can simulate abnormal flow states. Signals from the motion of the cardiac walls can simulate an abnormality by generating (*a*) red areas as the wall aproaches the transducer and (*b*) blue areas as it recedes (24). Valve motion also can create ghost images and may simulate mild valvular incompetence. These potentially confounding signals are most pronounced during exercise.

Artifacts can be differentiated from flow signals, especially by careful frame-by-frame analysis of the videotaped images. New filters that prevent or minimize artifacts have been developed also, and further refinements can be anticipated. Even with the current technical problems, Doppler color flow mapping shows great promise for improving the sensitivity and specificity of exercise echocardiography.

REFERENCES

1. Tennant R, Wiggers CJ: The effect of coronary occlusion on myocardial contraction. *Am J Physiol* 112:351–361, 1935.
2. Battler A, Froelicher VF, Gallagher KP, Kemper WS, Ross J: Dissociation between regional myocardial dysfunction and ECG changes during ischemia in the conscious dog. *Circulation* 62:735–744, 1980.
3. Wann LS, Faris JV, Childress RH, Dillon JC, Weyman AE, Feigenbaum H: Exercise cross sectional echocardiography in ischemic heart disease. *Circulation* 60:1300–1308, 1979.
4. Morganroth J, Chen CC, David D, Sawin HS, Naito M, Parrotto C, Meixell L: Exercise cross-sectional echocardiographic diagnosis of coronary artery disease. *Am J Cardiol* 47:20–26, 1981.
5. Visser CA, van der Wieken RL, Kan G, Lie KI, Busemann-Sokele E, Meltzer RS, Durrer D: Comparison of two-dimensional echocardiography with radionuclide angiography during dynamic exercise for the detection of coronary artery disease. *Am Heart J* 106:528–534, 1983.
6. Robertson WS, Feigenbaum H, Armstrong WF, Dillon JC, O'Donnell J, McHenry PW: Exercise echocardiography: A clinically practical addition in the evaluation of coronary artery disease. *J Am Coll Cardiol* 2:1085–1091, 1983.
7. Maurer G, Nanda NC: Two dimensional echocardiographic evaluation of exercise-induced left and right ventricular asynergy: Correlation with thallium scanning. *Am J Cardiol* 48:720–727, 1981.
8. Heng MK, Simard M, Lake R, Udhoji VH: Exercise two-dimensional echocardiography for diagnosis of coronary artery disease. *Am J Cardiol* 54:502–507, 1984.
9. Jaarsma W, Visser CA, Kupper ADF, Res JCJ, VanEenige MJ, Roos JP: Usefulness of two-dimensional exercise echocardiography shortly after myocardial infarction. *Am J Cardiol* 57:86–90, 1986.
10. Ginzton LE, Conant R, Brizendine M, Lee F, Mena I, Laks MM: Exercise subcostal two-dimensional echocardiography: A new method of segmental wall motion analysis. *Am J Cardiol* 53:805–811, 1984.
11. Zwehl W, Gueret P, Meerbaum S, Holt S, Corday E: Quantitative two-dimensional echocardiography during bicycle exercise in normal subjects. *Am J Cardiol* 47:866–873, 1981.
12. Crawford MH, Amon KW, Vance WS: Exercise 2-dimensional echocardiography: Quantitation of left ventricular performance in patients with severe angina pectoris. *Am J Cardiol* 51:1–6, 1983.
13. Limacher MC, Quinones MA, Poliner LR, Nelson JG, Winters WL Jr, Waggoner AD: Detection of coronary artery disease with exercise two-dimensional echocardiography: Description of a clinically applicable method and comparison with radionuclide ventriculography. *Circulation* 67:1211–1218, 1983.
14. Crawford MH, Petru MA, Amon KW, Sorensen SG, Vance WS: Comparative value of two-dimensional echocardiography and radionuclide angiography for quantitating changes in left ventricular performance during exercise limited by angina pectoris. *Am J Cardiol* 53:42–46, 1984.
15. Rushmer RF, Watson N, Harding D, Baker D: Effects of acute coronary occlusion on performance of right and left ventricles in intact unanesthetized dogs. *Am Heart J* 66:522–531, 1963.
16. Noble MIM, Trenchard D, Guz A: Left ventricular ejection in conscious dogs: 1. Measurement and significance of the maximum acceleration of blood from the left ventricle. *Cardiovasc Res* 29:139–147, 1966.
17. Jewitt D, Gabe I, Mills C, Maurer B, Thomas M, Shillingford J: Aortic velocity and acceleration measurements in the assessment of coronary heart disease. *Eur J Cardiol* 113:299–305, 1974.
18. Loeppky JA, Greene ER, Hoekenga DE, Caprihan A, Luft UC: Beat-by-beat stroke volume assessment by pulsed Doppler in upright and supine exercise. *J Appl Physiol* 50:1173–1182, 1981.
19. Bennett ED, Barclay SA, Davis AL, Mannering D, Mehta N: Ascending aortic blood velocity and acceleration using Doppler ultrasound in the assessment of left ventricular function. *Cardiovasc Res* 18:632–638, 1984.
20. Labovitz AJ, Buckingham RA, Habermehl, K, Nelson J, Kennedy HL, Williams GA: The effects of sampling site on the two-dimensional echo-Doppler determination of cardiac output. *Am Heart J* 109:327–332, 1985.
21. Daley PJ, Sagar KB, Wann LS: Doppler echocardiographic measurement of flow velocity in the ascending aorta during supine and upright exercise. *Br Heart J* 54:562–567, 1985.
22. Bryg RJ, Labovitz AJ, Mehdirad AA, Williams GA, Chaitman BR: Effect of coronary artery disease on Doppler-derived parameters of aortic flow during upright exercise. *Am J Cardiol* 58:14–19, 1986.
23. Zachariah ZP, Hsiung MC, Nanda NC, Kan MN, Gatewood RP Jr: Color Doppler assessment of mitral regurgitation induced by supine exercise in ischemic heart disease. *Am J Cardiol* 59:1266–1270, 1987.
24. Switzer DF, Nanda NC: Doppler color flow mapping. *Ultrasound Med Biol* 11:403–416, 1985.

14

Supine Stress Exercise Echocardiogram: Technique and Usefulness in the Evaluation of Patients with Coronary Artery Disease

Donald V. Mahony, M.D.

Each year, many people with no clinical symptoms of coronary artery disease (CAD) suffer cardiac death secondary to severe coronary atherosclerosis. Clinicians have used a variety of diagnostic techniques in an attempt to identify these patients, and the exercise stress electrocardiogram (ECG) has long played an important role in this process. However, regional myocardial dysfunction is thought to occur soon after the onset of ischemia and before changes on the surface ECG become evident. Consequently, there is considerable interest in increasing the sensitivity of exercise stress testing to detect these patients. This has led to combining echocardiography or radionuclide angiography with exercise stress testing to assess left ventricular (LV) function and detect the effects of exercise-induced ischemia.

Although several studies have shown that both stress exercise echocardiography (exercise echo) and radionuclide imaging are specific and highly sensitive for detection of CAD (1–14), exercise echo enjoys several advantages: (a) the patient is not exposed to radiation; (b) the patient does not require intravenous injections; and (c) multiple tomographic views of the heart are available for evaluation of regional wall motion.

A potential disadvantage of exercise echo is the perceived difficulty of obtaining a technically satisfactory study on an exercising patient with exaggerated respiratory effort and tachycardia. However, computerized imaging systems have

become available allowing slow motion replay of a single cardiac cycle as a continuous loop, as well as side-by-side playback of resting and exercise cycles (Nova-MicroSonics CAD 888 digital analyzer, ATL Nova-MicroSonics Corporation, Mahwah, New Jersey). By effectively removing exercise-associated artifacts, these systems greatly improve recognition of wall motion abnormalities.

INDICATIONS FOR EXERCISE ECHOCARDIOGRAPHY

The decision to recommend exercise echo testing for a given patient must be left to the patient's physician and depends on many factors. These include clinical history, presence of cardiac risk factors, occupation, and results of other examinations. However, our laboratory has found exercise echo testing to be particularly helpful in the evaluation and management of the following patients.

1. *Patients with angina or atypical chest pain and an abnormal resting or exercise ECG study.* Information gained regarding LV function and the presence or absence of CAD will be quite helpful in planning the timing and extent of further diagnostic tests.

2. *Patients requiring evaluation of cardiovascular status prior to various surgical procedures.* It is our experience that many patients who have evidence of severe LV dysfunction by exercise echo testing and who have severe CAD verified

310

by coronary angiography may have no (or very minimal) symptoms suggesting CAD.

3. *Patients about to enter an exercise program.* Exercise echo testing may identify asymptomatic patients who are at risk for sudden cardiac death because of silent CAD. An autopsy study performed on 60 patients who died suddenly while playing squash showed that 51 had had severe CAD (15). More than 50% of these patients had had no known heart disease, and 25% had been entirely asymptomatic.

4. *Patients who undergo streptokinase therapy and angioplasty.* Exercise echo tests may be performed pre- and poststreptokinase therapy and angioplasty to evaluate changes in LV function.

5. *Patients receiving adriamycin (and similar drugs).* Serial exercise echo testing will allow close follow-up of LV function during treatment. The ability to evaluate the response of the LV to exercise may allow earlier detection of drug-induced LV dysfunction.

6. *Patients who have had a myocardial infarction or coronary artery bypass graft(s).* Exercise echo testing allows evaluation of cardiovascular reserve and exercise ability. This could be used to stratify postinfarction patients into risk groups

to aid in determining the need for further diagnostic testing. Patients with normal exercise echo tests would be classified as low risk, be managed medically, and undergo repeat exercise testing at least yearly. Patients with abnormal tests at low levels of exercise (<100 W (Watts) would be classified as high risk, would probably have significant LV dysfunction, and should be referred for coronary artery angiography. Patients with abnormal tests at high levels of exercise (>100 W) would be classified as intermediate risk. If these patients showed wall motion abnormalities or an abnormal ejection fraction (EF), they would be referred for coronary artery angiography. Patients with no wall motion abnormalities and a normal EF would be managed medically with close follow-up.

The role of exercise echo testing in completely asymptomatic patients is less well defined. The presence of cardiac risk factors, an age of >40 yr, and employment in particular occupations (e.g., airline pilots, police officers, and fire fighters) certainly would justify the use of exercise echo as a screening test for CAD in asymptomatic patients. The increased sensitivity and specificity over the standard exercise stress ECG would appear to make exercise echo the preferred screening test to identify silent CAD for disability and insurance evaluation programs.

TECHNIQUE

Exercise Echo Protocol

At the St. Jude Hospital and Rehabilitation Center in Fullerton, California, which is a private community hospital, all patients are exercised in the noninvasive laboratory.[a] Exercise is performed with patient in the supine position on a Pickler-Cambridge table (model #8420). The angle of inclination of this table can be varied to obtain the optimal degree of left lateral position for the best two-dimensional echocardiographic views. A bicycle ergometer is positioned at the end of the table (Fig. 14.1).

Supine bicycle exercise testing is our choice for exercise echo tests for several reasons. First, in some patients, LV function abnormalities occur only during exercise and return to normal or near-normal immediately after exercise. Any testing that is done only before and after exercise could miss these patients. At best, it would detect only

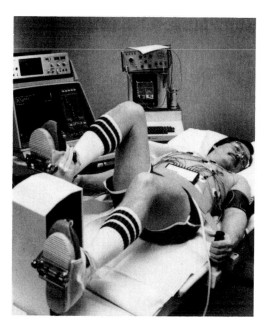

Figure 14.1. View of the two-dimensional echocardiographic equipment, Pickler-Cambridge inclined table, and bicycle ergometer as arranged in the author's laboratory.

[a]These studies were done during the time I was Director of the Non Invasive Laboratory.

minor abnormalities that would be difficult to evaluate. Second, supine posture is an important potentiator of exercise-induced myocardial ischemia. Currie et al. (16) exercised 40 patients with known CAD and compared supine and erect graded bicycle exercise. Twenty-eight patients (70%) developed S-T segment depression in the erect position, and 40 (100%) developed S-T segment depression in the supine position. Supine echo exercise allows detection of more subtle abnormalities. In addition, constant monitoring of wall motion during exercise increases safety, since the test can be stopped immediately if significant abnormalities develop. There have been no deaths or serious clinical problems in 146 exercise echo tests performed in our laboratory.

The supine position also allows recording of better echo images from several different locations. This is especially true for patients who must be placed in a left lateral position on a tilt table to obtain adequate images. In our experience, 25–30% of all patients must be imaged from the left lateral position. Ninety-eight percent of all patients tested in the supine position were imaged, although views at rest, at peak exercise, and immediately after exercise were obtained in only 95%.

Blood pressure, measured with a cuff sphygmomanometer, and a 12-lead ECG are recorded immediately before exercise, once each minute during exercise, and for 5 min after exercise. The systolic blood pressure ratio is calculated by dividing the mean of the systolic blood pressure taken each minute for 3 min after exercise by the peak systolic blood pressure measured during exercise (7). A normal ratio is less than 0.8.

Two-dimensional echocardiography is performed with a hand-held transducer before exercise, at peak exercise, immediately after exercise, and 5 min after exercise. All patients are studied with a Hewlett Packard (model #77020 AL) echocardiograph with a 2.25 MHz transducer. All standard views (long-axis, short-axis, apical four-chamber, two-chamber apical long-axis, and subxiphoid views) are recorded, if possible. The patient's feet are placed on the bicycle pedals for preexercise echo views and maintained there for the peak exercise and immediately postexercise studies.

Exercise starts at 45–60 rpm. Stress work load begins at 30 W and increases 25 W every 3 min, depending on patient response. In patients who have difficulty with increased levels of exercise, we find that the combination of increasing the revolutions per minute and slightly decreasing the stress work load usually produces a heart rate increase equal to at least 85% of the calculated maximum heart rate. The patient is told to give 30 sec notice before stopping exercise so that peak exercise echo views can be obtained. The majority of our patients are able to cooperate with this instruction, but a few have stopped exercise suddenly. Recording all echo views every 3 min usually provides enough data for an adequate exercise study, even in this group of patients.

Continuous monitoring of the heart during exercise will often show onset of marked regional wall contraction abnormalities before either the ECG shows any significant change or angina develops. We usually will discontinue the exercise test at this time, as the development of new regional wall contraction abnormalities dictates further diagnostic studies, such as coronary artery angiography.

Approximately 5% of patients are difficult to image. In this group it is not possible to obtain all standard views, especially at peak exercise. We image these patients in the extreme left lateral position before and immediately after exercise, using an apical view.

Analysis of Exercise Echo Data

The MicroSonics CAD 888 digital analyzer was used to evaluate our exercise echo data. This system contains a large-memory frame grabber that digitizes the videotape images in real time during review. The best cardiac cycles are selected for each patient, then held in digital memory to be replayed in a cine-type continuous loop. These cycles are compared in side-by-side or quad screen continuous loops, are synchronized to the ECG, and thus are free from motion artifact. Once in digital memory, all required measurements are made easily, and the images and data are stored on disk for further use. Regional wall motion is evaluated by comparing end-systolic and end-diastolic images of the LV during various phases of the exercise protocol. Since changes in heart views may affect calculation of LV variables, it is critical to obtain similar echo views during the entire test.

In addition to evaluating regional wall motion, we calculate several variables that describe LV function. These include EF, end-systolic volume index (ESVI) (end-systolic volume (ESV) divided by body surface area (BSA), ml^3/m^2, and the ratio between the peak systolic pressure (PSP) as measured by cuff sphygmomanometer and the ESVI (PSP/ESVI, mm Hg/ml^3m^{-2}). These variables are calculated routinely before exercise, at peak exercise, and immediately after exercise. In our experience, fewer than 10% of patients show increased LV dysfunction after exercise than before or during exercise. In these patients, LV function variables also are calculated at 5 min after exercise.

Interpretation of Exercise Echo Studies

An exercise echo always is considered abnormal and indicative of LV dysfunction if regional wall motion abnormalities develop or persist during or immediately after exercise. Also, an absolute increase in EF of fewer than 5 percentage points at peak exercise is considered abnormal. An increase in the ESVI at peak exercise also is considered an abnormal response, as long as the examiner thinks the echo images are satisfactory and are obtained in similar planes throughout the various phases of the exercise test. The test is normal if wall motion is normal and EF and ESVI responses to exercise are normal; the test is considered borderline if there is an abnormal response to exercise in four or more of the eight LV function variables listed below. Otherwise, the test is read as normal.

The following criteria are used to define normal responses to exercise for the additional LV function variables:

1. EF > 0.7 at peak exercise;
2. EF > 0.7 immediately after exercise;
3. EF increase of >20% immediately after exercise or >15% if resting EF is >0.65;
4. ESVI < 13 at peak exercise;
5. ESVI decrease of >32% at peak or immediately after exercise if resting ESVI < 0.7;
6. PSP/ESVI > 15 at peak exercise;
7. PSP/ESVI > 15 immediately after exercise;
8. Systolic blood pressure ratio < 0.8.

Our exercise echo studies are reported in three parts: (*a*) results of the stress ECG examination; (*b*) visual impression of the echo views; and (*c*) computer calculation of LV function variables and an accompanying test summary (Fig. 14.2). Computer calculations are done in our laboratory by technicians. After some experience, only 15–30 min are required to complete the calculations, depending on the quality of echo views obtained.

Accurate results depend on close attention to detail by both the physician and technician. After viewing the tape, the physician will have a fairly accurate impression of the test. Sometimes the calculated LV function variables show subtle changes that are not apparent on visual review of the tape because of respiratory interference or

other causes. A complete review of the test is conducted if the visual review and the LV function variable data do not agree.

Experience has shown that one-third of the tests are grossly very normal and one-third are obviously abnormal. Calculation of LV function variables by computer might not be needed for a qualitative impression in these cases, but are imperative about one-third of the time when motion artifact obscures subtle changes. In addition, calculation of LV function variables produces data that can be compared with information produced by other cardiac imaging techniques. Serial measurements of LV function variables also can be used to identify changes produced either by progression of disease or by various treatment modalities.

RESULTS OF PATIENT STUDIES

From July 1, 1984, through January 31, 1987, 1467 patients underwent exercise echo studies. These patients usually were referred by private physicians because of previous positive exercise ECG tests, chest pain syndromes, or the presence of a heart murmur or as part of a physical examination. From this sample we studied 132 consecutive patients in whom coronary artery angiography showed significant CAD. This was defined as 50% or more diameter obstruction in one or more coronary vessels.

Patients ranged in age from 36 to 77 yr and comprised 111 males and 21 females. Twenty-two of these patients were treated with β-adrenergic blocking agents, and 23 were treated with calcium channel-blocking agents. We selected 36 age-matched normal patients in order to determine normal values and to examine differences in LV function variables between normal and CAD patients. The ages of the normal patients ranged from 50 to 81 yr and comprised 25 males and 11 females. Differences between patient groups were examined using student's *t* test and the Mann-Whitney *U* test. A *p* value of 0.02 was considered significant.

The exercise echo test was normal in all patients without CAD and abnormal in 129 (97%) of the patients with CAD. One false-negative test was in a patient on β-adrenergic blocking agents who could perform only a submaximal amount of exercise. Six months later, this patient had a mild myocardial infarction. A coronary angiogram revealed triple-vessel disease with fairly good collateral circulation. The other two false-negative tests were in patients with 50–60% obstruc-

*** STRESS ECHO ANALYSIS ***

**ST. JUDE HOSPITAL
FULLERTON, CA**

Height: 172.72 cms.   Weight: 82 kgs.   BSA: 1.954 m^2
Age: 57.0 years.   HR: 68 bpm.   BP: 118/95 (s/d)

Apical 4 Chamber

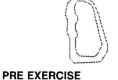

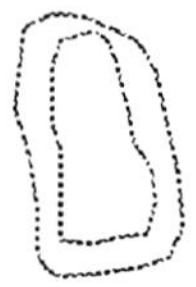

PRE EXERCISE

BP (s/d) 118/95	
Heart Rate 68	
EF 66	
ESV 32.6 ml	
ESVI 16.7 ml/m^2	
EDV 96.2 ml	
EDVI 49.2 ml/m^2	
PSP / ESVI 7.1	

PEAK EXERCISE

	% Change
BP (s/d) 235/120	99/ 26%
Heart Rate 131	93%
EF 75	12.86%
ESV 22.7 ml	-30.46%
ESVI 11.6 ml/m^2	-30.46%
EDV 89.2 ml	-7.25%
EDVI 45.6 ml/m^2	-7.25%
PSP / ESVI 20.2	186.40%

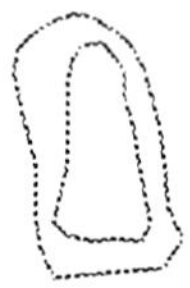

IMM POST

		% Change
BP (s/d) 207/110		75/ 16%
Heart Rate 130		91%
EF 76		14.80%
ESV 20.4 ml		-37.57%
ESVI 10.4 ml/m^2		-37.57%
EDV 84.3 ml		-12.30%
EDVI 43.1 ml/m^2		-12.30%
PSP / ESVI 19.9		180.97%
PSP ratio 0.0		
+1 min SP 213		
+2 min SP 171		
+3 min SP 157		

Figure 14.2. Example of computer printout obtained from MicroSonic CAD 888 digital analyzer. The LV function is normal. The following abbreviations are used throughout Figures 14.2–14.6: *BP*, blood pressure; *BSA*, body surface area; *EF*, ejection fraction; *EDV*, end-diastolic volume, *EDVI*, end-diastolic volume index; *ESV*, end-systolic volume; *ESVI*, end-systolic volume index; *HR*, heart rate; *PSP*, peak systolic pressure; *PSP/ESVI*, ratio of peak systolic pressure to end-systolic volume index; *SP*, systolic pressure.

tion of secondary coronary arteries (marginal). This would probably not result in LV dysfunction.

All patients with CAD showed abnormalities of regional wall motion during exercise. There were significant differences in LV function variables between normal patients and patients with CAD (Table 14.1). Differences were noted not only at rest but also during and after exercise. In addition, there were striking differences between patient groups in the percentage change in EF and ESVI during and after exercise.

LIMITATIONS

Exercise echo is a sensitive test for the evaluation of LV function. However, it is not always

Table 14.1. LV Function Variables

| | Patients | | |
| | Normal (n = 36) | CAD (n = 132) | p Value |
Variable			
Age (yr)	61.4 ± 7.1[a]	60.3 ± 8.1	0.45
EF (%)			
Rest	61 ± 5	55 ± 10	<0.001
Peak exercise	72 ± 5	54 ± 12	<0.001
% change	18 ± 9	0 ± 21	<0.001
After exercise	76 ± 5	56 ± 13	<0.001
% change	26 ± 11	3 ± 21	<0.001
ESVI (ml³/m²)			
Rest	16.4 ± 4.5	21.6 ± 9.2	<0.002
Peak exercise	11.6 ± 2.5	22.9 ± 14.5	<0.001
% change	− 27.5 ± 13.3	6.8 ± 31.5	<0.001
After exercise	10.7 ± 2.8	21.5 ± 12.0	<0.001
% change	− 32.9 ± 16.4	4.5 ± 33.1	<0.001
PSP:ESVI (mm Hg:ml³·m⁻²)			
Rest	8.1 ± 2.3	6.9 ± 2.6	<0.02
Peak exercise	16.9 ± 3.7	9.4 ± 4.0	<0.001
After exercise	17.8 ± 4.8	9.0 ± 4.0	<0.001
Systolic BP ratio	0.79 ± 0.08	0.87 ± 0.10	<0.001

[a]All values are mean ± SD. "After exercise" measurements were obtained immediately after exercise.

specific for CAD, and the following conditions may produce an abnormal exercise echo test:

1. Concentric LV hypertrophy;
2. Idiopathic hypertrophic subaortic stenosis;
3. Left bundle-branch block;
4. Congestive cardiomyopathy;
5. Valvular heart disease;
6. Mitral valve prolapse;
7. Small vessel CAD;
8. LV dysfunction of unknown etiology;
9. Treatment with β-adrenergic blocking agents or calcium channel-blocking antagonists.

Our laboratory has performed exercise echo tests on a small group of patients who have normal coronary artery angiograms, but who also exhibit anginal type chest pain, abnormal resting, or exercise ECG findings and abnormal exercise echo tests. We believe that we are now identifying patients with abnormal LV function unrelated to significant CAD and of unknown etiology.

Schofield (17) studied a similar group of 187 patients with angina who were found to have normal coronary artery angiograms. Sixty-six patients (35%) had wall motion abnormalities noted on the LV angiogram. Many patients in this group had evidence of systolic and diastolic dysfunction manifested by increased LV end-diastolic pressure and EF changes. The major cardiac risk factor present in this group of patients was smoking.

Physicians should watch for this type of patient so that prognostic information can be obtained. These patients probably represent less than 5% of the population being tested in any echocardiographic laboratory.

Patients who cannot exercise because of physical limitations, such as musculo-skeletal disease or marked peripheral vascular disease, are not candidates for exercise echo testing. Echo imaging following IV dipyridamole has been used with some success in these clinical situations. Patients who perform a submaximal exercise test may not reach the level of exercise necessary to demonstrate underlying CAD. This is especially true for patients who are taking β-adrenergic blocking agents.

Individuals with breast implants, cor pulmonale, thick chest walls, or obesity challenge the technician to produce usable echocardiographic images. An exercise echo test can be done if a resting echo was obtained. Suboptimal echocardiographic views are obtained in approximately 10–15% of these patients. Fortunately, manipulation of the views by the computer equipment usually provides diagnostic results.

SETTING UP A STRESS EXERCISE ECHOCARDIOGRAM LABORATORY

The following suggestions, based on empirical experience, are intended to help one set up a stress exercise echocardiogram laboratory and ensure that accurate data are obtained.

1. *Decide which method of exercise echo testing will be used in the laboratory.* Possibilities include pre- and posttreadmill and upright versus supine bicycle and the use of IV dipyridamole.

2. *Be sure that competent and dedicated ultrasound technicians are available for training.*

3. *Choose ultrasound equipment that will obtain and record the best possible echocardiographic images.* This information may be obtained from persons who already are experienced with exercise echo testing. Considerable time and accuracy will be wasted if the ultrasound equipment cannot penetrate a thick chest wall and produce optimal images.

4. *Obtain an off-line or on-line computer to perform necessary calculations and evaluate regional wall function.* Most laboratories will find it unsatisfactory to use the same computer to obtain the echocardiographic study and perform calculations. The number of off-line computer systems to choose from is growing very rapidly. Consideration should be given to the reputation and track record of each company in availability of service, down time of equipment in various laboratories, length of time in business, actual number of systems in clinical use, type of training programs provided to customers, and financial stability. The least expensive system may not be cheapest in the long run. At times, more expensive equipment will produce better results, require less technician time, and be more reliable for day-to-day use.

5. *Visit a laboratory with an active exercise program in order to see the technique in use.* This helps determine how to set up the laboratory and what ancillary personnel will be needed.

6. *Perform 20–30 exercise echo tests on normal patients to gain experience with the technique and to determine the normal range for the laboratory.* A significant deviation from published normal results should be investigated thoroughly to make sure there is no error in technique or calculations.

7. *Do exercise echo tests in 30–50 patients scheduled for coronary angiography because of suspected CAD.* It is essential that the exercise echo be performed before the catheterization, so that unbiased results are obtained. Comparison of regional wall contraction abnormalities between these procedures will establish the accuracy of the exercise echo test. Although the gold standard of coronary angiography has become somewhat tarnished over the past few years, it must

be used by any new exercise echo laboratory. As time goes by, the exercise echo test often will be helpful in evaluating some ambiguous coronary angiographic studies. Major epicardial vessels with 50% diameter obstruction are considered a significant finding and usually will cause an abnormal exercise echo test.

8. *Keep a log of all exercise echo tests and follow-up results of coronary angiographic studies, if done.* This will help assess the diagnostic accuracy of the laboratory. False-positive and false-negative results should be investigated in order to correct any possible errors in either test performance or the final diagnosis by the physician. There will be a learning curve for every laboratory, as there is in cardiac Doppler or coronary angiography.

9. *Attend exercise echo testing seminars and meetings in order to learn the current uses, limitations, and values from experts in the field.* This information may not be published in the medical literature for a year or so after it has been presented. By attending these meetings, new ideas, results, and expectations can be brought back to your laboratory immediately.

COMMENT

Comparison of Exercise Echo with Stress ECG Testing

Physicians are trying continuously to improve their noninvasive diagnostic techniques to detect CAD. The majority of practitioners rapidly changed from the Master's two-step exercise test to treadmill stress ECG testing because of its greater diagnostic ability. It soon became apparent that the routine stress treadmill test had many limitations. False-positive and false-negative tests occur, especially in female patients. False-positive treadmill tests may be caused by LV hypertrophy, anemia, abnormal resting S-T segments, drug therapy, electrolyte changes, idiopathic hypertrophic subaortic stenosis, left bundle-branch block, right ventricular hypertrophy, valvular heart disease, or Wolff-Parkinson-White syndrome.

A report on exercise ECG testing by the joint task force of the American College of Cardiology and the American Heart Association suggests a sensitivity of approximately 50% and a specificity of 90% in detecting myocardial ischemia in apparently healthy individuals (18). Different predictive values are observed in populations with different CAD prevalences. In our laboratory, results of the exercise ECG portion of the exercise echo test showed that of 132 patients with

CAD, the exercise ECG was positive in 78 (60%), normal in 37 (28%), and borderline in 17 (12%). Exercise echo sensitivity was 97% in this same group of patients. Heng et al. (19) reported 100% sensitivity and 93% specificity for detecting CAD by exercise echo. Quinones (2) found exercise echo to have a sensitivity of 92% and a specificity of 88%. Armstrong et al. (12) reported 100% sensitivity and 75% specificity. These data suggest that the exercise echo is a much better diagnostic test for CAD than is the exercise ECG.

Although exercise echo testing is more costly than stress ECG testing (Table 14.2), the increased sensitivity of exercise echo (>90% versus 65%) means that exercise echo testing costs less per patient for a correct diagnosis. In addition to being a cost-effective procedure, exercise echo also allows evaluation of valvular heart disease, including mitral valve prolapse, and diagnosis of conditions such as idiopathic hypertrophic subaortic stenosis.

Exercise Echo: Comparison to Thallium and Radionuclide Angiography

One reason for the growth of exercise echo tests has been physicians' disappointment with the results of radionuclide exercise studies. Berman and Maddahi (20) reported that visually interpreted stress-redistribution thallium-201 scintigraphy has approximately 85% sensitivity and 90% specificity in detecting CAD. Quantitative analysis has led to little change in the overall sensitivity and specificity of thallium, while the sensitivity of exercise wall motion studies is approximately 90%, and the specificity is roughly 80%. Exercise echo has been compared to radionuclide exercise tests in several reviews (2, 14, 21). These two procedures produced similar results in the early years of exercise echo tests, but exercise echo was somewhat less satisfactory in those times because of the inability to image all patients. The new echocardiographic equipment and computer techniques now make it possible to image over 95% of patients with suspected CAD.

Table 14.2. Approximate Cost of Exercise Tests at St. Jude Hospital (1989)

Test	Cost
Stress ECG	$ 333
Thallium scan with exercise	$1,100
Isotope wall motion study	$ 900
Exercise echo	$ 600

Our laboratory was able to image 98% of all patients studied in recent years. The current sensitivity and specificity for exercise echo test are as good as, and often better than, nuclear studies. Exercise echo is able to image multiple planes and obtain instantaneous data at various stages of exercise. Combined with the ease of serial testing, lack of radiation exposure, and lower cost of the procedure, the popularity of exercise echo among physicians, hospitals, clinics, and private offices should increase. The cost of setting up an exercise echo laboratory rather than a nuclear laboratory is much less, and the overhead of a stress echocardiogram laboratory should be less than that of a nuclear facility. It is a fact of life that physicians tend to use diagnostic facilities that they control. Since internists and cardiologists already are engaged heavily in echocardiographic diagnostic techniques, it is likely that they will develop exercise echo programs as soon as they are convinced that exercise echo is equal to or better than nuclear studies. In several areas where nuclear testing competes with a competent exercise echo program, exercise echo testing has increased at the expense of nuclear procedures.

Exercise echo is only about 60% as costly as radionuclide angiographic procedures (Table 14.2) and appears to be more sensitive to CAD. Thus, exercise echo is clearly a more cost-effective procedure.

Future Directions

Significant progress in exercise echo testing has been made in the past few years, particularly in the development of sophisticated computer techniques for analyzing LV function variables. There is no question that computer techniques for both imaging and analyzing data from exercise echo studies will continue to improve.

Determination of right ventricular function and diastolic function and easier ways to evaluate muscle thickening will add to the diagnostic ability of the exercise echo test. The exercise echo also will be helpful in evaluating the results of coronary angioplasty. It can provide noninvasive follow-up data on possible restenosis of previously dilated arteries by evaluating a patient for development of new wall motion abnormalities. Exercise echo testing may help select those patients who would benefit from repeat angiography and possible repeat coronary angioplasty.

The federal government, insurance companies, and other health providers are all trying vigorously to reduce their health care expenditures. A possibility is that they will try to limit the number of coronary artery angiogram studies performed because of the expense of these procedures. The exercise echo test could help decrease the number of coronary artery angiographic studies performed by selecting patients with demonstrated LV dysfunction who would most benefit from an angiogram. Exercise echo testing is no longer experimental—it can now be considered an alternative to or replacement for other forms of exercise stress testing (22).

EXERCISE ECHO CASE STUDIES

The value of exercise echo studies is demonstrated through a brief history and MicroSonic computer printout of several interesting patients. End-systole and end-diastolic outlines are presented for the apical four-chamber or the apical two-chamber views. EF, ESV, ESVI, EDV (end-diastolic volume), EDVI (end-diastolic volume index), and PSP/ESVI are listed for views taken at rest, at peak exercise, and immediately after

*** STRESS ECHO ANALYSIS ***

ST. JUDE HOSPITAL
FULLERTON, CA

Height: 185.42 cms.   Weight: 75 kgs.   BSA: 1.983 m^2
Age: 69.0 years.   HR: bpm.   BP: /   (s/d)

Apical 4 Chamber

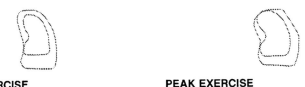

PRE EXERCISE		PEAK EXERCISE		% Change
BP (s/d) 159/88		BP (s/d) 178/104		12/18%
Heart Rate	62	Heart Rate	102	65%
EF	66	EF	60	-8.43%
ESV	27.3 ml	ESV	41.4 ml	51.76%
ESVI	13.7 ml/m^2	ESVI	20.9 ml/m^2	51.76%
EDV	79.8 ml	EDV	104.2 ml	30.51%
EDVI	40.3 ml/m^2	EDVI	52.6 ml/m^2	30.51%
PSP / ESVI	11.6	PSP / ESVI	8.5	-26.23%

IMMEDIATE POST

		% Change
BP (s/d) 174/100		9/14%
Heart Rate	102	65%
EF	56	-15.35%
ESV	39.2 ml	43.79%
ESVI	19.8 ml/m^2	43.79%
EDV	88.6 ml	10.92%
EDVI	44.7 ml/m^2	10.92%
PSP / ESVI	8.8	-23.89%
PSP ratio	1.0	
+1 min SP	174	
+2 min SP	170	
+3 min SP	180	

exercise. Regional wall contraction may be visualized in all views.

Case 1

A 69-year-old male had a single-vessel graft to the right coronary artery 6 months before this examination (Fig. 14.3). The left anterior descending coronary artery was reported to have only 20% diameter obstruction at that time. The patient continued to have atypical anterior left chest pain, and a recent thallium examination was within normal limits. An exercise echo was done to evaluate the patient's LV function.

During the first minute of exercise, the patient developed hypokinesis and akinesis of the septum and apex, and this became progressively worse postexercise. The test was discontinued after 3 min of exercise because of marked regional wall motion abnormalities. A repeat coronary angiogram revealed 90% obstruction of the left anterior descending coronary artery. Note the abnormal EF response, increased ESVI, abnormal

*** STRESS ECHO ANALYSIS ***

ST. JUDE HOSPITAL
FULLERTON, CA

Height: 172.72 cms.   Weight: 86 kgs.   BSA: 1.995 m^2
Age: 60.0 years.   HR: bpm.   BP: /   (s/d)

Apical 4 Chamber

PRE EXERCISE

BP (s/d) 128/86	
Heart Rate	74
EF	58
ESV	38.7 ml
ESVI	19.4 ml/m^2
EDV	92.7 ml
EDVI	46.5 ml/m^2
PSP / ESVI	6.6

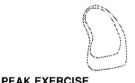

PEAK EXERCISE

		% Change
BP (s/d) 156/106		22/ 23%
Heart Rate	133	80%
EF	52	-11.19%
ESV	62.1 ml	60.50%
ESVI	31.1 ml/m^2	60.50%
EDV	128.7 ml	38.80%
EDVI	64.5 ml/m^2	38.80%
PSP / ESVI	5.0	-24.07%

IMMEDIATE POST

		% Change
BP (s/d) 136/84		6/ -2%
Heart Rate	133	80%
EF	54	-7.66%
ESV	50.5 ml	30.50%
ESVI	25.3 ml/m^2	30.50%
EDV	109.3 ml	17.88%
EDVI	54.8 ml/m^2	17.88%
PSP / ESVI	5.4	-18.58%
PSP ratio	1.0	
+1 min SP	154	
+2 min SP	158	
+3 min SP	138	

55 SECONDS POST EXERCISE

		% Change
BP (s/d) 154/94		20/ 9%
Heart Rate	105	42%
EF	61	5.19%
ESV	43.7 ml	12.87%
ESVI	21.9 ml/m^2	12.87%
EDV	112.9 ml	21.70%
EDVI	56.6 ml/m^2	21.70%
PSP / ESVI	7.0	6.59%

PSP/ESVI ratio response, and onset of hypokinesis and akinesis in the septal and apical regions that developed with exercise.

Case 2

A 60-year-old male who had had a possible myocardial infarction 13 years ago was now having occasional episodes of chest tightness with and without exercise (Fig. 14.4). A recent treadmill exercise test in his family physician's office was said to be normal. The patient was referred for an exercise echo test because of what was thought to be atypical chest pain. Early during exercise, he developed extensive wall motion abnormalities involving hypokinesis and akinesis of the septum and apex. The ECG also showed ischemic changes. Note the abnormal EF, ESVI, and onset of hypokinesis and akinesis involving the septum and apex at peak exercise. The abnormal findings rapidly returned to the resting level after peak exercise and, by 45 sec after exercise, were just about back to resting levels.

*** STRESS ECHO ANALYSIS ***

ST. JUDE HOSPITAL
FULLERTON, CA

Height: 154.94 cms. Weight: 54 kgs. BSA: 1.510 m^2
Age: 65.0 years. HR: bpm. BP: / (s/d)

Apical 4 Chamber

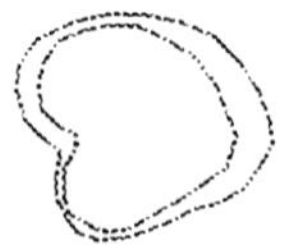

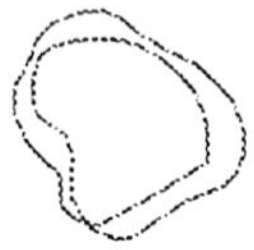

PRE EXERCISE

BP (s/d)	120/84
Heart Rate	72
EF	43
ESV	42.4 ml
ESVI	28.1 ml/m^2
EDV	74.7 ml
EDVI	49.5 ml/m^2
PSP / ESVI	4.3

PEAK EXERCISE

		% Change
BP (s/d)	140/90	17/ 7%
Heart Rate	120	67%
EF	53	22.37%
ESV	26.1 ml	-38.63%
ESVI	17.3 ml/m^2	-38.63%
EDV	55.2 ml	-26.07%
EDVI	36.6 ml/m^2	-26.07%
PSP / ESVI	8.1	90.10%

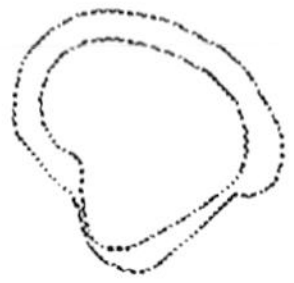

IMMEDIATE POST

		% Change
BP (s/d)	140/90	17/ 7%
Heart Rate	120	67%
EF	52	19.88%
ESV	39.0 ml	-8.09%
ESVI	25.8 ml/m^2	-8.09%
EDV	80.8 ml	8.25%
EDVI	53.6 ml/m^2	8.25%
PSP / ESVI	5.4	26.94%
PSP ratio	0.9	
+1 min SP	140	
+2 min SP	112	
+3 min SP	110	

Figure 14.5. Patient in Case 3 (see text).

This case illustrates that unless the patient is examined at peak exercise, valuable information will be lost, and significant pathology can be missed. A coronary artery angiogram study showed severe triple-vessel disease with an 80% left main coronary artery lesion.

Case 3

A 65-year-old female with mitral valve prolapse was referred for exercise echo testing because of a history of intermittent left anterior chest pain radiating down the left arm with and without exercise (Fig. 14.5). The patient had a markedly positive exercise ECG portion of the examination with 3 mm S-T segment depression and frequent ventricular extrasystoles with brief episodes of ventricular tachycardia. The patient had normal EF, ESVI, and regional contraction responses to exercise. The PSP/ESVI ratio showed a decreased response to exercise, suggesting LV dysfunction. Left atrial size increased with exercise. It was thought that the patient could not have significant

*** STRESS ECHO ANALYSIS ***

**ST. JUDE HOSPITAL
FULLERTON, CA**

Height: 182.88 cms.   Weight: 91 kgs.   BSA: 2.130 m^2
Age: 36.0 years.   HR: bpm.   BP: / (s/d)

Apical 4 Chamber

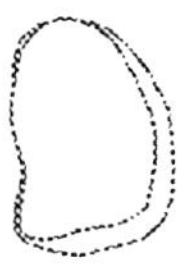

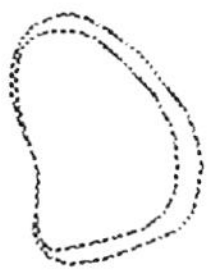

PRE EXERCISE		**PEAK EXERCISE**		**% Change**
BP (s/d)	98/82	BP (s/d)	148/98	51/20%
Heart Rate	95	Heart Rate	143	51%
EF	30	EF	31	2.05%
ESV	111.2 ml	ESV	114.9 ml	3.26%
ESVI	52.2 ml/m^2	ESVI	53.9 ml/m^2	3.26%
EDV	159.7 ml	EDV	166.4 ml	4.19%
EDVI	75.0 ml/m^2	EDVI	78.1 ml/m^2	4.19%
PSP / ESVI	1.9	PSP / ESVI	2.7	46.26%

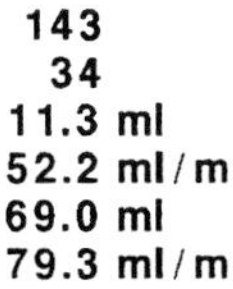

IMMEDIATE POST

		% Change
BP (s/d)	143/80	46/ -2%
Heart Rate	143	51%
EF	34	12.52%
ESV	111.3 ml	0.05%
ESVI	52.2 ml/m^2	0.05%
EDV	169.0 ml	5.83%
EDVI	79.3 ml/m^2	5.83%
PSP / ESVI	2.7	45.84%
PSP ratio	0.9	
+1 min SP	120	
+2 min SP	140	
+3 min SP	132	

Figure 14.6. Patient in Case 4 (see text).

CAD with a normal regional wall contraction response to exercise. The normal regional wall contraction response to exercise and abnormal LV function were believed to be probably due to mitral valve prolapse. The coronary artery angiogram study showed normal coronary arteries and marked mitral valve prolapse with mitral insufficiency. The patient did well after mitral valve replacement.

This case shows how exercise echo testing was helpful in separating LV dysfunction due to valvular disease from dysfunction caused by CAD and also suggested that the markedly positive stress ECG was a false-positive study.

Case 4

A 36-year-old male with a known lipid disorder and a history of three myocardial infarctions and one coronary artery bypass surgery was referred for evaluation of LV function (Fig. 14.6). He was not having any significant anginal pain. Coronary artery angiography 2 months earlier showed patent grafts to the right coronary artery and a 70% blockage in an internal mammary graft to the left anterior descending coronary artery. The patient was able to exercise for 9 min, reaching 80% of his maximal calculated heart rate with normal blood pressure and heart rate responses. The test was discontinued because of patient fatigue, and no angina was noted. The ECG at rest showed evidence of myocardial scarring with 1 mm S-T segment depression in some leads.

No ECG evidence of ischemic response developed with exercise. The resting echocardiogram showed decreased ventricular function with an EF of 30% increased ESVI, and a very low PSP:ESVI ratio. Abnormalities persisted with exercise. The apical two-chamber views suggested that the right coronary artery was the only artery able to respond to exercise, as increased contraction was noted during peak exercise at the inferior surface of the heart. One month after the exercise test, the patient developed unstable angina and expired while waiting for a cardiac transplant. The exercise echo study gave a much better picture of the patient's severe LV dysfunction than the exercise ECG.

This case suggests that it may be helpful to use exercise echo testing to stratify postmyocardial patients into risk categories. This could help determine which patients should be considered for more aggressive investigation and treatment of their CAD.

REFERENCES

1. Wann LS, Faris JV, Childress RH, Dillon JC, Weyman AE, Feigenbaum H: Exercise cross-sectional echocardiography in ischemic heart disease. *Circulation* 60:1300–1308, 1979.
2. Quinones MA: Exercise two-dimensional echocardiography. *Echocardiography* 1:151–163, 1984.
3. Morganroth J, Chen CC, David D: Exercise cross-sectional echocardiographic diagnosis of coronary artery disease. *Am J Cardiol* 47:20–26, 1981.
4. Mauer G, Nanda NC: Two-dimensional echocardiographic evaluation of exercise-induced left and right ventricular asynergy: Correlation with thallium scanning. *Am J Cardiol* 48:720–727, 1981.
5. Limacher MC, Quinones MA, Lawrence PR, Poliner LR, Nelson JG, Winters WL Jr, Waggoner AD, et al: Detection of coronary artery disease with exercise two-dimensional echocardiography: Description of a clinically applicable method and comparison with radionuclide ventriculography. *Circulation* 67:1211–1218, 1983.
6. Visser CA, van der Wieken RL, Kan G, et al: Comparison of two-dimensional echocardiography with radionuclide angiography during dynamic exercise for the detection of coronary artery disease. *Am Heart J* 106:528–533, 1983.
7. Crawford MH, Amon KW, Vance WS: Exercise two-dimensional echocardiography: Quantitation of left ventricular performance in patients with severe angina pectoris. *Am J Cardiol* 51:1–6, 1983.
8. Crawford MH, Petru MA, Amon KW, Vance WS, et al: Comparative value of two-dimensional echocardiography and radionuclide angiography for quantitating changes in left ventricular performance during exercise limited by angina pectoris. *Am J Cardiol* 53:42–54, 1984.
9. Robertson WS, Feigenbaum H, Armstrong WF, Dillon JC, O'Donnell J, McHenry PW: Exercise echocardiography: A clinically practical addition in the evaluation of coronary artery disease. *J Am Coll Cardiol* 2:1085–1091, 1983.
10. Iskandrian AS, Hakki A-H, Kane-Marsch S: Exercise thallium-201 scintigraphy in men with non-diagnostic exercise electrocardiograms. *Arch Intern Med* 146:2189–2193, 1986.
11. Kaul S, Boucher CA, Newell JB, Chesler DA, Greenberg JM, Okada RD, Strauss HW, Dinsmore RE, Pohost GM: Determination of the quantitative thallium imaging variables that optimize detection of coronary artery disease. *J Am Coll Cardiol* 7:527–537, 1986.
12. Armstrong, WF, O'Donnell J, Dillon JC, McHenry PL, Morris SN, Feigenbaum H: Complementary value of two-dimensional exercise echocardiography to routine treadmill exercise testing. *Ann Intern Med* 105:829–835, 1986.
13. Iskandrian AS, Hakki, A-H, Segal BL, Frankl WS, Kane-Marsch S, Unger J: Role of exercise thallium 201 imaging in decision making. *Arch Intern Med* 146:1098–1100, 1986.
14. Schneider RM, Weintraub WS, Klein LW, Seelaus P, Katz RI, Agarwal JB, Helfant RH: Multistage analysis of exercise radionuclide angiography in coronary artery disease. *Am J Cardiol* 58:36–41, 1986.

15. Northcote RJ, Flannigan C, Ballantyne D: Sudden death and vigorous exercise—A study of 60 deaths associated with squash. *Br Heart J* 55:198–203, 1986.
16. Currie PJ, Kelly MJ, Pitt A: Comparison of supine and erect bicycle exercise electrocardiography in coronary heart disease: Accentuation of exercise induced ischemic ST depression by supine posture. *Am J Cardiol* 52:1167–1173, 1983.
17. Schofield PM: Left ventricular dysfunction in patients with angina and normal coronary angiogram. *Br Heart J* 56:327–333, 1986.
18. Schlant RC, Blomquist CG, Brandenburg RO, DeBusk R, Ellestad MH, Fletcher GH, Froelicher VF, Hall RJ, McCallister BD, McHenry PL, Ryan TJ, Sheffield LT, Fisch C, DeSanctis RW, Dodge HT, Reeves TJ, Weinberg SL: Guidelines for exercise testing—A report of the Joint American College of Cardiology/American Heart Association Task Force on Assessment of Cardiovascular Procedures (Subcommittee on Exercise Testing). *Circulation* 74:653A–667A, 1986.
19. Heng MK, Simard M, Lake R, Udhoji VH: Exercise two-dimensional echocardiography for diagnosis of coronary artery disease. *Am J Cardiol* 54:502–507, 1984.
20. Berman DS, Maddahi I: Which patients need exercise nuclear cardiology tests? A Bayesian approach. Learning Center Highlights (American College of Cardiology). 1:1–5, 1986.
21. Applegate RJ, Crawford MH: Exercise echocardiography. *Echocardiography* 3:333–354, 1986.
22. Armstrong WF: Exercise Echocardiography: Ready, Willing and Able. *J Am Coll Cardiol* 11:1359–1361, 1988.

15

Two-Dimensional Echocardiography in Acute Coronary Care

Enrique Ostrzega, M.D.
Yzhar Charuzi, M.D.
Hiroshi Honma, M.D.

INTRODUCTION

The high prevalence of coronary artery disease and the potential life-threatening nature of acute ischemic syndromes make early diagnosis and assessment extremely important.

More than 50 years ago, coronary occlusion was shown to result in immediate reduction of segmental contraction (1). The ability of two-dimensional echocardiography (2DE) to detect regional wall motion abnormalities (2–9) has led to its use in acute manifestations of ischemic heart disease.

Two-dimensional echocardiography is particularly suited to rapid assessment of acutely ill patients. Due to its mobility, studies can be performed at the patient's bedside in the emergency room or coronary care unit. Visual interpretation of the studies can be done immediately either during the acquisition of data or by instantaneous replay. These data can have a crucial impact on the diagnosis and treatment of patients with suspected acute ischemic syndromes.

Evaluation of Acute Chest Pain Syndromes by 2DE

Patients presenting to an emergency room complaining of acute onset of chest pain often pose a diagnostic dilemma. When a typical history of retrosternal pain is accompanied by S-T segment elevation, a diagnosis of acute, evolving myocardial infarction can be made readily. However, coronary artery occlusion often can be electrocardiographically nonspecific or even silent.

Electrocardiographic studies during acute, evolving myocardial infarction show S-T segment elevation in fewer than 50% of patients on their initial electrocardiogram (10). Furthermore, acute myocardial infarction resulting from left circum-flex coronary artery occlusion is often undetected by the ECG (11). It is in these patients who present to an emergency room with acute chest pain and a nondiagnostic ECG that 2DE has a unique role (9, 12).

Sasaki et al. (9) performed 2DE studies on 46 patients without prior myocardial infarction who were admitted to the hospital for assessment of acute chest pain shortly after the onset of symptoms. On admission, all patients had a normal or nondiagnostic ECG and normal or nonsignificant elevation of serum creatinine phosphokinase (CK) activity. The data suggest that wall motion abnormalities can differentiate reliably between patients with myocardial ischemia or early infarction and patients with nonischemic chest pain when 2DE studies are done during an episode of chest pain. Furthermore, patients with regional wall motion abnormalities on 2DE performed after the resolution of pains were later diagnosed as having myocardial infarction.

Oh et al. (13) studied patients admitted to the emergency room with acute chest pain. A high correlation was found between left ventricular regional wall motion abnormalities and a subsequent diagnosis of myocardial infarction.

Detection, Localization, and Sizing of Myocardial Infarction

Transmural acute myocardial infarction is characterized by the rapid development of akinesis or dyskinesis (14). A high correlation has been found between the location of segmental wall motion abnormalities by 2DE and the diagnosis and localization of transmural infarction by electrocardiography (6). The extent of myocardial infarction determined by 2DE has been shown to correlate with peak serum CK (15).

A good correlation has also been found when pathologic data from postmortem studies were used for comparison. Weiss et al. (16) visually assessed wall motion abnormalities on 2DE in 20 patients who underwent subsequent postmortem examinations. Regional wall motion abnormalities were found in 90% of pathologically infarcted segments. However, wall motion abnormalities were also observed in 46% of morphologically normal segments, a finding in accordance with other investigators (17, 18). In an experimental study, Lieberman et al. (19) found that wall motion abnormalities alone led to overestimation of infarct size. Also, wall motion abnormalities were less precise than wall thickening in discriminating between infarcted and noninfarcted zones. Tethering of normal myocardium adjacent to ischemic areas is thought to cause echocardiographic overestimation of infarct size (19–21).

There is some controversy regarding the incidence of echocardiographic wall motion abnormalities in patients with nontransmural myocardial infarction. Loh et al. (22) correctly identified 10 of 12 patients with a non-Q wave infarction, using severe hypokinesis rather than akinesis as the criterion for wall motion abnormality. However, others found wall motion abnormalities in fewer than 30% of patients with nontransmural myocardial infarction (23).

Segmental Wall Motion Abnormalities in Acute Myocardial Infarction and Its Relationship to the Artery of Infarction

Analysis of segmental wall motion abnormalities in patients with acute myocardial infarction can help predict the involved coronary vessel (24–26) (Fig. 15.1). Stamm et al. (25) correlated echocardiographic and angiographic findings in patients with acute myocardial infarction and single-vessel disease. Myocardial infarction involving the left anterior descending coronary artery resulted in asynergy of the anterior, septal, and apical segments. In 95% of these patients, accurate prediction of left anterior descending artery disease proximal or distal to the first septal perforator could be determined by asynergy in the basal anterior or basal septal segments. An overlap was found between asynergic segments in infarcts resulting from occlusion of right or left circumflex coronary arteries (Fig. 15.2). In a recent study (27), a detailed 2DE assessment of ventricular septal wall motion was performed in 42 patients with a first acute myocardial infarction. Overall, 36 of these patients (85%) showed

septal involvement. Patients with anterior myocardial infarction due to left anterior descending artery occlusion showed asynergy of the anterior and distal ventricular septal segments. In patients with inferior myocardial infarction, the inferior and proximal septal segments were involved. Left circumflex and right coronary artery disease could not be individualized due to overlap of septal segments with wall motion abnormalities.

Thrombolytic Therapy in Acute Myocardial Infarction: Role of 2DE

The ability to perform serial studies in acutely ill patients makes 2DE a very useful technique for noninvasively monitoring the response of patients to treatment in acute myocardial infarction. This is particularly useful in assessing reperfusion with thrombolytic agents (i.e., streptokinase, recombinant tissue plasminogen activator) during

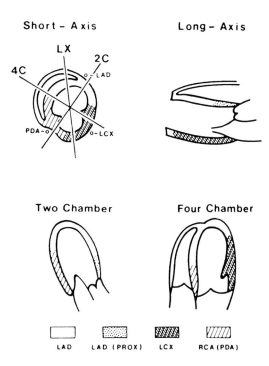

Figure 15.1. Diagram illustrating the relationship between two-dimensional echocardiographic views and coronary artery perfusion. *4C* = four-chamber view; *LX* = long-axis view, *2C* = two-chamber view, *LAD* = left anterior descending artery, *LCX* = left circumflex artery, *RCA* = right coronary artery, *PDA* = posterior descending artery. (From Feigenbaum H: *Echocardiography*, ed. 4. Philadelphia, Lea & Febiger, 1986, pp 465–468.)

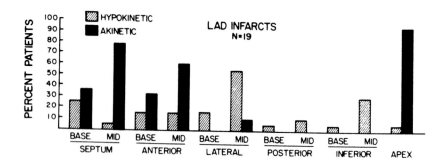

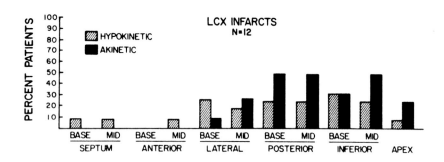

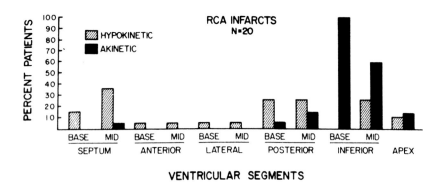

VENTRICULAR SEGMENTS

Figure 15.2. Frequency and distribution of asynergy after single-vessel infarction. The percentage of single-vessel stenosis patients with hypokinetic and akinetic or dyskinetic motion is calculated for each segment. *LAD* = left anterior descending artery, *LCX* = left circumflex artery, *RCA* = right coronary artery. (From Stamm RB, et al: Echocardiographic detection of infarction: Correlation with the extent of angiographic coronary disease. *Circulation* 67:233, 1983. By permission of the American Heart Association, Inc.)

the evolving phase of acute myocardial infarction (28–31).

Charuzi et al. (32) showed significant improvement in regional and global left ventricular function in patients who underwent successful intracoronary thrombolysis within 3 hr of the onset of chest pain. Studies were analyzed both quantitatively and qualitatively (Fig. 15.3). Improve-

ment of left ventricular function was noted on the tenth day study but not on the immediate post-thrombolysis study. No improvement was seen in patients with unsuccessful thrombolysis or in a group of patients treated conventionally.

Topol et al. (33) reported similar findings in a series of patients with acute myocardial infarction undergoing thrombolysis with recombinant tissue

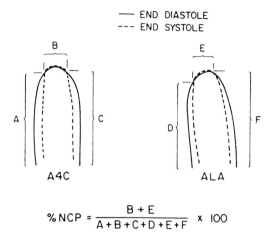

$$\% NCP = \frac{B + E}{A + B + C + D + E + F} \times 100$$

Figure 15.3. Calculation of the percentage of noncontractile perimeter (%*NCP*). *A, C, D,* and *F* indicate the length of the end-diastolic outline where inward motion occurred during systole. *B* and *E* indicate the length of the end-diastolic outline that was akinetic or dyskinetic during systole. *A4C* = apical four-chamber view, *ALA* = apical long-axis view. (From Charuzi Y, et al: Improvement in regional and global left ventricular function after intracoronary thrombolysis: Assessment with two-dimensional echocardiography. *Am J Cardiol* 53:662, 1984).

plasminogen activator. In this study, functional recovery was more pronounced in patients who had coronary artery balloon angioplasty following successful thrombolysis.

It has been postulated that stunned myocardium or prolonged postischemic ventricular dysfunction (34–37) may account for the lack of early improvement shown in these studies.

Prognostic Value of 2DE in Acute Myocardial Infarction

The prognosis for patients with acute myocardial infarction is related primarily to infarct size and functional status of the remaining noninfarcted myocardium (8, 15, 38–40). Because of its ability to determine global and regional ventricular function, 2DE is suited ideally for determining early and late prognosis in patients with acute myocardial infarction. When performed early in the course of myocardial infarction, 2DE can help stratify high- and low-risk groups (38). Wall motion indices used to measure global left ventricular function correlated highly with clinical indexes of ventricular function (41, 42). This

method predicted hemodynamic deterioration including cardiogenic shock and other inhospital complications (8, 15, 43, 44). Similarly, the usefulness of predischarge 2DE as a prognostic indicator for long-term follow-up has been demonstrated. These studies identify a subset of patients at increased risk of complications after myocardial infarction (40, 45).

Two-dimensional echocardiography is also very useful for detecting and evaluating complications that occur during the course of an acute myocardial infarction.

Left Ventricular Aneurysm

Left ventricular aneurysm is a relatively common complication of acute myocardial infarction. Its incidence ranges from 3.5% to 38% (46–50). It is associated frequently with congestive heart failure, systemic embolization, and arrhythmia.

Left ventricular aneurysm develops through dilatation and thinning of the infarcted segment (i.e., infarct expansion) (51). Eventually the aneurysm turns into fibrous tissue, commonly interlaced with residual muscle fibers. The most common sites for aneurysms are the left ventricular apex and anterior wall. However, aneurysms can also occur in other left ventricular segments (Figs. 15.4 and 15.5).

Two-dimensional echocardiography has been recognized as the technique of choice to detect and assess left ventricular aneurysm (49, 52–55). Echocardiographically, an aneurysm is seen as a dilated and dyskinetic segment that remains dilated during diastole (52). The orifice or neck of an aneurysm is wide, with a diameter usually comparable to the maximal diameter of the aneurysm (56). The neck is the transition between the dyskinetic aneurysm and the more normally contracting myocardium. The presence of a wide neck makes the diagnosis of left ventricular aneurysm much easier.

Serial echocardiographic studies have shown that aneurysm is seen between the first and fourteenth day following infarction. Once formed, aneurysms tend to dilate further. Thus, the size of an aneurysm in the early stage after acute myocardial infarction is either equal to or smaller than an aneurysm during the chronic stage (57).

Myocardial Infarct Expansion

Myocardial expansion is the thinning and dilatation of the infarct zone (51, 58, 59) resulting from passive stretching and slippage of freshly necrotic muscle fibers (60, 61) (Fig. 15.6). This

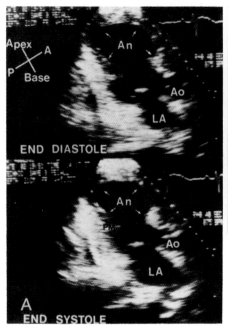
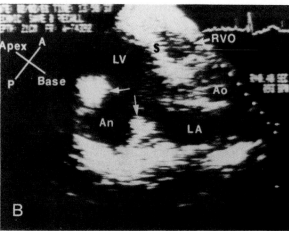

Figure 15.4. *A,* Apical long-axis views showing a large apical aneurysm (*An*) in diastole (*upper panel*) and systole (*lower panel*). *B,* Parasternal long-axis view showing an aneurysm (*An*) with a broad neck (*arrows*) of the posterior basilar segment of the left ventricle (*LV*). *A* = anterior, *P* = posterior, *Ao* = aorta, *LA* = left atrium, *PM* = posteromedial papillary muscle, *S* = interventricular septum, *RVO* = right ventricular outflow tract. (Adapted from Hagan AD, et al: Two-dimensional echocardiography. Clinical-pathological correlations in adult and congenital heart disease. In: *Coronary Artery Disease.* Boston, Little, Brown, 1983, pp 163.)

is more common in myocardial infarction due to left anterior descending artery occlusion (62) and is associated with a high incidence of cardiac rupture (63).

Infarct expansion occurs early following acute myocardial infarction. Serial 2DE studies showed that infarct expansion can be detected within 24–72 hrs in 30% of patients with acute myocardial infarction (59, 64, 65). Infarct expansion may contribute to chronic progressive ventricular enlargement. This is due to lengthening of both the infarcted and the normal myocardium (66, 67) and is thought to be the precursor of true left ventricular aneurysm (51, 68).

Pseudoaneurysms

In contrast to true aneurysm, pseudoaneurysm is a rare complication of acute myocardial infarction (69–71). Pseudoaneurysm develops when a left ventricular free wall rupture is contained by the pericardial sac, preventing a sudden hemopericardium. Pseudoaneurysms can vary in size from small to very large.

Unlike true aneurysms, which usually occur at the apex, pseudoaneurysms have no preferential distribution. The wall of the pseudoaneurysm is usually thin and is at high risk of rupture (69, 70, 72). Pseudoaneurysms typically have a narrow neck, which is the site of sharp discontinuity of endocardial images (56, 73). The ratio between the maximal width of the neck and the maximal diameter of the aneurysmal sac does not exceed 0.5. This ratio has been found useful in differentiating pseudoaneurysms from true ventricular aneurysms and ranges from 0.9 to 1.0 (56). Pseudoaneurysms are usually filled with blood clots, which are easy to visualize by 2DE (Fig. 15.7).

Eccentrically located pseudoaneurysms (originating in the posterior or posterolateral walls) may be missed because of lung attenuation of the echo beam (73–75).

Acquired Ventricular Septal Defect

Transmural rupture of the ventricular septum is a rare complication of acute myocardial infarction (76), but prompt recognition is essential

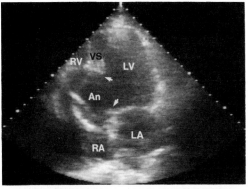

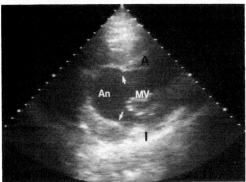

Figure 15.5. Apical four-chamber view (*top*) and parasternal short-axis view (*bottom*) showing a large ventricular septal aneurysm (*An*) with a broad neck (*arrows*). This patient had a surgical repair of a ventricular septal rupture secondary to acute inferior myocardial infarction. The aneurysm developed in the remainder of the infarcted septum not covered by the synthetic patch. *A* = anterior, *I* = inferior, *MV* = mitral valve, *LV* = left ventricle, *LA* = left atrium, *RV* = right ventricle, *RA* = right atrium, *VS* = ventricular septum.

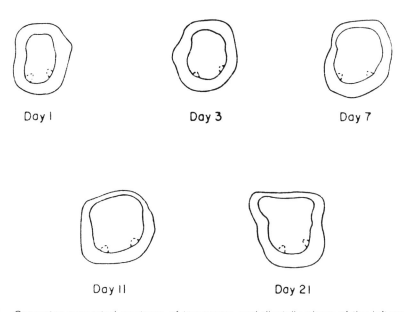

Figure 15.6. Computer-generated contours of transverse end-diastolic views of the left ventricle from serial echocardiographic studies of a patient with an anterior transmural infarction. Papillary-muscle locations recorded as radial coordinates are represented by *dotted lines*. Progressive development of regional dilatation and thinning in the infarcted area is apparent by the seventh day. (Adapted from Eaton LW, et al: Regional cardiac dilatation after acute myocardial infarction: Recognition by two-dimensional echocardiography. *N Engl J Med* 300:57, 1979.)

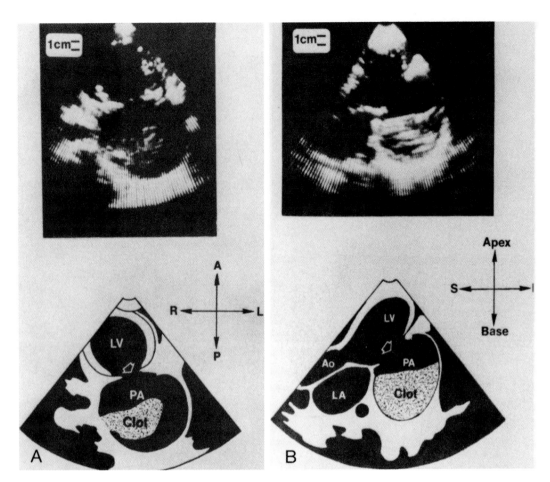

Figure 15.7. *A*, Two-dimensional echocardiographic short-axis view (*top*) with labeled diagram (*bottom*) of a patient with a pseudoaneurysm (*PA*) of the inferior wall of the left ventricle (*LV*) with a narrow neck (*open arrow*) and intracavitary echoes suggestive of thrombus. *B*, Two-chamber apical long-axis view in a different patient, demonstrating a large saccular pseudoaneurysm (*PA*) communicating with the left ventricular cavity (*LV*) at the zone of myocardial discontinuity (*open arrow*). Dense echoes suggestive of clot are noted in the false chamber. The systolic frame is accompanied by a labeled idealized diagram. *Ao* = aorta, *LA* = left atrium, *S* = superior, *I* = inferior, *A* = anterior, *P* = posterior, *R* = right, *L* = left. (Adapted from Catherwood E, et al: Two-dimensional echocardiographic recognition of left ventricular pseudoaneurysm. *Circulation* 62:294, 1980. By permission of the American Heart Association, Inc.)

because of its high mortality and the potential for surgical repair (76–80). Acquired ventricular septal defects usually occur within 1 week after the onset of acute myocardial infarction (76–81) and can be located in the anterior or inferior ventricular septal segment (82, 83). The site of rupture is either inside a septal aneurysm or in the transition between infarcted and normal septal tissue.

The septal defect can be seen frequently by 2DE as discontinuity of myocardial echoes (Fig. 15.8). The sensitivity of 2DE in detecting the site of the rupture frequently depends on meticulous screening of the ventricular septum. The most useful views for visualization of an acquired ventricular septal defect are the apical four-chamber, subcostal long-axis, and to a lesser extent, the parasternal short-axis views (83). When the actual tear cannot be visualized, contrast echocardiography can be used (83–85). Echo contrast inside the right ventricle is washed out during systole by noncontrast blood entering from the left ventricle. In diastole, echo contrast can be seen crossing from the right into the left ventricle, indicating bidirectional flow (Fig. 15.9). Doppler echocardiography combined with 2DE has been shown to be very useful in diagnosing and assessing acquired ventricular septal defects (86–89).

Ventricular Free Wall Rupture

Ventricular free wall rupture usually occurs within the first week of acute myocardial infarction. Its incidence in hospitalized patients who die of acute myocardial infarction varies between 4% and 24% (90–93). The rupture of the wall leads to acute hemopericardium, causing cardiac tamponade and rapid death. On rare occasions, when the rupture is less abrupt and the leakage of blood into the pericardial sac is slower, 2DE may indicate the actual site of the rupture (Fig. 15.10).

Even without direct visualization of the wall tear, regional dilatation and a thin ventricular wall persisting throughout the cardiac cycle, in association with pericardial effusion, can be indications of imminent rupture (94).

Ventricular Thrombi

Left ventricular thrombi are a common complication of acute myocardial infarction. Autopsy studies have found left ventricular thrombi in 20–60% of transmural myocardial infarctions (47, 95–98). The incidence of systemic embolization associated with left ventricular thrombi ranges from 0.6% to 6.4% in clinical studies, but has been reported in up to 20% of cases in autopsy studies (47, 48, 99, 100).

Two-dimensional echocardiography is highly sensitive and specific in detecting left ventricular thrombi, which tend to develop on akinetic or dyskinetic segments (101–104). The overwhelming majority of thrombi are located in the left ventricular apex, probably because of sluggish blood flow associated with apical infarction (96, 105, 106). Left ventricular thrombi may also be present in other segments with severe wall motion abnormalities (Figs. 15.11 and 15.12). Thrombi may be mural, may be adherent to the left ventricular wall, or may protrude into the left ventricular cavity. They may have smooth, multilobulated, or ragged intracavitary borders. Echo density of a clot is usually higher than that of adjacent myocardial tissue (107, 108). However, distinction between the thrombus and the underlying tissue may be difficult. At times when it cannot be directly identified, a "normal" wall

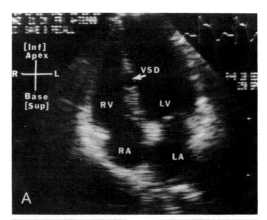

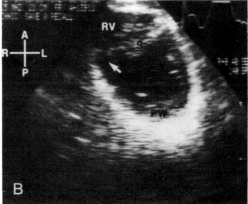

Figure 15.8. A, Apical four-chamber view showing a ventricular septal defect (*VSD*) (*arrow*) secondary to rupture from an extensive posteromedial myocardial infarction. B, Parasternal short-axis view of the same patient as in A, showing the rupture site (*arrow*) of the posterior portion of the interventricular septum (*S*). *LV* = left ventricle, *RV* = right ventricle; *LA* = left atrium, *RA* = right atrium, *PW* = posterior wall, *A* = anterior, *P* = posterior, *R* = right, *L* = left. (Adapted from Hagan AD, et al: Two-dimensional echocardiography. Clinical-pathological correlations in adult and congenital heart disease. In: *Coronary Artery Disease.* Boston, Little, Brown, 1983, pp 163.)

thickness in an aneurysmatic segment would suggest the presence of a mural thrombus (109). Echo density of the thrombus varies in each case, probably due to its histologic composition (110). Thrombi can appear homogeneous, speckled, or layered. Occasionally, low-density, swirling echoes can be detected next to an akinetic wall (Fig. 15.11C). This phenomenon is thought to repre-

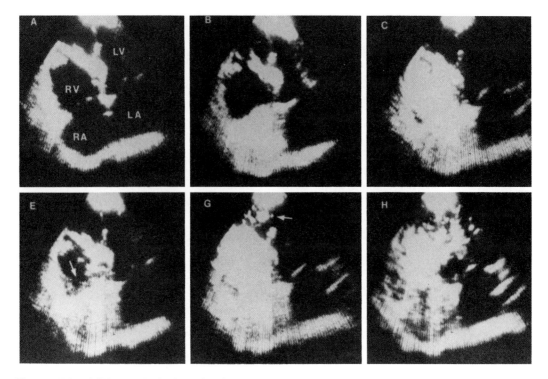

Figure 15.9. Still frames in the four-chamber view of a patient with a ventricular septal defect, before and after saline contrast injection. After injection, microbubbles fill the right atrium (*RA*) (*B*) and right ventricle (*RV*) (*C*). In the next systole, they are completely washed out of the right ventricle from the apex to base (*E*). During the next diastole, microbubbles again fill the right ventricle (*G*) and spill over into the left ventricle *LV*) through the ventricular septal defect at the apex of the interventricular septum (*arrow, panels G* and *H*). *LA* = left atrium. (Adapted from Drobac M, et al: Ventricular septal defect after myocardial infarction: Diagnosis by two-dimensional contrast ecohcardiography. *Circulation* 67:335, 1983. By permission of the American Heart Association, Inc.)

sent stagnant blood that becomes echogenic (110, 111).

Accurate diagnosis of thrombi requires ruling out artifacts: reverberations or confounding structures like trabeculae, papillary muscles, chordae tendineae, endocardial bridges, or intracardiac tumors (110). False diagnosis of ventricular thrombi can be minimized by visualizing the thrombus in more than one view.

Serial 2DE studies are necessary to monitor changes in size and shape of a left ventricular thrombus, especially during anticoagulation therapy (112–115).

Mitral Regurgitation

Mitral regurgitation is a relatively common complication of acute myocardial infarction. This is caused by a spectrum of abnormalities, pri-

marily related to disruption of the subvalvular apparatus.

Papillary muscle dysfunction is the most common cause of mitral regurgitation in acute myocardial infarction. Echocardiographically, one or both leaflets fail to reach the normal systolic position in relation to the mitral valve ring (116) (Fig. 15.13). Also, dyskinesis or akinesis at the base of at least one of the papillary muscles usually is seen (116–118). These echocardiographic findings are not specific for papillary muscle dysfunction secondary to acute myocardial infarction and can be observed in other conditions associated with left ventricular dilatation (119).

Papillary muscle rupture is a rare complication of acute myocardial infarction (120–122) and usually occurs within 1 week following the infarction (Fig. 15.14). Rupture is associated with severe mitral regurgitation and cardiac failure

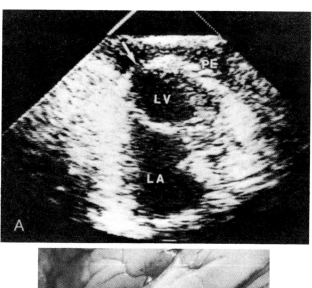

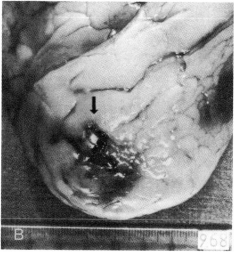

Figure 15.10. *A,* Two-dimensional echocardiographic subcostal two-chamber view showing a defect across the free wall of the left ventricle (*arrow*). The heart is surrounded by a characteristic contour of echo-free pericardial effusion. *LV* = left ventricle, *LA* = left atrium, *PE* = pericardial effusion. *B,* Pathologic specimen showing anterior myocardial infarction with rupture of the heart. The rupture represents a laceration in the anterior wall of the infarcted left ventricle (*arrow*). (Adapted from Desoutter, P et al: Two-dimensional echographic visualization of free ventricular wall rupture in acute anterior myocardial infarction. *Am Heart J* 108:1360, 1984.)

(120). The posteromedial papillary muscle is involved more frequently than the anterolateral papillary muscle, probably because of its single blood supply (120, 123, 124).

There are several forms of rupture. In the incomplete form, a residual piece of papillary muscle maintains the anatomic continuity with the mitral valve. In complete rupture, there is detachment of either one head or the whole papillary muscle. On echocardiography, in addition to marked hyperdynamic motion of the normal myocardium, a flail mitral leaflet can be observed (Fig. 15.15). There is loss of normal coaptation, and the tip of the affected leaflet can be seen protruding into the left atrium during systole. The detached head of the papillary muscle may also be visualized.

Right Ventricular Infarction

Evidence of right ventricular myocardial infarction is a common finding in inferior wall myocardial infarction and is rather specific for right

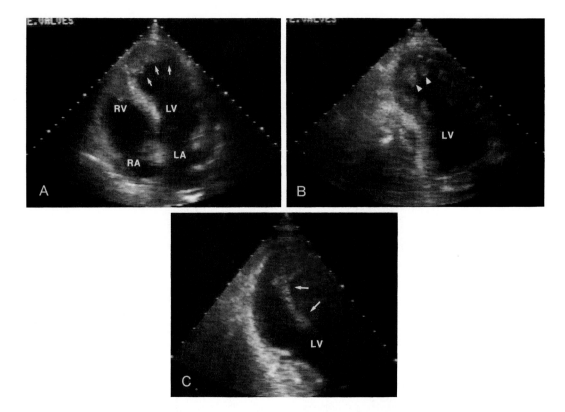

Figure 15.11. Two-dimensional echocardiographic images from a patient with acute anterior myocardial infarction. *A,* Apical four-chamber view showing a large mural thrombus (*arrows*) in an apical aneurysm. *B,* Apical long-axis view showing two protruding thrombi (*arrowheads*). *C,* Magnified apical four-chamber view taken 1 week later. The streak of dense echoes from the apex directed toward the center of the cavity seen on this still frame (*arrows*) represents swirling echoes on real-time display. *LV* = left ventricle, *LA* = left atrium, *RV* = right ventricle, *RA* = right atrium.

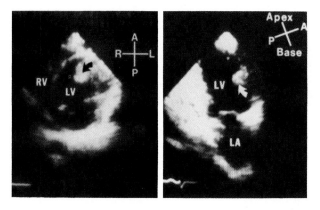

Figure 15.12. Parasternal short-axis view (*left panel*) and apical long-axis view (*right panel*) demonstrating a large thrombus (*arrows*) attached to an akinetic anterolateral wall. Any target suggestive of mass or thrombus should be reproducible in two tomographic planes 90° to each other to confirm whether the target is an actual mass. Abbreviations are the same as for Figure 15.8. (Adapted from Hagan AD, et al: Two-dimensional echocardiography. Clinical-pathological correlations in adult and congenital heart disease. In: *Coronary Artery Disease.* Boston, Little, Brown, 1983, pp 163.)

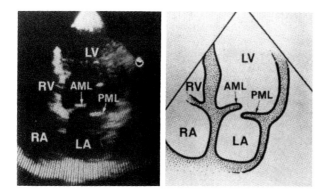

Figure 15.13. Still frame in the four-chamber view taken at end-systole of a patient with incomplete mitral leaflet closure and the corresponding schematic diagram. At end-systole, the anterior mitral leaflet (*AML*) fails to reach the atrioventricular ring, suggesting incomplete systolic closure of the mitral valve. *LV* = left ventricle, *LA* = left atrium, *RV* = right ventricle, *RA* = right atrium, *PML* = posterior mitral leaflet. (From Godley RW, et al: Incomplete mitral leaflet closure in patients with papillary muscle dysfunction. *Circulation* 63:565, 1981. By permission of the American Heart Association, Inc.)

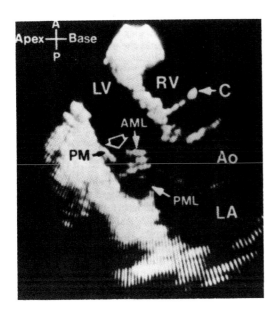

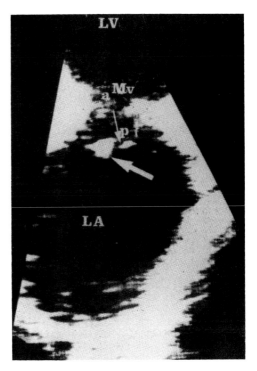

Figure 15.14. A low sternal border parasternal long-axis view showing the rupture site (*open arrow*) of the posterior papillar muscle (*PM*) with prominent reflectance caused by the tip of the papillary muscle and chordae tendineae attached to the anterior mitral leaflet (*AML*). *LV* = left ventricle, *RV* = right ventricle, *LA* = left atrium, *Ao* = aorta, *PML* = posterior mitral leaflet, *C* = catheter, *A* = anterior, *P* = posterior. (From Mintz GS, et al: Two-dimensional echocardiographic identification of surgically correctable complications of acute myocardial infarction. *Circulation* 64:91, 1981. By permission of the American Heart Association, Inc.)

Figure 15.15. Apical view (systolic frame) of a patient with severe mitral regurgitation due to a ruptured papillary muscle. The flail posterior (*p*) mitral leaflet (*thin arrow*) overshoots the anterior leaflet (*a*) and lies within the left atrium (*LA*). The increased thickness of the tip of the flailing segment (*large arrow*) is suggestive of a mass lesion—in this case, the head of the papillary muscle. *LV* = left ventricle, *Mv* = mitral valve. (From Donaldson RM, et al: Echocardiographic visualization of the anatomic causes of mitral regurgitation resulting from myocardial infarction. *Postgrad Med J* 58:257, 1982.)

coronary artery occlusion (125, 126). Isolated right ventricular infarction is very rare (127). Right ventricular infarction becomes clinically significant when a proximal right coronary artery occlusion causes ischemia in a significant portion of the ventricle. Right ventricular myocardial infarction may be associated with arterial hypotension, cardiogenic shock (128), atrioventricular (A-V) block (126, 129), ventricular tachyarrhythmias (130, 131), tricuspid regurgitation (132), and right-to-left shunt through a patent foramen ovale (133). Right ventricular thrombi are a rare finding in the course of acute myocardial infarction (126, 134).

Two-dimensional echocardiography has become a reliable technique for detecting and assessing segmental right ventricular wall motion abnormalities (132, 135). Segments of the right ventricle can be visualized in almost every stand-

ard view and also in special right ventricular views (132). Right ventricular wall motion abnormalities can either persist (133, 136) or show spontaneous improvement (137–140). In addition to assessment of wall motion, 2DE can detect complications of right ventricular myocardial infarction effectively. These include right ventricular dilatation with or without paradoxical septal motion (132, 136, 141), right ventricular aneurysm (132) (Fig. 15.16), and thrombus (142). For assessment of tricuspid regurgitation and right-to-left shunt, contrast echo may be useful (132, 143), although echo-Doppler can offer a more clear and definite diagnosis.

SUMMARY

The greatest problem in obtaining technically adequate 2DE studies in the acute stage is that patients may be too ill to cooperate. The oper-

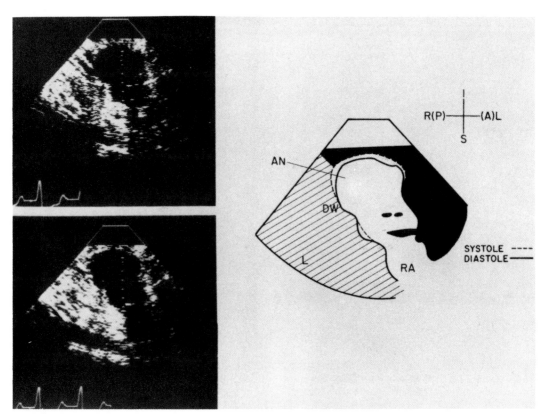

Figure 15.16. Right ventricular aneurysm. The right-heart apical two-chamber view shows a large aneurysm that involves the apical region. Labeled diagram on the *right. AN* = aneurysm, *DW* = diaphragmatic wall, *L* = liver, *RA* = right atrium, *I* = inferior, *R* = right, *P* = posterior, *S* = superior, *A* = anterior, *L* = left. (From D'Arcy B, et al: Two-dimensional echocardiographic features of right ventricular infarction. *Circulation* 65:167, 1982. By permission of the American Heart Association, Inc.)

ator's skill and observer's experience also are crucial elements in obtaining adequate 2DE studies. In spite of its limitations, 2DE is probably the most useful and versatile diagnostic tool for the evaluation of patients in different stages of acute coronary care.

REFERENCES

1. Tennant R, Wiggers CJ: The effect of coronary occlusion on myocardial contraction. *Am J Physiol* 112:351, 1935.
2. Kerber RE, Abboud FM: Echocardiographic detection of regional myocardial infarction. *Circulation* 47:997, 1973.
3. Feigenbaum H, Corya BC, Dillon JC, Weyman AE, Rasmussen S, Black MJ, Chang S: Role of echocardiography in patients with coronary artery disease. *Am J Cardiol* 37:775, 1976.
4. Kisslo JA, Robertson D, Gilbert BW, von Ramm O, Behar VS: A comparison of real-time, two-dimensional echocardiography and cineangiography in detecting left ventricular asynergy. *Circulation* 55:134, 1977.
5. Kerber RE, Marcus ML, Abboud FM: Echocardiography in experimentally induced myocardial ischemia. *Am J Med* 63:21, 1977.
6. Heger JJ, Weyman AE, Wann LS, Dillon JC, Feigenbaum H: Cross-sectional echocardiography in acute myocardial infarction: Detection and localization of regional left ventricular asynergy. *Circulation* 60:531, 1979.
7. Visser CA, Lie KI, Kan G, Meltzer R, Durrer D: Detection and quantification of acute, isolated myocardial infarction by two dimensional echocardiography. *Am J Cardiol* 47:1020, 1981.
8. Charuzi Y, Davidson RM, Barrett MJ, Beeder C, Marshall LA, Loh LK, Prause JA, Meerbaum S, Corday E: Simultaneous assessment of segmental and global left ventricular function by two-dimensional echocardiography in acute myocardial infarction. *Clin Cardiol* 6:255, 1983.
9. Sasaki H, Charuzi Y, Beeder C, Sugiki Y, Lew AS: Utility of echocardiography for the early assessment of patients with nondiagnostic chest pain. *Am Heart J* 112:494, 1986.
10. Rude RE, Poole WK, Muller JE, Zoltan T, Rutherford J, Parker C, Roberts R, Raabe DS, Gold HK, Stone PH, Willerson JT, Braunwald E, and the MILIS Study Group: Electrocardiographic and clinical criteria for recognition of acute myocardial infarction based on analysis of 3697 patients. *Am J Cardiol* 52:936, 1983.
11. Blanke H, Cohen M, Schlueter GU, Karsch KR, Rentrop KP: Electrocardiographic and coronary arteriographic correlations during acute myocardial infarction. *Am J Cardiol* 54:249, 1984.
12. Oh JK, Miller FA, Shub C, Reeder GS, Tajik AJ: Evaluation of acute chest pain syndromes by two-dimensional echocardiography: Its potential application in the selection of patients for acute reperfusion therapy. *Mayo Clin Proc* 62:59, 1987.
13. Oh JK, Shub C, Miller FA Jr, Evans WE, Tajik AJ: Role of two-dimensional echocardiography in

the emergency room. *Echocardiography* 2:217, 1985.
14. Horowitz RS, Morganroth J, Parrotto C, Chen CC, Soffer J, Pauletto FJ: Immediate diagnosis of acute myocardial infarction by two-dimensional echocardiography. *Circulation* 65:323, 1982.
15. Gibson RS, Bishop HL, Stamm RB, Crampton RS, Beller GA, Martin RP: Value of early two-dimensional echocardiography in patients with acute myocardial infarction. *Am J Cardiol* 49:1110, 1982.
16. Weiss JL, Bulkley BH, Hutchins GM, Mason SJ: Two-dimensional echocardiographic recognition of myocardial injury in man: Comparison with postmortem studies. *Circulation* 63:401, 1981.
17. Weyman AE, Franklin TD, Egenes KM, Green D: Correlation between extent of abnormal regional wall motion and myocardial infarct size in chronically infarcted dogs (Abstr). *Circulation* 55 (Suppl III):III-72, 1977.
18. Wyatt HL, Meerbaum S, Heng MK, Rit J, Gueret P, Corday E: Experimental evaluation of the extent of myocardial dyssynergy and infarct size by two-dimensional echocardiography. *Circulation* 63:607, 1981.
19. Lieberman AN, Weiss JL, Jugdutt BL, Becker LC, Bulkley BH, Garrison JB, Hutchins GM, Kallman CA, Weisfeldt ML: Two-dimensional echocardiography and infarct size: Relationship of regional wall motion and thickening to the extent of myocardial infarction in the dog. *Circulation* 63:739, 1981.
20. Force T, Kemper A, Perkins, L. Gilfoil M, Cohen C, Parisi A: Overestimation of infarct size by quantitative two dimensional echocardiography: The role of tethering and of analytic procedures. *Circulation* 73:1360, 1986.
21. Gillam LD, Guyer DE, Franklin TD, Hogan RD, Weyman AE: The mechanism of abnormal wall motion in infarct border zones (Abstr). *J Am Coll Cardiol* 1:620, 1983.
22. Loh IK, Charuzi Y, Beeder C, Marshall LA, Ginsburg JH: Early diagnosis of nontransmural myocardial infarction by two-dimensional echocardiography. *Am Heart J* 104:963, 1982.
23. Henschke, CI, Risser TA, Sandor T, Hanlon WB, Neumann A, Wynne J: Quantitative computer-assisted analysis of left ventricular wall thickening and motion by two-dimensional echocardiography in acute myocardial infarction. *Am J Cardiol* 52:960, 1983.
24. Feigenbaum H: *Echocardiography*, ed 4 Philadelphia, Lea & Febiger, 1986, pp 465–468.
25. Stamm RB, Gibson RS, Bishop HL, Carabello BA, Beller GA, Martin RP: Echocardiographic detection of infarction: Correlation with the extent of angiographic coronary disease. *Circulation* 67:233, 1983.
26. Pierard LA, Sprynger M, Carlier J: Echocardiographic prediction of the site of coronary artery obstruction in acute myocardial infarction. *Eur Heart J* 8:116, 1987.
27. Y. Sugitzi, personal communication.
28. Van De Werf F, Ludbrook PA, Bergmann SR, Tiefenbrunn AJ, Fox KAA, de Geest H, Verstraete M, Collen D, Sobel BE: Coronary throm-

bolysis with tissue-type plasminogen activator in patients with evolving myocardial infarction. *N Engl J Med* 310:609, 1984.

29. The TIMI Study Group: The thrombolysis in myocardial infarction (TIMI) trial: Phase I findings. *N Engl J Med* 312:932, 1985.

30. Verstraete M, Bernard R, Bory M, Brower RW, Collen D, de Bono DP, Erbel R, Huhmann W, Lennane RJ, Lubsen J, Mathey D, Meyer J, Michels HR, Rutsch W, Schartl M, Schmidt W, Uebis R, von Essen R: Randomized trial of intravenous recombinant tissue-type plasminogen activator versus intravenous streptokinase in acute myocardial infarction. *Lancet* 1:842, 1985.

31. Verani MS, Roberts R: Preservation of cardiac function by coronary thrombolysis during acute myocardial infarction: Fact or myth? *J Am Coll Cardiol* 10:470, 1987.

32. Charuzi Y, Beeder C, Marshall LA, Sasaki H, Pack NB, Geft I, Ganz W: Improvement in regional and global left ventricular function after intracoronary thrombolysis: Assessment with two-dimensional echocardiography. *Am J Cardiol* 53:662, 1984.

33. Topol EC, Weiss JL, Brinker JA, Brin KP, Gottlieb SO, Becker LC, Bulkley BH, Chandra N, Flaherty JT, Gerstenblith G, Gottlieb SH, Guerci AD, Ouyang P, Llewellyn MP, Weisfeldt ML, Shapiro EP: Regional wall motion improvement after coronary thrombolysis with recombinant tissue plasminogen activator: Importance of coronary angioplasty. *J Am Coll Cardiol* 6:426, 1985.

34. Braunwald E, Kloner RA. The stunned myocardium: Prolonged, postischemic ventricular dysfunction. *Circulation* 66:1146, 1982.

35. Murphy ML, Peng CF, Kane JJ, Straub KD: Ventricular performance and biochemical alteration of regional ischemic myocardium after reperfusion in the pig. *Am J Cardiol* 50:821, 1982.

36. Lang TW, Corday E, Gold H, Meerbaum S, Rubin S, Costantini C, Hirose S, Osher J, Rosen V: Consequences of reperfusion after coronary occlusion. Effects on hemodynamic and regional myocardial metabolic function. *Am J Cardiol* 33:69, 1974.

37. Kloner RA, Ellis SG, Lange R, Braunwald E: Studies of experimental coronary artery reperfusion: effect on infarct size, myocardial function, biochemistry, ultrastructure and microvascular damage. *Circulation* 68 (SupplI):I-8, 1983.

38. Horwitz RS, Morganroth J: Immediate detection of early high-risk patients with acute myocardial infarction using two dimensional echocardiographic evaluation of left ventricular wall motion abnormalities. *Am Heart J* 103:814, 1982.

39. Abrams, DS, Starling MR, Crawford MH, O'Rourke RA: Value of noninvasive techniques for predicting early complications in patients with clinical class II acute myocardial infarction. *J Am Coll Cardiol* 2:818, 1983.

40. Nishimura RA, Reeder GS, Miller FA, Ilstrup DM, Shub C, Seward JB, Tajik AJ: Prognostic value of predischarge two dimensional echocardiogram after acute myocardial infarction. *Am J Cardiol* 53:429, 1984.

41. Shiina A, Tajik AJ, Smith HC, Lengyel M, Se-

ward JB: Prognostic significance of regional wall motion abnormality in patients with prior myocardial infarction: A prospective correlative study of two-dimensional echocardiography and angiography. *Mayo Clin Proc* 61:254, 1986.

42. Van Reet RE, Quinones MA, Poliner LR, Nelson JG, Waggoner AD, Kanon D, Lubetkin SJ, Pratt CM, Winters WL Jr: Comparison of two-dimensional echocardiography with gated radionuclide ventriculography in the evaluation of global and regional left ventricular function in acute myocardial infarction. *J Am Coll Cardiol* 3:243, 1984.

43. Heger JJ, Weyman AE, Wann S, Rogers EW, Dillon JC, Feigenbaum H: Cross-sectional echocardiographic analysis of extent of left ventricular asynergy in acute myocardial infarction. *Circulation* 61:1113, 1980.

44. Nishimura RA, Tajik AJ, Shub C, Miller FA, Ilstrup DM, Harrison CE: Role of two dimensional echocardiography in the prediction of in-hospital complications after acute myocardial infarction. *J Am Coll Cardiol* 4:1080, 1984.

45. Kloner RA, Parisi AF: Acute myocardial infarction: Diagnostic and prognostic applications of two-dimensional echocardiography. *Circulation* 75:521, 1987.

46. Schlichter J, Hellerstein HK, Katz LN: Aneurysm of the heart: A correlative study of 102 proved cases. *Medicine* 33:43, 1954.

47. Abrams DL, Edelist A, Luria MH, Miller AJ. Ventricular aneurysm: A reappraisal based on a study of 65 consecutive autopsied cases. *Circulation* 27:165, 1963.

48. Dubnow MH, Burchell HB, Titus JL. Postinfarction ventricular aneurysm. A clinicomorphologic and electrocardiographic study of 80 cases. *Am Heart J* 70:753, 1965.

49. Visser CA, Kan G, David GK, Lie KI, Durrer D: Echocardiographic-cineangiographic correlation in detecting left ventricular aneurysm: A prospective study of 422 patients. *Am J Cardiol* 50:337, 1982.

50. Visser CA, Kan G, Meltzer RS, Koolen JJ, Dunning AJ, Van Corler M, DeKoning H: Incidence, timing and prognostic value of left ventricular aneurysm formation after myocardial infarction: A prospective, serial echocardiographic study of 158 patients. *Am J Cardiol* 57:729, 1986.

51. Weisman HF, Healy B: Myocardial infarct expansion, infarct extension and reinfarction: Pathophysiologic concepts. *Progr Cardiovasc Dis* 30:73, 1987.

52. Weyman AE, Peskoe SM, Williams ES, Dillon JC, Feigenbaum H: Detection of left ventricular aneurysms by cross-sectional echocardiography. *Circulation* 54:936, 1976.

53. Barrett MJ, Charuzi Y, Corday E: Ventricular aneurysm: cross-sectional echocardiographic approach. *Am J Cardiol* 46:1133, 1980.

54. Baur HR, Daniel JA, Nelson RR: Detection of left ventricular aneurysm on two dimensional echocardiography. *Am J Cardiol* 50:191, 1982.

55. Wong M, Shah PM: Accuracy of two dimensional echocardiography in detecting left ventricular aneurysm. *Clin Cardiol* 6:250, 1983.

56. Gatewood RP, Nanda NC: Differentiation of left

ventricular pseudoaneurysm from true aneurysm with two-dimensional echocardiography. *Am J Cardiol* 46:869, 1980.

57. Matsumoto M, Watanabe F, Goto A, Hamano Y, Yasui K, Minamino T, Abe H, Kamada T: Left ventricular aneurysm and the prediction of left ventricular enlargement studied by two-dimensional echocardiography: Quantitative assessment of aneurysm size in relation to clinical course. *Circulation* 72:280, 1985.

58. Hutchins GM, Bulkley BH: Infarct expansion versus extension: Two different complications of acute myocardial infarction. *Am J Cardiol* 41:1127, 1978.

59. Eaton LW, Weiss JL, Bulkley BH, Garrison JB, Weisfeldt ML: Regional cardiac dilatation after acute myocardial infarction: Recognition by two-dimensional echocardiograph. *N Engl J Med* 300:57, 1979.

60. Weisman H, Bush D, Kallman C, Weisfeldt M, Bulkley B: Cellular mechanism of infarct expansion: stretch vs slippage (Abstr). *Circulation* 68 (Suppl III):III-253, 1983.

61. Erlebacher JA, Richter RC, Alonso DR, Devereux RB, Gay WA: Early infarct expansion: Structural or functional? *J Am Coll Cardiol* 6:839, 1985.

62. Pirolo JS, Hutchins GM, Moore W: Infarct expansion: Pathologic analysis of 204 patients with a single myocardial infarct. *J Am Coll Cardiol* 7:349, 1986.

63. Schuster EH, Bulkley BH: Expansion of transmural myocardial infarction: A pathophysiologic factor in cardiac rupture. *Circulation* 60:1532, 1979.

64. Merzlish JL, Berger HL, Plankey M, Errico D, Levy W, Zaret BL: Functional left ventricular aneurysm formation after acute anterior transmural myocardial infarction: Incidence, natural history and prognostic implications. *N Engl J Med* 311:1001, 1984.

65. Pierard LA, Albert A, Gilis F, Sprynger M, Carlier J, Kulbertus HE: Hemodynamic profile of patients with acute myocardial infarction at risk of infarct expansion. *Am J Cardiol* 60:5, 1987.

66. Erlebacher JA, Weiss JL, Weisfeldt ML, Bulkley BH: Early dilation of the infarcted segment in acute transmural myocardial infarction: Role of infarct expansion in acute left ventricular enlargement. *J Am Coll Cardiol* 4:201, 1984.

67. Erlebacher JA, Weiss JL, Kallman C, Weisfeldt ML, Bulkley BH: Late effects of acute infarct dilation of heart size. *Am J Cardiol* 49:1120, 1982.

68. Hochman JS, Bulkley BH: The pathogenesis of left ventricular aneurysm: An experimental study in the rat model. *Am J Cardiol* 50:83, 1982.

69. Van Tassel RA, Edwards JE: Rupture of the heart complicating myocardial infarction; analysis of 40 cases including nine examples of left ventricular false aneurysms. *Chest* 61:104, 1972.

70. Vlodaver Z, Coe JJ, Edwards JE: True and false aneurysms: Propensity for the latter to rupture. *Circulation* 51:567, 1975.

71. Roberts WC, Morrow AG: Pseudoaneurysm of the left ventricle: An unusual sequel of myocardial infarction and rupture of the heart. *Am J Med* 43:639, 1967.

72. Ersek RA, Chesler E, Korns ME, Edwards JE: Spontaneous rupture of a false left ventricular aneurysm following myocardial infarction. *Am Heart J* 77:677, 1969.

73. Catherwood E, Minz GS, Kotler MN, Parry WR, Segal BL: Two-dimensional echocardiographic recognition of left ventricular pseudoaneurysm. *Circulation* 62:294, 1980.

74. Levy R, Rozanksi A, Charuzi Y, Childs W, Waxman A, Corday E, Berman DS: Complementary roles of two-dimensional echocardiography and radionuclide ventriculography in ventricular pseudoaneurysm diagnosis. *Am Heart J* 102:1066, 1981.

75. Saner HE, Asinger RW, Daniel JA, Olson J: Two-dimensional echocardiographic identification of left ventricular pseudoaneurysm. *Am Heart J* 112:977, 1986.

76. Sanders RJ, Kern WH, Blount SG: Perforation of the interventricular septum complicating myocardial infarction. A report of eight cases. *Am Heart J* 81:736, 1956.

77. Giulianai ER, Danielson GK, Pluth JR, Odyneic NA, Wallace RB: Post-infarction ventricular septal rupture: Surgical considerations and results. *Circulation* 49:455, 1974.

78. Donahoo JS, Brawley RK, Taylor D, Gott VL: Factors influencing survival following post-infarction ventricular septal defects. *Ann Thorac Surg* 19:648, 1975.

79. Kaplan MA, Harris CN, Kay JH, Parker DP, Magidson O: Postinfarctional ventricular septal rupture. Clinical approach and surgical results. *Chest* 69:734, 1976.

80. Selzer A, Gerbode F, Kerth WJ: Clinical, hemodynamic, and surgical considerations of rupture of ventricular septum after myocardial infarction. *Am Heart J* 78:598, 1969.

81. Vlodaver Z, Edwards JE: Rupture of ventricular septum or papillary muscle complicating myocardial infarction. *Circulation* 55:815, 1977.

82. Minz GS, Victor MF, Kotler MN, Parry WR, Segal BL: Two-dimensional echocardiographic identification of surgically correctable complications of acute myocardial infarction. *Circulation* 64:91, 1981.

83. Bishop HL, Gibson RS, Stamm RB, Beller GA, Martin RP: Role of two dimensional echocardiography in the evaluation of patients with ventricular septal rupture postmyocardial infarction. *Am Heart J* 102:965, 1981.

84. Farcot JC, Boisante L, Rigand M, Bardet J, Bourdarias JP: Two-dimensional echo sector angiographic diagnosis of ventricular septal defect after acute anterior myocardial infarction. *Am J Cardiol* 45:370, 1980.

85. Drobac M, Gilbert B, Howard R, Baigrie R, Rakowski H: Ventricular septal defect after myocardial infarction: Diagnosis by two-dimensional contrast echocardiography. *Circulation* 67:335, 1983.

86. Keren G, Sherez J, Roth A, Miller H, Laniado S: Diagnosis of ventricular septal rupture from acute myocardial infarction by combined 2-dimensional and pulsed doppler echocardiography. *Am J Cardiol* 53:1202, 1984.

87. Recusani F, Raisaro A, Sgalambro A, Tronconi L, Venco A, Salerno Ardissino D: Ventricular

septal rupture after myocardial infarction: Diagnosis by two-dimensional and pulsed Doppler echocardiography. *Am J Cardiol* 54:277, 1984.

88. Miyatake K, Okamoto M, Kinoshita N, Park Y-D, Nagata S, Izumi S, Fusejima K, Sakakibara H, Nimura Y: Doppler echocardiographic features of ventricular septal rupture in myocardial infarction. *J Am Coll Cardiol* 5:182, 1985.

89. Panidis IP, Mintz GS, Goel I, McAllister M, Ross J: Acquired ventricular septal defect after myocardial infarction: Detection by combined two-dimensional and Doppler echocardiography. *Am Heart J* 111:427, 1986.

90. Naeim F, de al Maza LM, Robbins SL: Cardiac rupture during myocardial infarction: A review of 44 cases. *Circulation* 45:1231, 1972.

91. Spiekerman RE, Brandenburg JT, Achor RWP, Edwards JE. The spectrum of coronary heart disease in a community of 30,000. A clinicopathologic study. *Circulation* 25:57, 1962.

92. Schechter DC: Cardiac structural and functional changes after myocardial infarction. III. Parietal rupture and pseudoaneurysm. *NY State J Med* 74:1011, 1974.

93. Bates RJ, Beutler S, Resenkov L, Anagnostopoulos CE: Cardiac rupture—Challenge in diagnosis and management. *Am J Cardiol* 40:429, 1977.

94. Hermoni Y, Engel PJ: Two-dimensional echocardiography in cardiac rupture. *Am J Cardiol* 57:180, 1986.

95. Graber JD, Oakley CM, Pickering BN, Goodwin JF, Raphael MJ, Steiner RE: Ventricular aneurysm: An appraisal of diagnosis and surgical treatment. *Br Heart J* 34:830, 1972.

96. Jordan RA, Miller RD, Edwards JE, Parker RL: Thrombi embolism in acute and healed myocardial infarction. I. Intracardiac mural thrombus. *Circulation* 6:1, 1952.

97. Phares WS, Edwards JE, Burchell HB: Cardiac aneurysms: Clinico-pathologic studies. *Mayo Clin Proc* 28:264, 1953.

98. Yater WM, Welsh PP, Stapleton JF, Clark ML: Comparison of clinical and pathological aspects of coronary artery disease in men of various age groups: A study of 950 autopsied cases from the Armed Forces Institute of Pathology. *Ann Intern Med* 34:352, 1951.

99. Hellerstein HK, Martin JW: Incidence of thromboembolic lesions accompanying myocardial infarction. *Am Heart J* 33:443, 1947.

100. Miller RD, Jordan RA, Parker RI, Edwards JE: Thromboembolism in acute and in healed myocardial infarction. II. Systemic and pulmonary artery occlusion. *Circulation* 65:7, 1952.

101. Friedman JF, Carlson K, Marcus FI, Woulfenden JM: Clinical correlations in patients with acute myocardial infarction and left ventricular thrombus detected by two-dimensional echocardiography. *Am J Med* 72:894, 1982.

102. Keating EC, Gross SA, Schlamowitz RA, Glassman J, Mazur JH, Pitt WA, Miller D. Mural thrombi in myocardial infarctions: Prospective evaluation by two-dimensional echocardiography. *Am J Med* 74:989, 1983.

103. Weinreich DJ, Burke JF, Pauletto FJ: Left ventricular mural thrombi complicating acute myocardial infarction. *Ann Intern Med* 100:789, 1984.

104. Ezekowitz MD, Kellerman DJ: Detection of active left ventricular thrombosis during acute myocardial infarction using In-111 platelet scintigraphy. *Chest* 86:35, 1984.

105. Garvin CF: Mural thrombi in the heart. *Am Heart J* 21:713, 1941.

106. Hamby RI, Wisoff BG, Davison ET, Hartstein ML: Coronary artery disease and left ventricular mural thrombi: Clinical, hemodynamic and angiocardiographic aspects. *Chest* 66:488, 1974.

107. Reeder GS, Tajik AJ, Seward JB: Left ventricular mural thrombus: Two-dimensional echocardiographic diagnosis. *Mayo Clin Proc* 56:82, 1981.

108. Stratton JR, Lighty GW, Pearlman AS, Ritchie JL: Detection of left ventricular thrombus by two dimensional echocardiography: Sensitivity, specificity and causes of uncertainty. *Circulation* 66:156, 1982.

109. DeMaria AN, Bommer W, Neumann A, Grehl T, Weinart L, deNardo S, Amsterdam E, Mason D: Left ventricular thrombi identified by cross-sectional echocardiography. *Ann Intern Med* 90:14, 1979.

110. Asinger RW, Mikell RL, Sharma B, Hodges M: Observations on detecting left ventricular thrombus with two-dimensional echocardiography: Emphasis on avoidance of false positive diagnosis. *Am J Cardiol* 47:145, 1981.

111. Mikell FL, Asinger RW, Eisperger J, Anderson WR, Hodges M: Regional stasis of blood in the dysfunctional left ventricle: Echocardiographic detection and differentiation from early thrombosis. *Circulation* 66:755, 1982.

112. Cabin HS, Roberts WC: Left ventricular aneurysm, intraaneurysmal thrombus and systemic embolus in coronary heart disease. *Chest* 77:586, 1980.

113. Takagi Y, Okumachi F, Yoshida K, Kato H, Yanagihara K, Yoshikawa J: Cross-sectional echocardiographic features of mobile left ventricular thrombi. *J Cardiography* 11:957, 1981.

114. Haugland JM, Asinger RW, Mikell FL, Elsperger J, Hodges M: Embolic potential of left ventricular thrombus detected by two dimensional echocardiography (Abstr). *Am J Cardiol* 47:471, 1981.

115. Meltzer RS, Visser CA, Kan G, Roelandt J: Two-dimensional echocardiographic appearance of left ventricular thrombi with systemic emboli after myocardial infarction. *Am J Cardiol* 53:1511, 1984.

116. Godley RW, Wann LS, Rogers EW, Feigenbaum H, Weyman AE: Incomplete mitral leaflet closure in patients with papillary muscle dysfunction. *Circulation* 63:565, 1981.

117. Rider CF, Taylor DEM, Wade JD: The effect of papillary muscle damage on atrioventricular valve function in the left heart. *Am Exp Physiol* 50:15, 1965.

118. Tsakaris AG, Rastelli GC, Amorim D, Titus JL, Wood EM: Effects of papillary muscle damage on mitral valve closure in infarct anesthetized dogs. *Mayo Clin Proc* 45:275, 1970.

119. Kinney EL, Frangi MJ: Value of two dimensional echocardiographic detection of incomplete mitral leaflet closure. *Am Heart J* 109:87, 1985.

120. Wei JY, Hutchins GM, Bulkley BH: Papillary muscle rupture in fatal acute myocardial infarction. A potentially treatable form of cardiogenic shock. *Ann Intern Med* 90:149, 1979.

121. Nishimura RA, Schaff HV, Shub C, Gersh BJ, Edwards WD, Tajik AJ: Papillary muscle rupture complicating acute myocardial infarction: Analysis of 17 patients. *Am J Cardiol* 51:373, 1983.

122. Barbour DJ, Roberts WC: Rupture of a left ventricular papillary muscle during acute myocardial infarction: Analysis of 22 necropsy patients. *J Am Coll Cardiol* 8:558, 1986.

123. Sanders RJ, Neubuerger KT, Ravin A: Rupture of papillary muscles: Occurrence of rupture of the posterior muscle in posterior myocardial infarction. *Dis Chest* 31:316, 1957.

124. Vlodaver Z, Edwards JE: Rupture of ventricular septum or papillary muscle complicating myocardial infarction. *Circulation* 55:815, 1977.

125. Wackers FJT, Lie KI, Sokole EB, Res J, van der Schoot JB, Durrer D: Prevalence of right ventricular involvement in inferior wall infarction assessed with myocardial imaging with thallium-291 and technetium-99 m pyrophosphate. *Am J Cardiol* 42:358, 1978.

126. Isner JM, Roberts WC: Right ventricular infarction complicating left ventricular infarction secondary to coronary heart disease. Frequency, location, associated findings and significance from analysis of 236 necropsy patients with acute or healed myocardial infarctions. *Am J Cardiol* 42:885, 1978.

127. Wartman WB, Hellerstein HK: The incidence of heart disease in 2000 consecutive autopsies. *Ann Intern Med* 28:41, 1948.

128. Gerwitz H, Gold HK, Fallon JT, Pasternak RC, Leinbach RC: Role of right ventricular infarction in cardiogenic shock associated with inferior myocardial infarction. *Br Heart J* 42:719, 1979.

129. Cohn JN, Guiha NH, Broder MI, Limas CJ: Right ventricular infarction. Clinical and hemodynamic features. *Am J Cardiol* 33:209, 1974.

130. Sclarovsky S, Zafrir N, Strasberg B, Kracoff O, Lewin RF, Arditi A, Rosen KM, Agmon J: Ventricular fibrillation complicating temporary ventricular pacing in acute myocardial infarction. Significance of right ventricular infarction. *Am J Cardiol* 48:1160, 1981.

131. Karagueuzian HS, Sugi K, Ohta M, Fishbein MC, Mandel WJ, Peter T: Inducible sustained ventricular tachycardia and ventricular fibrillation in conscious dogs with isolated right ventricular infarction. Relation to infarct structure. *J Am Coll Cardiol* 7:850, 1986.

132. D'Arcy B, Nanda NC: Two-dimensional echocardiographic features of right ventricular infarction. *Circulation* 65:167, 1982.

133. Marmor A, Geltman EM, Biello DR, Sobel BE, Siegel BA, Roberts R: Functional response of the right ventricle to myocardial infarction: Dependence on the site of left ventricular infarction. *Circulation* 64:1005, 1981.

134. Stowers SA, Leiboff RH, Wasserman AG, Katz R, Bren G, Hsu I: Right ventricular thrombus formation in association with acute myocardial infarction: Diagnosis by 2-dimensional echocardiography. *Am J Cardiol* 52:912, 1983.

135. Lopez-Sendon J, Garcia-Fernandez MA, Coma-Canella I, Yanguela MN, Banuelos F: Segmental right ventricular function after acute myocardial infarction: Two-dimensional echocardiographic study in 63 patients. *Am J Cardiol* 51:390, 1983.

136. Jugdutt BI, Sussex BA, Sivaram CA, Rossall RE: Right ventricular infarction: Two-dimensional echocardiographic evaluation. *Am Heart J* 107:505, 1984.

137. Klein HO, Tordjman T, Ninio R, Sareli P, Oren V, Lang R, Gefen J, Pauzner C, DiSegni E, David D, Kaplinsky E: The early recognition of right ventricular infarction: Diagnostic accuracy of the electrocardiographic V_4R lead. *Circulation* 67:558, 1983.

138. Legrand V, Rigo P, Smetts JP, Demoulin JC, Collignon P, Kulbertus HE: Right ventricular myocardial infarction diagnosed by 99-m technetium pyrophosphate scintigraphy: Clinical course and follow-up *Eur Heart J* 4:9, 1983.

139. Schofer J, Stritzke P, Becher H, Montz R, Bleifeld W, Mathey G: Scintigraphic evidence that right ventricular myocardium tolerates ischemia better than left ventricular myocardium. *Circulation* 68 (Suppl III):392, 1983.

140. Bellamy GR, Rasmussen HH, Nasser FN, Wiseman JC, Cooper RA: Value of two-dimensional echocardiography, electrocardiography, and clinical signs in detecting right ventricular infarction. *Am Heart J* 112:304, 1986.

141. Panidis ID, Kotler MN, Mintz GS, Ross J, Ren JF, Herling J, Kutalek S: Right ventricular function in coronary artery disease as assessed by two-dimensional echocardiography. *Am Heart J* 107:1187, 1984.

142. Friedman HZ, Buda AJ: Biventricular thrombus formation in association with acute myocardial infarction: Diagnosis by two-dimensional echocardiography. *J Clin Ultrasound* 14:315, 1986.

143. Manno BV, Bemis CE, Carver J, Mintz GS: Right ventricular infarction complicated by right to left shunt. *J Am Coll Cardiol* 1:554, 1983.

16

Evaluation of Cardiomyopathies

Robert E. Fowles, M.D.
Robert A. Quaife, M.D.

INTRODUCTION

Cardiomyopathies are suited ideally for study by ultrasound. These myocardial disorders of various and unknown causes are at this point probably best understood and described in practical anatomic and functional terms, rather than by specific pathophysiologic concepts. Several classification schemes for cardiomyopathies have been developed. Myocardial disease may be classified by etiology, such as viral, toxic, or ischemic causes. However, in the strictest sense, the term *cardiomyopathy* should be reserved for heart muscle ailments of unknown cause.

Cardiomyopathies are often grouped according to pathophysiology, resulting in the terms congestive, obstructive, or restrictive. Morphologic classification is based upon anatomic abnormalities, as in dilated, hypertrophic, or obliterative. Since echocardiography excels in capturing the anatomic and geometric patterns of the heart, ultrasound examination of cardiomyopathies is best suited to the morphologic classification system.

Dilated cardiomyopathy lends itself particularly well to both clinical and research applications of echocardiography. After all, in its simplest analysis, echocardiography reveals the hallmark features of dilated cardiomyopathy—an enlarged, diffusely hypocontractile left ventricle. Cardiac ultrasound is a reliable, safe, and relatively inexpensive imaging technique that can provide the following information regarding structure and function in dilated cardiomyopathy:

1. Measurement of cardiac dimensions and contractile performance;
2. Description of geometric features;
3. Differentiation of dilated cardiomyopathy from other heart muscle disorders, such as hypertrophic cardiomyopathy;
4. Exclusion of other primary cardiac abnormalities such as valvular disease;
5. Serial follow-up of cardiac status with regard to either clinical deterioration or evaluation of various treatments;
6. Detection of certain complications of cardiomyopathy;
7. Determination of several hemodynamic correlates, such as venous and pulmonary hypertension, systolic function, cardiac output changes, and diastolic filling patterns.

ECHOCARDIOGRAPHIC FEATURES OF DILATED CARDIOMYOPATHY

Morphologic Patterns

Echocardiographic features of dilated cardiomyopathy are distinct. Morphologic and geometric patterns are easily evident on two-dimensional echocardiography (1). For example, the usually ellipsoid, cross-sectional, long-axis shape of the left ventricle becomes more spherical (Fig. 16.1). Left ventricular dilation may be so extensive that the chamber's internal minor axis diameter can increase by 50–100% (2, 3). End-systolic dimensions are elevated markedly and differ little from end-diastolic measurements, reflecting diffuse reduction of contractile performance. Within the cavernous left ventricle, the mitral leaflets are separated markedly from the septal and posterior endocardial surfaces.

Mitral valve anterior leaflet-septal separation is a sign of both global ventricular dilation and hypokinesis (4). End-diastolic absolute thicknesses of the anteroseptal and free posterior left ventricular walls most often are normal or only mildly increased, but relative to the degree of chamber dilation they appear quite thinned. However, total left ventricular mass is significantly greater than normal, due to the combi-

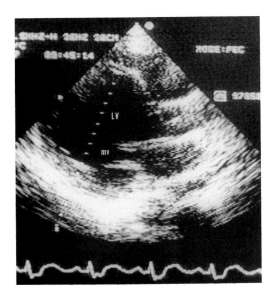

Figure 16.1. Dilated cardiomyopathy, parasternal long-axis view. The left ventricle (*LV*) is round rather than ellipsoid, and the minor axis diameter measures almost 10 cm. The mitral valve (*mv*) and its leaflet excursion are dwarfed by the left ventricular dilation, but left atrial size is normal.

nation of profound chamber dilation and compensatory hypertrophy (5). Pericardial effusion is uncommon and, if present, is typically very small and is not a significant influence on left ventricular function. Left atrial volume may range from normal to markedly increased, but is usually proportionately less than that of the left ventricle. Right ventricular and right atrial enlargement vary, depending on duration and severity of disease, and reflect right heart failure (Fig. 16.2).

M-Mode versus Two-Dimensional Echocardiography

M-mode echocardiography is still highly useful in dilated cardiomyopathy, especially for measurement of various dimensions and indices. One of the strengths of M-mode recording is its relatively exact portrayal of dynamically changing events along a geometrically unidimensional axis, displayed with respect to time. Examples include fractional shortening (FS) and mitral E-point-septal separation (MEPSS). The time-dependent aspects of these parameters are appreciated more easily on M-mode echograms.

The development of two-dimensional echocardiography extended, rather than replaced, M-mode

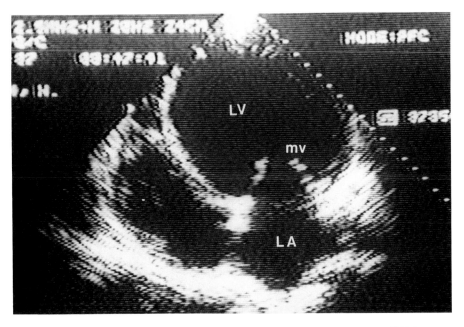

Figure 16.2. Dilated cardiomyopathy, apical four-chamber view. The left ventricle (*LV*) is extremely enlarged, with a minor axis diameter of 10 cm. Note the round shape of the left ventricle and the relatively smaller appearing mitral valve (*mv*) and left atrium (*LA*).

recording. The major strength of two-dimensional scanning is spatial representation. Two-dimensional imaging can direct the M-mode beam through optimally chosen segments, enhancing the quality of unidimensional, time-swept data. Also, two-dimensional imaging can detect and clarify certain anatomic and functional features of dilated cardiomyopathy better than does M-mode recording (1). These features include the spherical, globular nature of dilation and other three-dimensional aspects; the shape and dilation of the mitral annulus; the extent and nature of hypertrophy; and endomyocardial topography, such as trabeculations. Other features include the presence of thrombus and the diffuseness of hypocontractility versus some elements of asynergy, which are seen sometimes in dilated cardiomyopathy.

Differentiating Types of Cardiomyopathy

Cardiomyopathies are diverse in pathophysiology and morphology. In attempts to grapple with this diversity as well as to explain the genesis of some myocardial diseases, cardiomyopathies have been organized according to various classification schemes. The system most compatible with echocardiography is morphologic classification. Thus, "congestive" cardiomyopathy is more aptly categorized as dilated, with the enlarged, hypokinetic left ventricle causing a range of symptoms, only some of which may be "congestive." Hypertrophic cardiomyopathy is just that—thickened ventricular walls without chamber dilation, with systolic performance usually normal or even excessive (6) (Fig. 16.3). As defined morphologically, even a freeze-frame, two-dimensional echocardiographic image will reveal these respective abnormalities in dilated and hypertrophic cardiomyopathy.

Other primary myocardial diseases are not quite as evident from two-dimensional images alone. Cardiomyopathies whose major pathophysiologic feature is reduction of ventricular filling are termed restrictive. This is typified hemodynamically by elevated end-diastolic pressure, often occurring relatively early in diastole. This results in a "square root" pattern in a pressure tracing. Restriction may be caused by a variety of pathologic conditions.

The physiologic flaw of restriction is a phenomenon that does not lend itself to echocardiographic imaging. Morphologically, ventricular size, ventricular shape, and systolic performance usually are normal, at least in early stages. This later progresses to dilation, though not as great as in dilated cardiomyopathy. However, some echocardiographic clues often are available. The ventricular abnormalities in restrictive cardiomyopathies may be revealed by careful examination of good quality ultrasonic imaging (Fig. 16.4).

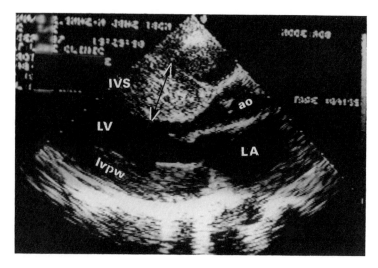

Figure 16.3. Asymmetric hypertrophic cardiomyopathy. In this long-axis parasternal view, the interventricular septum (*IVS*) measures 3.5 cm, and the left ventricular posterior wall (*lvpw*) measures 1 cm. Left ventricular (*LV*) cavity diameter at end-diastole is small at 3 cm, and left atrial size is slightly increased with a diameter of 4.5 cm, especially in relation to the aorta (*ao*).

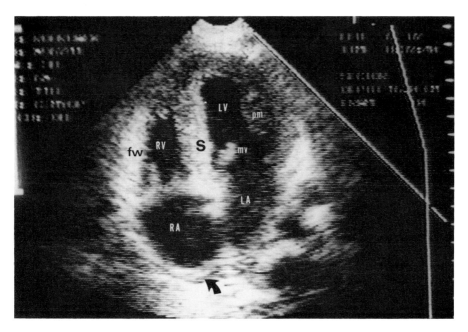

Figure 16.4. Restrictive cardiomyopathy. Cardiac amyloidosis is shown in this four-chamber view. Both left ventricular (*LV*) and right ventricular (*RV*) cavity sizes are normal. The right atrium (*RA*) is enlarged, as is the left atrium (*LA*) (not fully open to view in this figure). Papillary muscle (*pm*), septum (*S*), and right ventricular free wall (*fw*) are all thickened. The mitral valve (*mv*) leaflets are thickened as well, and a small pericardial effusion is indicated around the right atrium by the *black arrow*.

The typical morphologic and functional distinctions between cardiomyopathies can be confounded occasionally by apparent overlaps between types. For example, congestive heart failure may present with diffuse hypocontractility but only mild left ventricular dilation. This condition, termed mildly dilated congestive cardiomyopathy, has been reported in a minority of patients requiring cardiac transplantation (7) and may be confused with restrictive cardiomyopathy. A new type of cardiomyopathy—called nondilated, nonhypertrophic—has been proposed to incorporate these cases, which can be identified by clinical and echocardiographic means. Just as nondilated hearts may on first inspection appear to mimic restrictive cardiomyopathy, dilated cardiomyopathy may in the course of disease manifest restrictive characteristics.

Infiltrative disorders causing restrictive cardiomyopathy can be divided into processes causing interstitial abnormalities or intracellular depositions. The interstitial abnormalities include amyloidosis, mucopolysaccharidosis, sarcoidosis, and fibrosis. Intracellular depositions include iron, glycogen, and lipids.

The most common restrictive cardiomyopathy in the United States is amyloidosis, in which relatively normal myocardial cells and fibers are encased in an infiltrating proteinaceous substance, preventing normal diastolic relaxation and other cardiac functions. Echocardiographically, amyloid may be recognized by its somewhat characteristic features: a relatively small or normal ventricular cavity size, thickened right and left ventricular walls, dilated atria, and often pericardial effusion. However, these features are not specific, and the same constellation may be seen in hypertrophic cardiomyopathies and renal disease. Furthermore, advanced cases may progress to ventricular dilation.

Ultrasonic inspection of myocardial amyloidosis reveals rather diffuse myocardial involvement as a rule. Impressive thickening is seen throughout, including the right ventricular free wall, papillary muscles atrial septum, and even valvular leaflets (8, 9). Many echocardiographers observe a subjective textural change, described as a "glistening" or "sparkling" quality, to the myocardial image (9). This rather vague, descriptive approach results from a current lack of more specific or objective means of describing the curious visual abnormality often produced by amyloid infiltration and rendered by video reproduction of ultrasonic output.

Other infiltrative cardiomyopathies have an even less characteristic echocardiographic appearance than amyloidosis. Myocardial sarcoidosis may be detected by echocardiography, but findings are nonspecific. The interventricular septum is commonly involved with sarcoid granulomas, leading to either increased thickness or thinning in the case of scarring. Left ventricular dilation and hypokinesis, as well as right ventricular changes, may occur when pulmonary involvement has led to cor pulmonale. Endocardial fibrosis may be revealed by increased reflectance along the cavity-myocardial interface (10). Cardiac hemochromatosis most often is accompanied by echocardiographic changes of left ventricular dilation, normal wall thickness, and decreased contractility. However, in early stages it may show less severe abnormalities. Perhaps the greatest value of echocardiography is the ability to examine left ventricular appearance and function as treatment proceeds, such as phlebotomy for iron removal in the case of hemochromatosis (11).

Storage disorders of glycogen and lipids, such as Pompe's, Cori's, and Fabry's disease, may be accompanied by profound but not necessarily diagnostic cardiac abnormalities. These include increased wall thickness, normal ventricular cavity diameters, and varying systolic function. Fabry's disease, an X-linked recessive defect in glycolipid metabolism, may manifest a granular, sparkling myocardial appearance similar to amyloidosis. For heritable myocardial diseases, echocardiography may serve as a noninvasive technique for screening kindred.

Restrictive cardiomyopathy may be produced by space-occupying lesions that reduce diastolic filling by infiltrating myocardial tissue and actually obliterating part of the ventricular cavity. The most prominent example of obliterative-restrictive cardiomyopathy is Loeffler's syndrome. These disorders are quite rare in temperate climes but have been detected and described echocardiographically (10, 12).

Valvular anatomy in restrictive cardiomyopathy is usually normal. However, the valvular supporting apparatus, annulus, or portions of leaflets themselves occasionally may be involved by the infiltrative process, sometimes affecting function. Independent of leaflet anatomic lesions, abnormal ventricular filling in restrictive cardiomyopathy may secondarily alter atrioventricular valve dynamics. The application of Doppler techniques to echocardiography has been particularly helpful in bridging the gap between ultrasonic imaging and physiology. Doppler echocardiography in dilated cardiomyopathy is described later in this chapter.

In the future, infiltrative myocardial disorders may be detected and differentiated better by the use of ultrasonic tissue characterization methods. If so, the horizon of echocardiography will be expanded from the gross world of whole organ morphology into the realm of myocardial composition. Most existing work on tissue characterization has been carried out in ischemic myocardial disease, such as acute, experimental ischemia (13), infarction and fibrosis (14), and reperfusion (15, 16). Reflection, or backscatter, of ultrasound from myocardium is dependent on many properties. The cardiac cycle itself affects backscatter, with maximum reflectance at end-diastole and the minimum at end-systole. Intrinsic contractility and elasticity are probably involved in this cycle dependence and are affected by either ischemia or cardiomyopathy. Calcification certainly increases backscatter, as does deposition of collagen or, probably, other substances such as amyloid. Recent application of quantitative ultrasonic tissue characterization to human patients has differentiated normal myocardium from that of dilated cardiomyopathy (17).

For several years qualitative observations have opened the door to ultrasonic tissue characterization in cardiomyopathies. Alterations in myocardial appearance have been reported in hypertrophic cardiomyopathy (a "ground glass" septal texture or "highly refractile echoes"), amyloidosis ("sparkling or "glistening"), and storage diseases and dilated cardiomyopathy. Lack of specificity limits the usefulness of such subjective, qualitative observations and points out the need for more quantiative methods. Quantitation of ultrasonically gathered data is the subject of currently active research and proceeds along two avenues: (a) measurement of directly obtained radio frequency acoustic parameters, such as backscatter, and statistical treatment and digital analysis of either radio frequency data, or (b) video image features.

NONINVASIVE EVALUATION OF SYSTOLIC FUNCTION IN DILATED CARDIOMYOPATHY

Echocardiographic Imaging and Measurement

Evaluating systolic performance is an important aspect of echocardiographic examination of the left ventricle. Echocardiography is useful in making the diagnosis of dilated cardiomyopathy, quantifying the severity of the disorder, and following its course. The advantages of ultrasonic examination of systolic performance are that it is noninvasive, easily repeatable, highly portable, and relatively inexpensive.

Measurement of left ventricular cavity dimensions in diastole and systole constitutes the foundation for echocardiographic observation of systolic function. As an ellipsoid three-dimensional shape, the left ventricular cavity's cyclically changing volume is most readily transected ultrasonically through its minor axis. That minor axis left ventricular internal diameter (LVID) is conventionally measured through midcavity just distal to the mitral leaflet tips. This usually encompasses the space between the left side of the anterior interventricular septum and the left ventricular posterior endocardium. Systolic fractional shortening (FS) is expressed as

$$FS\ (\%) = \frac{(LVID_{ed} - LVID_{es})}{LVID_{ed}} \times 100 \quad 16.1$$

where ed and es = end-diastolic and end-systolic measurements of LVID. FS is the simplest and most direct M-mode echocardiographic parameter expressing systolic function. Obviously, for FS to accurately represent the general state of the whole left ventricle, diffusely uniform contraction must be present. This is the case in most cardiomyopathies.

With progressive left ventricular enlargement in dilated cardiomyopathy, the chamber becomes more globular or rounded. This increased sphericity may magnify discrepancies between M-mode echocardiographically measured FS and angiographically determined ejection fraction (EF) (18). In general, however, if left ventricular volume overload disorders such as valvular regurgitation are excluded, agreement between echocardiographic FS and angiographic EF is good ($r = 0.82$) (18).

Clinically, left ventricular EF is the most universally used parameter to characterize left ventricular systolic performance. Echocardiographic measurement of EF demands a three-dimensional approach or set of assumptions, since

$$EF = \frac{\begin{array}{c}\text{End-diastolic volume} \\ - \text{ end-systolic volume}\end{array}}{\text{End-diastolic volume}} \quad 16.2$$

A few methods have been developed to estimate left ventricular cavity volume from M-mode echocardiographically measured dimensions (19, 20). Two-dimensional echocardiography allows a more comprehensive approximation of volume, usually calculated as a rotation of cross-sectional area from one or more planes of examination.

Other parameters may have certain advantages in measuring systolic function. By including left ventricular ejection time (determined from either phonocardiography or M-mode aortic valve echocardiography), one can calculate velocity of circumferential fiber shortening (V_{CF}) (21), which can be a theoretically superior index. Still other systolic performance parameters can be derived from M-mode measurement, including the maximal rate of displacement of the posterior left ventricular endocardial echo (3) and normalized mean rates of systolic wall thickening (22–24). Some of these parameters appear to allow distinction between ischemic myocardial disease and dilated cardiomyopathy. M-mode echocardiographic studies have found early systolic closure of the aortic valve to be more pronounced in patients with dilated cardiomyopathy than in normal subjects, indicating yet another approach to examining systolic function (25). Exercise may enhance the ability of M-mode measurements to discriminate between various types of myocardial impairment (26).

M-mode-derived or unidimensional measurements have been used in dilated cardiomyopathy to assess the interrelationship between chamber size or shape and left ventricular mechanics. An example is the calculation of left ventricular mass as well as meridional wall stress from simultaneous measurements of M-mode dimensions and left ventricular or systemic pressures (27). As encouraging as these methods are in assessing ejection fraction and fractional shortening, in examining systolic performance it is desirable to detect changes in intrinsic myocardial contractility as accurately as possible, apart from varying loading conditions. Myocardial contractility appears to be well represented in a relatively preload-independent fashion by the left ventricular end-systolic wall stress-velocity of fiber shortening relation (28). This sensitive contractility index is obtained noninvasively by combining M-mode echocardiographic and carotid pulse tracings of the subject at rest. Varying afterload is incorporated into the index as end-systolic meridional wall stress. An apparently depressed level of contractility can be distinguished from normal performance burdened by increased afterload, as the above relationship relates the appropriateness of V_{CF} for given wall stress. The index appears to be useful in situations of varying preload.

A good example of the sensitivity of wall stress-myocardial shortening relations has been reported in patients receiving the cardiotoxic antineoplastic agent doxorubicin (29). Otherwise inapparent depression of intrinsic myocardial contractility was detected in approximately one-half of the patients with low-normal fractional shortening (28–30%) by examining the end-systolic wall stress-fractional shortening relation. This deterioration in contractility had been offset by reduced afterload as reflected by reduced meridional wall stress, leading to values for fractional shortening in the low-normal range. The slope value of the end-systolic pressure-dimension relation and the position of the left ventricular end-systolic wall stress-percent fractional shortening relation are noninvasively obtainable, reproducible, and sensitive indices of intrinsic contractility. They appear to be independent of preload and afterload and allow serial comparison over time between patients of differing age and size.

Doppler echocardiography gives further means for measuring left ventricular systolic performance. Blood flow can be examined across a cross-sectional area of left ventricular outflow tract, aortic valve or annulus, or proximal ascending aorta. Measurable parameters include peak flow velocity, acceleration time, average acceleration, ejection time, flow velocity integral, deceleration time, and average deceleration. These values are obtained from the Doppler velocity waveform and represent various facets of left ventricular performance. Angiographic left ventricular ejection fraction correlates well ($r = 0.77$) with continous wave Doppler-derived peak flow velocity and still better with peak acceleration (30). Peak aortic flow velocity and aortic flow velocity integral have been shown to clearly identify dilated cardiomyopathy patients whose values for these parameters are one-half those of normal subjects (31).

Relatively straightforward Doppler echocardiographic methods can yield accurate measurements of stroke volume. For each systolic cycle, or stroke, the flow velocity integral (FVI) can be measured as the area under the Doppler velocity profile, expressed as (cm/sec) $\times$ sec = cm. Multipled by the cross-sectional area (A) (in cm^2) across which systolic flow occurs, FVI (cm) $\times$ A (cm^2) becomes stroke volume (cm^3). Using M-mode echocardiographic measurement of aortic leaflet early systolic separation as the diameter of a circular cross-sectional outflow area, the above product, FVI $\times$ A, correlates impressively ($r = 0.95$) with thermodilution-obtained stroke volume (32). Since cardiomyopathy patients are usually free of aortic leaflet disease, such methods are simple and apparently accurate, noninvasive ways to measure cardiac output. The Doppler method may underestimate peak velocity, since obliquity between the interrogating beam and blood flow will diminish measured velocity as the cosine of the angle between beam and flow. Several ultrasonic windows are used to find the maximum velocity. Doppler echocardiographic measurement is sensitive to changes in stroke volume that may result from interventions such as afterload reduction (32–34).

NONINVASIVE EVALUATION OF DIASTOLIC DYNAMICS IN DILATED CARDIOMYOPATHY

Relationships between left ventricular diastolic filling parameters and symptoms of congestive or dilated cardiomyopathies have been reemphasized recently. Patients with dilated cardiomyopathies have abnormal diastolic function determined by invasive measurement of left ventricular pressure-volume relationships, reduced negative dp/dt, and prolonged time constant of pressure curves. Such data have supported the notion of impaired diastolic ventricular relaxation in dilated cardiomyopathies (35, 36). Until now, assessment of left ventricular filling dynamics required invasive procedures. Doppler echocardiography combined with two-dimensional echocardiography affords noninvasive investigation of volume-pressure relationships necessary for characterization of diastolic function (37).

Just as Doppler echocardiography measures systolic function, or left ventricular outflow, it can quantitate various parameters of inflow or filling. Formerly, left ventricular cineangiography was required to measure diastolic function. Combined Doppler echocardiography and two-dimensional ultrasonic imaging at the mitral valve annulus yields the following:

1. Peak filling rate (ml/sec): the product of early diastolic filling velocity and cross-sectional area of mitral annulus.
2. Normalized filling rate (sec^{-1}): the ratio of peak filling rate to end-diastolic volume, EDV (EDV = $(3.42 \times L \times D_{max}) - 6.44$, where L is the greatest diastolic long-axis measurement from the apical four-chamber view, and D_{max} is the greatest diastolic minor axis diameter measured from apical or parasternal views);
3. Half-filling fraction: the time velocity integral (TVI) over the first half of the diastolic filling period, divided by the total diastolic TVI;
4. Volume/time curves, from which instantaneous slope can be derived to give time-dependent or peak dV/dt.

Comparative studies such as that by Rokey et al. (38), in which these parameters were measured, have shown the combination of two-dimensional and Doppler echocardiography to be comparable in accuracy to invasive catheterization and angiography. Reduced early diastolic filling usually is accompanied by increased atrioventricular inflow velocity, causing a reversal of the usual E and A amplitudes (35, 38, 39).

The primary limitations of combined two-dimensional and Doppler techniques rest in the accuracy of determining cross-sectional mitral annulus area and left ventricular end-diastolic volume (38, 40). Also, pathologic sources of ventricular filling, such as shunts or aortic regurgitation, may introduce error (35, 38, 40).

Diastolic function may be assessed by Doppler echocardiography without two-dimensional imaging. Doppler waveform analysis shows that the E wave amplitude or early diastolic peak velocity and the duration of Doppler early flow correlate with early, passive ventricular filling as determined by radionuclide angiography (41). The ratio (E/A) of early diastolic filling velocity (E) to atrial filling velocity (A) correlates with similar radionuclide-measured (37) and catheterization-determined parameters (42). Other Doppler-determined values correlate even better with radionuclide measurements, including diastolic filling period and interval from end-systole to peak early diastolic flow (37).

Dilated cardiomyopathy patients make up only a fraction of the subjects in most of the afore-mentioned studies. Takenaka et al. evaluated 33 patients with dilated cardiomyopathy, using pulsed Doppler echocardiography (35, 39). Early diastolic peak mitral flow velocity, atrial flow velocity, and the ratio (E/A) of the two were assessed. Dilated cardiomyopathy patients without mitral regurgitation had significantly lower early diastolic peak flow velocity and E/A ratio compared to normal subjects. The presence of mitral regurgitation seems to obscure this distinction (35, 39).

Noninvasive evaluation of diastolic function can be accomplished on a beat-to-beat basis and yields acceptable correlation with the invasive gold standards, catheterization and angiography, as well as with other techniques such as radionuclide studies (35–37, 39, 41). Doppler echocardiography is essential to successful determination of diastolic function, since M-mode echocardiography, apex cardiography, and phonocardiography appear to be insensitive in both ischemic myocardial disease and dilated cardiomyopathy (36).

Ventricular diastolic function is a complex phenomenon determined by many factors, including intrinsic myocardial properties, loading conditions, and ventricular relaxation. The accuracy of two-dimensional and Doppler echocardiography in assessing diastolic function depends on imaging quality and may be compromised by valvular regurgitation, tachycardia, pericardial disease, and right ventricular compression. However, current interest in diastolic properties of cardiomyopathies and in the effects of various interventions, especially pharmacologic, promises to enhance noninvasive examination even further.

PATHOLOGICAL CONDITIONS ASSOCIATED WITH CARDIOMYOPATHY
Thrombi

In dilated cardiomyopathy the enlarged, hypocontractile chambers constitute a prothrombotic milieu. Left ventricular thrombi can be seen by echocardiography in most cases (Fig. 16.5). The classic appearance of a distinct, rounded mass attached to the left ventricular wall and protruding into the cavity is practically diagnostic on two-dimensional echocardiography and is superior to the usually vague "filling defect" sometimes seen with contrast ventriculography.

Since clots adhere to the endocardial surface, sometimes differentiation between mural thrombus and myocardium may be difficult. This is especially true if the clot does not protrude much

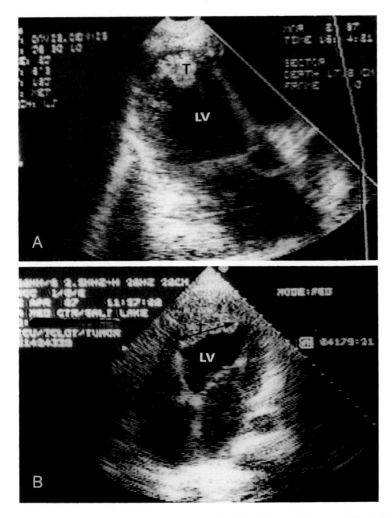

Figure 16.5. Mural thrombi in dilated cardiomyopathy. *A*, Apical long-axis view of the left ventricle (*LV*), in which a discrete globular thrombus (*T*) is seen in the apex. *B*, A different case, with a mural-adherent left ventricular (*LV*) thrombus (*T*) that lies along 5 cm of the apical and septal segments in this four-chamber view.

into the chamber cavity, the thrombus has undergone some degree of organization, or increased wall trabeculation is present. Often, clots form in the apex, where they may be detected less easily but should still be distinguishable from anatomic variations seen even in normal hearts. These normal variants include accessory chordae tendineae and muscular bands or bridges. Two-dimensional echocardiography has (*a*) a high predictive value for the absence of clots and (*b*) good sensitivity and specificity for left ventricular thrombi. Left atrial clots are visualized less easily.

The prevalence of thrombus formation has not been clearly defined in dilated cardiomyopathy.

Results from a limited series of echocardiographically studied patients suggest variable percentages of thrombosis in dilated cardiomyopathy (43, 44). However, likelihood of thromboembolic events in dilated cardiomyopathy is substantial enough to warrant consideration of prophylactic systemic anticoagulation, based on an estimated equivalent of a 3.5% yearly incidence (45). Once their presence is detected, disappearance of thrombi may also be observed by ultrasound (46).

New developments in cardiac ultrasound promise to improve our ability to detect thrombus or the setting in which thrombosis is more likely to occur. By analyzing the radio frequency ultrasound backscatter or by statistically processing the video image, tissue signature techniques may allow more certain differentation between thrombus and myocardium (47). Low velocity blood flow, reflecting relative stagnation within a dilated cardiac chamber, can be detected ultrasonically. In two-dimensional imaging, localized stasis may produce a curious pattern of swirling echo reflectances that are clearly differentiable from formed thrombus (48). The enhanced dynamic and spatial imaging afforded by color flow Doppler techniques may also identify low velocity flow conditions more favorable to thrombosis in the left ventricle (49).

Ventriculoatrial Regurgitation

Mitral regurgitation is a common accompaniment to dilated cardiomyopathy. Leaflet appearance is usually unremarkable, without prolapse of chordal abnormalities. Doppler pulsed wave mapping and color flow display disclose relatively mild regurgitation in proportion to the degree of left ventricular dilation and hypokinesis (Fig. 16.6). Mitral annular dilation appears to be a component of the mechanism of valvular insufficiency, which is secondary or functional (50).

Tricuspid insufficiency accompanies right ventricular dilation, and the mechanism is probably the same as for secondary mitral regurgitation. As in the case of mitral insufficiency, current Doppler techniques allow semiquantitative estimation of severity.

Pulmonary Hypertension

An additional bonus in the case of tricuspid insufficiency is the ability of Doppler echocardiography to estimate right ventricular and, hence, pulmonary, systolic peak pressures (51). This is performed using the simplified Bernoulli equation:

$$P_{grad} = 4v^2 \qquad 16.3$$

where P_{grad} = pressure gradient across a defined orifice and v^2 = peak velocity of blood flow across that orifice. Peak right ventricular systolic pressure (and hence that of the pulmonary artery in the absence of pulmonic stenosis) is the pressure gradient across the tricuspid valve plus estimated or measured right atrial/central venous pressure. As interventions are applied, the detection and quantification of pulmonary hypertension in dilated cardiomyopathy and heart failure may be clinically highly useful.

Pericardial Effusion

Significant pericardial effusion is rare in dilated cardiomyopathy. Small amounts of pericardial fluid are not unusual, but moderate to large effusions should raise suspicion of complicating factors or specific etiology.

Specific Disorders

The term *dilated cardiomyopathy*, speaking strictly, is reserved for myocardial disease of unknown origin. Practically considered, many may avoid this purist approach, since exact diagnosis in the case of a large, poorly contractile left ventricle appears much less important than therapy, which is the same for almost all such cases anyway. However, it is important to rule out disorders that are otherwise potentially treatable,

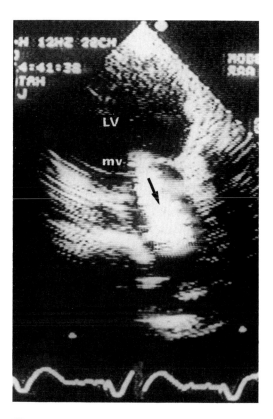

Figure 16.6. Mitral regurgitation in dilated cardiomyopathy. In this apical view of the dilated left ventrilce (*LV*) retrograde flow across the mitral valve (*mv*) is shown by the *arrow*. In black and white, the color flow Doppler image of the regurgitation is a white cloud almost filling the left atrium. Normally, the extent of mitral regurgitation in dilated cardiomyopathy is less than that shown here.

making especially thorough use of the noninvasive survey provided by ultrasound.

Ischemic heart disease is a common cause of left ventricular dilation and dysfunction. Most often recognizable by history, coronary syndromes are not usually diagnostic challenges. In younger patients, diabetics, and others, ischemic myocardial disease may present without angina or defined myocardial infarction and resemble dilated cardiomyopathy. This resemblance is compounded by the fact that dilated cardiomyopathy often displays elements of asynergy, with better contraction in the basilar segments than in the others. The echocardiographic distinguishing features of ischemic disease include marked asynergy, wall thinning, aneurysms, and occasionally papillary muscle fibrosis/dysfunction.

Myocarditis may be found in dilated cardiomyopathy and is thought to be the inflammatory response to viral or other stimuli. Its exact role in the genesis of dilated cardiomyopathy is not yet defined; myocarditis has been shown to cause or evolve into a dilated cardiomyopathy but to be treatable with immunosuppressive drugs (52). The diagnosis must be made by endomyocardial biopsy, but ultrasound is helpful in revealing the ventricular hypokinesis (with or without extreme dilation) typical of severe myocardial inflammation. Patients with myocarditis may present acutely with pulmonary edema and shock or may have a more indolent course. In either case, echocardiography is an efficient means of screening for possible biopsy, as well as following left ventricular function (53).

Volume overload conditions may deteriorate to a state of ventricular dilation and dysfunction identical to dilated cardiomyopathy. Examples include end-stage mitral or aortic regurgitation and interchamber shunting.

ECHOCARDIOGRAPHIC GUIDANCE OF HEART BIOPSY

Endomyocardial biopsy is a relatively new technique for investigation of histopathology in various myocardial diseases. Cardiac biopsy has been reviewed widely and has become increasingly common in the United States in recent years (54). The full extent of its usefulness has not yet been realized (55), but heart biopsy is essential in diagnosing cardiac allograft rejection. The technique has found wide acceptance in determining severity of anthracycline- (adriamycin) induced myocardial damage and in diagnosing various myocardial conditions. These conditions include amyloidosis, myocarditis, hemochromatosis, and Fabry's disease. Biopsy is useful in dilated cardiomyopathy to rule out specific myocardial diseases and may be effective in assessing prognosis. The percutaneous transvascular approach is safer than needle biopsies of other solid organs and permits tissue examination of severely ill patients.

Endomyocardial biopsy is performed percutaneously, via either the venous or arterial system, by passing a catheter bioptome into the right or left ventricle. The procedure is performed under local anesthesia and often is done at the same time as cardiac catheterization or angiography. Consequently, fluoroscopy originally was used for anatomic visualization. Two-dimensional echocardiography is also an effective means for guidance of the bioptome (Fig. 16.7). Ultrasound usually does not replace fluoroscopy, unless the biopsy is performed in a setting where echocardiography is more convenient, desirable, or the only imaging method available. For example, biopsy can be performed using ultrasound at the bedside in the intensive care unit. Most often, however, echocardiography is supplementary to fluoroscopy. The two-dimensional apical or subcostal view allows good visualization in 90% of all cases, revealing the exact site of bioptome-endocardial contact and confirming tissue sampling. Since it is desirable to sample several sites for adequate histologic examination, two-dimensional echocardiography can be a valuable anatomic guide. The fluoroscopic view may not be as accurate, because echocardiography can pinpoint the bioptome tip more readily.

The right ventricle is by far the most common chamber biopsied. It is not always easy to confirm by fluoroscopy that the bioptome is actually in the right ventricle. Traditionally, the provocation of ventricular extrasystoles has been an additional sign of correct placement. It is possible to place the bioptome erroneously into the coronary sinus or to fail to cross the tricuspid valve. Also, the chordae tendineae potentially can be injured by inadvertent application of the biopsy forceps. Finally, the right ventricular free wall should be avoided as a site of biopsy due to its relative thinness—often 2 mm—and attendant risk of perforation. Echocardiography usually can locate the bioptome tip very accurately, probably better than fluoroscopy. For these reasons, adjunctive two-dimensional imaging may be desirable.

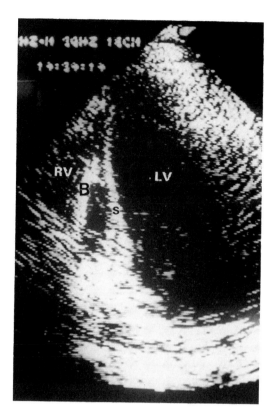

Figure 16.7. Percutaneous transvenous endomyocardial right ventricular biopsy. This two-dimensional echocardiogram was made during biopsy, showing the bioptome (*B*) within the right ventricle (*RV*). The bioptome is positioned against the interventricular septum (*s*) toward the apex. This site is judged to be safer than the free wall due to risk of perforation. Since most myocardial processes are diffuse, the septal endocardium of the right ventricle is sampled due to ease and safety. The left ventricle (*LV*) is dilated.

Echocardiographic Correlates of Prognosis in Dilated Cardiomyopathy

Assessing the likelihood of survival in patients with dilated cardiomyopathy has become even more important as new pharmacologic interventions emerge to accompany the definitive form of surgical therapy—transplantation. Although long-term survival in dilated cardiomyopathy is generally poor, the disease affects a diverse population with many subsets. Not only are multiple causes probably involved, but mortality may vary widely within the subsets.

The severity of left ventricular enlargement does not appear to be a totally reliable predictor of mortality. Systolic and diastolic function appear to be the major physiologic determinants of survival as mechanical characteristics. Electrical phenomena such as arrhythmias and conduction block complete the picture (56). Echocardiographic studies have shown that approximately two-thirds of dilated cardiomyopathy patients display some degree of segmental wall motion abnormalities. The one-third with completely diffuse hypokinesis tend to have a worse prognosis (57). Pathologic studies have suggested that dilated cardiomyopathy patients with thinner left ventricular walls also have lower survival rates. This finding may be confirmed on echocardiography (58), which is a sensitive and reliable method for measuring wall thickness.

ECHOCARDIOGRAPHY IN THE TRANSPLANT PROGRAM

The tremendous recent success of heart transplantation represents a remarkable advance in modern cardiovascular care. In the late 1960s, transplantation was a desperate experimental procedure with a relatively dismal outcome. However, in the ensuing years the technique has become well accepted as an aggressive but effective step in rescuing patients with end-stage cardiac dysfunction. Approximately one-half of all heart transplant recipients receive the operation for severe dilated cardiomyopathy. Current 1-year survival rates can exceed 90%. This level of success can be attributed to long series of paintstaking advances in transplantation. These include the development of cardiac biopsy; better understanding of rejection immunology; careful donor selection and recipient preparation; improved surgical techniques, and new antirejection treatments, including cyclosporine.

Currently, endomyocardial biopsy is the sole method for accurate detection and grading of allograft rejection. Biopsy is performed frequently during the early postoperative period. In the late postoperative period, follow-up rejection certainly can occur, but less frequently, so biopsy is extended to approximately 3-month intervals.

Biopsy subjects the patient to small but finite risk. For these reaons it is desirable to develop more convenient, noninvasive methods for detecting rejection. Sensitive, specific immunologic markers, including radiolabeling, are under investigation. Likewise, ultrasound is becoming more useful as a means of rejection surveillance.

Echocardiographic signs can accompany the pathophysiologic changes caused by rejection (perivascular and interstitial inflammatory cellular infiltration, immunoglobulin and complement deposition, and myocardial edema). M-mode echocardiography can detect rejection-associated acute increases in left ventricular wall thickness and mass, probably secondary to edema (59). M-mode measurements have also revealed acute reductions in the rate of posterior left ventricular diastolic wall thinning and cavity lengthening in rejection (60). These reversible echocardiographic abnormalities during acute rejection are accompanied by shortening of the isovolumic relaxation time (IVRT). This parameter is obtained by combined electrocardiography, phonocardiography, and echocardiography. It is probably indicative of earlier mitral opening, possibly due to increased atrial pressure, typical for rejection (61). Systolic function usually deteriorates relatively late in rejection. However, the foregoing indicators of diastolic function are more sensitive.

Careful Doppler echocardiographic anaylsis of atrioventricular inflow reveals significant reduction in mitral pressure half-time that correlates with histologically graded severity of rejection (62). These diastolic parameter changes are unaccompanied by alterations in Doppler echocardiographic indices of systolic function, such as peak aortic velocity.

Echocardiography has become valuable not only for following recipients, but also for screening potential heart transplant donors. Donor availability is a limiting step for any transplant program, so widespread referral networks are desirable. Careful exclusion of abnormal allografts is crucial, especially since many potential donor hearts result from trauma. The possibility of injury or dysfunction before transplantation must be considered, since trauma is often associated with chest injury, hypotension, hypoxia, sepsis, or catecholamine infusions. Convenient, rapid, noninvasive echocardiographic screening enhances evaluation of donor hearts, making operative inspection much less likely to uncover defects prohibiting allografting. Echocardiographic screening can be effective in avoiding exclusion of donor hearts, the suitability of which would otherwise be questionable based solely on history of serious chest trauma, hypotension, cardiac arrest, or intense pressor administration (63). Echocardiography detects abnormalities that are subsequently confirmed at autopsy or excision, thus improving the potential for good allograft function posttransplantation.

SUMMARY

Modern cardiovascular diagnosis and treatment demand techniques that can detect and quantify pathophysiology. Expensive or invasive procedures must be preceded by reliable screening. Ultrasound fulfills the need for accurate, relatively inexpensive, quick, and safe diagnostic imaging and quantitative assessment. Nowhere is this more apparent than in the field of cardiomyopathies, the clinical symptoms and physical signs of which may confound the most experienced physician. Ultrasound has a crucial place in the diagnosis, categorization, and assessment of cardiomyopathies upon presentation. However, it is just as important a tool for detecting complications and following deterioration or improvement as the natural course of the illness is treated. The application of more quantitative methods to ultrasound as well as the incorporation of Doppler echocardiography assures continued and growing usefulness for diagnosing and managing myocardial disease.

REFERENCES

1. DeMaria AN, Bommer W, Lee G, et al: Value and limitations of two-dimensional echocardiography in assessment of cardiomyopathy. *Am J Cardiol* 46:1224, 1980.
2. Abbasi AS, Chahine RA, MacAlpin RN, et al: Ultrasound in the diagnosis of primary congestive cardiomyopathy. *Chest* 63:1973, 1973.
3. Corya B, Feigenbaum H, Rasmussen S, et al: Echocardiographic features of congestive cardiomyopathy compared with normal subjects and patients with coronary artery disease. *Circulation* 49:1153, 1974.
4. Massie BM, Schiller NB, Ratshin RA, et al: Mitral-septal separation: New echocardiographic index of left ventricular function. *Am J Cardiol* 39:1008, 1977.
5. Devereux RB, Reichek N: Echocardiographic determination of left ventricular mass in man. *Circulation* 55:613, 1977.
6. Martin RP, Rakowski H, French J, et al: Idiopathic hypertrophic subaortic stenosis viewed by wide-angle, phased array echocardiography. *Circulation* 59:1206, 1979.
7. Keren A, Billingham ME, Weintraub D, et al: Mildly dilated congestive cardiomyopathy. *Circulation* 72:302, 1979.
8. Child JS, Krivokapich J, Abbasi AS: Increased right ventricular wall thickness on echocardiography in amyloid infiltrative cardiomyopathy. *Am J Cardiol* 44:1391, 1979.
9. Cueto-Garcia L, Reeder GS, Kyle RA, et al: Echocardiographic findings in systemic amyloidosis:

Spectrum of cardiac involvement and relations to survival. *J Am Coll Cardiol* 6:737–743, 1985.

10. Acquatella H, Schiller NB, Puigbo JJ, et al: Value of two-dimensional echocardiography in edomyocardial disease with and without eosinophilia: A clinical and pathological study. *Circulation*. 67:1219, 1983.
11. Candell-Riera J, Lu L, Seres L, et al: Cardiac hemochromatosis: Beneficial effects of iron removal therapy: An echocardiographic study. *Am J Cardiol* 52:824–829, 1983.
12. Presti C, Ryan T, Armstrong WF: Two-dimensional and Doppler echocardiographic findings in hypereosinophilic syndrome. *Am Heart J* 114:172–175, 1987.
13. Schnittger I, Vieli A, Heiserman JE, et al: Ultrasonic tissue characterization: Detection of acute myocardial ischemia in dogs. *Circulation* 72:193–199, 1985.
14. Hoyt RH, Collins SM, Skorton DJ, et al: Assessment of fibrosis in infarcted human hearts by analysis of ultrasonic backscatter. *Circulation* 71:740–744, 1985.
15. Glueck RM. Mottley JG, Sobel BE, Perez JE: Effects of coronary artery occlusion and reperfusion on cardiac cycle-dependent variation of ultrasonic backscatter. *Circ Res* 56:683–689, 1985.
16. Fitzgerald PJ, McDaniel MD, Rolett EL, et al: Two-dimensional ultrasonic tissue characterization: Backscatter power, endocardial wall motion, and their phase relationship for normal, ischemic, and infarcted myocardium. *Circulation* 76:850–859, 1987.
17. Vered Z, Barzilai B, Mohr GA, et al: Quantitative ultrasonic tissue characterization with real-time integrated backscatter imaging in normal human subjects and in patients with dilated cardiomyopathy. *Circulation* 76:1067–1073, 1987.
18. Boudoulas H, Ruff PD, Fulkerson PK, et al: Relationship of angiographic and echographic dimensions in chronic left ventricular dilatation. *Am Heart J* 106:356–362, 1983.
19. Fortuin NJ, Hood WP Jr, Sherman E, et al: Determinations of left ventricular volumes by ultrasound. *Circulation* 44:575, 1971.
20. Teichholtz LE, Kreulen T, Herman MV, Gorlin R: Problems in echocardiographic volume determinations: Echocardiographic-angiographic correlations in the presence or absence of asynergy. *Am J Cardiol* 37:7, 1976.
21. Cooper RH, O'Rourke RA, Karliner JS, et al: Comparison of ultrasound and cineangiographic measurements of the mean rate of circumferential shortening in man. *Circulation* 46:914, 1972.
22. Rossen RM, Goodman DJ, Ingham RE, Popp RL: Ventricular systolic septal thickening and excursion in idopathic hypertrophic subaortic stenosis. *N Engl J Med* 291:1317–1319, 1974.
23. Watanabe K, Oda H, Tsuda T, Shibata A: Evaluation of response to dopamine in idiopathic dilated cardiomyopathy by echocardiography and thallium-201 myocardial scintigraphy. *Jap Heart J* 26:379–389, 1985.
24. Fujiwara T, Taramuto T, Kudo K, et al: Echocardiography of ischemic heart disease simulating dilated cardiomyopathy, with special reference to ab-

normal wall movement on the short axis. *J Cardiogr* 13:89–101, 1983.
25. Gardin JM, Tommaso CL, Talano JV: Echographic early systolic partial closure (notching) of the aortic valve in congestive cardiomyopathy. *Am Heart J* 107:135–142, 1984.
26. Sugishita Y, Matsuda M, Ito I, Koseki S: Evaluation of left ventricular reserve in left ventricular diseases: Non-invasive analysis of its determinants by dynamic exercise echocardiography. *Acta Cardiol (Brux)* 38:103–113, 1983.
27. Laskey WK, Sutton MS, Zeevi G, et al: Left ventricular mechanics in dilated cardiomyopathy. *Am J Cardiol* 54:620–625, 1984.
28. Colan SD, Borow KM, Neumann A: The left ventricular end systolic wall stress-velocity of fiber shortening relation: A load-independent index of myocardial contractility. *J Am Coll Cardiol* 4:715, 1984.
29. Borow KM, Henderson C, Neumann A: Assessment of left ventricular contractility in patients receiving doxorubicin. *Ann Intern Med* 99:750, 1983.
30. Sabban HN, Khaja F, Brymer JF, et al: Noninvasive evaluation of left ventricular performance based on peak aortic blood flow acceleration measured with a continuous wave Doppler velocity meter. *Circulation* 74:323, 1986.
31. Gardin JM, Iseri LT, Elkayam U, et al: Evaluation of dilated cardiomyopathy by pulsed Doppler echocardiography. *Am Heart J* 106:1057–1065, 1983.
32. Bouchard A, Blumlein S, Schiller NB, et al: Measurement of left ventricular stroke volume using continuous wave Doppler echocardiography of the ascending aorta and M-mode echocardiography of the aortic valve. *J Am Coll Cardiol* 9:75–83, 1987.
33. Rose JS, Nanna M, Rahimtoola SH, et al: Accuracy of determination of changes in cardiac output by transcutaneous continuous wave Doppler computer. *Am J Cardiol* 54:1099, 1984.
34. Elkayam V, Gardin JM, Berkley R, et al: The use of Doppler flow-velocity measurement to assess the hemodynamic response to vasodilators in patients with heart failure. *Circulation* 67:377, 1983.
35. Takenaka K, Dabestani A, Gardin JM, et al: Pulsed Doppler echocardiographic study of left ventricular filling in dilated cardiomyopathy. *Am J Cardiol* 58:143–147, 1986.
36. Rahko PS, Shaver JA, Salerni R, Uretsky BF: Noninvasive evaluation of systolic and diastolic function in severe coronary artery disease or idiopathic dilated cardiomyopathy. *Am J Cardiol* 57:1315–1322, 1986.
37. Friedman BJ, Drinkovic N, Miles H, et al: Assessment of left ventricular diastolic function: Comparison of Doppler echocardiography and gated blood pool scintigraphy. *J Am Coll Cardiol* 8:1348–1354, 1986.
38. Rokey R, Kuo LC, Zoghbi WA, et al: Determination of parameters of left ventricular diastolic filling with pulsed Doppler echocardiography: Comparison with cineangiography. *Circulation* 71:543–550, 1985.
39. Palomo AR, Quinones MA, Waggoner AD, et al: Echophonocardiographic determination of left atrial and left ventricular filling pressures with and with-

out mitral stenosis. *Circulation* 61:1043—1047, 1980.

40. DeMaria AN, Wisenbaugh T: Identification and treatment of diastolic dysfunction: Role of transmitral recordings. *J Am Coll Cardiol* 9:1106–1107, 1987.

41. Spirito P, Maron BJ, Bonow RO: Noninvasive assessment of left ventricular diastolic function: Comparative analysis of Doppler echocardiographic and radionuclide angiographic techniques. *J Am Coll Cardiol* 7:518–526, 1986.

42. Channer KS, Culling W, Wilde P, Jones JV: Estimation of left ventricular end-diastolic pressure by pulsed Doppler ultrasound. *Lancet* 1:1005–1007, 1986.

43. Reeder GS, Tajik AJ, Seward JB: Left ventricular mural thrombus: Two-dimensional echocardiographic diagnosis. *Mayo Clin Proc* 56:82–86, 1981.

44. Gottdiener JS, Gay JA, VanVoorhees L, et al: Frequency and embolic potential of left ventricular thrombus in dilated cardiomyopathy. *Am J Cardiol* 52:1281–1285, 1983.

45. Fuster V, Gersh BJ, Guilliani ER, et al: The natural history of idopathic dilated cardiomyopathy. *Am J Cardiol* 47:525–531, 1981.

46. Gould L, Gopalaswamy C, Chandy F, Kim BS: Congestive cardiomyopathy and left ventricular thrombus. *Arch Intern Med* 143:1472, 1983.

47. Shung KK, Fei DY, Ballard JO: Further studies on ultrasonic properties of blood clots. *J Clin Ultrasound* 14:269–275, 1986.

48. Mikell FL, Asinger RW, Elsperger KJ, et al: Regional stasis of blood in the dysfunctional left ventricle: Echocardiographic detection and differentiation from early thrombosis. *Circulation* 66:775, 1982.

49. Dittrich H, Holt B, Sahn D: Spatial patterns of mitral flow in patients with congestive cardiomyopathy determined by real-time two-dimensional echo Doppler color flow mapping. *J Am Coll Cardiol* 5:426, 1985.

50. Boltwood CM, Tei C, Wong M, Shah PM: Quantitative echocardiography of the mitral complex in dilated cardiomyopathy: The mechanism of functional mitral regurgitation. *Circulation* 68:498–508, 1983.

51. Yock PG, Popp RL: Noninvasive estimation of right ventricular systolic pressure by Doppler ultrasound in patients with tricuspid regurgitation. *Circulation* 70:657, 1984.

52. Mason JW, Billingham ME, Ricci DR: Treatment of acute inflammatory myocarditis assisted by endomyocardial biopsy. *Am J Cardiol* 45:1037–1044, 1980.

53. Fujii J, Sato H, Sawada H, et al: Echocardiographic assessment of left ventricular wall motion in myocarditis. *Heart Vess* (Suppl) 1:116–121, 1985.

54. Fowles RE, Mason JW: Role of cardiac biopsy in the diagnosis and management of cardiac disease. *Progr Cardiovac Dis* 27:153–172, 1984.

55. Mason JW: Endomyocardial biopsy: The balance of success and failure. *Circulation* 71:185–188, 1985.

56. Unverferth DV: Etiologic features, pathogenesis, and prognosis of dilated cardiomyopathy. *J Lab Clin Med* 106:349, 1985.

57. Wallis DE, O'Connell JB, Henkin RE, et al: Segmental wall motion abnormalities in dilated cardiomyopathy: A common finding and good prognostic sign. *J Am Coll Cardiol* 4:647–649, 1984.

58. Hayakawa M, Inoh T, Fukuzaki H: Dilated cardiomyopathy. An echocardiographic follow-up of 50 patients. *Jap Heart J* 25:955–968, 1984.

59. Billingham ME: Endomyocardial biopsy detection of acute rejection in cardiac allograft recipients. *Heart Vess* 1:86, 1985.

60. Paulsen W, Magid N, Sagar K, et al: Left ventricular function of heart allografts during acute rejection: An echocardiographic study. *Heart Transplant* 5:525–529, 1985.

61. Dawkins KD, Oldershaw PJ, Billingham SE, et al: Changes in diastolic function as a noninvasive marker of cardiac allograft rejection. *Heart Transplant* 3:286, 1984.

62. Valantine HA, Fowler MB, Hunt SA, et al: Changes in Doppler echocardiographic indexes of left ventricular function as potential markers of acute cardiac rejection. *Circulation* 76 (Suppl 5):V-86, 1987.

63. Gilbert EM, Krueger SK, Murray JL, et al: Echocardiographic evaluation of potential cardiac transplant donors. *J Thorac Cardiovasc Surg* (in press).

17

Doppler Assessment of Systolic Cardiac Function

Robert J. Bryg, M.D.
Arthur J. Labovitz, M.D.

INTRODUCTION

Since its introduction in clinical cardiology, Doppler echocardiography has been utilized primarily for the noninvasive evaluation of valvular and congenital heart diseases. However, these conditions represent only a small fraction of cardiovascular disease. A much wider application for Doppler echocardiography would be in the assessment of left ventricular systolic function.

The first reported use of cardiac Doppler was for the assessment of aortic flow velocity, a measure of left ventricular systolic function. In 1969, Light (1) demonstrated that aortic velocity could be obtained easily and noninvasively from the suprasternal notch with pulsed Doppler echocardiography. Six years later, Boughner et al. (2) showed the aortic flow pattern, also obtained from the suprasternal notch, was different in patients with hypertrophic cardiomyopathy than in normal subjects. Also in 1975, Huntsman demonstrated the reliability of determining aortic blood flow velocity by transcutaneous Doppler ultrasound. During the next 5 years, the emphasis shifted to the use of Doppler for evaluating valvular disease. Only recently has there been a resurgence of interest in aortic flow patterns in a variety of disease states.

EVALUATION OF BASAL CARDIAC FUNCTION

Left ventricular systolic function can be evaluated using several different Doppler measurements. These include peak ejection velocity, acceleration time (time from onset of systolic flow to the peak velocity), left ventricular ejection time, flow velocity integral (area under the velocity curve), and the peak and mean aortic acceleration (Fig. 17.1).

Over the past few years a number of reports have validated the use of Doppler echocardiography to calculate stroke volume and cardiac output (3–12). With Fick and thermodilution outputs used as gold standards, these studies have shown that Doppler measurements from a variety of sites throughout the heart and great vessels can be used to calculate cardiac output noninvasively. These sites include each of the four cardiac valves as well as flow in the ascending and descending aorta.

The basic principle for determining these values remains the same in each case. In the absence of significant valvular stenosis, the area under the Doppler flow velocity curve (flow velocity integral) is directly proportional to the stroke volume. This flow velocity integral is used to calculate stroke volume by multiplying it by the cross-sectional area of the vessel or valve through which the blood is flowing. The product of the stroke volume and heart rate is the cardiac output.

The formula for the Doppler calculation of cardiac ouput (Fig. 17.2) is:

$$\text{Cardiac output} = \text{Flow velocity integral} \times \text{cross-sectional area} \times \text{heart rate.} \quad 17.1$$

It is important to recognize the limitations in measuring each of these components, most importantly the cross-sectional area, before clinically applying these principles.

The factor most sensitive to error is the diameter of the vessel or valve. In measuring the diameter of flow for the aortic region, investigators have used a variety of measurements. These include A-mode measurement of the ascending aorta, M-mode measurement of the aorta, and two-dimensional echocardiographic measure-

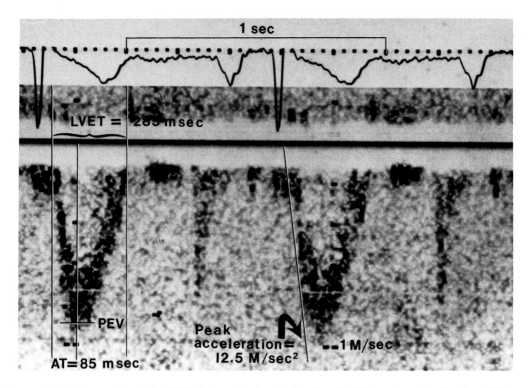

Figure 17.1. The peak velocity (*PEV*), left ventricular ejection time (*LVET*), and acceleration time (*AT*) are demonstrated. Peak acceleration is the steepest slope of the velocity curve. The mean acceleration is the peak velocity divided by the acceleration time (*PEV/AT*). In this example, the mean acceleration is 10.6 m/sec².

ment of the diameter of the aorta and left ventricular outflow tract (3–8).

The most reliable measurements, both taken from a two-dimensional, parasternal long-axis view, are the left ventricular outflow tract and the ascending aorta just distal to the sinus of Valsalva. Gardin et al. (5) demonstrated a poor correlation between thermodilution measurements and the Doppler calculations used in M-mode-derived aortic root measurement. This study found the best measurement to be from inner wall to inner wall of the ascending aorta and the best view to be the long-axis view above the sinus of Valsalva. Labovitz et al. (6) used both the long-axis view of the left ventricular outflow tract and the ascending aorta above the sinus of Valsalva and found similar correlations for both measures. Other investigators, using A-mode measurement, have had mixed results (3, 4, 13, 14).

Although aortic flow has been the flow most commonly used to determine cardiac output, all of the valves have been studied. Fisher validated

a model for calculating cardiac output from mitral valve flow. Using M-mode measurement of mitral valve motion, this method calculates cardiac output from a constant integration of the width of the mitral valve opening and Doppler mitral valve flow. Other investigators have reported good correlations between Doppler-derived and thermodilution cardiac outputs for all the valves (9–12). However, calculating the area of flow through these other valves is often fraught with error. The pulmonic valve area is difficult to obtain in adults. In the atrioventricular (AV) valves the difficulty is in determining the area of flow across the valve through diastole.

The other variable in calculating cardiac output that is subject to error is the flow velocity integral obtained by integrating the spectral tracing over time. Rather than using an approximation to describe the area under the curve, most investigators are now doing the integration themselves.

Determining the area under the curve is a much smaller source of variation. One study showed only a 3% variation when one observer measured the same tracing twice, and only a 5% variation between observers (15).

Numerous studies have resulted in a wide variety of validated methods for calculating cardiac output (4–14). However, the best method uses aortic flow and measures the aortic root dimensions from inner wall to inner wall. This measurement is made from the parasternal long-axis view either at the aortic annulus or above the sinus of Valsalva. The flow velocity integral is digitized using the modal velocity (the darkest part of the curve) obtained by pulsed Doppler.

Calculation of cardiac output by Doppler remains controversial despite the apparently good results (16, 17). Two main controversies involve determination of the diameter of flow and the use of thermodilution as a gold standard. In addition, an incident angle of more than 20° between the Doppler beam and the blood flow can cause a significant systematic error in the calculation of stroke volume and cardiac output.

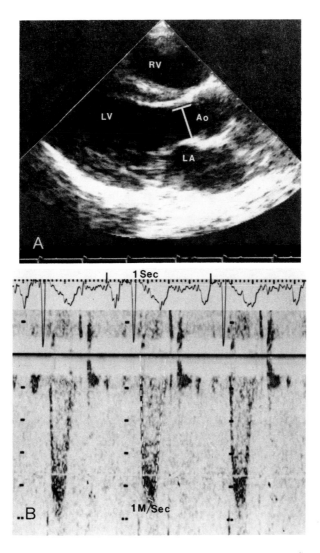

Figure 17.2. Calculation of cardiac output. The diameter of the left ventricular outflow tract is demonstrated in the parasternal long-axis view (Figure 17.2A). The area under the velocity curve, or flow velocity integral (FVI), is illustrated. Cardiac output = FVI × area of aorta × heart rate. *Ao* = aorta, *LA* = left atrium, *LV* = left ventricle, *RV* = right ventricle.

Not only are there problems in calculating cardiac output by Doppler, there are no significant differences in cardiac output among normal subjets, coronary artery disease patients, and congestive cardiomyopathy patients. Consequently, the isolated Doppler determination of cardiac output often provides little useful information about cardiac function.

Some investigators have suggested that the flow velocity integral or the stroke distance would be better indicators of function. Gardin et al. (18) demonstrated lower peak velocities and flow velocity integrals in patients with congestive cardiomyopathies than in normal subjects. However, there were no significant differences in cardiac output due to the increased heart rate in patients with congestive cardiomyopathy. As a result, the focus of recent research has been on the measurement of serial changes in Doppler measurements as a result of therapeutic interventions.

Acceleration of blood flow is another measurement that can be used to evaluate left ventricular function. In 1964, Rushmer (19) suggested that maximal blood acceleration would describe left ventricular function accurately. Subsequent studies, using velocity catheters, demonstrated a decrease in maximal acceleration after acute coronary occlusions (20) and acute myocardial infarction (21). The acceleration of blood flow is the first derivative of the velocity curve and can be calculated from the velocity curve (22). A good correlation between maximal acceleration and ejection fraction at rest has been reported by Sabbah et al. (23) This study also showed a good correlation between peak ejection velocity and ejection fraction.

REGURGITANT FRACTIONS AND SHUNTS

The methodology that allows us to measure cardiac output by Doppler echocardiography can also be used to measure differences in volumes in certain pathologic states. These include intracardiac shunts and valvular regurgitant lesions. A regurgitant volume is calculated by measuring the volume across a regurgitant valve and subtracting from that the volume of a remote, normally functioning valve. For instance, in mitral regurgitation one calculates the stroke volume across the mitral valve as the product of the mitral velocity integral and the cross-sectional area of the mitral valve annulus. The volume of flow in a normal valve, say the aorta, would be calculated the same way. Again, this would be the product of flow velocity integral and the cross-sectional area. The difference between the mitral and aortic volumes is the mitral regurgitant volume. Dividing this value by the calculated mitral volume provides an estimate of the mitral regurgitant fraction. Several investigators validated the accuracy of these calculations of regurgitant volumes across the mitral, aortic, and pulmonic valves (24–26).

Similarly, the ratio of pulmonary to systematic blood flow (Qp:Qs) can be determined by measuring the right ventricular stroke volume at the pulmonic valve and the left ventricular stroke volume at the aorta. However, the inherent problems in Doppler-calculated stroke volumes and cardiac outputs must be considered before using these techniques clinically (27, 28)

EFFECTS OF DRUG ADMINISTRATION

There are differences in Doppler-derived measurements of aortic flow even when basal cardiac function is being evaluated. This appears to be due to variations in the overall contractility of the ventricle and systematic vascular resistance. Consequently, Doppler echocardiography can be used to study the effects of various drug interventions on overall cardiac function and vascular tone.

A study by Elkayam et al. (29) examined the effects of vasodilators on Doppler aortic blood flow measurements. Thirteen patients underwent a total of 18 drug interventions. Peak flow velocity, left ventricular ejection time, and flow velocity integral were determined with each intervention.

There was a good overall correlation between the thermodilution-derived stroke volume and the Doppler-derived flow velocity integral ($r = 0.88$). There was also a decrease in Doppler peak flow velocity when the thermodilution-derived systemic vascular resistance increased. On the other hand, there was no correlation at baseline between either stroke volume or systematic vascular resistance and absolute values for peak flow velocity, flow velocity integral, or left ventricular ejection time.

The flow velocity integral accurately reflected the changes in stroke volume and the inverse relationship between vascular resistance and peak flow velocity. Therefore, the changes in aortic flow caused by vasodilators can be measured accurately noninvasively by Doppler echocardiography.

Although Doppler-derived measurements are affected by changes in vascular resistance, they are altered even more dramatically by changes in the inotropic state. Wallmeyer et al. (30) studied the effects of positive and negative inotropes in an animal model. With preload and afterload held constant, a positive inotrope (dobutamine) increased the peak aortic flow velocity and mean acceleration. Both were decreased when a negative inotrope (propranolol) was administered. Invasive measurements have confirmed the Doppler observations, and other studies have shown similar results. Peak flow velocity decreased 33% from baseline in the study by Wallmeyer et al. (30), after 1 mg/kg of propranolol was given and increased 50% in the study by Elkayam et al. (29) when dobutamine was given.

A substantial body of data now exists regarding the effects of inotropes, daily variation in Doppler-derived measurements, and observer variability of these measurements. Consequently, we can define any change greater than 15% in peak flow velocity or flow velocity integral occurring after an intervention as likely being caused by that intervention.

EVALUATION OF CARDIAC PACING

With the advent of dual-chamber, multiprogrammable pacemakers has come controversy regarding how to determine the best type of pacing to use. Some patients would benefit most from a ventricular demand pacemaker (VVI), while others would be best served by maintaining A-V synchrony with a dual-chamber pacemaker (DDD). Doppler echocardiography has shown promise in assessing the efficacy of dual-chamber pacemaker modes.

Using Doppler echocardiography to determine cardiac output, Stewart et al. (31) studied the changes in hemodynamics occurring when pacing is changed from VVI to DDD. He also tested whether intact ventriculoatrial (V-A) conduction or global left ventricular function could predict which patients would benefit from DDD pacing. Stewart found that changes in pacemaker modes were instantaneously reflected in beat-to-beat changes in Doppler-derived aortic flow patterns. In patients with intact V-A conduction or in patients who had the pacemaker syndrome during VVI pacing, DDD pacing produced a 30% increase in cardiac output over VVI pacing. In the remaining subjects, the mean increase in cardiac output was only 14%. Global left ventricular function, assessed by ejection fraction, did not predict who would derive hemodynamic benefit from dual-chamber pacing.

In a similar study, Labovitz et al. (32) assessed the effects of loss of A-V synchrony on changes in stroke volume (Fig. 17.3). He found that patients with a normal left atrial size had a 32% decrease in the flow velocity integral going from DDD to VVI pacing. In patients with left atrial enlargement, defined as a left atrial size larger than 2.2 cm/M², there was only an 11% change

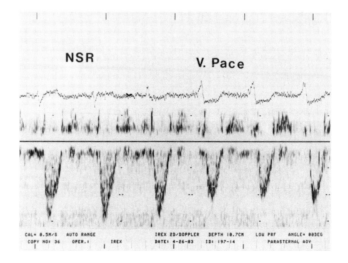

Figure 17.3. The change in Doppler aortic flow when going from normal sinus rhythm (*NSR*) to VVI pacing (*V. Pace*) mode is illustrated. (Reprinted with permission from the American College of Cardiology and Labovitz AJ, et al: Noninvasive assessment of pacemaker hemodynamics by Doppler echocardiography: Importance of left atrial size. *J Am Coll Cardiol* 6:198, 1985.)

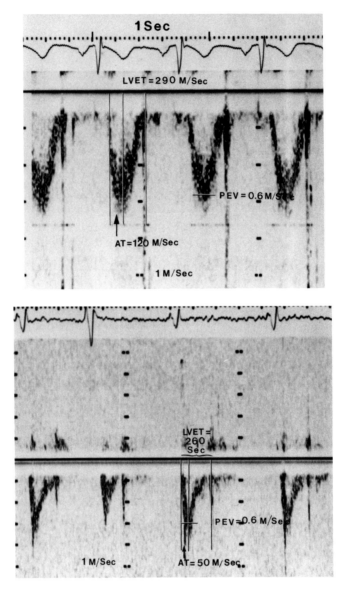

Figure 17.4. Typical pulmonary artery systolic flow profiles seen in patients with normal (*left*) and elevated pulmonary artery pressure (*right*). The patient with elevated pulmonary artery pressure has a much shorter acceleration time (50 msec) than the normal subject (120 msec). *AT* = acceleration time, *LVET* = left ventricular ejection time, *PEV* = peak velocity.

in the flow velocity integral. This latter change might not be significant due to the interobserver variability of Doppler measurements. As in the study by Stewart et al. (31), global left ventricular function was not predictive of changes in stroke volume. Both these studies were performed with the patients supine, so this does not rule out differences in responses when the patient is in an upright position.

Another possible application for Doppler echocardiography is determining the optimal A-V interval with dual-chamber pacemakers. Two preliminary reports have assessed changes in A-V intervals to maximize cardiac output (33, 34). Both studies documented patient-to-patient differences in the optimal A-V delay. Some patients required short delays, while others required long delays to maintain the best cardiac output. Both authors expressed the opinion that Doppler could be very useful in the initial programming of a dual-chamber pacemaker.

EVALUATION OF PULMONIC FLOW

Several investigators have studied forward pulmonic flow using pulsed Doppler (35, 36). These studies established that normal peak velocity in the main pulmonary artery is approximately 63 cm/sec, as opposed to 92 cm/sec in the ascending aorta. Ejection time is slightly longer in the pulmonary artery (331 msec) than in the ascending aorta (294 msec). Mean acceleration time for pulmonic flow is 160 msec as opposed to 100 msec for aortic flow (Fig. 17.4).

Since acceleration time decreases as pulmonary artery pressure increases, some studies suggest using acceleration time to estimate pulmonary artery pressure (37–39). A good correlation has been reported between pulmonary artery acceleration time and peak systolic pulmonary artery pressure in children with pulmonary hypertension due to congenital heart disease. This correlation was weakened when acceleration time was corrected for the right ventricular ejection time. However, there was also a good correlation between the mean pulmonary artery pressure and both acceleration time and corrected acceleration time.

Mahan et al. (38) found this same correlation in adults and developed an equation to estimate mean pulmonary artery pressure (PAP):

$$\text{Mean PAP} = (-0.45)(\text{AT}) + 79 \quad 17.2$$

where AT = acceleration time. However, Mahan found considerable differences in the mean pulmonary artery pressures for similar acceleration times. As a result, his laboratory uses pulmonary artery acceleration time primarily as a simple screening procedure to differentiate normal from increased pulmonary artery pressues (J. M. Gardin, personal communication).

Other investigators have produced similar results using a variety of equations to calculate peak pulmonary artery pressure (38). All these methods suffer from the same problem: a variation in acceleration time for a given pulmonary artery pressure.

Still, Doppler echocardiography may be useful in gauging changes in pulmonary artery pressure in response to therapy. In a preliminary report on seven patients, Dabestani et al. (39) demonstrated an increase in pulmonic peak velocity,

flow velocity integral, and average acceleration following administration of a vasodilator. Catheter-obtained pulmonary vascular resistance decreased and cardiac output increased. Mean pulmonary artery pressure did not change, and the issue of changes in acceleration time was not addressed.

AORTIC FLOW PATTERNS IN HYPERTROPHIC CARDIOMYOPATHY

One of the first reported uses of Doppler echocardiography was in the noninvasive assessment of aortic flow in hypertrophic obstructive cardiomyopathy. The initial report showed that aortic flow peaked earlier in systole and sometimes ceased in midsystole. More recently, several carefully designed studies have evaluated aortic flow in hypertrophic obstructive cardiomyopathy.

A National Institutes of Health study demonstrated a continuum of flow patterns in the ascending aorta, with nonobstructed hearts maintaining a normal ascending aortic flow pattern (40). The flow pattern is shortened progressively in patients with moderate obstruction. This is followed by a bifid flow pattern where flow stops in midsystole before having a secondary peak. Other researchers have demonstrated this cessation of flow in midsystole occuring at approximately the same time that the mitral valve touches the septum, due to systolic anterior motion. Flow cessation also happens when the maximal gradient occurs in the left ventricular outflow tract (41–43).

CONCLUSION

Systolic cardiac function can be analyzed using a variety of invasive and noninvasive techniques. Doppler echocardiography has unique advantages in certain areas, most notably in serial determination of the effects of therapy, noninvasive measurement of regurgitant fractions and shunts, evaluation of cardiac pacing, and measurement of cardiac output.

REFERENCES

1. Light LH: Non-injurious ultrasonic technique for observing flow in the human aorta. *Nature* 224:1119–1121, 1969.
2. Boughner DR, Schuld RL, Persaud JA: Hypertrophic obstructive cardiomyopathy: Assessment by echocardiographic and Doppler ultrasound techniques. *Br Heart J* 37:917–923, 1975.
3. Chandraratna PA, Nanna M, McKay C, Nimalasuriya A, Swinny R, Elkayam U, Rahimtoola SH: Determination of cardiac output by transcutaneous

continuous-wave Doppler computer. *Am J Cardiol* 53:234–237, 1984.

4. Rose JS, Nanna M, Rahimtoola SH, Elkayam U, McKay C, Chandraratna PAN: Accuracy of determination of changes in cardiac output by transcutaneous continuous-wave Doppler computer. *Am J Cardiol* 54:1099–1101, 1984.

5. Gardin JM, Tobis JM, Dabestani A, Smith C, Elkayam U, Castleman E, White D, Allfie A, Henry WL: Superiority of two-dimensional measurement of aortic vessel diameter in Doppler echocardiographic estimates of left ventricular stroke volume. *J Am Coll Cardiol* 6:66–74, 1985.

6. Labovitz AJ, Buckingham TA, Habermehl K, Nelson J, Kennedy HL, Williams GA: The effect of sampling site on the two-dimensional echo Doppler determination of cardiac output. *Am Heart J* 109:327–332, 1985.

7. Stewart WJ, Jiang L, Mich R, Pandian N, Guerrero JL, Weyman AE: Variable effects of changes in flow rate through the aortic, pulmonary, and mitral valves in valve area and flow velocity: Impact on quantitative Doppler flow calculations. *J Am Coll Cardiol* 6:653–662, 1985.

8. Lewis JF, Kuo LC, Nelson JG, Limacher MC, Quinones MA: Pulsed Doppler echocardiographic determination of stroke volume and cardiac output: Clinical validation of two new methods using the apical window. *Circulation* 70:425–431, 1984.

9. Goldberg SJ, Sahn DJ, Allen HD, Valdes-Cruz IM, Hoenecke H, Carnahan Y: Evaluation of pulmonary and systematic blood flow by 2-dimensional Doppler echocardiography using fast Fourier transform spectral analysis. *Am J Cardiol* 50:1394–1400, 1982.

10. Fisher DC, Sahn DJ, Friedman MJ, Larson D, Valdes-Cruz IM, Horowitz S, Goldberg SJ, Allen HD: The mitral valve orifice method for non-invasive two-dimensional echo Doppler determination of cardiac output. *Circulation* 67:872–877, 1983.

11. Meijboom EJ, Horowitz S, Valdes-Cruz IM, Sahn DJ, Larson DF, Limo CO: A Doppler echocardiographic method for calculating volume flow across the tricuspid valve: Correlative laboratory and clinical studies. *Circulation* 71:551–556, 1984.

12. Loeber CP, Goldberg SJ, Allen HD: Doppler echocardiographic comparison of flows distal to the four cardiac valves. *J Am Coll Cardiol* 4:268–272, 1984.

13. Waters J, Kwan OL, Kerns G, Takeda P, Low R, Booth D, DeMaria A: Limitiations of Doppler echocardiography in the calculation of cardiac output (Abstr). *Circulation* 66:II-122, 1982.

14. Waters JS, Kwan OL, DeMaria AN: Sources of error in the measurement of cardiac output by Doppler techniques (Abstr). *Circulation* 68:III-229, 1983.

15. Gardin JM, Dabestani A, Martin K, Allfie A, Russell D, Henry WL: Reproductibility of Doppler aortic blood flow measurement studies on intraobserver, intraobserver and day-to-day variability in normal subjects. *Am J Cardiol* 54:1092–1098, 1984.

16. Sahn DJ: Determination of cardiac output by echocardiographic Doppler methods: Relative accuracy of various sites for measurement. *J Am Coll Cardiol* 6:663–664, 1985.

17. Schuster AH, Nanda NC: Doppler echocardiographic measurement of cardiac output: Comparison with a non-golden standard. *Am J Cardiol* 53:257–259, 1984.

18. Gardin JM, Iseri LT, Elkayam U, Tobis J, Childs W, Burn CS, Henry WL: Evaluation of dilated cardiomyopathy by pulsed Doppler echocardiography. *Am Heart J* 106:1057–1065, 1983.

19. Rushmer RF: Initial ventricular impulse—a potential key to cardiac evaluation. *Circulation* 29:268–283, 1964.

20. Noble MI, Trenchard D, Guz A: Left ventricular ejection fraction in conscious dogs—measurement and significance of the maximum acceleration of blood from the left ventricle. *Circ Res* 19:139–147, 1966.

21. Kezdi P, Stanley EL, Marshall WJ, Kordenat RK: Aortic flow velocity and acceleration as an index of ventricular performance during myocardial infarction. *Am J Med Sci* 257:61–71, 1969.

22. Kolettis M, Jenkins BS, Webb-Peploe MM: Assessment of left ventricular function by indices derived from aortic flow velocity. *Br Heart J* 38:18–31, 1976.

23. Sabbah HN, Khaja F, Brymer JF, McFarland TRM, Albert DE, Snyder JE, Goldstein S, Stein PD: Noninvasive evaluation of left ventricular performance based on peak aortic blood acceleration measured with a continous-wave Doppler velocity meter. *Circulation* 74:323–329, 1986.

24. Blumlein S, Bouchard A, Schiller B, Dae M, Byrd BF, Ports T, Botvinick EH: Quantitation of mitral regurgitation by Doppler echocardiography. *Circulation* 74:306–314, 1986.

25. Ascah KJ, Stewart WJ, Jiang L, Guerrero JL, Newell JB, Gillam JD, Weyman AE: A Doppler two-dimensional echocardiographic method for quantitation of mitral regurgitation. *Circulation* 72:377–383, 1985.

26. Goldberg SJ, Allen HD: Quantitative assessment by Doppler echocardiography of pulmonary or aortic regurgitation. *Am J Cardiol* 56:131–135, 1985.

27. Meijboom EJ, Valdes-Cruz IM, Horowitz S, Sahn DJ, Larson DF, Young KA, Lima CO, Goldberg SJ, Allen HD: A two-dimensional Doppler echocardiographic method for calculation of pulmonary and systemic blood flow in a canine model with a variable-sized left-to-right extracardiac shunt. *Circulation* 68:437–445, 1983.

28. Valdes-Cruz IM, Horowitz S, Mesel E, Sahn DJ, Fisher DC, Larson D: A pulsed Doppler echocardiographic method for calculating pulmonary and systemic blood flow in atrial level shunts: Validation studies in animals and initial human experience. *Circulation* 69:80–86, 1984.

29. Elkayam U, Gardin JM, Berkley R, Hughes CA, Henry WL: The use of Doppler flow velocity measurement to assess the hemodynamic response to vasodilators in patients with heart failure. *Circulation* 67:377–383, 1983.

30. Wallmeyer K, Wann LS, Sagar KB, Kalbfleisch J, Klopfenstein HS: The influence of preload and heart rate on Doppler echocardiographic indexes of left ventricular performance: Comparison with invasive indexes in an experimental preparation. *Circulation* 74:181–186, 1986.

31. Stewart WJ, Dicola VC, Harthorne JW, Gillam

LD, Weyman AE: Doppler ultrasound measurement of cardiac output in patients with physiologic pacemakers: Effects of left ventricular function and retrograde ventriculoatrial conduction. *Am J Cardiol* 54:308–312, 1984.

32. Labovitz AJ, Williams GA, Redd RM, Kennedy HL: Noninvasive assessment of pacemaker hemodynamics by Doppler echocardiography: Importance of left atrial size. *J Am Coll Cardiol* 6:196–200, 1985.

33. Haskel RJ, French WJ: Optimum AV interval in dual chamber pacemakers. *PACE* 9:670–675, 1986.

34. Forfang K, Otterstad JE, Ihlen H: Optimal atrioventricular delay in physiologic pacing determined by Doppler echocardiography. *PACE* 9:17–20, 1986.

35. Gardin JM, Burns CS, Childs WJ, Henry WL: Evaluation of blood flow velocity in the ascending aorta and main pulmonary artery of normal subjects by Doppler echocardiography. *Am Heart J* 107:310–319, 1984.

36. Goldberg SJ, Sahn DJ, Allen HD, Valdes-Cruz IM, Hoenecke H, Carnahan Y: Evaluation of pulmonary and systemic blood flow by two-dimensional Doppler echocardiography using fast Fourier transform spectral analysis. *Am J Cardiol* 50:1394–1400, 1982.

37. Kosturakis D, Goldberg SJ, Allen HD, Loeber C: Doppler echocardiographic prediction of pulmonary arterial hypertension in congenital heart diseae. *Am J Cardiol* 53:1110–1115, 1984.

38. Mahan G, Dabestani A, Gardin J, Allfie A, Burn C, Henry W: Estimation of pulmonary artery pressure by pulsed Doppler echocardiography (Abstr). *Circulation* 68:III-367, 1983.

39. Dabestani A, Mahan G, Johnston W, Russell D, Burn C, Henry W: Pulsed Doppler evaluation of vasodilator therapy in pulmonary hypertension (Abstr). *Circulation* 68:III-134, 1983.

40. Maron BJ, Gottdiener JS, Arle J, Rosing DR, Wesley YE, Epstein SE: Dynamic subaortic obstruction in hypertrophic cardiomyopathy: Analysis by pulsed Doppler echocardiography. *J Am Coll Cardiol* 6:1–5, 1985.

41. Yock PG, Hatle L, Popp RL: Patterns and timing of Doppler detected intracavitary and aortic flow in hypertrophic cardiomyopathy. *J Am Coll Cardiol* 8:1047–1058, 1986.

42. Gardin JM, Dabestani A, Glasgow GA, Butman S, Burn CS, Henry WL: Echocardiography and Doppler flow observations in obstructed and nonobstructed hypertrophic cardiomyopathy. *Am J Cardiol* 56:614–621, 1985.

43. Bryg RJ, Pearson A, Williams GA, Labovitz AJ: Left ventricular systolic and diastolic flow abnormalities in hypertrophic obstructive cardiomyopathy: evaluation by Doppler echocardiography. *Am J Cardiol* 59:925–931, 1987.

18

Echo-Doppler in Hypertrophic Cardiomyopathy

Robert J. Siegel, M.D., Peter C. D. Pelikan, M.D.,
Howard N. Allen, M.D., John Michael Criley, M.D.

INTRODUCTION

The purpose of this chapter is to review the functional anatomy and physiology of the heart in patients with hypertrophic cardiomyopathy as revealed by echocardiographic and Doppler examination. We discuss the cardiac anatomy, noninvasive diagnosis of hypertrophic cardiomyopathy (HCM) by echocardiographic criteria, parameters of systolic function, evidence supporting diastolic dysfunction, and significance and mechanism of left ventricular (LV) outflow tract pressure gradients.

ANATOMY

Hypertrophic cardiomyopathy as a distinct pathologic entity (Table 18.1) was first described by Teare (1) in 1958 during postmortem examination of eight young patients who died suddenly. His studies documented an unusual thickening of the interventricular septum (asymmetrical septal hypertrophy (ASH)) as well as septal myofiber disarray. He thought that the unusually thick septum might represent a cardiac hamartoma, but did not postulate a mechanism to explain sudden death in these patients. Subsequent postmortem investigations confirmed Teare's findings in many patients. The pathognomonic characteristic of this disorder is idiopathic left ventricular hypertrophy (LVH). In up to 20–30% of cases, this may be concentric and therefore without ASH (2). Of 42 patients with HCM studied in our laboratories, 29 had ASH and 12 had concentric LVH. LVH may be localized. For example, in Japan, apical hypertrophy is frequent (3). Maron and coworkers (4) documented additional patterns of hypertrophy: (a) hypertrophy confined to the anterior segment of the basal septum; (b) hypertrophy of the anterior and posterior septum; (c) hypertrophy of the septum and free wall; and (d) hypertrophy of the posterior septum, the anterolateral free wall, or the apical portion of the left ventricle.

In addition to idiopathic LVH, characteristic findings include a small- or normal-sized LV cavity, left atrial dilatation, LV mural endocardial plaque in the outflow tract and beneath the posterior mitral leaflet, mitral valve thickening, mitral annular calcification, and disproportionate elongation of the mitral leaflets (5–7).

Microscopic examination of the ventricular myocardium reveals myocyte hypertrophy and variable degrees of myofiber disarray (8, 9). Although epicardial coronary arteries are frequently large and widely patent (although not immune from atherosclerosis), abnormal thickening of the intima and media of the intramural coronary segments has been reported in 50–80% of patients (10). Patchy interstitial fibrosis and even large areas of myocardial scarring have been reported in the absence of atherosclerotic disease (11, 12).

ETIOLOGY

Echocardiographic screening of family members has shown a distinct genetic basis for the inheritance of HCM in 50–60% of cases (13). The transmission is most consistent with autosomal dominant inheritance with variable penetrance. The hypertrophy frequently becomes manifest during the accelerated growth phase of puberty (14), although some cases of HCM are seen in infancy (15). It should be stressed that even in the absence of genetic factors, patients with this disorder develop LVH without left ventricular pressure overload as caused by systemic hypertension, aortic valve disease, or aortic coarctation. Furthermore, intracavitary pressure gradients in HCM do not appear to cause progressive

Table 18.1. Pathological Anatomy of HCM

Morphologic Criteria for Diagnosis

I. Idiopathic primary ventricular hypertrophy
  A. Usually asymmetrical
    1. Left ventricle > right ventricle
    2. Septum > free wall
    3. Regional variants (including apical)
  B. Nondilated ventricular cavities
  C. "Crowded" and traumatized mitral valve
    1. Disproportionate elongation of leaflets
    2. Thickened leaflets
    3. Impact endocardial lesions (plaques)
      a. Septal (opposite anterior leaflet)
      b. Mural (beneath posterior leaflet)
    4. Calcified annulus
II. Atrial dilatation (left atrium > right atrium)
III. Microscopic features
  A. Focal myofiber disarray
  B. Myocyte hypertrophy
  C. Interstitial fibrosis
  D. Thickened intramural coronary arteries

hypertrophy (14, 16). The severity of the LVH is not related to the presence or magnitude of a left ventricular outflow tract (LVOT) pressure gradient. Moreover, progression of LVH generally does not occur in adults, even when a significant LV outflow tract pressure gradient is present (15).

Primary HCM thus exists without a known etiology. There are secondary forms, however, which can anatomically and functionally mimic primary HCM. These include hypertensive HCM (17); growth hormone-mediated LVH (e.g., acromegaly) (18); LVH due to aortic valve disease with intracavitary LV outflow pressure gradients developing after aortic valve replacement (19); and catecholamine-induced LVH associated with pheochromocytoma (20).

PHYSIOLOGY

The left ventricle in HCM exhibits abnormal function in both systole and diastole (Table 18.2).

Systole

Left ventricular contraction is hyperdynamic with rapid emptying and increased ejection fraction (21–30). Ejection fractions are frequently so high as to cause almost complete emptying of the ventricle (cavity obliteration). The high ejection fraction and rapid emptying frequently are associated with dynamic intracavitary pressure gradients (25, 28, 29). When groups of HCM patients are compared, those with the highest ejection fractions (92% ± 6%) have resting pressure gradients; those with the lowest (76% ± 9%, $p < 0.001$) have no pressure gradients; and those with

inducible gradients have intermediate ejection fractions (85% ± 9%; $p < 0.05$) (25). When gradients are provoked by standard maneuvers (Valsalva maneuver, sodium nitroprusside or isoproterenol infusion, or a postextrasystolic beat), the ejection fraction and rate of emptying increase as compared to those in the baseline nongradient state. These relationships suggest that the pressure gradient results from the hyperdynamic emptying of the left ventricle rather than the impediment of outflow tract obstruction.

Mitral regurgitation (MR) is present frequently (22, 25, 27, 31, 32). This occurs predominantly in midsystole and late systole, at a time when the mitral apparatus is compressed and distorted in the contracted ventricular cavity. Systolic contraction of the mitral annulus is greatly exaggerated in the HCM ventricle, and this further puckers and distorts the leaflets, interfering with competent coaptation. The relationship between the size of the ventricle and the incompetence of the mitral valve is similar to that seen in mitral prolapse; as the ventricle becomes smaller, the valve becomes more incompetent ("ventriclovalvular disproportion") (33).

Another form of systolic mitral valve dysfunction is systolic anterior motion (SAM) of the mitral apparatus. SAM is seen in M-mode echocardiograms as a multilayered "rainbow" occupying the space between the inward moving posterior wall and the relatively inert septum (Fig. 18.1). In those instances where two-dimensional echocardiograms reveal that the anterior or both mitral leaflets move toward the ventricular septum during systole, it has been proposed that the leaf-

Table 18.2. Pathophysiology of HCM

I. Systolic features
  A. "Hyperdynamic" ventricular contractions
    1. Increased ejection fraction (degree of emptying)
    2. Increased rate of ventricular emptying
      a. Ventricle "empty" by midsystole
      b. Aortic valve "preclosure"
    3. Sustained contraction (after emptying)
    4. Intracavitary pressure gradients
    5. Brisk aortic upstroke (increased dP/dT)
  B. Mitral valve dysfunction
    1. Mitral regurgitation
      a. Holosystolic
      b. Late systolic augmentation
    2. Systolic anterior motion
II. Diastolic features
  A. Delayed rate of isovolumic relaxation
  B. Decreased diastolic compliance
  C. Increased atrial transport function ("atrial kick")

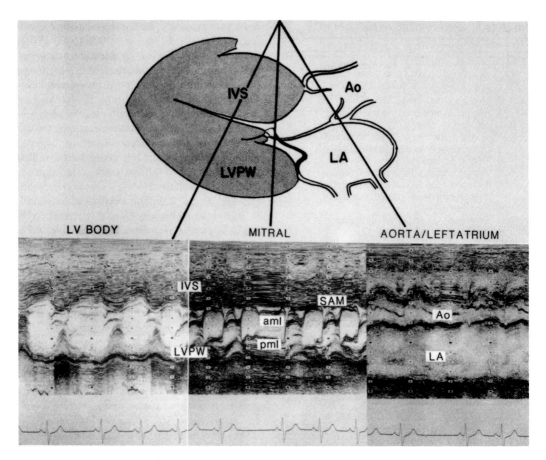

Figure 18.1. Schematic of the obliterated LV cavity based on the parasternal long-axis cross-sectional echocardiogram of a patient with hypertrophic cardiomyopathy. The three M-mode echoes are aligned to the appropriate two-dimensional beam angles. The *left panel* demonstrates asymmetric septal hypertrophy and increased fractional shortening with hyperdynamic wall motion. The *center panel* demonstrates SAM of the mitral apparatus. In the *right panel*, left atrial enlargement and aortic valve preclosure are present. *aml* = anterior mitral leaflet; *Ao* = aorta; *IVS* = interventricular septum; *LA* = left atrium; *LVPW* = left ventricular posterior wall; *pml* = posterior mitral leaflet.

lets are drawn forward by the negative pressure associated with the high early systolic ejection velocity in the outflow tract (34, 35). On apical two- and four-chamber views, a "hockey stick" or "crossed swords" appearance of the anterior and posterior mitral leaflets identifies SAM. Other two-dimensional echocardiographic studies have demonstrated that the subvalvular apparatus (chordae tendineae, papillary muscles, and distal valve tips), not the main portion of the leaflets, comprises SAM (36–38). Of the patients with HCM and SAM evaluated in our laboratories, most (67%) had subvalvular SAM present on two-dimensional echocardiography (Tables 18.3 and 18.4).

There is a long-standing controversy about the significance of SAM and its relationship to the dynamic intracavitary pressure gradients in HCM. The prevailing theory holds that SAM obstructs the egress of blood through the outflow tract and is responsible for the pressure gradient (39). This concept is supported by the *temporal* correlation of the intracavitary pressure gradient with echocardiographic SAM (34, 39). Furthermore, duration of SAM-septal contact correlates positively with the magnitude of the intracavitary gradient (40).

It is, however, difficult to reconcile "obstruction" to outflow with the supernormal ejection fraction and the rapidity with which ejection oc-

Table 18.3. Echocardiographic Characteristics of HCM

I. Hypertrophic, nondilated left ventricle in the absence of inciting cause (e.g., aortic stenosis, hypertension, coarctation)
II. Abnormal thickening of LV wall in the absence of myocardial infarction
  A. Asymmetrical septal hypertrophy (ASH)
  B. Disproportionate upper septal thickening (DUST)
  C. Apical hypertrophy
  D. Other regional
  E. Concentric
III. Hyperdynamic left ventricle with obliteration of submitral cavity
  A. Increased percentage of fractional shortening
  B. Increased inward excursion of posterior LV wall
  C. "Sessile" interventricular septum (by M-mode)
IV. Mitral valve
  A. Prolonged diastolic septal apposition
  B. M-mode: reduced E–F slope and prominent B shoulder
  C. Anterior position of mitral valve apparatus
  D. Systolic anterior motion (SAM) with or without SAM-septal contact
    1. "Hockey stick"
    2. "Crossed swords"
  E. Thickened leaflets
  F. Annular calcification
V. Aortic valve
  A. Systolic fluttering
  B. Systolic preclosure
  C. Reduced diastolic slope (M-mode) of aorta
VI. Left atrial enlargement

curs. Dynamic gradients can be provoked in normal human and experimental animal ventricles under a variety of stimuli that have in common increased contractility, decreased filling, and/or decreased arterial impedance (21, 23, 25, 41–46). The similarity of HCM gradients and the intracavitary pressure gradients occurring in nonobstructed, hyperdynamic normal ventricles have formed the basis for questioning the validity of outflow tract obstruction in HCM. In addition, when a latex model of the ventricle, which is designed to be incapable of obstruction, is caused to empty rapidly and completely by the above provocations, the generation of dynamic gradients can be reproduced (42, 47, 48) (Fig. 18.2). In the model ventricle, as in hypertrophic cardiomyopathy, the phenomenon responsible for these dynamic gradients has been termed *cavity obliteration*. As the ventricle rapidly empties, there are two pressure zones within the ventricle: high pressure in the obliterating body and lower pressure in the noncontractile outflow tract. The tran-

sition between the high and low pressure zones occurs at the interface between the obliterated body and the noncontractile outflow tract. When the cavity of the model ventricle is explored with micromanometer pressure transducers, catheter-mounted velocity probes, and echo-Doppler interrogation, the measured intracavitary pressure gradients correlate with the Doppler estimates ($r = 0.98$), and the highest velocity is recorded at the basal portion of the obliterated ventricle at its interface with the noncontractile outflow tract (47, 48).

In the human or experimental animal ventricle, augmented contractions obliterate the entire submitral cavity, similar to the ventricle in HCM (41, 42, 44–48). In each of these settings, the interface between the obliterated cavity and the widely patent outflow tract occurs at the level of the mitral valve. The body of the left ventricle up to the mitral valve is contractile and capable of obliterating. The anterior leaflet of the mitral valve forms the posterior boundary of the low pressure outflow tract, while the underside of the mitral valve (principally the inflated ventricular aspect of the posterior mitral leaflet) resides in the high pressure zone within the obliterating ventricular cavity. This pressure difference within the obliterating ventricle could *result in* SAM, rather than SAM causing the pressure difference.

Our echocardiographic findings are consistent with SAM being generated by the hyperdynamic ejection observed in HCM. Ninety-five percent of patients with SAM that we studied by two-dimensional echocardiography had cavity obliteration. Moreover, the duration of SAM-septal

Table 18.4. Echocardiographic Findings in 42 Cases of HCM with SAM

	Present N (%)	Absent N (%)
ASH	29 (71)	12 (29)
Aortic valve preclosure	26 (65)	14 (35)
Mitral annular calcification	18 (43)	24 (57)
Reduced mitral diastolic slope	37 (88)	5 (12)
Mitral valve diastolic septal contact	36 (90)	4 (10)
Septal plaque	24 (57)	18 (43)
Subvalvular SAM	25 (68)	12 (32)
Left atrial enlargement	29 (69)	13 (31)
Cavity obliteration	38 (95)	2 (5)

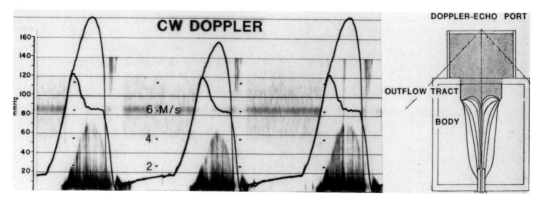

Figure 18.2. Doppler-pressure gradient correlates in an experimental cavity obliteration ventricular model. A simple latex model of the ventricle has been placed in a plastic box and exposed to phasic pneumatic pressure, which permits filling and emptying of the ventricle. The conical ventricle has been designed without valves and tapers from the cylindrical rigid outflow collar to the pointed apex. The body of the ventricle was obliterated with application of pneumatic pressure, while the rigid outflow tract remained as a "dead space." Micromanometer catheters in the obliterating body and patent outflow tract recorded a pressure drop of 60–100 mm Hg during "pulsus alternans," induced by varying the magnitude of the applied pneumatic pressure. Ultrasonic recording through a fluid-filled chamber adjacent to the outflow tract (*Doppler-echo port*) permitted imaging and Doppler velocity recording. The pressure gradient is 93 mm Hg, and the Doppler velocity is 5 m/sec (equivalent to 100 mm Hg). In the second complex, the pressure gradient is 70 mm Hg, and the Doppler velocity is 4.3 m/sec (74 mm Hg). When a wide range of gradients was induced by greater and lesser applications of pneumatic pressure, the correlation coefficient (*R*) between manometric and Doppler-estimated gradients was 0.98. *CW Doppler* = continuous wave Doppler.

contact was highly correlated with the percentage of fractional shortening ($R = 0.66$ $p < 0.001$), an index of contractility; in addition, the smaller the LV end-systolic volume, the greater the duration of SAM-septal contact ($R = 0.65$, $p < 0.001$).

Thus, the echocardiographic data support that SAM could result from rapid and complete emptying, as opposed to serving as an impediment to LV emptying.

Diastole

There is a reduced rate of diastolic relaxation and decreased distensibility (compliance) of the HCM ventricle, variously explained by hypertrophy, ischemia, myofiber disarray, fibrosis, and/or abnormal calcium flux within the myocardial elements (22, 49–57). This diastolic dysfunction results in elevated LV filling pressure, delayed onset and/or reduced rate of early diastolic passive mitral inflow, and increased atrial transport function ("atrial kick") (Fig. 18.3). Left atrial dilatation results from the additive effects of diastolic dysfunction and mitral regurgitation. Dyspnea and orthopnea in HCM are related to diastolic dysfunction and resulting pulmonary ve-

nous hypertension. Limitations in cardiac output, which become manifest during exertion, tachycardias, or loss of atrial kick, result from the reduced ventricular filling volume. Diastolic dysfunction explains the presence of congestive symptoms in the setting of supernormal ventricular emptying better than does "outflow tract obstruction" (52, 57). Furthermore, patients without pressure gradients are frequently symptomatic and have a significant risk of premature death (49, 58).

ECHOCARDIOGRAPHIC CRITERIA FOR THE DIAGNOSIS OF HCM

The gross morphology and functional physiology described above provide groundwork for the echocardiographic recognition of HCM. The sine qua non for HCM is the presence of LVH in the absence of known causative factors (2, 5, 22, 30, 49). The echocardiographic characteristics of HCM are listed in Table 18.3. Wall thickness, the echocardiographic manifestation of hypertrophy, is most precisely measured by M-mode echocardiography (2–4). The localization of hypertrophy and the typical features of left ventricular ejection dynamics are appreciated better with two-

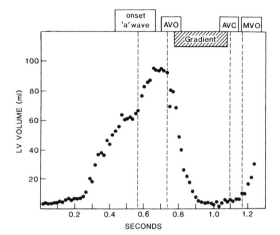

Figure 18.3. The atrial kick, identified by "onset A wave," contributes over 30 ml (>30%) to the LV end-diastolic volume. These volumes were calculated from cineangiograms during left ventriculography in a patient with HCM. Each *dot* identifies a volumetric measurement calculated from an individual angiographic frame. A complete cardiac cycle is shown. Diastole starts at time 0. Gradient refers to the onset and offset of the LVOT gradient. Isovolumetric relaxation time occurs from aortic valve closure (*AVC*) to mitral valve opening (*MVO*). *AVO* = aortic valve opening.

dimensional echocardiography. Echocardiographic findings seen in 42 of our cases of HCM with SAM are listed in Tables 18.4 and 18.5.

TWO-DIMENSIONAL ECHOCARDIOGRAPHY

The dynamic images generated by two-dimensional echocardiography provide a comprehensive functional-anatomic depiction of the abnormalities in HCM. The patient illustrated in Figures 18.4–18.6 had typical HCM and died suddenly during exertion. He had sustained an exercise-induced cardiac arrest 29 months previously but was successfully defibrillated by paramedics. He underwent five echo-Doppler studies between the two cardiac arrests, with remarkably similar findings of massive ASH, SAM (with brief duration of SAM-septal contact), and outflow tract velocities of 1.5–2 m/sec. Thus, evidence of significant outflow tract gradients was not present.

The two-dimensional images are shown in the parasternal long-axis (*A1–A6*) and parasternal short-axis projections at the level of the mitral valve (*B1–B6*) and body of left ventricle (*C1–C2*) (Fig. 18.5). The heart has been cut to represent the long-axis view. Selected diastolic and systolic two-dimensional frames are arranged in Table 18.6, with *asterisks* representing frames depicted in the line drawings in Figure 18.4:

The early diastolic frames demonstrate that the circumference of the mitral sleeve occupies the entire circumference of the LV inflow tract in early diastole (*B1*); the contact between the anterior mitral leaflet and the interventricular septum is seen clearly in *A1*. The irregular cavity of the submitral left ventricle increases in size between *C1* and *C2*, as the anterior mitral leaflet floats dorsally (i.e., *A1–A2, B1–B2*). With the onset of ventricular systole, the mitral valve closes (*A3, B3*), followed by aortic valve opening (*A4*). The mitral valve sleeve becomes puckered and distorted as the LV walls thicken and the endocardium moves centripetally (i.e., *B3–B5*). SAM-septal contact is seen in *A5* and *B5*, while cavitary obliteration of the submitral cavity is seen in *A5* and *C5*.

The composition of SAM can be appreciated best by integrating the M-mode and two-dimensional findings. In the M-mode depiction (Fig. 18.6) a multilayered or laminated texture can be appreciated in systole, and the two-dimensional frames demonstrate the posterior mitral leaflet engulfing the anterior leaflet in *B5* and projecting anterior to the anterior mitral leaflet (in *A5*). Thus, echocardiographic SAM depicts ventral movement of the interdigitating corrugations of the anterior and posterior mitral leaflets as well as the chordae tendineae. In late systole, as LV contraction abates and LV pressure declines, there is retrograde movement of blood from the patent

Table 18.5. M-Mode Echocardiographic Measurements in 42 Cases of HCM

	Mean ± Standard Deviation	Range
Ventricular septal thickness (mm)	21.8 ± 4.8	14–34
LV posterior wall thickness (mm)	14.6 ± 3.4	11–27
LV internal diameter at end-systole (mm)	20.6 ± 7.3	5–37
LV internal diameter at end-diastole (mm)	40.9 ± 7.5	20–57
Left atrial dimension (mm)	45.1 ± 9.2	30–70
Fractional shortening (%)	51.3 ± 15.4	18–88

Table 18.6.

	1 early	2 mid	3 isovolumic	4 early	5 mid	6 late
		DIASTOLE		SYSTOLE		
	(E point)	(F point)	(MV closed)[a]	(AV open)[a]	(SAM)	
Long axis	A1	A2*	A3	A4	A5*	A6
Short axis	B1	B2*	B3	B4	B5*	B6
Short axis	C1	C2*	C3	C4	C5*	C6

[a]MV = mitral valve, AV = aortic valve.
The timing of the above numbered frames is represented on the M-mode echocardiogram by *vertical lines* in Figure 18.6.

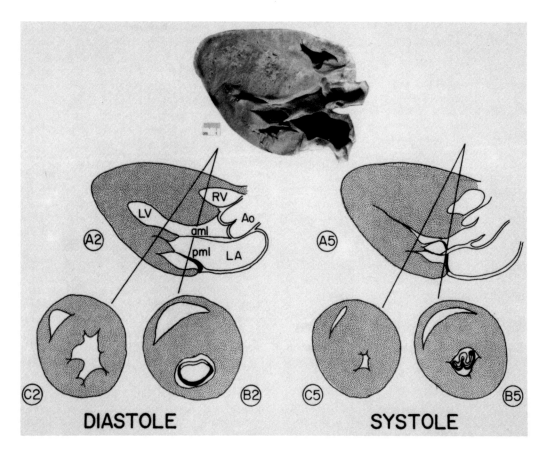

Figure 18.4. HCM heart related to two-dimensional echocardiographic image planes. A postmortem specimen from a patient dying with HCM has been cut along the long axis, allowing comparison with echocardiographic views. There is massive asymmetrical hypertrophy of the heart, principally involving the interventricular septum. The ventricular cavities are pathologically small, and the mitral valve is crowded. *A2, A5*, etc. refer to the antemortem two-dimensional echocardiographic images displayed in Figure 18.5. The diagrams depict middiastole in long-axis (*A2*) and two short-axis planes, ventricular body (*C2*) and mitral region (*B2*). The midsystolic counterparts are shown on the *right*. The mitral sleeve, best seen in diastole in *A2* and *B2*, consists of one-third of the anterior mitral leaflet (*aml*) in white and two-thirds of the posterior leaflet (*pml*) in black. Systolic anterior motion of the mitral apparatus is depicted in *A5* and *B5*. The anterior and posterior mitral leaflets seem to decussate in *A5*; in the short-axis plane (*B5*), the mitral sleeve is collapsed like a closed umbrella, with the posterior leaflet engulfing the anterior leaflet. Thus the posterior leaflet projects ventral to the anterior leaflet to give the appearance of crossing or "punching through" the anterior leaflet. *Ao* = aorta, *LA* = left atrium, *LV* = left ventricle.

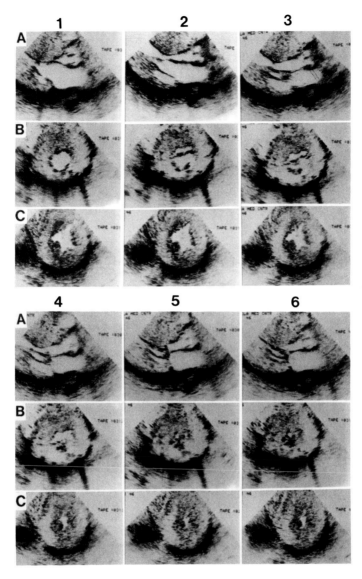

Figure 18.5. Two-dimensional echocardiogram obtained 8 months premortem in 16-year-old patient with HCM. These echocardiographic frames depict the heart in parasternal long-axis (*A1–A6*), short-axis mitral region (*B1–B6*), and short-axis ventricular body (*C1–C6*) planes. The diagrams in Figure 18.3 relate to the *numbered frames*. The timing of the frames in each plane, *1–6*, corresponds to the *vertical lines* in the M-mode echo of the mitral region in Figure 18.5. *Frames 1* and *2* are early diastolic and middiastolic, while frames *3–6* were obtained at 100 msec intervals from the onset of systole, encompassing the onset, offset, and duration of systolic anterior motion.

subaortic chamber (aortic vestibule) apically toward the obliterated ventricular cavity. This retrograde movement of blood causes reversal of SAM as the mitral leaflets move dorsally.

Although not demonstrated in the patient in Figs. 18.4–18.6, many patients with HCM have "preclosure" of the aortic valve during systole, as shown in Fig. 18.7. Preclosure occurs at a time when outflow from the left ventricle is waning or absent and the left ventricle has achieved its "dead space" or minimum systolic volume (49). Studies of the fluid mechanics of the aortic valve in normal people have shown that decelerating blood in the ascending aorta results in eddies that cause

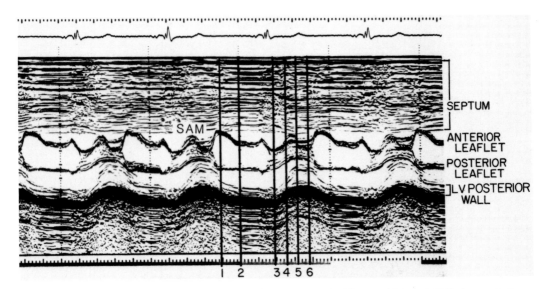

Figure 18.6. M-mode echocardiogram of the same patient as in Figures 18.4 and 18.5 demonstrates a 5 cm "sessile" septum and crowded mitral apparatus with diastolic and systolic contact between the mitral valve and septum. The posterior wall thickens markedly during its 2 cm systolic inward excursion. The *horizontal time markers* occur at 0.04 and 0.2 sec, and the vertical dimensional calibration is in 0.2 and 1 cm increments. The *solid numbered lines* refer to the timing of the frames in Figures 18.4 and 18.5.

aortic valve closure to begin, even though LV ejection is not complete (59, 60). Thus, in addition, to reduce flow by midsystole, eddies created by deceleration of ascending aortic flow could also promote preclosure, even though there is still some forward flow.

ECHO-DOPPLER INDICES OF DIASTOLIC ABNORMALITIES IN HCM

Diastolic compliance in patients with HCM is reduced as a result of the increased wall thickness (53). This causes a shift of the diastolic pressure volume relationship upward and to the left (Fig. 18.8). LV diastolic relaxation is slower, LV filling pressure is increased, and the volume of LV filling is reduced (50–57). These factors very likely cause symptoms due to pulmonary venous hypertension (dyspnea) and reduced cardiac output (fatigue and syncope). Additionally, impaired relaxation in combination with increased LV mass may result in coronary supply-demand imbalance, myocardial ischemia, and chest pain (61, 62). The functional and hemodynamic consequences of diastolic abnormalities are evident on echocardiographic and Doppler examination.

M-mode echocardiography is well suited for evaluating the diastolic time period due to a rapid sampling rate (1000/sec), which allows careful

measurement of changes in the rates of diastolic posterior aortic root movement, anterior mitral leaflet middiastolic closure (E-F slope), changes in LV dimensions, endocardial wall motion, wall thinning, and rate of posterior wall diastolic excursion. Decreased diastolic aortic root movement ("left-atrial emptying-index") implies reduced diastolic left atrial emptying and therefore abnormal LV diastolic filling (63, 64) (Figs. 18.7–18.9). A flat mitral valve E-F slope reflects prolonged early to middiastolic transmitral flow due to decreased LV compliance and/or relaxation. In addition, left atrial enlargement often reflects chronic elevation of LV end-diastolic pressure, although in HCM it may also reflect the presence of mitral regurgitation.

For more precise evaluation, computer digitization of the M-mode echocardiogram allows analysis of diastole by the assessment of diastolic LV posterior wall thinning, time-to-peak LV internal dimension, peak velocity of circumferential fiber change, and time-to-peak circumferential fiber change (65–68). By digitizing M-mode echocardiograms, Spirito et al. (53) found abnormalities in 80% of patients with HCM. In these patients, increased LV wall thickness correlated directly with reduction in rate of diastolic filling and with prolongation of the duration of LV fill-

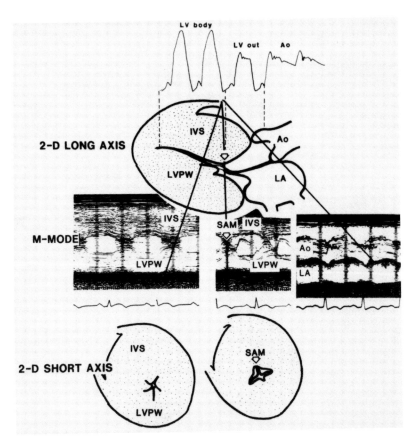

Figure 18.7. Hemodynamic and echocardiographic correlations in HCM. *Upper panel:* A diagrammatic depiction of a withdrawal pressure recording *(top)* demonstrating an intracavitary pressure gradient is aligned with a long-axis, two-dimensional *(2-D)* echocardiogram in midsystole. *Central panels:* Below the long-axis figure are three M-mode panels representing the ventricular body, mitral valve, and aortic-left atrial regions of the left heart. *Bottom panels:* The two-dimensional *(2-D)* short-axis views of the midsystolic LV body and mitral valve regions are aligned with the M-mode panels of the same regions immediately above. The high pressure zone bounded by the *left* and *center dashed lines* is within the obliterating submitral LV body *(LV body)*. The low pressure zone exists in the subaortic vestibule *(LV out)*, bounded apically by the compressed mitral apparatus and basally by the aortic valve leaflets. This region of the left ventricle is largely membranous and therefore does not contract or obliterate; it shares the same systolic pressure as the aortic root with which it is in open communication during systole. SAM *(arrows)* is composed of an amalgam of leaflet tips, chordae, and submitral apparatus. Preclosure of the aortic valve is seen in the *right-hand* M-mode *panel. Ao* = aorta, *IVS* = interventricular septum, *LA* = left atrium, *LVPW* = left ventricular posterior wall.

ing, as measured by the isovolumic relaxation time (IVRT = time from the peak systolic excursion of the LV posterior wall to the time of mitral valve opening). Additional symptoms were more frequent in those patients with more extensive LVH and the greater extent of abnormal diastolic wall motion (53). DeCoodt et al. (69) used digitized M-mode echocardiography to assess the three phases of diastole: (*a*) early, rapid filling; (*b*) middiastolic, slow filling ("diastasis"); and (*c*) atrial "kick". Whereas normally early rapid filling causes 73% of total LV diameter increase, this percentage change was reduced to 55% in HCM patients. In addition, the atrial contribution to LV diameter increase was nearly double that seen in normal subjects (28% in HCM versus 15% in normal subjects).

Echocardiographic evidence of improved dia-

Figure 18.8. *Line AC* identifies a normal ventricular pressure-volume curve. *Curve AB* is representative of the abnormal shift of the pressure-volume relationship upward and to the left, which may be seen in HCM due to abnormal ventricular compliance and relaxation.

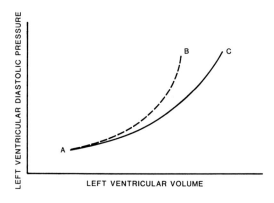

stolic function in HCM, with decreases in IVRT and increases in rate of posterior wall thinning, have been found using the calcium channel-blockers nifedipine (70), verapamil (71), and diltiazem (72). Hanrath and coworkers (71) showed improvement in LV isovolumic relaxation (IVRT), rate of LV posterior wall thinning, and an increase in LV dimension after the acute administration of verapamil. In patients on chronic ver-

apamil therapy, Hasin et al. (73) did not find such changes in IVRT or posterior wall thinning but did demonstrate an increase in the mitral E-F slope and a slight reduction in left atrial dimension. Suwa et al. (72), also using M-mode echocardiography to monitor therapeutic efficacy in HCM patients, found the calcium channel-blocker diltiazem to be effective in increasing diastolic filling velocity and decreasing the time to the oc-

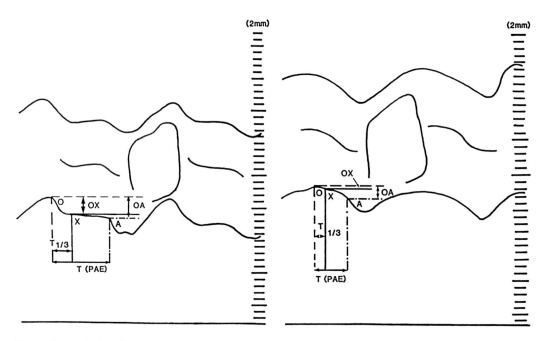

Figure 18.9. Left atrial emptying index (LAEI) in a normal subject (*left panel*) and an abnormal patient (*right panel*). The LAET is calculated by measuring the posterior movement of the posterior aortic wall during the first one-third of passive atrial emptying ($T_{1/3} = O - X$ points) divided by the excursion of the posterior aortic wall during total passive atrial emptying (*T (PAE)*) (*preatrial contraction O − A*). In the normal patient, most of passive atrial emptying occurs early, and the LAEI is therefore nearly equal to 1. In the presence of delayed left atrial emptying, which can be due to reduced LV diastolic compliance, impaired LV relaxation, or mitral stenosis, the LAEI is markedly reduced.

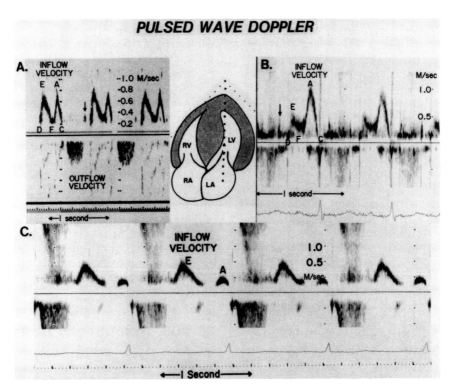

PULSED WAVE DOPPLER

Figure 18.10. *Center* (between *panels A* and *B*): Schematic of apical four-chamber two-dimensional echocardiogram, demonstrating pulse wave Doppler sample volume just below the mitral valve annulus. *LA* = left atrium, *LV* = left ventricle, *RA* = right atrium, *RV* = right ventricle. In *panels A–C*, diastolic Doppler inflow patterns are shown from three different patients with hypertrophic cardiomyopathy. The *arrow* indicates the aortic closure (A_2) sound. Pertinent measurements include: A_2 (*arrow*) to D, reflecting the time interval from aortic closure to the onset of the mitral inflow velocity; D–F, the early diastolic flow duration; E-F slope, reflecting the rate of early diastolic filling; the E:A ratio is indicative of the relative atrial contribution to filling. In *panel A*, the early Doppler flow (*E*) and late flow due to the atrial kick (*A*) are of similar magnitude. In *panel B*, the duration from aortic closure (*arrow*) to E is increased, the E-F slope is flat, reflecting slow deceleration of early diastolic flow velocity, and there is increased late diastolic filling due to atrial contraction (reflected by the prominent A wave). In *panel C*, the deceleration rate of the early diastolic peak (E-F slope) is reduced and D–F duration is increased; however, the atrial contribution is reduced (not increased) in this patient who had marked left atrial enlargement (7.0 cm).

currence of peak velocity of circumferential fiber change in diastole. Suwa et al. did not observe these changes with use of propranolol at low doses (60–120 mg/day). However, Bourmayan et al. (74) studied higher doses of propranolol (mean dose: 390 mg/day) and did find decreased IVRT reflecting enhanced diastolic relaxation. Pharmacologic improvement in LV diastolic filling in patients with HCM has been shown to be associated with enhanced exercise tolerance (57).

Doppler, radionuclide, and contrast angiographic assessment of LV diastolic function have been shown to correlate well with one another (75, 76). Spirito et al. (75) found an 84% agreement in differentiating normal from abnormal diastolic function and a 100% concordance on the patients with normal diastolic LV function. Doppler-echocardiographic LV diastolic function is assessed by measuring the ventricular filling from an apical four-chamber view. The pulse wave Doppler cursor is placed to detect the sample LV inflow velocities at about 1 cm below the mitral annulus (Fig. 18.10). The cursor is adjusted to get the sample volume with the highest inflow velocities. The cycles with the best signal:noise ratio and highest E and A peaks should be chosen for evaluating parameters of LV diastolic function (75–77).

Diastolic Doppler indices that can be used to evaluate LV diastolic function include: (*a*) time interval from aortic valve closure to the onset of mitral valve inflow (isovolumic relaxation); (*b*) duration of early diastolic flow, defined by the time from the onset of early mitral flow (D point on Doppler flow pattern) to the time of middiastolic diastasis (F point); (*c*) early maximal flow velocity measured by the height of the E point; (*d*) deceleration of flow velocity in early diastole (E-F slope); (*e*) maximal late diastolic flow velocity (A wave height); and, (*f*) relative contribution of early (E) and late (A) diastolic flow to LV filling (ratio of heights of E:A waves) (75–77) (Fig. 18.10).

Assessing such indices of LV diastolic function reveals a number of pulsed wave Doppler patterns in HCM (Fig. 18.10*A–C*). Reduced E:A ratio and reduced early diastolic deceleration rate have been demonstrated in HCM by a number of investigators (75, 77, 78). However, the E:A ratio may be misleading and insensitive in HCM. In one study, the magnitude of the atrial contribution as well as the E:A ratio was found to be abnormal in only about 20% of HCM patients (78). The E:A ratio in HCM is increased by the augmented early inflow in mitral regurgitation (MR). Since significant MR results in an increased left atrial-left ventricular early diastolic pressure gradient, a higher E point, due to early transmitral flow, may occur and thus cause "pseudonormalization" of the E:A ratio. A further increase in the E:A ratio may result from the loss of atrial kick that occurs in a massively dilated atrium (Figs. 18.1 and 18.10*C*).

By Doppler methods, patients with HCM also have prolonged isovolumic relaxation times, prolonged duration of early diastolic filling, reduced early maximal velocity of filling, and increased atrial contribution to filling (77–81). Diastolic filling abnormalities are extremely common in patients with HCM (Table 18.7). As previously described for digitized M-mode echo, diastolic dysfunction is found by Doppler in about 80% of HCM patients (78). The most frequent abnormal Doppler parameters of LV filling are the prolongation of the isovolumic relaxation period and the duration of early diastolic peak flow. In addition, there are reductions in the deceleration rate and in the maximal flow velocities (Fig. 18.10, Table 18.7). In a comprehensive study of HCM patients, Ma-

ron and coworkers (78) documented that Doppler parameters of diastolic dysfunction frequently are present in symptomatic as well as asymptomatic patients. It has been hypothesized by Wigle (39) that the "subaortic stenosis may act as a contraction load" that impairs LV diastolic filling. This hypothesis is not supported by the frequent presence of abnormal diastolic function in the absence of an LV outflow tract gradient in HCM patients. Moreover, patients without outflow tract gradients in Maron's series were equally likely to have evidence of abnormal diastolic function (78). This finding implicates the inordinate amount of LVH and its consequences rather than a contraction load as the cause of abnormal LV diastolic function. Furthermore, abnormal right ventricular diastolic function has also been demonstrated by Doppler echocardiography in a group of HCM patients (82).

DOPPLER SYSTOLIC FLOW PATTERNS

In an attempt to characterize *systolic* flow patterns and LV ejection dynamics, Maron and coworkers (83) used pulsed wave Doppler to study 50 patients with HCM. In patients with left ventricular outflow tract (LVOT) gradients (mean: 75 mm Hg) (N = 20), termed "obstructive" HCM, LV ejection was characterized by very early and rapid emptying. In these HCM patients with outflow gradients, 76% ± 14% of the aortic flow velocity occurred in the first one-third of systole, compared with 37% ± 5% for normal subjects and 39% ± 7% for HCM patients without gradients. Furthermore, in the gradient group there was a significantly greater fraction of the integral of aortic flow velocity curve (91% ± 10%) occurring in the first one-half of systole, compared to 63% ± 5% for normal subjects and 65% ± 8% for HCM patients without LVOT gradients (see Table 18.8). Such findings are consistent with the more rapid than normal LV emptying in HCM patients with gradients reported by investigators using other techniques, including intraoperative aortic flow probes, catheter-mounted flow probes, and angiographic volumetric studies (49). Although in 7 of 20 of the HCM patients with gradients studied by Maron, there was a small second peak of aortic flow velocity, a second peak in aortic flow was not found by investigators using invasive methods to quantitate aortic flow, such as circumferential aortic flow probe or angiographic volumetric methods (21, 23–26, 31, 45, 49).

Table 18.7. Diastolic Indices Assessed by Doppler Echocardiography in 111 Patients with Hypertrophic Cardiomyopathy and 86 Control Subjects[a]

	Patients with Hypertrophic Cardiomyopathy	Control Subjects	p Value
RR interval (msec)	994 ± 193	1,039 ± 131	NS
$A_2 - D$ (msec)	94 ± 24	78 ± 12	< 0.001
D − F (msec)	244 ± 55	220 ± 28	< 0.001
E − F slope (m/sec²)	3.4 ± 1.4	4.9 ± 1.3	< 0.001
E (m/sec)	0.5 ± 0.2	0.6 ± 0.1	< 0.001
A (m/sec)	0.4 ± 0.3	0.3 ± 0.1	< 0.001
E:A	1.4 ± 0.8	2.1 ± 0.9	< 0.001

[a]From Maron BJ, Spirito P, Green KJ, Wesley YE, Bonow RO, Arce J: Noninvasive assessment of left ventricular diastolic function by pulsed Doppler echocardiography in patients with hypertrophic cardiomyopathy. *J Am Coll Cardiol* 10:733–742, 1987.
[b]A = maximal late flow velocity (due to atrial contraction); A_2–D = isovolumic relaxation; D–F = duration of early peak of flow velocity; *E* = maximal diastolic flow velocity; E:A = ratio of maximal flow velocity in early diastolic to maximal flow velocity in late diastole; E–F slope = rate of decrease (deceleration) of flow velocity in early diastole.

Yock and coworkers (59) also studied HCM patients with pulse wave Doppler but did not find a consistent "second" aortic flow peak pattern as recorded in seven of the twenty patients studied by Maron et al. (83). They noted that in different locations, single, double, or triple positive "flow peaks" could be recorded in the aorta during systole (59). Yock et al. (59) demonstrated that the high degree of heterogeneity in the aortic velocity contours is mostly likely indicative of late systolic eddies of flow moving in different directions within the aorta. They concluded that the second aortic flow peaks recorded in HCM patients with LVOT gradients are due to either reflected pressure waves secondary to rapid initial ejection or rapid aortic flow deceleration—not a result of a second wave of forward blood flow (59).

In the pulsed wave mode, Doppler can be used to assess the relative LV emptying rate, the LV filling rate, and the degree of mitral regurgitation. In the continuous wave mode, Doppler can be used to study the magnitude of LVOT pressure gradients. Transducer angulation is critical to identifying accurately the magnitude of the LVOT gradient, and care must be taken to avoid the inappropriate recording of the LV-left atrial gradient resulting from MR instead of the LVOT

(LV-aortic) gradient. Differentiating the LVOT and mitral regurgitation CW tracings can be facilitated by pulsed wave mapping between the left atrium and LVOT. Furthermore, the MR jet appears somewhat earlier than the LVOT jet, the MR jet has a higher peak velocity (as LV gradient from left-ventricle left atrium is greater than left ventricle (LVOT), and the contour of the LVOT tracing differs from the MR tracing. The LVOT velocity signal generally shows: (*a*) an initial gradual rise followed by (*b*) an abrupt increase in velocities, resulting in (*c*) a concave appearance to the LVOT velocity and (*d*) a reduced signal intensity at the late systolic LVOT velocities (Fig. 19.2 and 18.11 *A–C*) (47, 48, 59). The reduced signal intensity on Doppler tracings indicates that the late systolic high velocity jets represent a small amount of late volumetric flow.

Color flow Doppler provides additional information in the evaluation of HCM patients. It is particularly useful in (*a*) assessing the severity of mitral regurgitation, (*b*) studying the direction of the mitral regurgitation jet (generally posterolateral); and (*c*) differentiating the elevated Doppler velocities due to the LVOT jet and the mitral regurgitation jet. Color flow studies have corroborated the high frequency of mitral regurgitation

Table 18.8. Fraction of the Integral of Aortic Flow Velocity Curve[a]

	First One-Third of Systole (%)	First One-Half of Systole (%)
Normal	37 ± 5	63 ± 5
HCM without LVOT gradient	39 ± 7	65 ± 8
HCM with LVOT gradient	76 ± 14	91 ± 10

[a]Data are from Maron BJ, Gottdiener JS, Arce J, Rosing DR, Wesley YE, Epstein SE: Dynamic subaortic obstruction in hypertrophic cardiomyopathy: Analysis by pulsed Doppler echocardiography. *J Am Coll Cardiol* 6: 1–15, 1985.

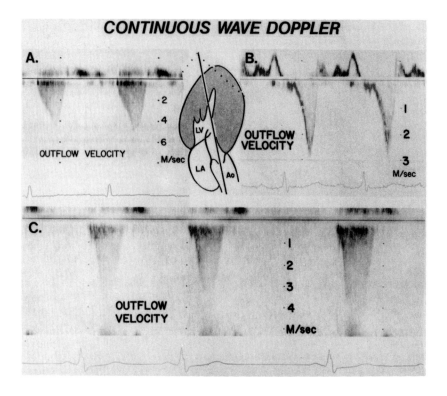

Figure 18.11. *Center* (between *panels A* and *B*): Schematic of apical long-axis view, demonstrating continuous wave sample volume across LVOT. *Ao* = aorta, LA = left atrium, *LV* = left ventricle. In *panels A–C*, outflow tract velocities from three different patients are shown. In *panel A*, the maximal LVOT velocity is 5 m/sec, reflecting a LVOT gradient of 100 mm Hg. The asymptotic or sigmoid shape of the continuous wave velocity are typical of HCM outflow tract velocities (> 3 m/sec) in which the early systolic gradual rise in velocity becomes accelerated terminally. In *panel B*, there is also terminal acceleration to 3 m/sec (LVOT gradient approximately 36 mm Hg), but the entire velocity pattern from early to end-systole has a concave pattern. In *panel C*, LVOT velocities exceed 4 m/sec (gradient of > 64 mm Hg), and the terminal high velocities show a decreased intensity consistent with little late volumetric flow at the time of the maximal outflow tract gradient.

detected in angiographic studies, but no significant correlation has been found between the degree of mitral regurgitation and the magnitude of the LVOT gradient (84, 85).

The preponderance of echo-Doppler findings in HCM indicates that LV diastolic function is impaired in most of these patients. Moreover, there is a general consensus that abnormal LV diastolic function is an important part of the pathophysiology of HCM and frequently accounts for the patient's symptoms. However, the significance of intraventricular pressure gradients in HCM has been the subject of great interest and controversy (22, 30, 39, 49). Review of the available data indicates there is reason to question the importance of HCM intracavitary gradients. Yock

and colleagues (59) proposed that the critical pathophysiologic question regarding elevated LVOT gradients was whether they result in abnormal LV stress and cause progressive LV hypertrophy. According to the law of Laplace, wall stress or tension (T) is determined by pressure (P), radius (R), and wall thickness (h) in the following manner:

$$T = (P \times R)/h. \qquad 18.1$$

Thus, LV systolic wall stress may not be increased due to the presence of LVH and the reduced LV systolic chamber size (86). Consistent with this thesis, the presence of LVOT gradients has not been observed to result in progressive LVH (14,

16); development of LVH is similarly independent of the presence of an LVOT gradient (14, 16). Such dynamic outflow tract gradients do *not* correlate with the severity of mitral regurgitation (25), the presence or severity of diastolic dysfunction (78), cardiac symptoms (49, 58), or the frequency of sudden death (58).

CONCLUSION

Echo-Doppler ultrasonography has become the most useful method for establishing the diagnosis and quantitating the dysfunction in patients with HCM. Echo-Doppler combines the ability to see the intracardiac structures with the assessment of aortic outflow, patterns of ventricular filling and emptying, mitral regurgitation, and LVOT gradients. Historically, it was the recognition of the outflow tract pressure gradient during cardiac catheterization that characterized this disease as a form of outflow tract obstruction. During the early years of discovery of the condition now known as hypertrophic cardiomyopathy, an indelible impression was established that gradient equaled obstruction and that this "obstruction" was responsible for associated signs, symptoms, morbidity, and mortality.

Recordings of dynamic images of the heart, not available in the early years following the discovery of HCM, revealed HCM to be a unique cardiac disorder in which the ventricle emptied more rapidly and completely than in the normal heart, unlike the obstructed (e.g., aortic stenosis) ventricle which demonstrated an impeded rate of emptying. These observations contradicted the equation

$$\text{Pressure gradient} = \text{Obstruction}, \quad 18.2$$

as did the lack of correlation of the presence of a pressure gradient with morbidity and mortality. It is now apparent that the combination of inordinate LV hypertrophy and related diastolic dysfunction better explains cardiac symptomatology.

Noninvasive imaging techniques now enable the cardiologist to characterize the functional anatomy patients with HCM and to follow the clinical course and response to therapy. This evolving technology permits a more intimate and thorough evaluation of the HCM patient than any previous diagnostic procedure(s). It is hoped that this chapter has served to emphasize the relevant features of HCM and will permit the reader to understand better the controversy about the relevance of "obstruction."

ACKNOWLEDGMENTS

The authors gratefully acknowledge the assistance of David Criley and Angelika Appleton for their help in the preparation of this manuscript and figures.

REFERENCES

1. Teare D: Asymmetrical hypertrophy of the heart in young adults. *Br Heart J* 20:1–8, 1957.
2. Shapiro LM, McKenna WJ: Distribution of left ventricular hypertrophy in hypertrophic cardiomyopathy: A two-dimensional echocardiographic study. *J Am Coll Cardiol* 2:437–444, 1983.
3. Yamaguchi H, Ishimura T, Nishiyama S, et al: Hypertropic nonobstructive cardiomyopathy with giant negative T waves (apical hypertrophy): Ventriculographic and echocardiographic features in 30 patients. *Am J Cardiol* 44:401–412, 1979.
4. Maron BJ, Gottdiener JS, Bonow RO, Epstein SE: Hypertrophic cardiomyopathy with unusual location of left ventricular hypertrophy undetectable by M-mode echocardiography: Identification by wide-angle two-dimensional echocardiography. *Circulation* 63:409–418, 1981.
5. Roberts WC: The structural basis of abnormal cardiac function: A look at coronary, hypertensive, valvular, idiopathic myocardial, and pericardial heart diseases. *Clin Cardiovasc Physiol*, 1–56, 1976.
6. Corday SR, Virmani R, Waller B, Shah PM: Necropsy evaluation of anterior mitral leaflet elongation in cardiomyopathies: Possible role in hypertrophic cardiomyopathy. *Circulation* 60 (Suppl):243, 1979.
7. Salazar AE, Edwards JE: Friction lesions of the ventricular endocardium. Relation to chordae tendineae of the mitral valve. *Arch Pathol* 90:364–376, 1970.
8. St John Sutton MG, Lie JT, Anderson KR, O'Brien PC, Frey RL: Histopathological specificity of hypertrophic obstructive cardiomyopathy: Myocardial fiber disarray and myocardial fibrosis. *Br Heart J* 44:433–443, 1980.
9. Van Der Bel-Kahn J: Muscle fiber disarray in common heart diseases. *Am J Cardiol* 40:355–364, 1977.
10. Maron BJ, Wolfson JK, Epstein SE, Roberts WC: Intramural ("small vessel") coronary artery disease in hypertrophic cardiomyopathy. *J Am Coll Cardiol* 8:545–557, 1986.
11. Tanaka M, Fujiwara H, Onodera T, Wu D-J, Hamashima Y, Kawai C: Quantitative analysis of myocardial fibrosis in normals, hypertensive hearts, and hypertrophic cardiomyopathy. *Br Heart J* 55:575–581, 1986.
12. Maron BJ, Epstein SE, Roberts WC: Hypertrophic cardiomyopathy and transmural myocardial infarction without significant atherosclerosis of the extramural coronary arteries. *Am J Cardiol* 43:1086–1102, 1979.
13. Henry WL, Clark CE, Epstein SE: Asymmetric septal hypertrophy: Echocardiographic identification of the pathognomonic anatomic abnormality of IHSS. *Circulation* 47:225–233, 1973.
14. Maron BJ, Spirito P, Wesley Y, Arce J: Development and progression of left ventricular hyper-

trophy in children with hypertrophic cardiomyopathy. *N Engl J Med* 315:610–614, 1986.

15. Maron BJ, Tajik AJ, Ruttenberg HD, et al: Hypertrophic cardiomyopathy in infants clinical features and natural history. *Circulation* 65:7–17, 1982.

16. Spirito P, Maron BJ: Absence of progression of left ventricular hypertrophy in adult patients with hypertrophic cardiomyopathy. *J Am Coll Cardiol* 9:1013–1017, 1987.

17. Topol EJ, Traill TA, Fortuin NJ: Hypertensive hypertrophic cardiomyopathy of the elderly. *N Engl J Med* 312:277–283, 1985.

18. Gilbert PL, Siegel RJ, Melmed S, Sherman CT, Fishbein MC: Cardiac morphology in rats with growth hormone-producing tumors. *J Mol Cell Cardiol* 17:805–811, 1985.

19. Thompson R, Ahmed M, Pridie R, Yacoub M: Hypertrophic cardiomyopathy after aortic valve replacement. *Am J Cardiol* 45:33–41, 1980.

20. Rutledge JC, Eng A, Silva J Jr: Malignant hypertension and asymmetric septal hypertrophy in a 43-year-old black man. *West J Med* 145:356–361, 1986.

21. Criley JM, Lewis KB, White RI Jr, Ross RS: Pressure gradients without obstruction: A new concept of "hypertrophic subaortic stenosis." *Circulation* 32:881–887, 1965.

22. Goodwin JF: The frontiers of cardiomyopathy. *Br Heart J* 48:1–18, 1982.

23. Murgo JP, Alter BR, Dorethy JF, Altobelli SA, McGranahan GM Jr: Dynamics of left ventricular ejection in obstructive hypertrophic cardiomyopathy. *J Clin Invest* 66:1369–1382, 1980.

24. Hernandez RR, Greenfield JC Jr, McCall BW: Pressure-flow studies in hypertrophic subaortic stenosis. *J Clin Invest* 43:401–407, 1964.

25. Siegel RJ, Criley JM: Comparison of ventricular emptying with and without a pressure gradient in patients with hypertrophic cardiomyopathy. *Br Heart J* 53:283–291, 1985.

26. Surgue DD, McKenna WJ, Dickie S, et al: Relation between left ventricular gradient and relative stroke volume ejected in early and late systole in hypertrophic cardiomyopathy: Assessment with radionuclide cineangiography. *Br Heart J* 52:602–609, 1984.

27. Chahine RA, Raizner AE, Ishimori T, Montero AC: Echocardiographic, haemodynamic and angiographic correlations in hypertrophic cardiomyopathy. *Br Heart J* 39:945–953, 1977.

28. Manyari DE, Paulsen W, Boughner DR, Purves P, Kostuk WJ: Resting exercise left ventricular function in patients with hypertrophic cardiomyopathy. *Am Heart J* 105:980–987, 1983.

29. Borer JS, Bacharach SL, Green MV, et al: Effect of septal myotomy and myectomy on left ventricular systolic function at rest and during exercise in patients with IHSS. *Circulation* 60 (Suppl 1):I-82–I-87, 1979.

30. Maron BJ, Bonow RO, Cannon RO III, Leon MB, Epstein SE: Hypertrophic cardiomyopathy: Interrelations of clinical manifestations, pathophysiology, and therapy (first of two parts). *N Engl J Med* 316:780–789, 1987.

31. Kinoshita N, Nimura Y, Okamoto M, Miyatake K,

Nagata S, Sakakibara H: Mitral regurgitation in hypertrophic cardiomyopathy: Non-invasive study by two dimensional Doppler echocardiography. *Br Heart J* 49:574–583, 1983.

32. Wigle ED, Adelman AG, Auger P, Marquis Y: Mitral regurgitation in muscular subaortic stenosis. *Am J Cardiol* 24:698–706, 1969.

33. Kramer DS, French WJ, Criley JM: The postextrasystolic murmur response to gradient in hypertrophic cardiomyopathy. *Ann Intern Med* 104:772–776, 1986.

34. Pollick C, Morgan CD, Gilbert BW, Rakowski H, Wigle ED: Muscular subaortic stenosis: The temporal relationship between systolic anterior motion of the anterior mitral leaflet and the pressure gradient. *Circulation* 66:1087–1094, 1982.

35. Spirito P, Maron BJ: Patterns of systolic anterior motion of the mitral valve in hypertrophic cardiomyopathy: Assessment by two-dimensional echocardiography. *Am J Cardiol* 54:1039–1046, 1984.

36. Ginzton LE, Criley JM: "Obstructive" systolic anterior motion of the mitral valve in cavity obliteration. *Circulation* 64 (Suppl IV):30, 1981.

37. Gehrke J, Goodwin JF: The significance of systolic anterior motion (SAM) on the mitral valve echo pattern in hypertrophic cardiomyopathy. *Clin Cardiol* 1:152–162, 1978.

38. Sahn D, Barratt-Boyes B, Graham K, Hill D, Kerr A: Clarification of the site of "mitral septal apposition" in idiopathic hypertrophic subaortic stenosis (IHSS) by intra-operative two-dimensional (2D) echocardiography. *Am J Cardiol* 49:1009, 1982.

39. Wigle ED: Hypertrophic cardiomyopathy: A 1987 viewpoint. *Circulation* 75:311–322, 1987.

40. Henry WL, Clark CE, Glancy DL, Epstein SE: Echocardiographic measurement of the left ventricular outflow gradient in idiopathic hypertrophic subaortic stenosis. *N Engl J Med* 288:989–993, 1973.

41. Gauer OH: Evidence in circulatory shock of an isometric phase of ventricular contraction following ejection. *Fed Proc* 9:47, 1950.

42. White RI Jr, Criley JM, Lewis KB, Ross RS: Experimental production of intracavity pressure differences: Possible significance in the interpretation of human hemodynamic studies. *Am J Cardiol* 19:806–817, 1967.

43. Shabetai R: A new syndrome in hypovolemic shock: Systolic murmur and intraventricular pressure gradient. *Am J Cardiol* 24:404–408, 1969.

44. Grose R, Maskin C, Spindola-Franco H, Yipintsoi T: Production of left ventricular cavity obliteration in normal man. *Circulation* 64:448–455, 1981.

45. Wilson WS, Criley JM, Ross RS: Dynamics of left ventricular emptying in hypertrophic subaortic stenosis: A cineangiographic and hemodynamic study. *Am Heart J* 73:4–16, 1967.

46. Braunwald E, Ebert PA: Hemodynamic alterations in idiopathic hypertrophic subaortic stenosis induced by sympathomimetic drugs. *Am J Cardiol* 10:475–488, 1962.

47. Criley JM, Siegel RJ: Obstruction is unimportant in the pathophysiology of hypertrophic cardiomyopathy. *Postgrad Med J* 62:515–529, 1986.

48. Siegel RJ, Ellis PS, Pelikan PCD, Maurer G, Criley

JM: Pressure, flow, and velocity studies of experimentally produced intracavitary pressure gradients. *Circulation* 70 (Suppl II):II-130, 1986.

49. Criley JM, Siegel RJ: Has "obstruction" hindered our understanding of hypertrophic cardiomyopathy? *Circulation* 72:1148–1154, 1985.

50. Sanderson JE, Gibson DG, Brown DJ, Goodwin JF: Left ventricular filling in hypertrophic cardiomyopathy: An angiographic study. *Br Heart J* 39:661–670, 1977.

51. Hanrath P, Mathey DG, Siegert R, Bleifeld W: Left ventricular relaxation and filling pattern in different forms of left ventricular hypertrophy: An echocardiographic study. *Am J Cardiol* 45:15–23, 1980.

52. Bonow RO, Rosing DR, Bacharach SL, et al: Effects of verapamil on left ventricular systolic function and diastolic filling in patients with hypertrophic cardiomyopathy. *Circulation* 64:787–796, 1981.

53. Spirito P, Maron BJ, Chiarella F, et al: Diastolic abnormalities in patients with hypertrophic cardiomyopathy: Relation to magnitude of left ventricular hypertrophy. *Circulation* 72:320–316, 1985.

54. Hess OM, Grimm J, Krayenbuehl HP: Diastolic function in hypertrophic cardiomyopathy: Effects of propranolol and verapamil on diastolic stiffness. *Eur Heart J* 4 (Suppl F):47–56, 1983.

55. Lorell BH, Paulus WJ, Grossman W, Wynne J, Cohn PF: Modification of abnormal left ventricular diastolic properties by nifedipine in patients with hypertrophic cardiomyopathy. *Circulation* 65:499–507, 1982.

56. Anderson DM, Raff GL, Ports TA, Brundage BH, Parmley WW, Chatterjee K: Hypertrophic obstructive cardiomyopathy: Effects of acute and chronic verapamil treatment on left ventricular systolic and diastolic function. *Br Heart J* 51:523–529, 1984.

57. Bonow RO, Dilsizian V, Rosing DR, Maron BJ, Bacharach LS, Green MV: Verapamil-induced improvement in left ventricular diastolic filling and increased exercise tolerance in patients with hypertrophic cardiomyopathy: Short and long-term effects. *Circulation* 72:853–854, 1985.

58. Frank S, Braunwald E: Idiopathic hypertrophic subaortic stenosis: Clinical analysis of 126 patients with emphasis on the natural history. *Circulation* 37:759–788, 1968.

59. Yock PG, Hatle L, Popp RJ: Patterns and timing of Doppler-detected intracavitary and aortic flow in hypertrophic cardiomyopathy. *J Am Coll Cardiol* 8;5:1047–1058, 1986.

60. Bellhouse BJ, Talbot L: The fluid mechanics of the aortic valve. *J Fluid Mech* 35:721–735, 1969.

61. Cannon RO III, Rosing DR, Maron BJ, et al: Myocardial ischemia in patients with hypertrophic cardiomyopathy: Contribution of inadequate vasodilator reserve, and elevated left ventricular filling pressures. *Circulation* 71:234–243, 1985.

62. Pasternac A, Noble J, Streulens Y, Elie R, Henschke C, Bourassa MG: Pathophysiology of chest pain in patients with cardiomyopathies and normal coronary arteries. *Circulation* 65:778–789, 1982.

63. Dougherty AH, Maccarelli GV, Gray EL, et al: Congestive heart failure with normal systolic function. *Am J Cardiol* 54:778–782, 1984.

64. Dreslinski GR, Frohlich ED, Dunn FG, Messerli FH, Suarez DH, Reisin E: Echocardiographic diastolic ventricular abnormality in hypertensive heart disease: Atrial emptying index. *Am J Cardiol* 47:1087–1090, 1981.

65. Sanderson JE, Gibson DG, Brown DJ, Goodwin JF: Left ventricular filling in hypertrophic cardiomyopathy. An echocardiographic study. *Br Heart J* 39:661–670, 1977.

66. Gibson DG, Sanderson JE, Traill TA, Brown DJ, Goodwin JF: Regional left ventricular wall movement in hypertrophic cardiomyopathy. *Br Heart J* 40:1327–1333, 1978.

67. Gibson DG, Traill TA, Hall RJC, Brown DJ: Echocardiographic features of secondary left ventricular hypertrophy. *Br Heart J* 41:54–59, 1979.

68. Hanrath P, Mathey DG, Siefert R, Bleifeld W: Left ventricular relaxation and filling pattern in different forms of left ventricular hypertrophy: An echocardiographic study. *Am J Cardiol* 45:15–23, 1980.

69. Decoodt P, Mathey D, Swan HJC: Assessment of left ventricular filling by echocardiography in normal subjects and in subjects with coronary artery disease and with asymmetric septal hypertrophy. *Acta Cardiol* 34:11–33, 1979.

70. Lorell BH, Paulus WJ, Grossman W, et al: Modification of abnormal left ventricular diastolic properties by nifedipine in patients with hypertrophic cardiomyopathy. *Circulation* 65:499–507, 1982.

71. Hanrath P, Mathey DG, Kremer P, et al: Effect of verapamil on left ventricular isovolumic relaxation time and regional left ventricular filling in hypertrophic cardiomyopathy. *Am J Cardiol* 45:1258–1264, 1980.

72. Suwa M, Hirota Y, Kawamura K: Improvement in left ventricular diastolic function during intravenous and oral diltiazem therapy in patients with hypertrophic cardiomyopathy: An echocardiographic study. *Am J Cardiol* 54:1047–1053, 1984.

73. Hasin Y, Lewis BS, Lewis N, Weiss AT, Gotsman MS: Long-term effect of verapamil in hypertrophic cardiomyopathy. *Int J Cardiol* 1:243–251, 1982.

74. Bourmayan C, Razavi A, Fournier C, Dussaule JC, Baragan J, Gerbaux A, Gay J: Effect of propranolol on left ventricular relaxation in hypertrophic cardiomyopathy: An echographic study. *Am Heart J* 109:1311–1316, 1985.

75. Spirito P, Maron BJ, Bonow RO: Noninvasive assessment of left ventricular diastolic function: Comparative analysis of Doppler echocardiographic and radionuclide angiographic techniques. *J Am Coll Cardiol* 7:518–526, 1986.

76. Rokey R, Kuo LC, Zoghbi WA, Limacher MC, Quinones MA: Determination of parameters of left ventricular diastolic filling with pulsed Doppler echocardiography: Comparison with cineangiography. *Circulation* 71:543–550, 1985.

77. Labovitz AJ, Pearson AC: Evaluation of left ventricular diastolic function: Clinical relevance and recent Doppler echocardiographic insights. *Am Heart J* 114:836–850, 1987.

78. Maron BJ, Spirito P, Green KJ, Wesley YE, Bonow

RO, Arce J: Noninvasive assessment of left ventricular diastolic function by pulsed Doppler echocardiography in patients with hypertrophic cardiomyopathy. *J Am Coll Cardiol* 10:733–742, 1987.

79. Oki T, Asai M, Takemura H, et al: Pulsed Doppler echocardiographic assessment of diastolic left ventricular hemodynamics in hypertrophic cardiomyopathy: Relationship between the mode of left ventricular filling and the distribution of left ventricular hypertrophy. *J Cardiogr* 13:523, 1983.

80. Kitabatake A, Inoue M, Asso M, et al: Transmitral blood flow reflecting diastolic behavior of the left ventricle in health and disease—A study by pulsed Doppler technique. *Jap Circ J* 46:92, 1982.

81. Takenaka K, Dabestani A, Gardin JM, et al: Left ventricular filling in hypertrophic cardiomyopathy: A pulsed Doppler echocardiographic study. *J Am Coll Cardiol* 7:1263, 1986.

82. Okamoto M, Kinoshita N, Miyatake N, et al: Diastolic filling of the right echocardiography. *J Cardiogr* 13:79, 1983.

83. Maron BJ, Gottdiener JS, Arce J, Rosing DR, Wesley YE, Epstein SE: Dynamic subaortic obstruction in hypertrophic cardiomyopathy: Analysis by pulsed Doppler echocardiography. *J Am Coll Cardiol* 6:1–15, 1985.

84. Nishimura RA, Tajik AJ, Reeder GS, Seward JB: Evaluation of hypertrophic cardiomyopathy by Doppler color flow imaging: Initial observations. *Mayo Clin Proc* 61:631–639, 1986.

85. Maurer G, Siegel RJ: Assessment of hypertrophic cardiomyopathy by color flow mapping continuous wave and high pulse repetition frequency Doppler. *Circulation* 70 (Suppl II):II-130, 1986.

86. Pouleur H, Rousseau MF, Van Eyll C, Brasseur LA, Charlier AA: Force velocity-length relations in hypertrophic cardiomyopathy: Evidence of normal or depressed myocardial contractility. *Am J Cardiol* 52:813–817, 1983.

19

Echocardiography of the Right Ventricle

Rodney A. Foale, M.D.
Petros Nihoyannopoulos, M.D.

INTRODUCTION

The inherent peculiarities of right ventricular anatomy limit assessment of structure and function by any presently developed imaging method, invasive or noninvasive. Therefore, this chamber has been relatively overlooked compared to the attention given the left ventricle in studies of heart disease. Also, disorders of right ventricular structure or function may be clinically silent. Left ventricular dysfunction results in increased left atrial and pulmonary venous pressure or in decreased stroke volume, and both events are revealed early by well-recognized clinical syndromes. With the right ventricle, however, similar manifestations of backward or forward failure may be relatively silent. Systemic venous congestion is easily absorbed in the compliant venae cavae and hepatic veins. The forces that govern forward output of the right ventricle are complex and strongly influenced by the left ventricle, which with its greater mass drives the circulation of blood through the heart. It is not until a major, acute insult is inflicted on the right ventricle that a fall in output may become clinically apparent.

For example, acute pressure load with the pulmonary circulation occluded by thrombus can be, and frequently has been, missed even when extensive. Similarly, the diastolic failure of right ventricular ventricular myocardial infarction can also be missed. To explore these phenomena we should perhaps look to the crescent shape of the right ventricle that allows such easy adaptability to changing pressure and volume load. This factor may account for the greater reserve with respect to right ventricular failure.

The central, retrosternal location of the right ventricle, coupled with its complex geometry, makes evaluation difficult by any imaging technique. Some imaging methods rely on external landmarks for orientation, such as magnetic resonance imaging, positron emission tomography, and computerized axial tomography. These techniques conventionally acquire images in a sagittal or transverse orientation. However, the right ventricle does not lie in this position in relation to the chest. Thus, planar images that are oblique to the true long or short axis of the chamber and its parts are unlikely to provide reproducible measurements of chamber size or wall thickness. Assessment of the right ventricle by gated blood pool imaging may be constrained by overlap from other chamber blood pool signals. Even contrast right ventricular angiography fails to provide an easy assessment of global or regional right ventricular function. This is due to its inherent dependence on a cavity silhouette, which comprises overlapping regions of right ventricular wall. The same constraints seriously limit the assessment of regional left ventricular function by this method.

Echocardiography offers some advantages over other methods. Reproducible M-mode measurements of right ventricular outflow tract and anterior wall thickness have been reported. These measurements were taken with the transducer applied to the anterior chest wall (1). This single dimension, afforded by M-mode echocardiography, cannot account for the complexities of right ventricular geometry and the variable pattern of the right ventricular wall as easily as it can assess the more symmetric left ventricular cavity. However, over the past decade a number of conceptual and technical advances have markedly enhanced the ability of echocardiography to record details of right ventricular chamber dimension.

This, in turn, has increased our understanding of the structure and function of this chamber.

First, abnormalities of right ventricular function frequently result in the early enlargement and rotation of the chamber, so that the lung is displaced and the right ventricle occupies less of a retrosternal position. Consequently, the right ventricle is more accessible to ultrasound examination. Also, advances in echocardiographic imaging have centered on development of two principles: (*a*) planar imaging with two-dimensional echocardiography, and (*b*) blood flow velocity measurements by Doppler echocardiography. Thus, diastolic and systolic performance can be assessed.

The necessity to orient images to internal cavity landmarks makes two-dimensional echocardiography well suited for evaluating the different orientations and the separate parts of the right ventricular cavity. At present, echocardiography is unique in its ability to assess the right ventricle in health and disease.

THE NORMAL RIGHT VENTRICLE

Right Ventricular Anatomy: Echocardiographic Considerations

The complexities of chamber shape and wall thickness are easily apparent following even casual examination of an autopsied heart. The right ventricular chamber lies anterior and inferior to the left and wraps, crescent-like, around the left ventricular bulk. The shape of the right ventricle is well suited to its function. Its characteristic anatomy has evolved to accommodate the physiologic extremes of circulatory need. At a moment, the right ventricle—'even on quiet respiration'—must be able to cope with fluctuations in venous return encouraged by phasic changes in intrathoracic pressures. In addition, the right ventricle must be able to accommodate a sudden increase in peripheral venous blood from exercise. Although these phasic changes are attenuated in the left ventricle by the capacious vessels of the lung, they can be accommodated by the right ventricle because of its shape. A crescent has the least efficient volume-to-area ratio. Thus, for a small and relatively effortless increase in transverse diameter, a disproportionate increase in volume will occur. These increases can be immediate, and the right ventricle accomplishes them virtually from beat to beat.

For the echocardiographic examination of the right ventricle, the chamber can be considered to have three anatomic parts: the inflow, outflow, and body (Fig. 19.1). The inflow is bound proximally by the tricuspid valve annulus and distally by the trabecular portion of the interventricular septum. The outflow tract extends from the crista supraventricularis through to the pulmonary valve annulus. The body consists of the trabecular portion of the interventricular septum and the free wall and apex (2).

Each portion of the right ventricle has a slightly different orientation. Therefore, it is impossible for any single-plane technique to encompass the entire cavity. Successful examination depends upon subtle orientation in three separate imaging planes.

Furthermore, the right ventricular free wall and the right side of the interventricular septum have variable trabecular patterns. The trabeculae toward the apex are often extensive. They may compound the difficulties in measuring true right ventricular wall thickness, just as the trabeculae of the right ventricular septal aspect may confuse the successful measurement of true interventricular septal thickness (3). The echocardiographic measurement of right ventricular free wall thickness should exclude cavity trabeculae.

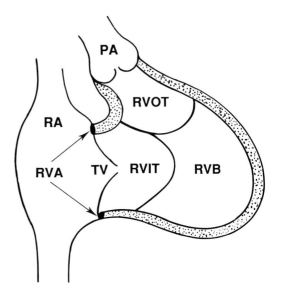

Figure 19.1. Schematic diagram of right ventricular anatomy, *RA* = right atrium, *RVA* = right ventricular annulus, *TV* = tricuspid valve, *RVIT* = right ventricular inflow tract, *RVB* = right ventricular body, *RVOT* = right ventricular outflow tract, *PA* = pulmonary artery.

Echocardiographic Study and Measurement of the Normal Right Ventricle

It follows that echocardiography, with obligatory reference to planar orientation on internal cavity landmarks, should provide a more reliable measurement of cavity size and wall thickness than techniques that create images of the right ventricular chamber without reference to that chamber's peculiar structure and oblique orientation.

We have built upon the experience of other groups (4–6) and proposed a systematic approach to the evaluation of right ventricular measurements of cavity size and free wall thickness that can be undertaken as part of a standardized examination protocol (Table 19.1). In this study (7), the three parts of the right ventricle were imaged and measured from several transducer positions used in a standard examination sequence. The measurement of these three parts are now considered separately.

Right Ventricular Inflow Tract

Detailed measurement of the right ventricular inflow tract can be performed from four different transducer locations (Figs. 19.2–19.5).

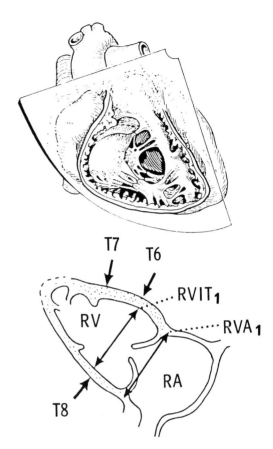

Figure 19.2. (Reproduced with permission from *British Heart Journal.*)

Table 19.1. Standardized Echocardiographic Examination (Including Right Ventricular Measurements)

Transducer Position	Axis	View[a]
Left parasternal edge	Long	Left ventricle
		Aorta
		RV inflow[b]
		RV outflow[b]
	Short	**Aorta**
		Mitral valve
		Tricuspid valve
		LV serial views[b]
Cardiac apex	Long	**Four chamber**
		Two chamber
Subcostal	Long	**Four chamber**
	Short	LV serial views[b]
		Mitral valve
		Aorta
Suprasternal (or upper sternal edge)	Long	Aortic arch
	Short	Aortic arch

[a]Bold type represents views from which ventricular measurements are made.
[b]LV, left ventricular; RV, right ventricular.

Parasternal Long-Axis Right Ventricular Inflow Tract View. This view (Fig. 19.2) is specific for the right ventricular inflow tract and may be obtained conveniently in sequence following the long-axis view of the left ventricle from the left parasternal transducer position (Table 19.1). The transducer is inclined from this left ventricular orientation inward beneath the sternum with caudal angulation. The transducer may be moved down one or two interspaces if too much of the right ventricular outflow tract or aortic root is in view. Also, the transducer location over the precordium usually will need to be a little more toward the cardiac apex, so that the appropriate landmarks are imaged.

The object of this manipulation, which can be difficult without experience (an excellent reason to incorporate the view in a standardized echocardiographic sequence) is to align the crescentic long-axis of the right ventricular inflow tract with

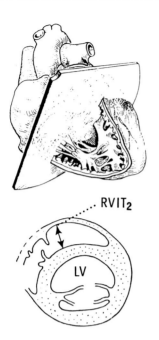

Figure 19.3. (Reproduced with permission from *British Heart Journal*.)

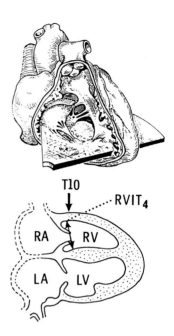

Figure 19.5. (Reproduced with permission from *British Heart Journal*.)

relationship to internal cavity landmarks, as shown in Fig. 19.1. Thus the right atrium and tricuspid valve annulus are aligned with the proximal part of the right ventricular body. Ideally, this includes

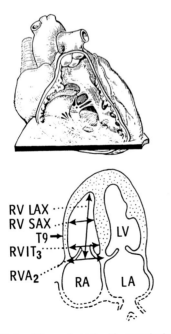

Figure 19.4. (Reproduced with permission from *British Heart Journal*.)

right ventricular papillary muscle but excludes any remnant of posterior interventricular septum. If the septum is displaced due to left ventricular disease, then the true alignment of the right ventricular inflow tract view can be difficult.

In the ideal view, the right ventricular diaphragmatic wall forms the inferior limit of the image. The anterior wall forms the superior aspect of the image. From this view the major axis of right ventricular inflow tract (RVIT 1), an important measure of right ventricular size, is obtained. This view also yields the tricuspid valve annular size (RVA) in addition to anterior and diaphragmatic wall thickness (Tables 19.2 and 19.3). The major axis measurement of the right ventricular inflow tract, RVIT 1, should be taken within one-third of the distance toward the cardiac apex, measured from below the tricuspid valve annulus. The tricuspid valve annulus RVA 1 is defined as the maximum separation of the tricuspid valve ring, itself measured by the points of attachment of the base of anterior and posterior valve leaflet to the atrioventricular junction.

Parasternal Short-Axis Right Ventricular Inflow Tract/Tricuspid Valve View. From the parasternal short-axis view of the mitral valve, slight medial tilt beneath the sternum will bring into the image more of the short-axis orientation of tricuspid valve leaflet tips and subtricuspid ap-

Table 19.2. Right Ventricular (RV) Chamber Size: Absolute Measurements from 41 Normal Subjects at End-Diastole[a]

	N (41)	Mean (cm)	2 SD	Range	Coefficient of Variation (within Measurements) (%)
RVIT 1	40	4.5	0.5	3.7–5.4	10.6
RVIT 2	29	3.0	0.3	2.4–3.9	12.2
RVIT 3	38	2.4	0.4	1.5–3.0	16.1
RVIT 4	29	5.1	0.5	4.0–7.0	11.2
RVOT 1	41	2.2	0.3	1.8–3.0	13.4
RVOT 2	41	2.3	0.3	1.8–2.9	13.0
RVOT 3	41	2.0	0.3	1.4–2.6	15.0
RVOT 4	41	2.7	0.2	2.0–3.2	10.1
RV LAX	40	7.6	0.5	6.9–8.9	5.9
RV SAX	40	3.0	0.3	2.4–3.7	10.2
RVA 1	41	3.4	0.3	2.5–4.0	9.5
RVA 2	41	2.4	0.3	1.6–3.1	14.1

[a]Reproduced with permission from *British Heart Journal*.
[b]Coefficient of variation (between measurements) mean (1 SD): 51 (12%); range: 36–72%.

paratus (Fig. 19.3). From this view, the crescent shape of the right ventricular inflow tract and body can be appreciated and the minor dimensions of the right ventricular inflow tract (RVIT 2) measured. This measurement is taken as the maximum perpendicular distance between the right side of the midinterventricular septum and the right ventricular free wall.

Apical Four-Chamber View. The cardiac apex is one of the principal landmarks in generating the image for the apical four-chamber view (Fig. 19.4). The other landmarks are the annuli of the tricuspid and mitral valves. Usually, attention is concentrated on the left heart structures. However, with slight medial angulation of the transducer, measurement of right ventricular inflow tract (RVIT 3) can be obtained orthogonal to that obtained from the right ventricular inflow tract view shown in Fig. 19.2. Furthermore, from this view the lateral and right ventricular free wall can be assessed and measured for wall thickness. In addition, the second measurement of tricuspid valve annulus (RVA 2) can be obtained orthogonal to that shown in Fig. 19.2.

Table 19.3. Right Ventricular (RV) Chamber Size: Measurements from 41 Normal Subjects at End-Diastole Corrected for Body Surface Area[a]

	N (41)	Mean (cm)	2 SD	Range	Coefficient of Variation (within Measurements) (%)
RVIT 1	40	2.6	0.3	2.0–3.3	11.8
RVIT 2	29	1.7	0.2	1.4–2.0	10.8
RVIT 3	38	1.4	0.2	1.0–1.8	16.1
RVIT 4	29	2.9	0.4	2.3–3.6	12.3
RVOT 1	41	1.3	0.2	1.0–1.7	12.6
RVOT 2	41	1.3	0.3	1.0–2.9	22.5
RVOT 3	41	1.1	0.1	0.9–1.4	12.4
RVOT 4	41	1.6	0.2	1.2–2.0	12.7
RV LAX	40	4.4	0.4	3.6–5.4	9.1
RV SAX	40	1.8	0.2	1.4–2.2	12.7
RVA 1	41	2.0	0.2	1.6–2.4	10.2
RVA 2	41	1.5	0.2	1.1–1.8	14.3

[a]Reproduced with permission from *British Heart Journal*.
[b]Coefficient of variation (between measurements) mean (1 SD): 51 (12%); range: 37–72%.

Subcostal Four-Chamber View. This projection yields a fourth perspective on right ventricular inflow tract dimensions (RVIT 4), as well as an important measurement of the right ventricular diaphragmatic wall thickness (Fig. 19.5). This view is valuable when employed as part of the standardized examination sequence. It is of particular use when parasternal or apical windows do not provide good quality echocardiographic images. As with the other inflow tract measurements, RVIT 4 should be taken within one-third of the distance from the tricuspid valve annulus toward the perceived cardiac apex and only after tilting of the transducer to and fro produces the maximum cavity dimensions.

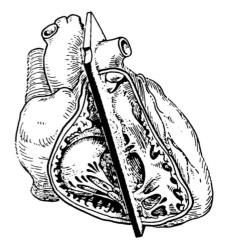

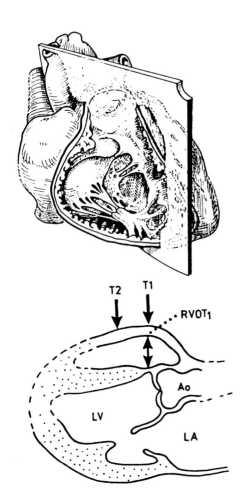

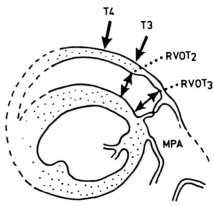

Figure 19.7. (Reproduced with permission from *British Heart Journal.*)

Right Ventricular Outflow Tract

The outflow tract of the right ventricle is, unlike its left-sided equivalent, quite different from the right ventricular inflow tract and body. Therefore, echocardiographic examination of this part of the right ventricle necessarily employs separate views and includes one view specific to the part (Figs. 19.6–19.8).

Parasternal Long-Axis of the Left Ventricle. From the commonly used echocardiographic plane, the right ventricular outflow tract is seen in an anterior location as it passes obliquely to the left of the aorta (Fig. 19.6). A measurement of the right ventricle at this level does not correlate to any identifiable major or minor axis measurement. However, it is the dimension obtained from M-mode echocardiography when the parasternal transducer position is used. There are

Figure 19.6. (Reproduced with permission from *British Heart Journal.*)

published data concerning right ventricular cavity size and wall thickness when measured from this location. Therefore, this is an important measurement to include in any assessment of the right ventricle for comparative reasons. In our study this measurement was designated RVOT 1 (7).

Parasternal Long-Axis of the Right Ventricular Outflow Tract. This view, specific to the right ventricular outflow tract, can be obtained by reference to cavity landmarks: the maximum dimension of the outflow tract, the pulmonary valve annulus, and the maximum possible distance in a distal direction of the main pulmonary artery, if possible, to the area of the bifurcation. From this view two outflow tract measurements can be made: RVOT 2 and RVOT 3, as illustrated in Figure 19.7.

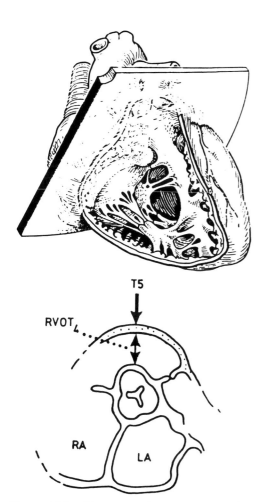

Figure 19.8. (Reproduced with permission from *British Heart Journal.*)

The outflow tract measurement RVOT 3 is taken just below the pulmonary valve annulus. A frequent mistake in the performance of this view is to use the short-axis projection of the aortic root as an internal cavity landmark. However, this view is "off axis" to the right ventricular outflow tract, which does not run at right angles to the aortic root short axis, but lies obliquely somewhere between the long- and short-axis orientation of the aorta. It therefore follows that to image the long axis of the right ventricular outflow tract properly, the echocardiographic plane must be oriented to internal cavity landmarks. These include the right ventricular outflow tract maximum dimension and pulmonary annulus.

The long axis of the right ventricular outflow tract may also be imaged from a subcostal transducer location. This may be especially useful in infants and children (8) or in patients with chronic obstructive airways disease.

Parasternal Short-Axis View of the Aortic Root. A further measurement of right ventricular outflow tract (RVOT 4) may be obtained for the standard parasternal short-axis view of the aortic root (Fig. 19.8). The measurement is taken anteriorly to the aortic root as the maximum dimension between the anterior wall and the right ventricular free wall endocardial signal. It is taken from the same region of the outflow tract as RVOT 1, except from a short-axis-orientated plane.

Right Ventricular Body

The body of the right ventricle lies anterior to the left ventricle and extends from the inflow tract toward the apex. The body may be conveniently viewed from the apical four-chamber transducer location. When careful measurement of the right ventricle is made, the view should be oriented medially away from the mitral annulus to concentrate most attention on the maximum dimensions of the right ventricle with reference to the apex and tricuspid annulus cavity landmarks.

Apical Four-Chamber View. The right ventricular body may be measured in long-axis (LAX) and short-axis (SAX) projection from the apical four-chamber view (Fig. 19.4). The long axis can be defined as the distance between the right ventricular apex and the midpoint of the tricuspid valve annulus. This measurement can present difficulties due to the imprecise identification of the apex. The short axis of the right ventricle, defined as lying at the midpoint between apex and annulus, is in a similar way difficult. Consequently, we measured the maximum short-axis diameter from the middle one-third of the right ventricle. The difficulties that trabeclulae present for the endocardial definition in the right ventricle also are compounded when this measurement is attempted, as the endocardial signals lie parallel to the interrogating ultrasound beam. These echoes may spread over 3–5 mm. Therefore, the midpoint of the endocardial echo signal should be taken as the point from which to measure the distance between the right ventricular septal endocardium and the right ventricular free wall.

Right Ventricular Chamber Size—Variation of the Measurement and Reproducibility

The coefficient variation for any measurement is defined as:

$$\frac{\text{Standard Deviation}}{\text{Mean}} \times 100\% \qquad 19.1$$

and can be taken as a measurement of the spread of a set of values about the mean.

When calculated for different measurements of chamber size or wall thickness *within* individuals, the coefficient of variation can be taken as an index of asymmetry of these two measurements. If calculated for the same measurement *between* individuals, it can be used to express the normal variability of the measurement within a population. However, if this measurement is likely to have small variation (an assumption that can be made for certain aspects of the right ventricle), the coefficient of variation also can be used to indicate the ease of standardization of the view from which the measurement was derived.

In our report (7) we used the coefficient of variation to assess the "ease of standardization" of the views described above in the measurement of the right ventricle. All right ventricular inflow tract measurements (RVIT 1–RVIT 4) had a low coefficient of variation (less than 20%). However, the easiest to obtain and most reproducible were RVIT 1 from the specific right ventricular inflow tract view and RVIT 3 from the apical four-chamber view. RVIT 2 and RVIT 4 were only obtained in approximately 70% of patients, and RVIT 2 had an unsatisfactory interobserver variability of 54%. This variability may be explained by the volume changes within the right ventricle expected from respiration. The diameter perhaps most affected by this change would be RVIT 2. In our study, measurements were not made in any specific time relationship within the respiratory cycle.

The right ventricular outflow tract measurements (RVOT 1–RVOT 4) also appear to be standardized satisfactorily, with coefficients of variation generally less than 20%. Also, these measurements were highly reproducible. In particular, the measurement of RVOT 1 from the parasternal long-axis projection, equivalent to the M-mode echocardiographic measurement, had a high degree of reproducibility and a low coefficient of variation. The equivalent measurement of the outflow tract taken from the parasternal short-axis projection, RVOT 4, was larger and less reproducible. These differences may be explained by differences in obtaining short-axis and long-axis images. A short-axis plane is more likely to pass obliquely through the area as there are no anatomic landmarks with which to orientate the image with precision.

Measurements of the right ventricular body, LAX and SAX, were equally acceptable from the viewpoint of standardization and reproducibility. Interobserver and intraobserver variation in the measurement of these dimensions, expressed as both the range of absolute difference and the percentage difference between the two measurements, are presented in Table 19.4.

Right Ventricular Wall Thickness— Methodology, Variation of the Measurement, and Reproducibility

Right ventricular wall thickness measurements can be obtained from each of the views described above (Figs. 19.2–19.8). We undertook measurements from ten points around the right ventricular free wall circumference. These were designated as T1–T10. Measurements of right ventricular free wall from the right ventricular outflow tract were designated T1–T5. T1 and T2 were taken from the parasternal view of the left heart, T3 and T4 from the right ventricular outflow tract view, and T5 from the parasternal short-axis view of the aortic root. T6 and T7 were also measurements of the free wall of the right ventricle from positions slightly toward the cardiac apex in the anterior wall. T6 and T7 were measured from the specific right ventricular inflow tract views. T8 was a measurement taken from the same view of the diaphragmatic wall of the right ventricle—the inferior wall of the right ventricle. T9 was a measurement of right ventricular free wall taken from the apical four-chamber view. T10 was a measurement similar to T9, but rather closer to the tricuspid valve annulus when imaged from a subcostal four-chamber projection.

Table 19.4. Interobserver and Intraobserver Variability of the Absolute Measurements of Right Ventricular (RV) Chamber Size[a]

	Interobserver				Intraobserver			
	Absolute Difference		Percentage of Difference		Absolute Difference		Percentage of Difference	
	Mean (cm)	2 SD	Mean	2 SD	Mean (cm)	2 SD	Mean	2 SD
RVIT 1	0.04	0.4	1.5	0.1	0.03	0.5	0.03	0.1
RVIT 2	1.0	0.4	54.0	0.4	0.08	0.4	2.4	0.1
RVIT 3	0.2	0.3	5.7	0.1	0.07	0.3	2.8	0.1
RVIT 4	0.1	0.7	0.8	0.1	0.2	0.7	4.5	0.1
RVOT 1	0.2	0.3	5.7	0.1	0.1	0.2	6.1	0.1
RVOT 2	0.3	0.3	14.0	0.1	0.3	0.2	13.0	0.1
RVOT 3	0.2	0.3	7.1	0.1	0.09	0.3	5.2	0.1
RVOT 4	0.2	0.4	12.0	0.2	0.05	0.2	1.4	0.1
RV LAX	0.3	0.6	3.8	0.1	0.3	0.5	3.8	0.1
RV SAX	0.2	0.7	10.0	0.3	0.04	0.4	1.1	0.2
RVA 1	0.06	0.5	0.6	0.1	0.2	0.2	5.9	0.1
RVA 2	0.2	0.3	6.0	0.1	0.1	0.3	3.0	0.1

[a]Reproduced with permission from *British Heart Journal.*

The results of these measurements are provided in Table 19.5. From this it can be seen that the range variations in a normal population may be up to 0.7 cm. In most cases, however, values did not exceed 0.4 cm. The higher values were recorded from the lateral wall of the apical four-chamber view and from the diaphragmatic wall of the subcostal view, areas more dense in trabeculation. While these measurements are being performed, every attempt should be made to ex-clude the trabecular patterns by careful review of the study in real time.

Additional factors may be that, particularly for the lateral wall of the ventricle measured from the apical four-chamber view, there is a spread of echocardiographic signal, and that these measurements may be near the resolution limits of echocardiographic systems.

Table 19.6 shows the interobserver and intraobserver variability of the absolute measure-

Table 19.5. Right Ventricular (RV) Wall Thickness: End-Diastolic Measurements from 41 Normal Subjects[a]

RV Wall Region	Absolute Values (cm)				Corrected for Body Surface Area (m²)			
	Mean	2 SD	Range	Coefficient of Variation (within Measurements) (%)	Mean	2 SD	Range	Coefficient of Variation (within Measurements) (%)
T1	0.3	0.07	0.2–0.5	20.7	0.2	0.04	0.1–0.3	22.4
T2	0.3	0.07	0.2–0.5	21.5	0.2	0.05	0.1–0.3	23.6
T3	0.3	0.05	0.3–0.5	15.9	0.2	0.04	0.1–0.3	20.1
T4	0.4	0.07	0.2–0.5	18.6	0.2	0.04	0.1–0.3	22.0
T5	0.3	0.08	0.2–0.5	21.8	0.2	0.05	0.1–0.3	25.8
T6	0.3	0.06	0.2–0.5	17.7	0.2	0.04	0.1–0.3	21.1
T7	0.4	0.07	0.3–0.5	20.2	0.2	0.05	0.1–0.3	24.1
T8	0.4	1.0	0.3–0.6	25.5	0.2	0.06	0.1–0.4	26.6
T9	0.4	0.07	0.3–0.6	16.7	0.2	0.05	0.1–0.3	21.1
T10	0.4	1.0	0.3–0.7	24.5	0.2	0.06	0.1–0.4	27.4

[a]Reproduced with permission from *British Heart Journal.*
[b]Coefficient of variation (between measurements) mean (1 SD): 17 (14%); range: 3–31% for absolute values; mean: 17 (14%); range: 8–35% for body surface area corrected values.

Table 19.6. Interobserver and Intraobserver Variability of the Absolute Measurements of Right Ventricular (RV) Wall Thickness

| RV Wall Region | Interobserver | | | | Intraobserver | | | |
| | Absolute Difference | | Percentage of Difference | | Absolute Difference | | Percentage of Difference | |
	Mean (cm)	2 SD	Mean	2 SD	Mean (cm)	2 SD	Mean	2 SD
T1	0.04	0.2	18	74	0.1	0.14	26	32
T2	0.01	0.12	6	21	0.02	0.16	4	48
T3	0.05	0.18	23	70	0.07	0.1	19	28
T4	0.02	0.18	11	52	0.05	0.1	13	26
T5	0.0	0.2	11	100	0.05	0.2	12	56
T6	0.02	0.2	15	41	0.04	0.14	9	38
T7	0.03	0.18	4	56	0.0	0.1	1	32
T8	0.06	0.2	9	64	0.01	0.2	8	58
T9	0.02	0.4	6	96	0.07	0.2	14	74
T10	0.09	0.18	19	36	0.04	0.1	13	32

ments of the right ventricular wall thickness. Like measurements of right ventricular cavity size, these also are expressed as the range of absolute difference and percentage difference between the two measurements. Values with a coefficient variation of more than 25% for different measurements *within* subjects confirms the morphologic description of a degree of asymmetry of right ventricular free wall thicknesses in normal individuals. However, the values for the coefficient of variation for the same measurement *between* subjects, also of mostly more than 20%, suggest that these measurements were less easy to standardize for reasons described above.

Doppler Assessment of Right Ventircular Hemodynamics

The velocity profile of blood flow across the tricuspid valve during diastole is influenced by several factors. These have been studied in more depth for the left ventricle than for the right ventricle but include right atrial pressure, right ventricular diastolic pressure, tricuspid valve morphology, and distensibility (compliance) of the right ventricular chamber. It is likely that this latter factor is considerably more complex than that studied for the left ventricle. Reasons for this are the eccentric shape of the right ventricle and, in part, the basic function of this chamber, which is to cope with widely varying diastolic filling conditions ranging from quiet respiration to sudden vigorous exercise. Because of this distensibility, atrial septal defect preferentially shunts to the more compliant right ventricle. This causes a left-

to-right direction of blood flow, limited only in early years by the size of the atrial septal defect.

The tricuspid valve diastolic velocity profile, as with so many other aspects of Doppler echocardiography, was first studied by Hatle et al. (9). Tricuspid valve flow can be measured best from the apical four-chamber position, either with continuous wave Doppler alone—the study being guided by the phasic change in respiration—or by simultaneous two-dimensional and Doppler mapping technique. In adults and infants beyond the first few days of life, tricuspid valve flow velocities are lower than those from the left heart. There also is considerable variation with respiration velocities increasing on inspiration as more blood passes through the right heart during that phase of the respiratory cycle. Also, the early diastolic decline, seen as the rapid filling phase of diastole, is much slower for the right ventricle than for the left ventricle. These differences in filling profiles between right and left ventricles are identified easily in adults and in normal children (Fig. 19.9).

Systolic outflow velocities may be recorded best from the parasternal edge and again can be guided easily by reference to simultaneous two-dimensional echocardiographic images. Alternatively, it can be guided by locating the pulmonary valve flow as being to the left and above the aortic flow, of course assuming normal arterial relations. The systolic flow can be recognized in the normal heart, and respiratory variations in peak velocity should be expected. Also, in some patients inspiration will be accompanied by forward flow in late diastole. This phenomenon is mimicked by the M-

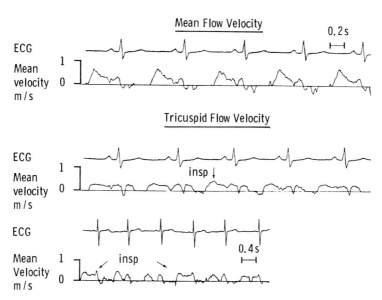

Figure 19.9. Mitral and tricuspid flow velocity curves from normal subjects recorded with pulsed Doppler. Mitral valve velocity is higher in early diastole and has a more rapid decline. Tricuspid flow velocity is lower, with a slower decline and with respiratory variation. Systolic flow velocity in the right ventricle is positive when transducer direction is toward the tricuspid valve area. (From Hatle L, Angelsen B: *Doppler Ultrasound in Cardiology.* Philadelphia, Lea & Febiger, 1982, 63–66. Reproduced with permission from Lea & Febiger.)

mode recording of an A wave dip of the pulmonary valve. This is caused by opening of the pulmonary valve leaflets as the result of right atrial systole effecting forward blood flow within the low pressure/high compliance ventricular chamber (10, 11).

Continuous wave Doppler assessment of right ventricular systolic pressure in the presence of tricuspid regurgitation has been described (12). From an apical transducer location, and probably best guided by reference to simultaneous two-dimensional echocardiographic imaging, the maximal velocities of the regurgitant jet directed away from the transducer are measured. An apical transducer location is best suited to this exercise as it will minimize the angle between the interrogating Doppler beam and the tricuspid regurgitant jet. When the peak velocity is recorded clearly, measurement of the pressure drop by the modified Bernoulli principle closely relates to the pressure drop from right ventricle to right atrium in systole.

For example, a peak velocity of 3.5 m/sec will correspond to a 49 mm Hg pressure drop during systole from the right ventricle to the right atrium. If right atrial pressure is assumed to be approximately 10 mm Hg, or can be measured from the jugular venous pressure directly, then the addi-

tion of the pressure drop to right atrial pressure will provide an estimate of right ventricular systolic pressure. In the example cited, right ventricular systolic pressure is estimated at 59 mm Hg. Correlations with cardiac catheterization measurements have been excellent.

In normal hearts, experience with color flow Doppler has taught us to expect a small amount of "physiological" tricuspid regurgitation in many normal subjects. However, the signals are of low intensity and unlike "true" tricuspid regurgitation. The usefulness of this Doppler method in direct measurement of abnormal right ventricular pressure or volume is considerable, principally due to the ready stretching of the tricuspid valve and the recurrence of functional tricuspid regurgitation in the early stages of any pressure or volume loading condition on the right heart. The general acceptance of this measurement by experienced echocardiographers attests to its reproducibility and clinical value.

THE ABNORMAL RIGHT VENTRICLE

Anatomic Adaption to Pressure and Volume Load

The right ventricle shares similar pressure and volume loading conditions to the left ventricle in utero and thus has similar cavity dimensions and wall thickness (13). Almost immediately following delivery, however, the right ventricle adapts to perinatal physiologic changes. Consequently, it achieves the shape and wall thickness proportions with respect to left ventricular measurements that characterize normal adult life. If systemic equivalent pressure or volume loading conditions persist due to abnormal cardiac anatomy, the right ventricle will remain hypertrophied. Examples of these conditions include perinatal pulmonary complications such as immature lung or meconium inhalation, the persistence of fetal circulation, right ventricular outflow tract obstructions, or cardiac shunt. These conditions maintain the right ventricle as a thick-walled, ellipsoid cavity. If the pressure load continues, so does increasing wall thickness. It appears that right ventricular pressure load at birth is not unlike pressure load of the left ventricle, producing increasing wall thickness and small ventricular cavities. Indeed, over time the right ventricle may hypertrophy from this condition to acquire pulmonary outflow atresia due to outflow tract muscle band thickening.

The child or adult who acquires an abnormal load on the right ventricle can show quite different adaptation of right ventricular cavity size and wall thickness. Although such changes depend in part upon the rate of development of abnormality, an early response to pressure or volume load is dilatation. Thus the first response of the right ventricle is to lose its crescent shape and dilate short-axis diameters. This is seen particularly in acute pressure or volume loading conditions accompanying acute pulmonary embolism or acquired ventricular septal defect as in septal rupture due to myocardial infarction. In either condition, the right ventricle immediately dilates from its crescent shape, a shape so efficient in low pressure conditions, by changing toward the more volume-efficient sphere. With uncontrolled volume load, such as septal rupture, or severe pressure load, as with acute obstruction of the pulmonary artery with thrombus, the chamber dilatation also stretches the tricuspid valve anulus. Furthermore, the leaflets of the tricuspid valve are tethered by caudal attachments to the right ventricular body. As the body dilates, the tricuspid leaflets are held into the right ventricular body and may fail to oppose during systole. Through these mechanisms, functional tricuspid regurgitation results. This event exacerbates volume load and adds to the problems the right ventricle may be experiencing in compensating for the initial insult.

If a more chronically acquired pressure load occurs, such as chronic pulmonary thromboembolic disease or pulmonary hypertension or cor pulmonale accompanying chronic obstructive airways disease, the right ventricle will first change shape rather than acquire wall hypertrophy as the left ventricle would do. It appears that the right ventricular hypertrophic response to pressure load is rather minimal compared to that of the left ventricle, which reacts to afterload pressure abnormality by an early increase in wall thickness and reduction in cavity dimension. Therefore, it may be that only the neonatal right ventricle behaves at birth like the left ventricle when exposed to pressure loading.

Echocardiography of the Right Ventricle in Congenital Heart Disease: Broad Principles

Chamber Identification

The echocardiographer presented with a patient diagnosed as having congenital heart disease may be perplexed by any number of potential connections and relationships of atria, ventricular chamber, or arteries. Adherence to a well-practiced protocol such as described earlier in this chapter (Table 19.1) should result in a complete anatomic and physiologic diagnosis in virtually all cases. This is true even in patients with marked chest wall deformities or postoperative scar in such cases. Subcostal transducer positions should furnish basic anatomic information. In patients with dextrocardia, mirror-image transducer location at the right sternal edge can be used.

The identification of correct ventricular morphology in congenital heart disease—particularly complex congenital heart disease—is mandatory to diagnosis. Frequently, this is the starting point from which the anatomic puzzle may be solved.

Fortunately, the right and left ventricles have several anatomic features that allow correct identification of appropriate chamber morphology. This is true even in the presence of severe distortion with pressure or volume load and even when initially there may appear to be only one chamber with large ventricular septal defect.

These features are listed in Table 19.7 and have been derived from a study of patients with complex congenital heart disease (14). Of these characteristics, chamber position, shape, wall thickness, and trabecular pattern may vary in accord with the embryologic blueprint that determines abnormalities of connection and relation. Many of these features will also vary with severe left- or right-sided pressure and volume loading conditions. The observation of moderator band may

Table 19.7. Morphologic Features Used in the Echocardiographic Recognition of a Right (RV) and Left Ventricular (LV) Morphology

Feature	LV	RV
Position	Left, posterior	Right, anterior
Shape	Ellipsoid	Crescentic/triangular
Wall thickness	≃1.0 cm	0.4–0.7 cm
Chamber		
Trabeculae	Smooth	Coarse
Moderator Band	−	+
"Strings"	+	−
Infundibulum	−	+
Associated AV[a] valve		
Leaflets	2	3
Attachment to crux	Superior	Inferior

[a]AV, atrioventricular.

also be subject to error when papillary muscle, septal, or trabecular structures are abnormally developed or positioned, a frequent occurrence in such abnormal anatomy.

Probably the most reliable echocardiographic marker of ventricular morphology is the identification of the associated atrioventricular valve. It follows that the observation of a three-cusped valve, attached inferiorly toward the cardiac apex at the crux by comparison to its neighbor, will correctly identify a morphologic tricuspid valve. Since "valves go with ventricles," the right ventricle is identified by association.

Of the features that correctly identify a tricuspid valve, the most consistent is its more inferior attachment to the crux of the heart, compared to the mitral valve. In complex abnormal anatomy, cusp number alone may be a less reliable criterion. The attachment of the valve base to the crux of the heart, however, is a reliable criterion even in the presence of large ventricular septal defects, although it can be ambiguous in atrioventricular canal defects. In the double-inlet ventricle, where by definition there is no inflow part of one potential second chamber, the attachment of the two atrioventricular valves is also ambiguous and may join at the same level at the crux of the heart (15). In these cases, main chamber morphology may be identified by trabecular pattern. It can also be identified by its position with respect to the outflow or rudimentary chamber associated usually with the anatomic complex.

Echo Appearances in Abnormal Loading Conditions

Pressure Load of the Right Ventricle. The right ventricular hypertrophy seen in the patients with congenital abnormalities present from fetal life is frequently very severe, measuring more than sev-eral millimeters, and is associated with a small cavity. The estimation of pressure load severity, although useful, may not be possible by measuring the degree of hypertrophy alone. This is because there is likely to be a nonlinear relationship between pressure load and the hypertrophic response. The systolic motion of the interventricular septum must be considered as a reflection of competing forces within the right and left ventricles. Thus it can be appreciated that, in normal subjects with normal pressure relationships, the configuration of the interventricular septum becomes concave toward the pressure dominant left ventricle as systole progresses. This is clearly in accord with hemodynamic principles. The low pressure right ventricular chamber remains crescentic in shape, apparently wrapped passively around the higher pressure left chamber.

Right ventricular pressure load, with systolic pressure levels approaching or exceeding those in the left, will affect interventricular septal motion. These effects were described by King et al. (16). With high right ventricular systolic pressures, the interventricular septum remains flattened and loses its concavity toward the left ventricular center. Reversal of septal shape during systole is best seen with right ventricular pressures that exceed systemic levels. In this situation, the interventricular septum becomes concave toward the center of the right ventricle. Experience has demonstrated the value of this sign as a guide to right ventricular systolic hypertension in children and also in a wider population of patients with pulmonary hypertension from a variety of causes (Fig. 19.10).

Volume Loading of the Right Ventricle. In conditions of right ventricular volume load, such as atrioseptal defect without pulmonary hypertension, the response of the right ventricle is to

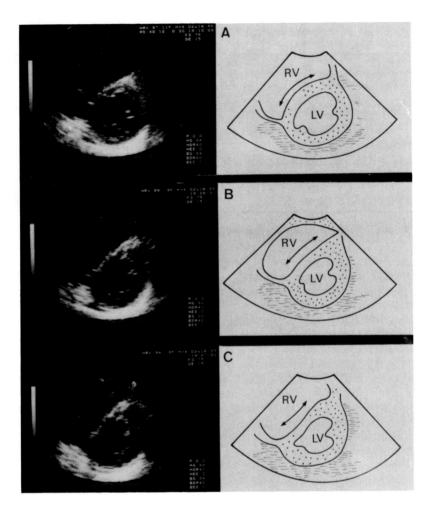

Figure 19.10. Right ventricular pressure load. Short-axis view of left (*LV*) and right ventricle (*RV*) showing end-diastolic to end-systolic progression (*A–C*) of septal concavity toward the right ventricle.

dilate and assume a more spheroidal shape. This response also affects septal motion and has been well described in early M-mode studies (17). The diastolic distortion of septal motion due to a volume-loaded right ventricle can easily be appreciated by two-dimensional echocardiography. The two-dimensional echo views are short-axis projections of the right and left ventricle from the parasternal transducer locations.

During systole, normal concave septal shape is seen toward the geometric center of the left ventricle. However, during diastole the right ventricle necessarily must accept the additional volume load placed upon it. Consequently, there is marked septal displacement with dominance by the right ventricle of left ventricular shape and marked dis-

tortion of the left ventricular cavity. The interventricular septum becomes concave toward the right ventricle during diastole. Right ventricular contraction then begins from a larger end-diastolic dimension and is necessarily enhanced in relationship to the severity of volume load.

Echocardiography of the Adult Right Ventricle in Pressure and Volume Load

The principles of pressure and volume load in relationship to interventricular septal motion also apply to acquired heart disease in the child or adult. The singular difference is the extent of right ventricular hypertrophy, which appears to be potentially far greater in patients whose abnormalities have been present in utero.

In utero, the right ventricle appears to react similarly to the left, when pressure loaded. Specifically, its mass increases and its end-diastolic and systolic cavity size is reduced. In acquired right ventricular pressure load, there appears to be more dilation and less hypertrophy. In hypertrophy of primary cause (hypertrophic cardiomyopathy, infiltrative heart disease) there is little cavity dilatation and, like the right ventricle with in-utero abnormalities, hypertrophy predominates.

Right Ventricular Pressure Load

Pulmonary Embolic Disease. Acute massive pulmonary embolism that survives until early echocardiographic study may show the effects of high right ventricular systolic pressures with systolic septal concavity toward the center of the right ventricle. More commonly, the appearances are dominated by a low cardiac output state, with a rather indeterminate septal wall motion and poor contractility of the right ventricle. The left ventricle may appear "volume starved" with impaired diastolic filling (18, 19). Invariably, right ventricular cavity dilatation and tricuspid regurgitation will be present in the early stages. Determination of systolic pressure by measurement of peak systolic velocities may be made difficult or even irrelevant by the low cardiac output state that complicates the acute condition.

Chronic thromboembolic disease of the lung may allow the right ventricle more time to develop a hypertrophic response. In the setting of normal left heart anatomy, a dilated and hypertrophied right heart discovered in isolation should raise the question of chronic thromboembolic pulmonary disease. In some cases of acute or chronic thromboembolic disease, residual clot may be seen within the right heart. Presumably, the "venous casts" embolizing to the lung may be caught with endocardial trabeculae of the atria or ventricle (Fig. 19.11).

Primary Pulmonary Hypertension. In patients with primary pulmonary hypertension, hypertrophy of the right ventricular free wall and septum usually dominates the echocardiographic picture. There may be little cavity dilatation seen in early stages. This perhaps suggests a slow evolution over a fairly long history, allowing time for the right ventricle to adapt to the acquired pressure load. Although this question has not been well studied, it is likely that the severity of hypertrophy relates to the severity and length of history. The onset of heart failure appears with

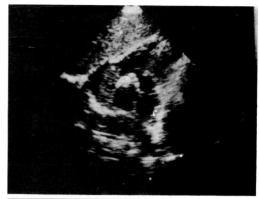

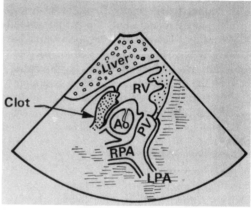

Figure 19.11. Clot within the right atrium imaged from a subcostal short-axis view of aorta. *Ao* = aorta, *LPA* = left pulmonary artery, *PV* = pulmonary vein, *RPA* = right pulmonary artery, *RV* = right ventricle.

cavity dilatation. The volume load, resulting in turn from functional tricuspid regurgitation, further burdens right ventricular systolic function, and systolic wall thickening may be reduced. In cases where pulmonary arterial pressures—and therefore right ventricular pressures—approach systemic levels, the septum will be concave toward the center of the right ventricular cavity during systole.

Pulmonary Hypertension Secondary to Left Heart Disease. In patients with pulmonary hypertension secondary to mitral valve disease, the most frequent finding is of cavity dilatation. Some increase in wall thickness may be seen. However, from our unpublished observations, this is less prominent than in patients with primary pulmonary hypertension. It may be that the development of secondary right ventricular hypertrophy depends upon the rate of development and time of exposure to the abnormal pressure load and not simply to severity. Many causes of left heart disease may show rapid deterioration, such as the development of atrial fibrillation in rheumatic mitral stenosis or the rupture of chordae in floppy mitral valve, causing severe mitral regurgitation. In these cases, pulmonary hypertension may develop acutely, and although the initial insult to the right ventricle is pressure, the early response is dilatation. This in itself leads to additional volume loading and right ventricular failure.

The echocardiographic consequences of pulmonary hypertension secondary to left heart disease are therefore of cavity dilatation with wall thickness measurements only 1 or 2 mm beyond normal values. The tricuspid valve ring stretches and results in incomplete closure of the tricuspid valve with tricuspid regurgitation. Right ventricular systolic pressure (and therefore pulmonary artery systolic pressure in the absence of outflow obstruction) may be estimated reliably by Doppler techniques as previously described.

Right Ventricular Volume Load

As tricuspid regurgitation is an almost invariable accompaniment of pressure load in acquired adult heart disease, much of the discussion above is relevant in the discussion of right ventricular volume load that follows.

Tricuspid Regurgitation. Volume loading in "primary" tricuspid regurgitation is most commonly seen in urban community hospitals in association with drug abuse. The echocardiographic abnormalities that result are of a generalized cavity dilatation but with vigorous right ventricular ejection. In these subjects, it will not be uncommon to find thickened, abnormal leaflets. This raises the question of whether hitherto unsuspected valve endocarditis is not responsible for the tricuspid regurgitation in this group. There are other causes, including reactive pulmonary hypertension due to injection of inert substances with the active compounds to which the abuser is addicted. However, often these patients will have treated themselves partially with varying antibiotic doses or have been prescribed such drugs for nonspecific symptoms. Right-sided endocarditis is itself often an elusive diagnosis and likely to present in a particularly nonspecific fashion in this population.

Of interest is the vigorous ejection seen in patients with "primary" tricuspid regurgitation unaccompanied by pulmonary hypertension. It seems from our experience that the right ventricle tolerates such volume load well.

Atrial Septal Defect. Most of the above considerations have applied to adult acquired disease. Atrial septal defect is present at birth, of course, but frequently presents in adolescent or adult life and so may be discussed appropriately in this section. It is this condition that provides the best example of right ventricular volume load. With volume loading from the interatrial communication present from birth, tricuspid valve leaflet growth and size appear to accommodate stretch of tricuspid annulus, and tricuspid regurgitation is not common. The ventricle therefore contracts vigorously in proportion to the magnitude of the interatrial shunt, itself correlated to the size of the atrial septal defect in patients who have normally compliant ventricular chambers. The cavity shows overall dilatation, and septal motion is grossly abnormal during diastole (20). This feature is less often seen in patients with pressure and volume load secondary to left heart disease. In this group, septal motion is the net effect of the right- and left-sided events.

Echocardiography of the Right Ventricle in Other Acquired Adult Heart Disease

Coronary Artery Disease. Just as in other conditions affecting the right side of the heart, right ventricular infarction is a subtle diagnosis when made by clinical, electrocardiographic, and other investigative means. However, its presence is important in determining prognosis in myocardial infarction. It is now well appreciated that right ventricular infarction often complicates inferoposterior or anteroseptal myocardial infarction. In particular, patients with inferoposterior left and right ventricular infarctions very poorly tolerate alterations to filling pressure, such as those induced by nitrates (21), and are particularly prone to cardiogenic shock and arrhythmia. Because of these factors, these patients as a group have a higher mortality than do patients with isolated left ventricular infarction alone (22–24).

Since the anatomic distribution of blood from left anterior descending and posterior descending arteries is to both right- and left-sided chambers, right heart infarction alone must be uncommon. Also, right ventricular infarction may not inevitably occur as a result of right coronary occlusion, even though blood supply to the right heart is interrupted. The explanation as to why, in right coronary occlusion, some patients develop infarction and others do not may lie in the recent observations by Forman et al. (25). In this study, patients with preexisting right ventricular hypertrophy from smoking-induced pulmonary disease were shown to be susceptible to hemodynamically important right ventricular infarction. Forman et al. measured right ventricular hypertrophy using M-mode guided by two-dimensional echocardiographic images. Two-dimensional echocardiography was used for the diagnosis of right ventricular infarction in this study, but its sensitivity for this diagnosis was believed to be poor. However, the failure to employ comprehensive two-dimensional echocardiographic views of the right ventricle, including specific right ventricular inflow tract views (which best image the inferior wall), may account for failure to show the benefit of the two-dimensional technique.

Given that right ventricular infarction may be difficult to diagnose using clinical and electrocardiographic criteria, echocardiography with the appropriate views can improve diagnostic accuracy. The specificity of subjective observer studies in the determination of regional wall motion abnormalities of the right ventricle have been poor. However, the sensitivity of the diagnosis is high (25–28). This is surprising until one considers the limitations of the methodology in each of these studies. This includes a lack of uniform "gold standard" for the diagnosis of infarction and the failure to employ views specific to the right ventricle.

Pathologic studies have suggested the presence of right ventricular infarction in 30–40% of patients with inferior infarction. In such cases, invariably there is involvement of the posterior interventricular septum and the posterior or inferior (diaphragmatic) wall of both right and left ventricles (Fig. 9.12). The extent of right ventricular infarction in inferior wall infarcts will depend on the right ventricular dominance of the vessel occluded. Clinical experience has taught that this is likely to be more of a problem with right coronary artery occlusion.

It has been our experience that in rupture of the septum in acute myocardial infarction, outcome may be determined by the residual contractility of right ventricular free wall. It appears from unpublished observations that the larger the associated right ventricular wall motion abnormality, the less likely the patient is to survive, irrespective of the extent of left ventricular involvement. It would further appear that the inferior wall of the right ventricle is of more hemodynamic importance than the anterior wall, which is frequently involved in infarction of the anterior and lateral wall of the left ventricle.

Having made these observations, it is quite clear that specific right ventricular views will contribute most to the assessment of regional wall motion abnormality in these areas. Regional wall analysis systems have not as yet been applied to the right ventricle. This is principally due to the complexities of right ventricular shape and the consequent difficulties of finding an appropriate center of mass around which to orient a radial analysis system. Nevertheless, "subjective observer" methods are of value and are deployed commonly in studies of left ventricular infarction and right ventricular infarction. However, most have not included the very views of the inflow and outflow tract that have the highest potential yield for the diagnosis. Therefore, it seems hardly surprising that the reported specificity of two-dimensional echocardiography for right ventricular infarctions is low.

In examining patients suspected of having right ventricular infarction, it should, in our opinion, be mandatory to employ specific right ventricular views. As previously described, these involve tilting the transducer in a medial and inferior orientation. In this way, specific images are obtained of the inferior circumference of the right ventricular diaphragmatic wall as it extends from the posterior septal groove toward the lateral right ventricular wall (Fig. 19.12). Having achieved these views, observations in real time will facilitate assessment of wall thickening characteristics during systole and inward endocardial excursion. These two features, when used with reference to neighboring right ventricular segments, will establish the diagnosis of regional wall abnormality. In the setting of clinical infarction, this means coronary artery occlusion. This is the method used in most laboratories and is practical in the assessment of left ventricular infarction. On theoretical grounds, it should be equally applicable to the right ventricular chamber if properly imaged. No doubt further studies will soon be forthcoming based upon improved methodology. It may be anticipated that two-dimensional echocardiography will be shown to be highly sensitive and specific for diagnosis of right ventricular infarctions.

The Right Ventricle in Hypertrophy and Cardiomyopathy

Hypertrophic Cardiomyopathy. The striking left ventricular abnormalities seen in primary heart muscle disease of the hypertrophic form often

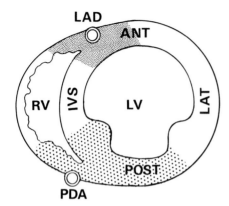

Figure 19.12. Right ventricular involvement in myocardial infarction. *ANT* = anterior, *IVS* = interventricular septum, *LAD* = left anterior descending coronary artery, *LAT* = lateral wall, *LV* = left ventricle, *PDA* = posterior descending coronary artery, *POST* = posterior wall, *RV* = right ventricle.

overshadows the echocardiographic findings in respect to the right ventricle. Given that the condition is defined by a finding of unexplained left ventricular hypertrophy, this is not particularly surprising. However, autopsy studies and, in particular, the report of sudden death in young adults with asymmetric left ventricular hypertrophy demonstrate that the majority had right as well as left ventricular involvement (29).

In a recent report of a consecutive group of patients with hypertrophic cardiomyopathy, systematic echocardiographic study was performed with particular attention directed to the right ventricle with specific right ventricular views (30). Thirty-two of the 73 patients studied (44%) had right ventricular hypertrophy with at least two wall thickness measurements exceeding 2 SD from the mean of normal subjects. In 15 of these 32 patients, all measurements of right ventricular wall thickness were abnormal, and obvious asymmetric right ventricular hypertrophy was observed in 6 patients.

Ten measurements of right ventricular wall thickness, as described in preceding sections, were performed on each patient in this group. An example from one patient with right ventricular abnormalities is provided in Figure 19.13. When the clinical correlations were examined, ventricular tachycardia, couplets, and supraventricular tachycardia were more common in the group with right ventricular hypertrophy. On echocardiographic assessment between mean and maximal

right ventricular wall thickness there was a strong correlation with measurements of regional and global left ventricular hypertrophy. Right ventricular hypertrophy, therefore, appeared to be a more common event in those patients with the more severe left ventricular abnormalities.

Hemodynamic measurements were also reported in approximately two-thirds of those patients with and without right ventricular hypertrophy. There appeared to be no correlation between the presence of right ventricular hypertrophy and pulmonary hypertension or pulmonary arteriolar resistance. In two patients with a pulmonary arteriolar resistance measuring greater than 265 dyne/sec/cm^{-5}, the right ventricular wall thickness was normal. Consequently, the underlying mechanism for right ventricular hypertrophy in hypertrophic cardiomyopathy would appear to be uncertain. There is no obvious secondary mechanism if the isolated hemodynamic measurements from this study can be accepted. Of course, isolated pressure measurement does not exclude the possibility of right ventricular hypertrophy being caused by consequences of left ventricular diastolic or systolic dysfunction. Monitoring of pressures in the right heart during exercise and normal daily life would have been preferred, although this is clearly impractical. The hemodynamic data available suggest that right ventricular hypertrophy was not secondary to right ventricular outflow tract obstructions. Presumably, therefore, the right ventricular hypertrophy present in this group is a primary hypertrophic response provoked by the unknown stimulus that causes left-sided hypertrophy. An echocardiographic finding of right ventricular hypertrophy in patients with left ventricular hypertrophy may favor the diagnosis of hypertrophic cardiomyopathy in the absence of any other obvious cause for the left ventricular hypertrophy. Clearly, the more severe the right ventricular hypertrophy in patients with unexplained left ventricular hypertrophy, the more likely the diagnosis represents primary cardiomyopathy.

The Right Ventricle and Other Causes of Right Ventricular Hypertrophy. The right ventricle frequently is involved in other conditions that cause severe "primary" left ventricular hypertrophy. For example, amyloid heart disease often shows marked increase in right ventricular wall thickness, and a characteristic sparkling echo may also be seen within the right ventricular wall, as with the left heart (Fig. 19.14). Similarly, glycogen storage disease produces severe left ventricular

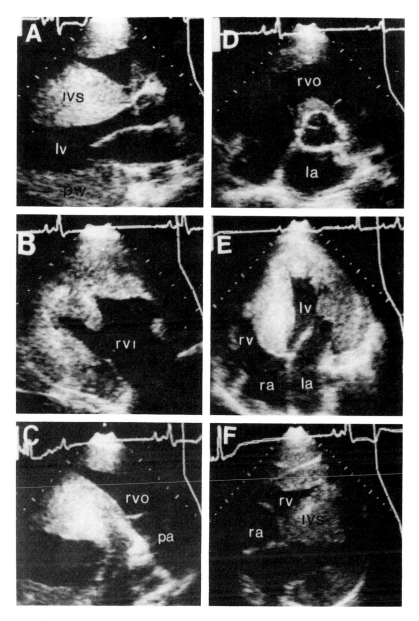

Figure 19.13. IVS = interventricular septum, *la* = left atrium, *lv* = left ventricle, *pa* = pulmonary artery, ra = right atrium, rv = right ventricle, rvi = right ventricular inflow, rvo = right ventricular outflow. (Reproduced with permission from the American College of Cardiology V.)

hypertrophy in the child and adolescent and primarily affects the right ventricle. These features may make differentiation of infiltrative heart muscle disease from severe hypertrophic cardiomyopathy difficult or impossible based on echocardiography alone.

Right ventricular hypertrophy as a possible consequence to left-sided diastolic or systolic dys-function in left-sided pressure load was examined by Gottdiener et al. (31). Right ventricular hypertrophy was reported in the majority of patients with left ventricular hypertrophy secondary to pressure load. Although in this study limited measurement of the right ventricular wall was performed, 64% of patients with aortic stenosis and 83% of those with hypertension had abnor-

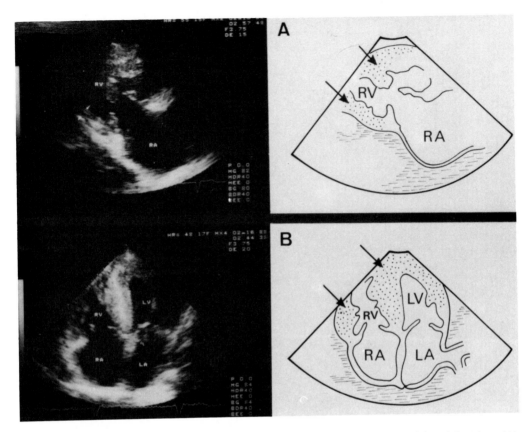

Figure 19.14. Amyloid infiltration of the heart with right ventricular hypertrophy. *LA* = left atrium, *LV* = left ventricle, *RA* = right atrium, *RV* = right ventricle.

mal right ventricular wall thickness. In these patients there was an association with pulmonary hypertension. However, the degree of hypertrophy in these patients was not comparable to that found in patients with hypertrophic cardiomyopathy.

From our own observations of patients with hypertension and aortic stenosis, a quite different pattern of right ventricular hypertrophy seems to occur when compared to the right ventricular hypertrophy of hypertrophic cardiomyopathy. The stimuli to right ventricular hypertrophy in patients with hypertrophic cardiomyopathy and pressure loading of the left ventricle are likely to be different and are as yet unknown. Answers may be forthcoming from analysis of cellular mechanisms as biopsy techniques and analysis of small muscle samples improve.

Right Ventricular Dysplasia and Dilated Cardiomyopathy. Recently, considerable interest has centered on the right ventricle as a potential source

of life-threatening arrhythmia in the young and in adults without coronary artery disease affecting the right ventricle. It is likely that a variety of conditions can be incriminated in this condition, including isolated right ventricular cardiomyopathy (32), Uhl anomaly (33), and arrhythmogenic right ventricular dysplasia (34–36). Furthermore, it is quite possible that these conditions may represent one end of a spectrum of heart muscle disease. In these patients, the right ventricle may represent the early signs of a progressive and potentially generalized myocardial disorder (35). Nevertheless, in a group of patients studied from our institution who presented with ventricular tachycardia of right ventricular origin (left bundle-branch block pattern), the group with adverse clinical and electrophysiologic features had generalized dilatation of the right ventricle (Fig. 19.15). In this "adverse group," four of the eight had marked additional regional wall motion abnormalities of the right ventricle. The appearances were consistent with arrhythmogenic right ventricular dysplasia. Our study suggested that surveillance of the right ventricle in patients presenting with serious arrhythmia and the presence of normal left heart anatomy may define right ventricular abnormalities, which in turn may identify patients at particularly high risk of sudden death (36).

Right Ventricular Restriction—Endomyocardial Disease. Restriction to filling of the heart has several causes, and in general the right ventricle is affected in a similar way as is the left ventricle. Primary restrictive cardiomyopathy may manifest with echocardiographic features typical of a restrictive physiology. These features are of small left and right ventricular chambers (which may appear hypertrophied) and substantial biatrial enlargement. One of the most common causes of restrictive cardiomyopathy, endomyocardial fi-

brosis (EMF), has echocardiographic features, which together with the general findings of a restrictive physiology will secure the correct diagnosis (Fig. 19.16). The specific feature affecting the right and left ventricles is an endocardial "shell" at the apex, with features suggesting adherent thrombus. Frequently, this fibrosis will involve the subvalvular apparatus of both tricuspid and mitral valves. The fibrosis at the apex or chordal level appears as a highly echo reflective signal with underlying normal wall thickness. This together with the small cavity sizes clearly differentiates the condition from mural thrombus adherent to 'the underlying scar of myocardial infarction or dilated cardiomyopathy.

The Right Ventricle and Tumors and Infection. The right ventricle may be involved with primary or particularly secondary tumors from any primary source. A mass seen within any part

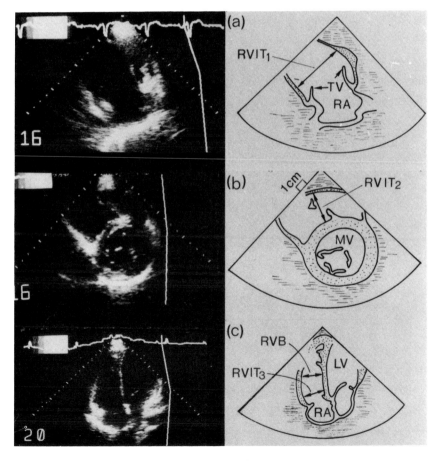

Figure 19.15. *LV* = left ventricle, RA = right atrium, *RVB* = right ventricular body, *TV* = tricuspid valve. (Reproduced with permission from *British Heart Journal.*)

Figure 19.16. Right and left ventricular involvement with endomyocardial fibrosis. Apical deposits from a four-chamber view. A = apex, LA = left atrium, LV = left ventricle, R = right, RA = right atrium, RV = right ventricle.

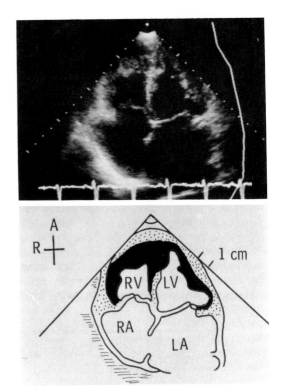

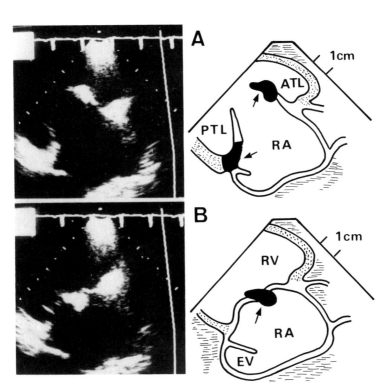

Figure 19.17. Patient in whom blood cultures with *S. faecalis* were thought to be associated with myocardial abscess and tricuspid valve infection. ATL = anterior tricuspid leaflet, EV = Eustachian valve, PTL = Posterior tricuspid leaflet, RA = right atrium, RV = right ventricle.

of the cavity should be regarded with great suspicion (37, 38). This is particularly true in patients of known primary source, especially large cell lymphoma, or in patients otherwise at risk of lymphoma, as in patients with HIV infection and the AIDS complex (39). Occasionally, the differentiation of right ventricular tumor mass may be difficult from that of infection. This is illustrated in Figure 19.17, which shows a patient in whom blood cultures with *Streptococcus faecalis* were thought to be associated with myocardial abscess and tricuspid valve infection. Subsequently, at autopsy, this patient was demonstrated to have lymphomatous infiltration of the heart.

CONCLUSION

The recent interest in the literature concerning the right ventricle expands our appreciation that right ventricular pathology may be the focus for many of the "difficult" treatment territories in cardiology. This includes sudden death in the young and heart failure and arrhythmia, particularly complicating acute cardiac infarction. In addition, an understanding of the pathophysiology of hypertrophy may be advanced by further studies of the right ventricle when affected by primary versus secondary factors.

These issues are difficult to study for a variety of reasons, not the least of which is the relative silence of the right ventricle when it comes to manifesting clinical features. Furthermore, it is resistant to investigation by standard noninvasive and invasive techniques. Consequently, its complex geometry and function cannot be studied by a single technique alone. Nevertheless, two-dimensional echocardiography with Doppler, if properly applied, may substantially advance our understanding of this key target of cardiology research.

REFERENCES

1. Fiegenbaum H: *Echocardiography*, ed 2. Philadelphia, Lea & Febiger, 1976, 255–266.
2. Hudson REB: *Cardiovascular Pathology*, London, Edward Arnold, 1965, vol 1, 15.
3. Keren A, Billingham ME, Popp RL: Echocardiographic recognition of parasternal structures. *J Am Coll Cardiol* 6:913–919, 1985.
4. Weyman AE: *Cross Sectional Echocardiography*. Philadelphia, Lea & Febiger, 1982, 497–504.
5. Report of the American Society of Echocardiography on Nomenclature and Standards in Two Dimensional Imaging. *Circulation* 57:583–587, 1978.
6. Schnittger I, Gordon EP, Fitzgerald PJ, Popp RL: Standardized intracardiac measurements of two dimensional echocardiography. *J Am Coll Cardiol* 2:934–938, 1983.
7. Foale R, Nihoyannopoulos P, McKenna W, Klienebenne A, Nadazdin A, Rowland E, Smith G: Echocardiographic measurement of the normal adult right ventricle. *Br Heart J* 56:33–44, 1986.
8. Lange LW, Sahn DJ, Allen HD, Goldberg SJ: Subxiphoid cross sectional echocardiography in infants and children with congenital heart disease. *Circulation* 59:513, 1979.
9. Hatle L, Angelsen B: *Doppler Ultrasound in Cardiology*. Philadelphia, Lea & Febiger, 1982, 63–66.
10. Weyman AE, Dillon JC, Feigenbaum H, Chang S: Echocardiographic patterns of pulmonary valve motion in valvular pulmonary stenosis. *Am J Cardiol* 34:644, 1974.
11. Foale R, King M, Weyman AE: The pulmonary valve. In Guiliani ER (ed): *Two Dimensional Real-Time Ultrasonic Imaging of the Heart*. Boston, Martinus Nijhoff, 1985, 101–114.
12. Skjaerae T, Hatle L: Diagnosis and assessment of tricuspid regurgitation with Doppler ultrasound. In: Lancee T (ed): *Echocardiology*. The Hague, Martinus Nijhoff, 1979, 233–235.
13. St John Sutton MG, Gewitz MH, Shah B, Cohen A, Reichek N, Gabbe S, Huff DS: Quantitative assessment of growth and function of the cardiac chambers in the normal human fetus: A prospective longitudinal echocardiographic study. *Circulation* 1984, 69:645–654, 1984.
14. Foale RA, Stephanini L, Rickards AF, Somerville J: Left and right ventricular morphology in complex congenital heart disease: Definition by two dimensional echocardiography. *Am J Cardiol* 49:93–99, 1982.
15. Foale RA, Donaldson R, Rickards AF, Somerville J: Double inlet ventricle: Two dimensional echocardiographic findings. *Circulation* 62:III-332, 1980.
16. King ME, Braun H, Goldblatt A, Liberthson RR, Weyman AE: Interventricular septal configuration as a predictor of right ventricular systolic hypertension in children: A cross sectional echocardiographic study. *Circulation* 80:68–75, 1983.
17. Feigenbaum H: *Echocardiography*, ed 2. Philadelphia, Lea & Febiger, 275–284.
18. Come PL, Riley MF, Carl LV, Nakao S: Echocardiographic findings in patients with proved pulmonary embolism. *Am Heart J* 112:1284–1290, 1986.
19. Jardin F, Dubourg O, Gueret P, Delorme G, Bourbarias JP: Quantitative two dimensional echocardiography in massive pulmonary embolism: Emphasis on ventricular interdependence and leftward septal displacement. *J Am Coll Cardiol* 10:1201–1206, 1987.
20. Ballester M, Pons G, Carreras F, Claddellas M: Reversed septal motion in right ventricular volume overload: False negative sign in the presence of increased septal thickness. *Clin Cardiol* 9:623–625, 1986.
21. Ferguson JJ, Diver DJ, Boldt M, Pasternak RC: Nitroglycerin induced hypotension with acute inferior myocardial infarction: A marker of right ventricular involvement? *Circulation* 72:III-460A, 1985.
22. Cohn JN, Grima NH, Broder MI, Limas CJ: Right ventricular infarction: Clinical and hemodynamic features. *Am J Cardiol* 33:209–214, 1974.

23. Lloyd EA, Gersh BT, Kenelly BM: Hemodynamic spectrum of "dominant" right ventricular infarction in 19 patients. *Am J Cardiol* 48:1016–1022, 1981.

24. Lorell B, Leinbach RC, Pohost GM, et al: Right ventricular infarction: Clinical diagnosis and differentiation from cardiac tamponade and pericardial constriction. *Am J Cardiol* 43:465–471, 1979.

25. Forman MB, Wilson BH, Sheller JR, Kopelman HA, Vaughn WK, Virmani R, Friesinger GC: Right ventricular hypertrophy is an important determinant of right ventricular infarction complicating acute inferior left ventricular infarction. *J Am Coll Cardiol* 10:1180–1187, 1987.

26. Darcy B, Nanda NC: Two dimensional echocardiographic features of right ventricular infarction. *Circulation* 65:167–173, 1982.

27. Dell'Italia LJ, Starling MR, Crawford MH, Boros BL, Chaudhuri TK, O'Rouke RA: Right ventricular infarction: Identification by hemodynamic measurements before and after volume loading and correlation with non-invasive techniques. *J Am Coll Cardiol* 4:931–939, 1984.

28. Baigrie RS, Haq A, Morgan CD, Rakowski H, Drobac M, McLaughlin P: The spectrum of right ventricular involvement in inferior wall myocardial infarction: A clinical, hemodynamic and non-invasive study. *J Am Coll Cardiol* 1:1396–1404, 1983.

29. Teare D: Asymmetric hypertrophy of the heart in young adults. *Br Heart J* 20:1–8, 1958.

30. McKenna WJ, Kleinebenne A, Nihoyannopoulos P, Foale R: Echocardiographic measurement of right ventricular wall thickness in hypertrophic cardiomyopathy: Relation to clinical and prognostic features. *J Am Coll Cardiol* 11:351–358, 1988.

31. Gottdiener, Gay JA, Maron BT, Fletcher RD: Increased right ventricular wall thickness in left ventricular pressure overload: Echocardiographic determination of hypertrophic response of the "non stressed" ventricle. *J Am Coll Cardiol* 6:550–555, 1985.

32. Fitchet DH, MacArthur CG, Oakley CM, Krikler DM, Goodwin JF: Right ventricular cardiomyopathy presenting with recurrent ventricular tachycardia. *Am J Cardiol* 47:402, 1981.

33. Child JS, Perloff JK, Francoz R, Yeatman LA, Henze G, Schelbert HR, Laks H: Uhl's anomaly (parchment right ventricle): Clinical, echocardiographic, radionuclear, hemodynamic and angiographic features in two patients. *Am J Cardiol* 53:635–637, 1984.

34. Rowland E, McKenna WT, Surgue D, Barclay R, Foale RA, Krikler DM: Ventricular tachycardia of left bundle branch block configuration in patients with isolated ventricular dilatation: Clinical and electrophysiological features. *Br Heart J* 51:15–24, 1984.

35. Rossi P, Massumi A, Gillette P, Hall RJ: Right ventricular dysplasia: Clinical features, diagnostic techniques and current management. *Am Heart J* 103:415–420, 1982.

36. Foale RA, Nihoyannopoulos P, Ribiero P, McKenna WJ, Oakley CM, Krikler DM, Rowland E: Right ventricular abnormalities in ventricular tachycardia of right ventricular origin: Relation to electrophysiological features. *Br Heart J* 56:45–54, 1986.

37. Carlin BW, Dianzumba SB, Wedel C, Jowner CR: Right ventricular inflow and outflow obstruction due to adrenal cell carcinoma. *Cathet Cardiovasc Diagn* 12:51–54, 1986.

38. Shrivastava S, Chopara P, Kumar AS: Fibrosarcoma of the right ventricle: A case report. *Int J Cardiol* 9:234–238, 1985.

39. Foale RA: Cardiac involvement with Aids, current opinions. *Cardiology* 3:245–248, 1988.

20

Role of Two-Dimensional Echocardiography in Infective Endocarditis

John G. Harold, M.D.
Eugenio Carmo, M.D.

The characteristic lesion of bacterial endocarditis is a friable verrucous vegetation attached to an endocardial surface most commonly overlying a heart valve (1). Vegetations can be large or small, sessile or pedunculated, circular or irregular. Although nonvalvular endocardial vegetations can occur, they are almost always associated with valvular vegetations. Infected vegetations are composed of clumps of bacteria, fibrin, platelet thrombi, and erythrocytes attached to the endocardial surface. Fungal vegetations are usually larger than their bacterial counterparts. In addition, fungal vegetations tend to embolize more easily and require surgical intervention more frequently.

Aortic vegetations usually are attached to the ventricular side of the valve, whereas mitral and tricuspid vegetations usually are attached to the atrial surface of the valve (2). Vegetations may produce diffuse thickening of the valve leaflets. In those cases the echocardiographic appearance is not specific for endocarditis, and differentiation from other pathologic processes is not always possible (3, 4).

Two-dimensional echocardiography is superior to M-mode echocardiography in the ability to detect and assess vegetations (Fig. 20.1). Masses must be approximately 3–4 mm in diameter before they can be appreciated by echocardiography. Vegetations appear on two-dimensional echocardiography as mobile, rapidly oscillating dense masses. These masses can involve a large portion of the valve leaflet or have more limited attachment, as in a polypoid lesion. In left-sided infectious endocarditis there is a higher compli-

cation rate associated with vegetations detected by echocardiography (e.g., embolization, congestive heart failure) than when vegetations are not visualized. However, there appears to be no direct correlation between the size, morphology, and location of a vegetation and the incidence of major complications or the need for valve replacement. Higher complication rates are seen (a) when vegetations involve more than one valve, (b) with associated mechanical lesions, such as a flail valve, and (c) with vegetations on other endocardial surfaces, such as mitral chordae tendineae.

The prognosis for right-sided endocarditis, even with echocardiographic visualization of a vegetation, is more favorable than for left-sided endocarditis. This is due to the fact that left-sided endocarditis usually is associated with a deformed valve, while right-sided endocarditis usually occurs on previously normal valves. Many patients with clinically proven infective endocarditis do not have identifiable vegetations by echocardiography. Thus, a negative echocardiographic study for vegetations does not rule out infective endocarditis.

Valvular abnormalities seen in conjunction with vegetations can be the result of previous damage to the valvular apparatus or recent damage due to an acute infective process (5). In the absence of sequential studies it is difficult to determine whether mechanical valvular abnormalities seen in conjunction with vegetations are old or a complication of a new infective process (6). Digital image processing of two-dimensional echocardiograms has been reported to have utility in dif-

Figure 20.1. Simultaneous M-mode and two-dimensional parasternal long-axis view in a patient with a large vegetation (v) on the mitral valve. The two-dimensional image helps to guide the M-mode beam, and the same depth resolution gives a better explanation of the findings. A large vegetation is attached to the posterior leaflet of the mitral valve. The distal part of the vegetation moves anteriorly during diastole, behind the anterior mitral valve (amv) leaflet. Ao = aorta, LA = left atrium, LV = left ventricle.

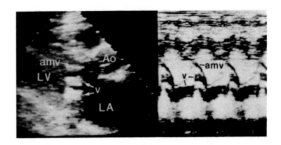

ferentiating active from chronic vegetations and may be useful in distinguishing active from cured infective endocarditis (7).

Two-dimensional and Doppler echocardiography are particularly useful in detecting the sequelae of infective endocarditis (8, 9). Hemodynamic data obtained from these methodologies assist in the clinical management of patients and in determining the need for valve replacement. Once diagnosed by two-dimensional echocardiography, vegetations are especially suitable for serial studies to determine their size and morphology (10). This information may be useful in assessing the efficacy of antimicrobial therapy and aiding in the determination of the timing of surgical intervention (11). A decrease in size of a vegetation, as seen by serial studies, would be consistent with the process of healing. However, a sudden disappearance of part or all of a vege-

tation is probably due to detachment and embolization. Vegetations may persist long after bacteriologic cure. An increase in size of a vegetation usually indicates a continuation of an active infective process. As stated, a negative echocardiographic study does not exclude the diagnosis of endocarditis, as small vegetations may not be visualized.

Two-dimensional echocardiography has clinical utility in detecting the localized complications of infectious endocarditis. These complications include: progression of the infection to adjacent structures, such as chordae tendineae; ring abscess; mitral valve aneurysm; progression to other valves; and the development of mechanical lesions, such as flail valve and ruptured chordae tendineae (12).

The most commonly used view for diagnosing mitral valve vegetations and associated compli-

Figure 20.2. Parasternal long-axis view during systole, demonstrating a moderate-sized mass (arrows) representing a vegetation within the mitral valve (MV). The vegetation protrudes into the left atrial cavity. AO = aortic root, LA = left atrium, LV = left ventricle, RV = right ventricle, A = anterior, P = posterior, Ba = base, Ap = apex.

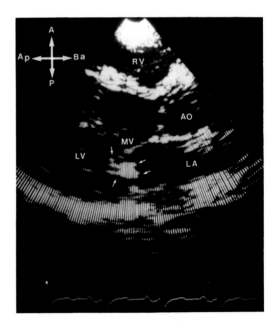

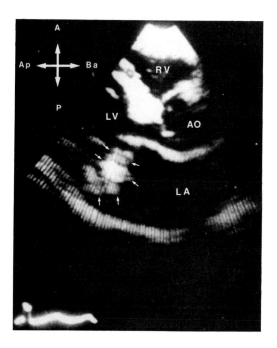

Figure 20.3. Parasternal long-axis view demonstrating a large irregular mass (*arrows*) representing a vegetation of the mitral valve. The valve itself cannot be identified on this still frame. The vegetation protrudes into the left atrium (*LA*). Abbreviations are the same as those identified in the legend to Figure 20.2.

cations is the parasternal long-axis view (Figs. 20.2 and 20.3). This view provides simultaneous visualization of the cavities adjacent to the mitral valve—the left atrium and the left ventricle—with their spatial relationship to the remainder of the mitral apparatus and the aortic valve. Complementary information should be obtained from any other view in which the mitral valve can be visualized (Figs. 20.4 and 20.5).

Mitral valve vegetations can be difficult to diagnose if they are small and superimposed on a previously distorted valve (13). In general, it is easier to diagnose a vegetation if it is large, especially if it prolapses into the left atrium during systole (Fig. 20.6*A* and *B*). Once diagnosis of a vegetation is made, the rest of the mitral valve apparatus should be explored (Fig. 20.7*A* and *B*). A localized thickening of the chordae tendineae

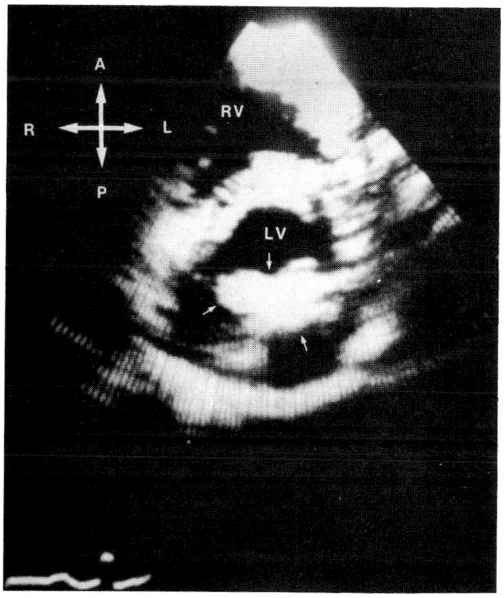

Figure 20.4. Short-axis view at the mitral valve level during systole. A large irregular mass (*arrows*) representing a vegetation is seen occupying almost the entire mitral valve orifice. *R* = right, *L* = left. Other abbreviations are the same as those identified in the legend to Figure 20.2.

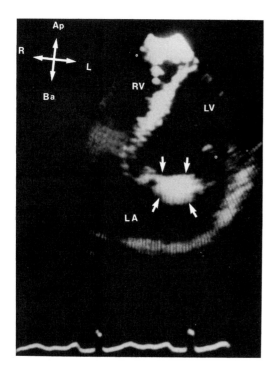

Figure 20.5. Apical four-chamber view of the patient illustrated in Figure 20.3, demonstrating a large irregular mass (*arrows*) representing a vegetation attached to the mitral valve. The vegetation protrudes into the left atrium (*LA*). *R* = right, *L* = left. Other abbreviations are the same as those identified in the legend to Figure 20.2.

would suggest chordal vegetations (Figs. 20.8–20.10). The diagnosis of superimposed vegetations is facilitated by the presence of high frequency oscillations on M-mode echocardiography. However, myxomatous degeneration of the mitral valve may cause valve thickening and multiple echoes of the anterior leaflet. When associated with mitral valve prolapse, these findings may mimic vegetative endocarditis with ruptured chordae tendineae. A gradual decrease in the size of a vegetation would suggest healing. However, vegetations may persist after the endocarditis has healed (Fig. 20.11*A* and *B*).

Localized complications of mitral valve endocarditis include destruction of the valve tissue and/or ruptured chordae tendineae. The latter is manifested echocardiographically by marked holosystolic protrusion of the valve into the left atrium, fine systolic fluttering, and coarse diastolic fluttering, usually of the anterior leaflet. The systolic prolapse of the flail valve into the left atrium can

simulate a left atrial myxoma or thrombus (Fig. 20.12). A complete two-dimensional echocardiographic study should be done to establish the correct diagnosis.

With the use of multiple views, the aortic valve is readily accessible for two-dimensional echocardiographic detection of vegetations and associated pathology (1). As with the mitral valve, the parasternal long-axis view is the most clinically useful view in the diagnosis of aortic valve vegetations (Fig. 20.13). However, the use of an additional view is required for a complete study.

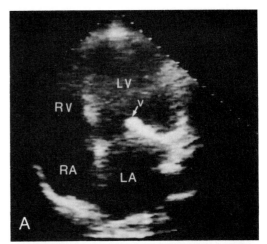

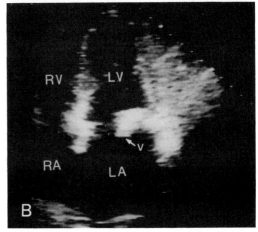

Figure 20.6. Apical four-chamber view of a patient with a large vegetation (*v*) attached to the posterior leaflet of the mitral valve. *A*, During diastole, the vegetation moves into the left ventricle (*LV*). *B*, During systole, the vegetation prolapses into the left atrium (*LA*). *RA* = right atrium, *RV* = right ventricle.

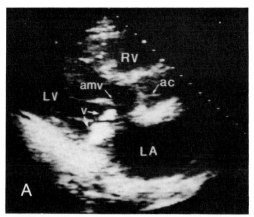

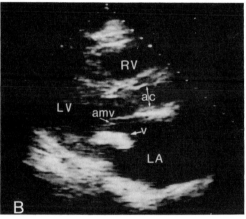

Figure 20.7. Parasternal long-axis view in a patient with a large vegetation (*v*) attached to the posterior leaflet of the mitral valve. *A,* During diastole, with the aortic cusps (*ac*) closed, the vegetation moves into the left ventricle (*LV*) behind the anterior mitral valve (*amv*) leaflet. *B,* During systole, with the aortic cusps opened, the vegetation prolapses into the left atrium (*LA*). *RV* = right ventricle.

Visualization of all three cusps is achieved by the use of the parasternal short-axis view. Aortic valve vegetations may prolapse into the left ventricular outflow tract during diastole. A decrease or diminution in size determined by serial studies would help to differentiate firm vegetations from valvular calcifications.

An occasional complication of aortic valve endocarditis is a flail valve. This diagnosis can be made by two-dimensional echocardiography. M-mode echocardiography is effective in demonstrating diastolic fluttering that results from aortic regurgitation and is seen with flail aortic leaflet (Figs. 20.14 and 20.15). Acute severe aortic regurgitation causes premature closure of the mitral valve which is best documented with M-mode echocardiography (15). Acute aortic regurgitation into a noncompliant left ventricle causes

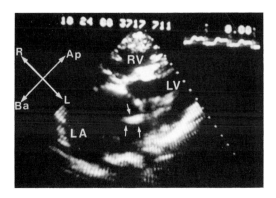

Figure 20.8. Subcostal long-axis view demonstrating a small mitral valve vegetation (*arrows*) protruding into a dilated left atrium (*LA*) during systole in a patient with chronic rheumatic valvulitis and bacterial endocarditis. *R* = right, *L* = left. Other abbreviations are the same as those identified in the legend to Figure 20.2.

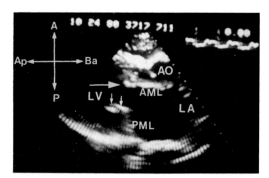

Figure 20.9. Parasternal long-axis view in end-diastole of the same patient as shown in Figure 20.8. A vegetation (*large arrow*) attached to the anterior mitral leaflet (*AML*) is seen in the left ventricular outflow tract. An elongated bright mass extending from the posterior mitral leaflet (*PML*) into the left ventricular (*LV*) cavity represents a vegetation attached to its chordae tendineae (*small arrows*). Abbreviations are the same as those identified in the legend to Figure 20.2.

a rapid rise of left ventricular diastolic pressure, which exceeds the left atrial pressure and leads to premature closure of the mitral valve. The more severe the aortic regurgitation, the more premature is the closure of the mitral valve. This finding in the setting of infective endocarditis has been reported as an indication for emergent aortic valve replacement (16). Doppler echocardiography is also useful in assessing the severity of aortic regurgitation (17).

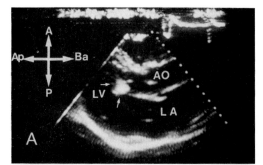

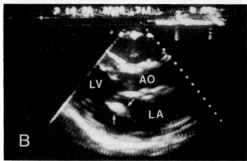

Figure 20.11. Diastolic (*A*) and systolic (*B*) frames of a parasternal long-axis view taken 3 years after recovery from infective endocarditis. A moderately sized healed vegetation (*arrows*) is seen prolapsing freely into the left atrium (*LA*) during systole. An identical two-dimensional echocardiographic pattern was seen in a study done 1 year before. Abbreviations are the same as those identified in the legend to Figure 20.2.

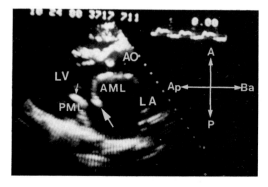

Figure 20.10. Parasternal long-axis view in systole of the patient illustrated in Figure 20.9. The flail anterior mitral leaflet (*AML*) and the vegetation attached to it (*large arrow*) prolapse into the left atrium (*LA*). The stiff posterior mitral leaflet (*PML*) and the vegetation attached to its chordae (*small arrow*) do not show any substantial positional change when compared to diastole. Abbreviations are the same as those identified in the legend to Figure 20.2.

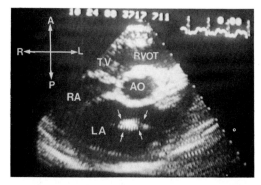

Figure 20.12. Parasternal short-axis view at the level of the aortic root (*AO*) taken during systole. An oval mass (*arrows*) is seen in the center of the left atrium (*LA*). In this view, the mass could be mistaken for a left atrial myxoma or a thrombus. However, the parasternal long-axis view (Figs. 20.8 and 20.10) supported the diagnosis of a vegetation. *TV* = tricuspid valve, *RVOT* = right ventricular outflow tract, *R* = right, *L* = left. Other abbreviations are the same as those identified in the legend to Figure 20.2.

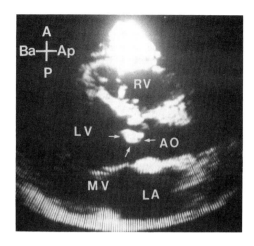

Figure 20.13. Parasternal long-axis view taken from a patient with infective endocarditis. An irregular mass (*arrows*) representing a vegetation is seen in the region of the aortic valve. *MV* = mitral valve. Other abbreviations are the same as those identified in the legend to Figure 20.2. Courtesy of Michael Barrett, M.D.

Aortic vegetations can cause a variety of ischemic syndromes, such as resting intermittent angina pectoris and/or myocardial infarction. These could occur due to partial or complete occlusion of the coronary ostia or coronary artery by an aortic vegetation (Fig. 20.16).

An unusual complication of aortic valve endocarditis is aortic ring abscess (Fig. 20.17). Determination of the size of the abscess and the discontinuity of the aortic valve and mitral valve require more than one echocardiographic view. The two best views are the parasternal short-axis view and parasternal long-axis view (18, 19). Other rare complications include mycotic aneurysms or sinus of Valsalva and myocardial abscess. An ab-

scess of the sinus of Valsalva may cause aneurysmal enlargement, and perforation may occur, creating a left-to-right shunt from the aorta to the right ventricle (20). Purulent pericarditis may occur as a result of extension of infection into the pericardial space by hematogenous seeding, rupture of a myocardial abscess, or perforation of a mycotic aneurysm (21).

The incidence of tricuspid valve endocarditis has increased in recent years due to intravenous drug abuse (22). This has led to a preponderance of tricuspid valve endocarditis involving anatomically normal valves. Right-sided endocarditis can be associated with multiple septic pulmonary emboli and pneumonia. Tricuspid valve vegetations

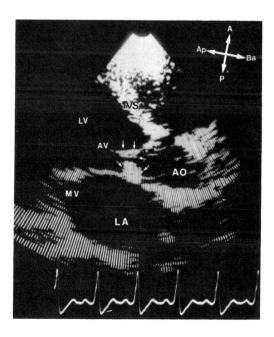

Figure 20.14. Parasternal long-axis view taken during diastole shows irregular masses (*small arrows*) representing vegetations attached to the right and noncoronary aortic valve (*AV*) cusps. The cusps and vegetations prolapse into the left ventricular cavity (*LV*) during diastole. The mitral valve (*MV*) appears normal. *IVS* = interventricular septum. Other abbreviations are the same as those identified in the legend to Figure 20.2.

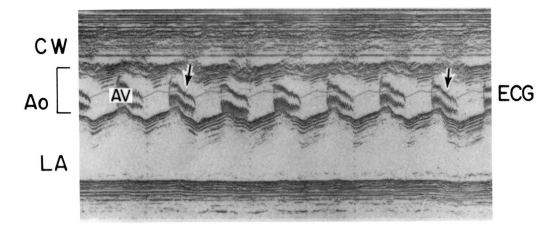

Figure 20.15. M-mode tracing of the aortic root (*Ao*) taken from the patient in Figure 20.14. During diastole the grossly thickened aortic cusps (*AV*) and their vegetations show marked separation and high frequency oscillation. *Arrows* = R wave of the QRS complex, *CW* = chest wall, *LA* = left atrium.

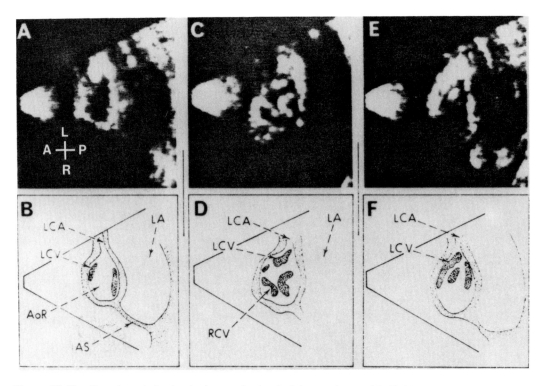

Figure 20.16. Parasternal short-axis view at the level of the aortic root (*AoR*). Vegetations are noted on all three cusps. The left coronary cusp vegetation (*LCV*) is moving into the orifice of the left main coronary artery (*LCA*) from its starting position in systole (*A, B*) through middiastole (*C, D*), and ending in late diastole (*E, F*). *AS* = interarterial septum, *RCV* = right coronary cusp vegetation, *LA* = left atrium. Other abbreviations are the same as those identified in the legend to Figure 20.4. (From Gilbert BW, Haney RS, Crawford F, McClellan J, Gallis HA, Johnson ML, Kisslo JA: Two-dimensional echocardiographic assessment and vegetative endocarditis. *Circulation* 55:346, 1977. With permission of the American Heart Association, Inc.)

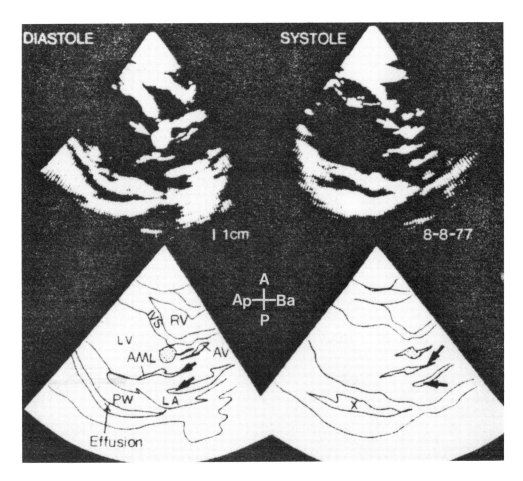

Figure 20.17. Parasternal long-axis view. The solid echo seen in the left ventricular outflow tract in diastole and in the aortic root during systole (*white arrows, hatched areas*) represents an aortic valve (*AV*) vegetation. A discontinuity between the anterior mitral leaflet (*AML*) and posterior aortic wall (*PW*) represents aortic ring abscess (*black arrows, bottom diagrams*). Echo-free space posterior to the left ventricular posterior wall represents pericardial effusion. *LA* = left atrium, *LV* = left ventricle, *RV* = right ventricle, *IVS* = interventricular septum. (From Mardelli TJ, Ogawa J, Hubbard FE, Dreifus LS, Meixell LL: Cross-sectional detection of aortic ring abscess in bacterial endocarditis. *Chest* 74:576, 1978.)

are usually larger than vegetations involving the mitral or aortic valves (Fig. 20.18). Two-dimensional echocardiography is useful in identifying tricuspid valve vegetations and differentiating them from true masses involving the tricuspid valve, such as a right atrial myxoma (23). In addition to the parasternal and apical views, the subcostal view may be an important view for consistent visualization of the tricuspid valve.

As with other valves, serial studies can be helpful in determining efficacy of treatment. Serial studies can document changes in the size of the vegetation and can detect the localized destruction of the leaflet and the appearance of a flail leaflet. Doppler echocardiography is useful in demonstrating the degree of tricuspid regurgitation.

, Infective endocarditis of the pulmonic valve is rare (24, 25). As is the case with the tricuspid valve, the presence of vegetations without a previous deformity of the pulmonic valve is not uncommon. The appearance of pulmonic valve vegetations is similar to the appearance of those on other valves (Fig. 20.19). Patients with ventricular septal defects may develop right-sided endocarditis at the site of the jet lesion on the endocardium of the right ventricular outflow tract, adjacent to the pulmonic valve.

Figure 20.18. Parasternal long-axis view of the right ventricle, demonstrating a vegetation, visualized as a large irregular mass (*small arrows*) attached to the tricuspid valve (*TV, large arrows*). *L* = left, *R* = right, *RA* = right atrium. Other abbreviations are the same as those identified in the legend to Figure 20.2.

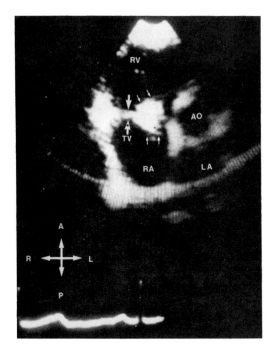

Prosthetic valve endocarditis carries an ominous prognosis. The ease of diagnosis depends on the type of prosthetic valve. The sewing ring and support structures of mechanical and bioprosthetic valves are strongly echogenic and may obscure the assessment of vegetations (26). The infectious process involving mechanical valves usually begins in the perivalvular area at the annular insertion site. Doppler echocardiography and color flow imaging may be useful in identifying perivalvular leaks. Necrosis of the supporting annular tissue may lead to loosening of sutures

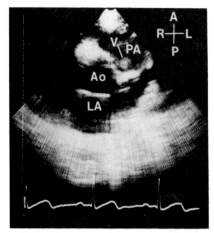 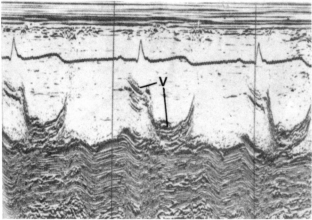

Figure 20.19. Parasternal short-axis view (*left*) through the aortic root (*Ao*) and the pulmonary artery (*PA*). A globular vegetation (*V*) is present on the pulmonic valve. An M-mode study (*right*) reveals multiple shaggy echoes on the pulmonic valve in systole and diastole, indicating a vegetation. *LA* = left atrium. Other abbreviations are the same as those identified in the legend to Figure 20.2. (From Berger M, Delfin LA, Jelveh M, Goldberg E: Two-dimensional echocardiographic findings in right-sided infective endocarditis. *Circulation* 61:855, 1980. With permission of the American Heart Association, Inc.)

and valvular dehiscence. This dehiscence may manifest as excessive rocking of the prosthesis. Flail leaflets occasionally may be seen in bioprosthetic valves.

Two-dimensional echocardiography and cardiac Doppler are powerful tools in the diagnosis and follow-up evaluation of patients with infective endocarditis. The complications of infectious endocarditis can be assessed in the majority of patients with minimal risk and discomfort.

REFERENCES

1. Roberts WC, Buchbinder NA: Healed left-sided infective endocarditis: A clinicopathological study of 59 patients. *Am J Cardiol* 40:867–888, 1977.
2. King ME, Weyman AE: Echocardiographic findings in infective endocarditis. In: Brest AN (ed): *Noninvasive Diagnostic Methods in Cardiology*. Philadelphia, FA Davis, 1983, vol 13, 147–165.
3. Wann LS, Dillon JC, Weyman AE, Feigenbaum H: Echocardiography in bacterial endocarditis. *N Engl J Med* 295:135–139, 1976.
4. Dillon JC, Feigenbaum H, Konecke LL, Davis RH, Chang S: Echocardiographic manifestations of valvular vegetations. *Am Heart J* 86:698–704, 1973.
5. Roy P, Tajik AJ, Giuliani ER, Schattenberg TT, Gau TT, Frye RL: Spectrum of echocardiographic findings in bacterial endocarditis. *Circulation* 53:474–482, 1976.
6. Markiewicz W, Peled B, Alroy G, Pollack S, Brook G, Rappaport J, Kerner H: Echocardiography in infective endocarditis. Lack of specificity in patients with valvular pathology. *Eur J Cardiol* 10:247–257, 1979.
7. Tak T, Rahimtoola SH, Kumar A, Gamage N, Chandraratna PAN: Value of digital image processing of two-dimensional echocardiograms in differentiating active from chronic vegetations in infective endocarditis. *Circulation* 78:116–123, 1988.
8. Stewart JA, Silimperi D, Harris P, Wise NK, Fraker TD, Kisslo JA: Echocardiographic documentation of vegetative lesions in infective endocarditis: Clinical implications. *Circulation* 61:374–380, 1980.
9. Martin RP, Meltzer RS, Chia BL, Stinson EB, Rakowski H, Popp RL: Clinical utility of two-dimensional echocardiography in infective endocarditis. *Am J Cardiol* 46:379–385, 1980.
10. Stafford A, Wann LS, Dillon JC, Weyman AE, Feigenbaum H: Serial echocardiographic appearance of healing bacterial vegetations. *Am J Cardiol* 44:754–760, 1979.
11. Davis RS, Strom JA, Frishman W, Becker R, Matsumoto M, LeJemtel TH, Sonnenblick EH, Frater RWM: The demonstration of vegetations by echocardiography in bacterial endocarditis. An indication for early surgical intervention. *Am J Med* 69:57–63, 1980.
12. Reid CL, Chandraratna PAN, Harrison EH, Kawanishi DT, Chandrasoma P, Nimalasuriya A, Rahimtoola SH: Mitral valve aneurysm: Clinical features, echocardiographic and pathologic correlations. *J Am Coll Cardiol* 2:460–464, 1983.
13. Boucher CA, Fallon JT, Myers GS, Hutler AM, Buckley MJ: the value and limitations of echocardiography in recording mitral valve vegetations. *Am Heart J* 94:37–43, 1977.
14. Berger M, Gallerstein PE, Benhuri P, Bhalla P, Goldberg E: Evaluation of aortic valve endocarditis by 2-dimensional echocardiography. *Chest* 80:61–67, 1981.
15. Meyer T, Sareli P, Pocock WA, Hadassah D, Epstein M, Barlow J: Echocardiographic and hemodynamic correlates of diastolic closure of mitral valve and diastolic opening of aortic valve in severe aortic regurgitation. *Am J Cardiol* 59:1144–1148, 1987.
16. Sareli P, Klein HO, Schamroth CL, Goldman AP, Antunes MJ, Pocock WA, Barlow JB: Contribution of echocardiography and immediate surgery to the management of severe aortic regurgitation from active infective endocarditis. *Am J Cardiol* 57:413–418, 1986.
17. Grayburn PA, Smith MD, Handshoe R, Friedman BJ, DeMaria AN: Detection of aortic insufficiency by standard echocardiography, pulsed Doppler echocardiography and auscultation. *Ann Intern Med* 104:599–605, 1986.
18. Mardelli TJ, Ogawa J, Hubbard FE, Dreifus LS, Meixell LL: Cross-sectional detection of aortic ring abscess in bacterial endocarditis. *Chest* 74:576–578, 1978.
19. Ellis SG, Goldstein J, Popp RH: Detection of endocarditis-associated perivalvular abscesses by two-dimensional echocardiography. *J Am Coll Cardiol* 5:647–653, 1985.
20. Incarvito J, Yang SS, Papa L, Fernandez J, Chang KS: Fungal endocarditis complicated by mycotic aneurysm of sinus Valsalva, interventricular septal abscess, and infectious pericarditis: Unique M-mode and two-dimensional echocardiographic findings. *Clin Cardiol* 4:34–38, 1981.
21. Weinstein L: Life-threatening complications of infective endocarditis and their management. *Arch Intern Med* 146:953–957, 1986.
22. Andy JJ, Sheikh MN, Ali N, Barnes BO, Fox LM, Curry CL, Roberts WC: Echocardiographic observations in opiate addicts with active infective endocarditis. *Am J. Cardiol* 40:17–23, 1977.
23. Come PC, Kurland GS, Vine HS: Two-dimensional echocardiography in differentiating right atrial and tricuspid valve mass lesions. *Am J Cardiol* 44:1207–1212, 1979.
24. Berger M, Delfin LA, Jelveh M, Goldberg E: Two-dimensional echocardiographic findings in right-sided infective endocarditis. *Circulation* 61:855–861, 1980.
25. Berger M, Wilkes HS, Gallerstein PE, Berdoff RL, Goldberg E: M-mode and two-dimensional echocardiographic findings in pulmonic valve endocarditis. *Am Heart J* 107:391–393, 1984.
26. Nagata S, Park YD, Nagae K, Beppu S, Kawazoe K, Tujita T, Sakakibara H, Nimura Y: Echocardiographic features of bioprosthetic valve endocarditis. *Br Heart J* 51:263–266, 1984.

21

Transesophageal Echocardiography

David J. Benefiel, M.D.
Michael F. Roizen, M.D.

Transesophageal echocardiography (TEE) is used at an ever-increasing number of medical centers in the United States. The subject of several reviews, it is used both inside and outside the operating room to diagnose acute and preexisting cardiac disease (1–6). In the intraoperative setting, regional myocardial ischemia is detected through the appearance of new segmental wall motion abnormalities (SWMA). Changes in preload, afterload, and contractility can be determined with accuracy. In addition, structural cardiac defects, both preexisting and acute, can be detected. The use of color flow, pulsed, and continuous wave Doppler enhances this capacity.

For monitoring during surgery, TEE overcomes the limitations of precordial M-mode and two-dimensional echocardiography (17–20). These limitations are incompatibility with surgical positioning, restrictions on placement of the transducer within the sterile field, the difficulty of maintaining precise orientation with tight skin contact, and frequent sound beam interference by lung tissue. This sound beam interference is exacerbated during controlled ventilation.

Transesophageal echocardiography can also offer advantages over precordial echocardiography in the nonsurgical setting to diagnose preexisting cardiac disease. Other uses include measurement of stroke volume, perfusion scanning of the myocardium, and intraoperative assessment of the repair of structural cardiac defects.

The transducer used is operationally identical to that used for precordial echocardiograms. However, it is miniaturized for insertion into the esophagus and usually is mounted at the tip of an endoscope (Fig. 21.1). The transducer is passed into the esophagus and thus is posterior to the heart and great vessels. The image obtained depends largely on the depth of insertion and rotation of the body of the endoscope. To a limited degree, it also depends on manipulation of the

tilt control of the endoscope. Once the desired image plane has been found, the controls can be locked and the image can be monitored continuously without constant attention to the transducer. There is no layer of air to obstruct the views, so image quality is good. Because the esophagus is close to the heart, higher frequency transducers with shorter range and better resolution can be utilized. The views are limited to those in a plane originating at the esophagus.

As the transducer is passed down the esophagus, imaging anteriorly toward the heart and great vessels yields views of the ascending aorta, aortic arch, and right and left pulmonary arteries. Then, as the transducer is advanced, imaging is blocked by the trachea until the carina is passed. Just below the carina, the ascending aorta, superior vena cava, and a portion of the pulmonary artery bifurcation can be seen (Fig. 21.2). The pulmonic valve and proximal coronary arteries often can also be seen. Rotating the probe from side to side will help to visualize the atrial appendages. Rotating the probe to the left approximately 90° should bring the descending aorta into view. The quality of this view depends on the location of the carina relative to these structures. As the transducer is passed inferior to the pulmonary artery, the left atrium becomes the structure closest to the esophagus. Now the aortic valve and right ventricular outflow tract can be visualized (Fig. 21.3). Further distally, a four-chamber view through the left atrium is obtained (Fig. 21.4). The atrioventricular valves, left ventricular outflow tract, atrial septum with the thin fossa ovalis, coronary sinus, atria, and ventricles can be visualized. This is an excellent view for Doppler assessment of the atrioventricular valves and the aortic valve. The axis of the transducer sound beam is almost parallel to the flow through the mitral valve, making quantitative Doppler evaluation possible. Below the atrioventricular groove, short-axis views of

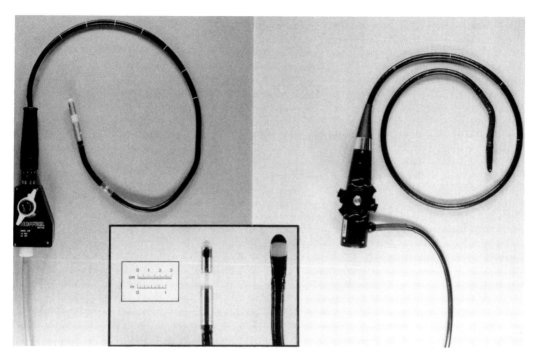

Figure 21.1. *Left:* A mechanical, 7.5 MHz probe (Hoffrel Instruments, Inc., S. Norwalk, CT). *Right:* A phased array, 3.5 MHz probe (Diasonics, Inc., Milpitas, CA).

the left ventricle are obtained (Figs. 21.5 and 21.6). Near this point the probe will enter the stomach. Care should be exercised if resistance to passage is felt. As the transducer is passed distally, the

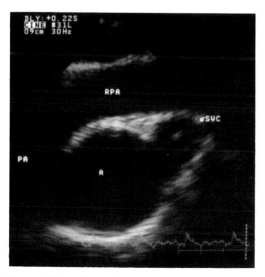

Figure 21.2. View of the aorta (*A*), pulmonary artery (*PA*) continuing into the right pulmonary artery (*RPA*), and superior vena cava (*SVC*) containing a pulmonary artery catheter.

base of the heart and mitral valve are seen first. The papillary muscles are seen next, and finally an apical short-axis view is obtained. Actually, the entire aorta from valve to the diaphragm can be visualized with TEE, except for a short segment above the aortic valve that is blocked by the tracheobronchial tree. The complete examination of the aorta should start at the aortic valve (Fig. 21.3). The probe is then withdrawn, and a short segment of the ascending aorta is seen (Fig. 21.2). Further withdrawing the probe temporarily obliterates the image because of the interposition of the tracheobronchial tree. Further withdrawing brings the ascending aorta into view. Then the probe is withdrawn, is rotated to the left, and is then advanced as the arch and descending aorta are visualized. These echocardiographic cross-sections have been verified through direct anatomic comparisons (21, 22). Although there is a potential for injury to the esophagus, no complications from use of two-dimensional TEE have occurred at our institutions in approximately 2000 uses.

ISCHEMIC HEART DISEASE

Acute myocardial ischemia produces a rapid decrease in myocardial performance that precedes the appearance of electrocardiographic

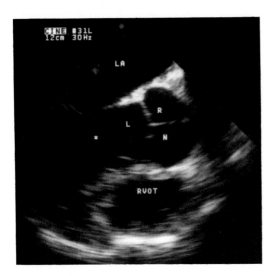

Figure 21.3. View of the aortic valve showing the left (*L*), right (*R*), and noncoronary (*N*) cusps, right ventricular outflow tract (*RVOT*), and the left atrium (*LA*). A small portion of the left ventricular outflow tract is shown (∗).

changes. Consequently, echocardiography is an excellent intraoperative technique to detect myocardial ischemia. During graded regional myocardial ischemia, the ischemic region rapidly develops SWMA that progress from dyssychronism to hypokinesia, akinesia, and ultimately dyski-

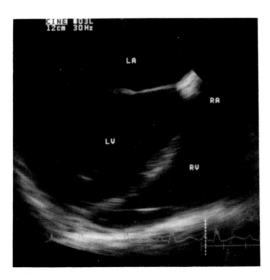

Figure 21.4. Tangential four-chamber view obtained at the level of the left atrium showing the left atrium (*LA*), right atrium (*RA*), left ventricle (*LV*), and right ventricle (*RV*).

nesia (23). Measurements from echocardiograms closely correspond with other accepted techniques, such as direct measurement (21) or measurement by sonomicrometers (24, 25).

Changes in wall thickness occurring during systole are a measure of contractility. In experiments on dogs, the echocardiogram has proved to be a precise indicator of contractility measured by systolic wall thickness (26). Precordial echocardiography has already been shown to measure cardiac function and SWMA reliably and reproducibly (27–30). Our investigators by interobserver comparison found that wall motion abnormalities can be detected reliably by TEE (31). Echocardiography also correlates well with angiography in the analysis of wall motion (32). The appearance of new intraoperative SWMA that persist throughout surgery predict postoperative myocardial infarction (MI).

Cahalan et al. (33) showed that SWMA could be detected reliably during surgery in 43 high-risk surgical patients. Seven had unresolved SWMA, and five of the seven had an MI. No patient without persistent SWMA suffered a MI. In patients with MI the area of persistent SWMA detected by TEE during surgery corresponded to the area of infarction indicated on the postoperative ECG. The two patients who had had persistent SWMA but no MI may have had prolonged postischemic myocardial dysfunction (34).

Smith et al. (35) compared intraoperative TEE with ECG for the detection of intraoperative myocardial ischemia. In 50 high-risk patients undergoing aortic or coronary surgery, 24 had intraoperative SWMA. Only six had S-T segment changes. All patients with S-T segment changes also had new SWMA. In three instances SWMA occurred before the S-T segment change, and in three instances they occurred simultaneously. All three patients with intraoperative MI also had persistent intraoperative SWMA. However, only one patient had S-T segment changes. In a control group of 10 healthy patients undergoing noncardiovascular surgery, no patient experienced SWMA, S-T segment changes, or MI. This demonstrated the superiority of two-dimensional TEE over electrocardiography for the intraoperative detection of myocardial ischemia. Furthermore, this confirmed the finding of Cahalan et al. that when new SWMA persist, MI is likely to have occurred. Shively et al. (36) also showed that the appearance of new SWMA during surgery that persist until skin closure are predictive of MI.

Immediate improvement of myocardial dys-

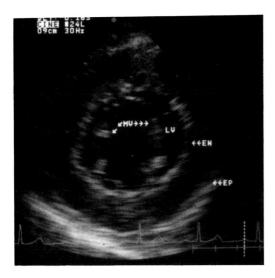

Figure 21.5. Short-axis view of the left ventricle at the level of the mitral valve shows mitral valve (*MV*) as a bright ring within the left ventricular cavity (*LV*) and the endocardium (*EN*) and epicardium (*EP*) as bright circular images separated by darker myocardium.

function following coronary revascularization can be demonstrated using two-dimensional TEE. Topol et al. (37) were able to demonstrate this improvement in patients undergoing coronary revascularization using intraoperative TEE. Transesophageal echocardiograms were recorded before and after coronary bypass surgery. By using

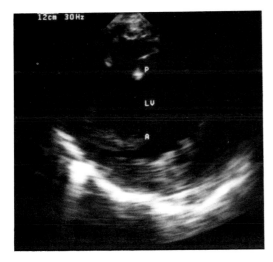

Figure 21.6. Short-axis view of left ventricle closer to the apex shows posteromedial papillary muscle (*P*), anterolateral papillary muscle (*A*), and left ventriclular cavity (*LV*).

a computer-aided contouring system, segmental systolic wall thickening was determined in 152 segments for each patient. Segments that demonstrated the most severe dysfunction prior to bypass were most likely to show sustained improvement following revascularization.

Roizen et al. (38) studied patients undergoing aortic reconstruction who experienced various levels of aortic occlusion (clamping) during surgery. In patients undergoing supraceliac clamping, 92% had either global hypokinesis or SWMA, 44% had SWMA, and 8% suffered MI. In patients with suprarenal clamping, 33% had abnormal wall motion, 17% had SWMA, and none suffered MI. In the infrarenal group, none had wall motion abnormalities or MI.

Two-dimensional echocardiography has been used reliably to diagnose acute MI and to predict complications in the post-MI period (39–42). Intraoperative persistent SWMA detected by TEE indicate a high likelihood of MI and identify patients at high risk for postoperative complications. This allows better prospective postoperative care.

The difference in acoustic properties of normal myocardium, ischemic myocardium, and infarcted myocardium can be detected. This provides a more promising method than qualitative SWMA analysis for differentiating these regions. Computer-assisted analysis of echo character may simplify and increase the reliability of the detection of myocardial ischemia (43). Ultimately, automated detection systems could reduce the amount of observer attention required to detect ischemia, making the more widespread use of TEE possible.

CARDIAC FUNCTION

The use of two-dimensional echocardiography in assessing cardiac performance is well established (44, 45). Transesophageal echocardiography's value in assessing cardiac performance has been demonstrated both intraoperatively (46–50) and in the nonsurgical setting (51–55).

Cardiac volumes and ejection fraction measured by echocardigraphy correlate well with values determined angiographically (56, 57) and in vitro (58). Beaupre et al. (59) studied the relationship between pulmonary artery occlusion pressure (PAOP) and left ventricular end-diastolic area determined by TEE. They found TEE to be a better measurement technique for preload than PAOP.

Stroke volume has been estimated with some

success by M-mode TEE (60). Cronnelly et al. used two-dimensional TEE to assess the effects of anesthetics (61) and volume loading (62) on hemodynamic variables during renal transplantation surgery.

Sudden changes in systemic vascular resistance are readily detectable by TEE. For example, in a patient being monitored with TEE who had an anaphylactic reaction to cefazolin sodium, Beaupre et al. (63) observed decreased left ventricular preload and afterload. Roizen et al. (64) also employed TEE in the anesthetic management of patients undergoing surgical resection of pheochromocytoma that was accompanied by sudden dramatic changes in systemic vascular resistance and contractility.

Serial visualization of the short-axis view of the left ventricle during surgery gives the anesthesiologist and surgeon an appreciation for changes in preload, afterload, and ventricular function which may be altered by the anesthetic, surgical manipulation, changes in rhythm, etc. (65–80).

STRUCTURAL DEFECTS

Precordial echocardiography is well established as a principal method of assessing structural cardiac defects. In some cases, it even supplants angiography (81).

Transesophageal echocardiography has become an important means of detecting cardiac and paracardiac lesions and space-occupying processes (82–95). It is especially useful in diagnosing atrial abnormalities (96–107). Also, TEE has been used to diagnose and aid in the interoperative removal of an intercardiac tumor (108).

Using a transesophageal echocardiographic probe with an integral Doppler transducer, Schlüter et al. (109) were able to determine flow across the mitral valve in patients with mitral valve insufficiency. Other investigators used Doppler TEE to assess the mitral valve (110–116), and congenital structural cardiac defects in children (117). Valvular function also can be assessed using microbubbles as a contrast medium (118).

Because of the close proximity of the aorta to the esophagus, dissection of the aorta is well visualized with TEE (119–128). Using color flow Doppler, true and false lumens and their relative contributions to blood flow can be determined.

In endocarditis, visualization of vegetations can be augmented with TEE, because of the close proximity of the atria to the esophagus. When a prosthetic mitral valve is present, TEE is the only method to adequately visualize the atrial side of the prosthesis to assess function (with Doppler) and look for vegetations (129–131).

Gas bubbles in suspension also can be used as contrast material to detect intracardiac right-to-left shunts. This technique has been used intraoperatively with TEE to detect ostium secundum atrial septal defects during surgery (132). Transesophageal echocardiography and contrast material have been used to identify patent foramen ovale during sitting posterior fossa craniotomy (133). Pediatric Doppler transesophageal echo probes recently have become available (117).

Gas bubbles can be used not only as contrast material within vascular channels but also for perfusion scanning. Intraaortic injection of hydrogen peroxide was used by Kemper et al. (134) as a contrast material in dogs. The bubbles entered the perfused myocardium, became lodged, and were visualized by echocardiography. Sonicated renografin has been used in humans to perfusion scan the myocardium (135).

UNWANTED INTRAVASCULAR AIR

Since gas in the circulation is visualized easily with echocardiography, TEE is useful for the detection of air embolism during surgery. Heretofore, the precordial Doppler transducer was used to detect air embolism. However, TEE was found to be at least as sensitive and probably more sensitive (136–142).

Air entering the systemic circulation after cardiopulmonary bypass can be detected by TEE, which can provide guidance in eliminating this potential source of organ damage (143–145). Two-dimensional echocardiography has also been used to detect postbypass-retained cardiac air (146). However, this technique is inferior to TEE, as surgery must be interrupted in order to monitor for air.

FUTURE USES
In the Operating Room

Transesophageal echocardiography has been established as an important experimental and clinical tool. What remains to be determined is how widespread its use will be in the near future. It may complement or supplant pulmonary artery catherization. If it does, under what circumstances will it compete with catheterization?

Cardiac size, contractility, and regional wall motion are more useful than filling pressures obtained from a pulmonary artery catheter. However, the pulmonary catheter provides a means of measuring cardiac output that is not obtainable from TEE at present. In addition, a pulmonary artery catheter provides a pulmonary venous pressure. Through its use we can prevent pulmonary venous congestion and pulmonary edema.

The issue of cost-effectiveness has not been resolved. At present the echocardiograph and probe cost about the same as a standard precordial system. In our experience, probes can be used approximately 100 times without repair. As use of the equipment increases, the cost may decrease. We believe that TEE eventually can be comparable in cost to monitoring techniques that are widely used at present.

As with any monitoring technique, the usefulness of TEE depends on the skill of the operator. When echocardiographic technique is more thoroughly integrated into the undergraduate medical curriculum, its use in the operating room naturally will expand.

Outside the Operating Room

Because of the availability of high resolution endoscopic transducers, TEE is an important advancement for precordial echocardiography. Its role in the assessment of the mitral valve prosthesis is undisputed. In the intensive care unit setting when patients are mechanically ventilated, TEE may be the only way to obtain echocardiograms.

Future uses will center around the need for high resolution imaging of structures adjacent to the esophagus, including the heart, lungs, aorta, and other great vessels. Since cardiologists are already familiar with the technique of echocardiography, they need only master the different tomographic planes and the use of the endoscope. The lack of complications with this procedure will help to foster its wide use. Now that pediatric probes (Aloka, Hoffrel) and biplane transducers (Aloka) are available, indications for use will extend more widely.

REFERENCES

1. Benefiel DJ, Roizen MF, Schiller NB: Monitoring with transesophageal echocardiography: A review. *Appl Cardiol* 14:9–14, 1986.
2. Kaplan JA: Transesophageal echocardiography. *Mt Sinai J Med (NY)* 51:592–594, 1984.
3. Schlüter M, Thier W, Hinrichs A, Kremers P, Siglow V, Hanrath P: Clinical use of transesophageal echocardiography. *Dtsch Med Wochenschr* 109 (18):722–727, 1984.
4. Hanrath P, Kremer P, Langenstein BA, Matsu-moto M, Bleifeld W: Transesophageal echocardiography: A new method for dynamic ventricle function analysis. *Dtsch Med Wochenschr* 106:523–525, 1981.
5. Goldman ME, Mindich BP, Nanda NC: Intraoperative echocardiography: Who monitors the flood gates are opened? *J Am Coll Cardiol* 11(6):1362–1364, 1988.
6. Frazin L, Talano JV, Stephanides L, Loeb HS, Kopel L, Gunnar RM: Esophageal echocardiography. *Circulation* 54:102–108, 1976.
7. Seward JB, Khandheria BK, Oh JK, Abel MD, Hughes RW Jr, Edwards WD, Nichols BA, Freeman WK, Tajik AJ: Transesophageal echocardiography: Technique, anatomic correlations, implementation, and clinical applications. *Mayo Clin Proc* 63(7):649–680, 1988.
8. Yock PG, Linker DT, Thapliyal HV, Arenson JW, Samstad S, Saether O, Angelsen BAJ: Real-time two-dimensional catheter ultrasound: A new technique for high-resolution intravascular imaging (Abstr). *J Am Coll Cardiol* 11(Suppl A):130A, 1988.
9. Hisanaga K, Hisanaga A, Nagata K, Yoshida S: A new transesophageal real-time two-dimensional echocardiographic system using a flexible tube and its clinical application. *Proc Jap Soc Ultrason Med* 32:43–44, 1977.
10. Hisanaga K, Hisanaga A, Nagata K, Ichie Y: Transesophageal cross-sectional echocardiography. *Am Heart J* 100:605–609, 1980.
11. Bertini A, Masotti L, Zuppiroli A, Cecchi F: Rotating probe for trans-oesophageal cross-sectional echocardiography. *J Nucl Med Allied Sci* 28:115–121, 1984.
12. DiMagno EP, Buxton JL, Regan PT, Hattery RR, Wilson DA, Suarez JR, Green PS: Ultrasonic endoscope. *Lancet* 1:629–631, 1980.
13. Souquet J, Hanrath P, Zitelli L, Kremer P, Langenstein BA, Schlüter M: Transesophageal phased array for imaging the heart. *IEEE Trans Biomed Eng* 29:707–712, 1982.
14. Schlüter M, Langenstein BA, Polster J, Kremer P, Souquet J, Engel S, Hanrath P: Transoesophageal cross-sectional echocardiography with a phased array transducer system: Technique and initial clinical results. *Br Heart J* 48:67–72, 1982.
15. Schlüter M, Hinrichs A, Thier W, Kremer P, Schröder S, Cahalan MK, Hanrath P: Transesophageal two-dimensional echocardiography: Comparison of ultrasonic and anatomic sections. *Am J Cardiol* 53:1173–1178, 1984.
16. Seward JB, Tajik AJ, DiMagno EP: Esophageal phased-array sector echocardiography: An anatomic study. In Hanrath P, Bleifeld W, Souquet J (eds): *Cardiovascular Diagnosis by Ultrasound: Transesophageal, Computerized, Contrast Doppler Echocardiography.* The Hague, Martinus Nijhoff, 1982, pp 270–279.
17. Shine KI, Perloff JK, Child JS, Marshall RC, Schelbert H: Noninvasive assessment of myocardial function. *Ann Intern Med* 92:78–90, 1980.
18. Popp RL, Rubenson DS, Tucker CR, French JW: Echocardiography: M-mode and two-dimensional methods. *Ann Intern Med* 93:844–856, 1980.

19. Reeder GS, Seward JB, Tajik AJ: The role of two-dimensional echocardiography in coronary artery disease: A critical appraisal. *Mayo Clin Proc* 57:247–258, 1982.

20. Henry WL: Evaluation of ventricular function using two dimensional echocardiography. *Am J Cardiol* 49:1319–1323, 1982.

21. Schlüter M, Hinrichs A, Thier W, Kremer P, Schröder S, Cahalan MK, Hanrath P: Transesophageal two-dimensional echocardiography: Comparison of ultrasonic and anatomic sections. *Am J Cardiol* 53:1173–1178, 1984.

22. Hinrichs A, Schlüter M, Kremer P, Becker K, Schröder S, Kloppel G, Hanrath P: Two-dimensional transesophageal echocardiography: Comparison of echocardiographic and anatomic section pictures. *Ultraschall Med* 4:243–247, 1983.

23. Forrester JS, Wyatt HL, de la Luz PL, Tyberg JV, Diamond GA, Swan HJC: Functional significance of regional ischemic contraction abnormalities. *Circulation* 54:64–70, 1976.

24. Pandian NG, Kerber RE: Two-dimensional echocardiography in experimental coronary stenosis: Sensitivity and specificity in detecting transient myocardial dyskinesis. Comparison with sonomicrometers. *Circulation* 66:597–602, 1982.

25. Pandian NG, Kieso RA, Kerber RE: Two-dimensional echocardiography in experimental coronary stenosis: Relationship between systolic wall thinning and regional myocardial perfusion in severe coronary stenosis. *Circulation* 66:603–611, 1982.

26. O'Boyle JE, Parisi AF, Nieminen M, Kloner RA, Khuri S: Quantitative detection of regional left ventricular contraction abnormalities by 2-dimensional echocardiography: Comparison of myocardial thickening and thinning and endocardial motion in a canine model. *Am J Cardiol* 51:1732–1738, 1983.

27. Heng MK, Wyatt HL, Meerbaum S, Hestenes J, Davidson R, Corday E, Woythaler J: An analysis of the reproducibility of 2-dimensional echocardiographic measurements (Abstr). *Am J Cardiol* 41:390, 1978.

28. Sahn DJ, DeMaria A, Kisslo JA, Weyman A: Interobserver variability in the quantitative evaluation of M-mode echocardiograms: Survey and recommendations (Abstr). *Am J Cardiol* 41:390, 1978.

29. Moynihan PF, Parisi AF, Feldman CL: Quantitative detection of regional left ventricular contraction abnormalities by two-dimensional echocardiography: Analysis of methods. *Circulation* 63:752–760, 1981.

30. Parisi AF, Moynihan PF, Folland ED, Feldman CL: Quantitative detection of regional left ventricular contraction abnormalities by two-dimensional echocardiography: Accuracy in coronary artery disease. *Circulation* 63:761–767, 1981.

31. Benefiel DJ, Byrd B, Lurz FW, Kremer P, Cahalan MK, Roizen MF, Beaupre PN, Smith J, Schiller N: Interobserver reliability in the interpretation of two-dimensional transesophageal echocardiograms. Society of Cardiovascular Anesth Annual Meeting, 1984.

32. Kisslo JA, Robertson D, Gilbert BW, von Ramm O, Behar VS: A comparison of real-time, two-dimensional echocardiography and cineangiography in detecting left ventricular asynergy. *Circulation* 55:134–141, 1977.

33. Cahalan MK, Kremer PF, Beaupre PN, Lurz FW, Roizen MF, Robinson S, Cohen NH, Hamilton WK, Schiller NB: Intraoperative myocardial ischemia detected by transesophageal two-dimensional echocardiography (Abstr). *Anesthesiology* 59:A164, 1983.

34. Braunwald E, Kloner RA: The stunned myocardium: Prolonged postischemic ventricular dysfunction. *Circulation* 66:1146–1149, 1982.

35. Smith JS, Cahalan MK, Benefiel DJ, Byrd BF, Lurz FW, Shapiro WA, Roizen MF, Bouchard A, Schiller NB: Intraoperative detection of myocardial ischemia in high-risk patients: Electrocardiography versus two-dimensional transesophageal echocardiography. *Circulation* 72:1015–1021, 1985.

36. Shively B, Watters T, Benefiel D, Cahalan MK, Botvinick EH, Schiller NB: The intraoperative detection of myocardial infarction by transesophageal echocardiography. *J Am Coll Cardiol* 7:2A, 1986.

37. Topol EJ, Weiss JL, Guzman PA, Dorsey-Lima S, Blanck TJ, Humphrey LS, Baumgartner WA, Flaherty JT, Reitz BA: Immediate improvement of dysfunction myocardial segments after coronary revascularization: Detection by intraoperative transesophageal echocardiography. *J Am Coll Cardiol* 4:1123–1134, 1984.

38. Roizen MF, Beaupre PN, Alpert RA, Kremer P, Cahalan MK, Schiller N, Cronnelly R, Lurz FW, Ehrenfeld WK, Stoney RJ: Monitoring with two-dimensional transesophageal echocardiography: Comparison of myocardial function in patients undergoing supraceliac, suprarenal, suprarenal-infraceliac, or infrarenal aortic occlusion. *J Vasc Surg* 1:300–305, 1984.

39. Horowitz RS, Morganroth J: Immediate detection of early high-risk patients with acute myocardial infarction using two-dimensional echocardiographic evaluation of left ventricular regional wall motion abnormalities. *Am Heart J* 103:814–822, 1982.

40. Gibson RS, Bishop HL, Stamm RB, Crampton RS, Beller GA, Martin RP: Value of early two-dimensional echocardiography in patients with acute myocardial infarction. *Am J Cardiol* 49:1110–1119, 1982.

41. Horowitz RS, Morganroth J, Parrotto C, Chen CC, Soffer J, Pauletto FJ: Immediate diagnosis of acute myocardial infarction by two-dimensional echocardiography. *Circulation* 65:323–329, 1982.

42. Eaton LW, Weiss JL, Bulkley BH, Garrison JB, Weisfeldt ML: Regional cardiac dilatation after acute myocardial infarction: recognition by two-dimensional echocardiography. *N Engl J Med* 300:57–62, 1979.

43. Skorton DJ, Collins SM, Nichols J, Pandian NG, Bean JA, Kerber RE: Quantitative texture analysis in two-dimensional echocardiography: Application to the diagnosis of experimental myocardial contusion. *Circulation* 68:217–223, 1983.

44. Quinones MA, Gaasch WH, Alexander JK: In-

fluence of acute changes in preload, afterload, contractile state and heart rate on ejection and isovolumic indices of myocardial contractility in man. *Circulation* 53:293–302, 1976.

45. Ruschhaupt DG, Sodt PC, Hutcheon NA, Arcilla RA: Estimation of circumferential fiber shortening velocity by echocardiography. *J Am Coll Cardiol* 2:17–84, 1983.

46. Beaupre PN, Cahalan MK, Kremer PF, Lurz FW, Schiller NB, Hamilton WK: Isoflurane, halothane, and enflurane depress myocardial contractility in patients undergoing surgery (Abstr). *Anesthesiology* 59:A59, 1983.

47. Roizen MF, Alpert RA, Beaupre PN, Kremer P, Cahalan MK, Schiller N, Stoney RH, Connelly R, Ehrenfeld WJ, Lurz F: Transesophageal echocardiography: Cardiovascular function after various levels of aortic occlusion (Abstr). *Anesthesiology* 59:A163, 1983.

48. Matsumoto M, Yasu O, Strom J, Frishman W, Kadish A, Becker RM, Frater RW, Sonnenblick EH: Application of transesophageal echocardiography to continuous intraoperative monitoring of left ventricular performance. *Am J Cardiol* 46:95–105, 1980.

49. Smith JS, Benefiel DJ, Beaupre PN, Sohn YJ, Lurz FW, Byrd BJ, Bouchard A, Schiller NB, Cahalan MK: Effect of phenylephrine on myocardial performance during carotid endarterectomy. *Anesthesiology* 61:A56, 1984.

50. Smith JS, Cahalan MK, Benefiel DJ, Lurz FW, Lampe GH, Byrd BJ, Schiller NB, Yee ES, Turley K, Ullyot DJ, Hamilton WK: Fentanyl versus fentanyl and isoflurane in patients with impaired left ventricular function. *Anesthesiology* 63:A318, 1985.

51. Terai C, Uenishi M, Sugimoto H, Shimazu T, Yoshioka T, Sugimoto T: Transesophageal echocardiographic dimensional analysis of four cardiac chambers during positive end-expiratory pressure. *Anesthesiology* 63:640–646, 1985.

52. Uenishi M, Sugimoto H, Sawada Y, Terai C, Yoshioka T, Sugimoto T: Transesophageal echocardiography during external chest compression in humans (Letter). *Anesthesiology* 60:618, 1984.

53. Matsumoto M, Hanrath P, Kremer P, Bleifeld W: Transesophageal echocardiographic evaluation of left ventricular function at and during dynamic exercise in aortic insufficiency. *J Cardiogr* 11:1147–1157, 1981.

54. Matsumoto M, Hanrath P, Kremer P, Tams C, Langenstein BA, Schlüter M, Weiter R, Bleifeld W: Evaluation of left ventricular performance during supine exercise by transesophageal M-mode echocardiography in normal subjects. *Br Heart J* 48:61–66, 1982.

55. Clements FM, de Bruijn NP, Kisslo JA: Transesophageal echocardiographic observations in a patient undergoing closed-chest massage. *Anesthesiology* 64:826–828, 1986.

56. Folland ED, Parisi AF, Moynihan PF, Jones DR, Feldman CL, Tow DE: Assessment of left ventricular ejection fraction and volumes by real-time, two-dimensional echocardiography: A comparison of cineangiographic and radionuclide techniques. *Circulation* 60:760–766, 1979.

57. Schiller NB, Acquatella H, Ports TA, Drew D,

58. Goerke J, Ringertz H, Silverman NH, Brundage B, Botvinick EH, Boswell R, Carlsson E, Parmley WW: Left ventricular volume from paired biplane two-dimensional echocardiography. *Circulation* 60:547–555, 1979.

58. Helak JW, Reichek N: Quantitation of human left ventricular mass and volume by two-dimensional echocardiography: In vitro anatomic validation. *Circulation* 63:1398–1407, 1981.

59. Beaupre PN, Cahalan MK, Kremer PF, Roizen MF, Cronnelly R, Robinson S, Lurz FW, Alpert R, Hamilton WK, Schiller NB: Does pulmonary artery occlusion pressure adequately reflect left ventricular filling during anesthesia and surgery (Abstr)? *Anesthesiology* 59:A3, 1983.

60. Oka Y, Moriwaki K, Hong Y, Frater RWM: Left ventricular stroke volume and systolic time interval determined by transesophageal aortic valve echogram (Abstr). *Anesthesiology* 59:A162, 1983.

61. Cronnelly R, Kremer PF, Beaupre PN, Cahalan MK, Salvatierra O, Feduska NJ: Hemodynamic response to anesthesia in patients with end-stage renal disease (Abstr). *Anesthesiology* 59:A47, 1983.

62. Cronnelly R, Kremer PF, Beaupre PN, Cahalan MK, Salvatierra O, Feduska NJ: Hemodynamic response to fluid challenge in anesthetized patients with end-stage renal disease (Abstr). *Anesthesiology* 59:A49, 1983.

63. Beaupre PN, Roizen MF, Cahalan MK, Alpert RA, Cassorla L, Schiller NB: Hemodynamic and two-dimensional transesophageal echocardiographic analysis of an anaphylactic reaction in a human. *Anesthesiology* 60:482–484, 1984.

64. Roizen MF, Hunt TK, Beaupre PN, Kremer P, Frimin R, Chang CN, Alpert RA, Thomas CJ, Tyrrell JB, Cahalan MK: The effect of alpha-adrenergic blockade on cardiac performance and tissue oxygen delivery during excision of pheochromocytoma. *Surgery* 94:941–945, 1983.

65. Cahalan MK, Lurz FC, Schiller NB: Transoesophageal two-dimensional echocardiographic evaluation of anesthetic effects on left ventricular function. *Br J Anaesth* 60(8 Suppl 1):99S–106S, 1988.

66. Abel MD, Nishimura RA, Callahan MJ, Rehder K, Ilstrup DM, Tajik AJ: Evaluation of intraoperative transesophageal two-dimensional echocardiography. *Anesthesiology* 66:64–68, 1987.

67. Gewertz BL, Kremser PC, Zarins CK, Smith JS, Ellis JE, Feinstein SB, Roizen MF: Transesophageal echocardiographic monitoring of myocardial ischemia during vascular surgery. *J Vasc Surg* 5:607–613, 1987.

68. Beaupre PN, Kremer PF, Cahalan MK, Lurz FW, Schiller NB, Hamilton WK: Intraoperative detection of changes in left ventricular segmental wall motion by transesophageal two-dimensional echocardiography. *Am Heart J* 107:1021–1023, 1984.

69. Schiller NB: Evaluation of cardiac function during surgery by transesophageal 2-dimensional echocardiography. In Hanrath P, Bleifeld W, Souquet J (eds): *Cardiovascular Diagnosis by Ultrasound: Transesophageal, Computerized, Contrast, Doppler Echocardiography*. The Hague, Martinus Nijhoff, 1982, pp 289–293.

70. Konstadt SN, Thys D, Mindich BP, Kaplan JA,

Goldman M: Validation of quantitative intra-operative transesophageal echocardiography. *Anesthesiology* 65:418–421, 1986.

71. Kremer P, Cahalan M, Beaupre P, Schröder E, Hanrath P, Heinrich H, Ahnefeld FW, Bleifeld W, Hamilton W: Intraoperative monitoring by two-dimensional echocardiography. *Anaesthesist* 34:111–117, 1985.

72. Kyo S, Takamoto S, Matsumura M, Asano H, Yokote Y, Motoyama T, Omoto R: Immediate and early postoperative evaluation of results of cardiac surgery by transesophageal two-dimensional Doppler echocardiography. *Circulation* 76(Suppl 5):V113–V121, 1987.

73. De Bruijn NP, Clements FM: *Transesophageal Echocardiography*. The Hague, Martinus Nijhoff, 1987.

74. Cahalan MK, Litt L, Botvinick EH, Schiller NB: Advances in noninvasive cardiovascular imaging: Implications for the anesthesiologist. *Anesthesiology* 66:356–372, 1987.

75. Yao FS: Intraoperative transesophageal two-dimensional echocardiography during cardiac anesthesia. *Ma Tsui Hsueh Tsa Chi* 24:156–159, 1986.

76. Koolen JJ, Visser CA, Wever E, Van Wezel H, Meyne NG, Dunning AJ: Transesophageal two-dimensional echocardiographic evaluation of bi-ventricular dimension and function during positive end-expiratory pressure ventilation after coronary artery bypass grafting. *Am J Cardiol* 59:1047–1051, 1987.

77. Kremer P, Schwartz L, Cahalan MK, Gutman J, Schiller NB: Intraoperative monitoring of left ventricular performance by transesophageal M-mode and 2-D echocardiography (Abstr). *Am J Cardiol* 49:956, 1982.

78. Clements FM, de Bruijn NP: Perioperative evaluation of regional wall motion by transesophageal two-dimensional echocardiography. *Anesth Analg* 66:249–261, 1987.

79. Matsumoto M, Oka Y, Strom J, Frishman W, Kadish A, Becker RM, Frater RWM, Sonnenblick EH: Application of transesophageal echocardiography to continuous intraoperative monitoring of left ventricular performance. *Am J Cardiol* 46:95–105, 1980.

80. Matsuzaki M, Matsuda Y, Ikee Y, Takahashi Y, Sasaki T, Toma Y, Ishida K, Yorozu T, Kumada T, Kusukawa R: Esophageal echocardiographic left ventricular anteriolateral wall motion in normal subjects and patients with coronary artery disease. *Circulation* 63:1085–1092, 1981.

81. Weyman AE, *Cross-Sectional Echocardiography*. Philadelphia, Lea & Febiger, 1982, 137–491.

82. Nellessen U, Daniel WG, Lichtlen PR: Importance of transesophageal echocardiography in the diagnosis of cardiac and paracardiac space-occupying processes. *Z Kardiol* 75:91–98, 1986.

83. Aschenberg W, Schlüter M, Kremer P, Schroder E, Siglow V, Bleifeld W: Transesophageal two-dimensional echocardiography for the detection of left atrial appendage thrombus. *J Am Coll Cardiol* 7:163–166, 1986.

84. Stern H, Erbel R, Borner N, Schreiner G, Meyer J: Spontaneous echocontrast, recorded by trans-esophageal echocardiography in type III aortic dissection. *Z Kardiol* 74:480–481, 1985.

85. Schreiner G, Erbel R, Mohr-Kahaly S, Kramer G, Henkel B, Meyer J: Detection of aneurysms of the atrial septum using transesophageal echocardiography. *Z Kardiol* 74:440–444, 1985.

86. Nellessen U, Daniel WG, Matheis G, Oelert H, Depping K, Lichtlen PR: Impending paradoxical embolism from atrial thrombus: Correct diagnosis by transesophageal echocardiography and prevention by surgery. *J Am Coll Cardiol* 5:1002–1004, 1985.

87. Borner N, Erbel R, Braun B, Henkel B, Meyer J, Rumpelt J: Diagnosis of aortic dissection by transesophageal echocardiography. *Am J Cardiol* 54:1157–1158, 1984.

88. Isaji F: Diagnosis of atrial septal defect (secundum type) with transesophageal echocardiography: Special reference to size and type of ASD. *Nippon Kyobu Geka Gakkai Zasshi* 32:37–49, 1984.

89. Thier W, Schlüter M, Kremer P, Hausdorf G, Krebber HJ, Schröder S, Hanrath P: Two-dimensional transesophageal echocardiography: A better presentation of intra-atrial structures. *Dtsch Med Wochenschr* 108:1903–1907, 1983.

90. Schlüter M, Langenstein BA, Thier W, Schmiegel WH, Krebber HJ, Kalmar P, Hanrath P: Transesophageal two-dimensional echocardiography in the diagnosis of cortriatriatum in the adult. *J Am Coll Cardiol* 2:1011–1015, 1983.

91. Kajita M, Nishiyama M, Tengan I, Shimarmura Y, Kei J, Kitaya T, Nishiwaki Y, Yano H, Kakinuma R, Matsuyama T: Transesophageal echocardiography for the diagnosis of lung cancer with left atrial involvement. *Kyobu Geka* 36:122–126, 1983.

92. Engberding R, Schulze-Waltrup N, Grosse-Heitmeyer W, Stoll V: Transthoracic and transesophageal 2-D echocardiography in the diagnosis of peri- and paracardial tumors. *Dtsch Med Wochenschr* 112:49–52, 1987.

93. Hofmann T, Behroz A, Köster W, Kasper W: Detection of intracardiac masses by two dimensional transesophageal echocardiography (Abstr). *Circulation* 76(Suppl 4):IV37, 1987.

94. Daniel WG, Schröder E, Nellessen U, Hausmann D: Diagnosis of intra- and extracardiac masses by echocardiography—comparison between the transthoracic and transesophageal approach (Abstr). *Circulation* 76(Suppl 4):IV38, 1987.

95. Thier W, Schlüter M, Krebber H-J, Polonius M-J, Klöppel G, Becker K, Hanrath P: Cysts in left atrial myxomas identified by transesophageal cross-sectional echocardiography. *Am J Cardiol* 51:1793–1795, 1983.

96. Gussenhoven EJ, Taams MA, Roelandt JC, Ligtvoet KM, McGhie J, van Herwerden LA, Cahalan MK: Transesophageal two-dimensional echocardiography: Its role in solving clinical problems. *J Am Coll Cardiol* 8:975–979, 1986.

97. Thier W, Schlüter M, Kremer P, Hausdorf G, Krebber HJ, Schröder S, Hanrath P: Transoesophageal 2-dimensional echocardiography: Better demonstration of intra-atrial structures. *Dtsch Med Wochenschr* 108:1903–1907, 1983.

98. Toma Y, Matsuda Y, Matsuzaki M, Anno Y, Uchida T, Hiroyama N, Tamitani M, Murata T, Yonezawa F, Moritani K, Katayama K, Ogawa H, Kusukawa R: Determination of atrial size by esophageal echocardiography. *Am J Cardiol* 52:878–880, 1983.

99. Morimoto K, Matsuzaki M, Tohma Y, Suetsugu M, Ono S, Anno Y, Okada K, Hiro J, Nishimura Y: Diagnosis and quantitative evaluation of atrial septal defect by transesophageal 2-D color Doppler echocardiography (Abstr). *Circulation* 76(Suppl 4):IV39, 1987.

100. Schreiner G, Erbel R, Mohr-Kahaly S, Krämer G, Henkel B, Meyer J: The detection of intraatrial septum aneurysms with the aid of transesophageal echocardiography. *Z Kardiol* 74:440–444, 1985.

101. Aschenberg W, Schlüter M, Kremer P, Schröder E, Siglow V, Bleifeld W: Transesophageal two-dimensional echocardiography for the detection of left atrial appendage thrombus. *J Am Coll Cardiol* 7:163–166, 1986.

102. Engberding R, Bender F, Schulze-Waltrup N, Grosse-Heitmeyer W: Improved ultrasonic diagnosis of peri- or paracardial tumors by transesophageal 2D-echocardiography (Abstr). *Circulation* 76(Suppl 4):IV38, 1987.

103. Isaji F: Diagnosis of atrial septal defect (secundum type) with transesophageal echocardiography: Special reference to size and type of ASD. *Nippon Kyobu Geka Gakkai Zasshi* 32:37–49, 1984.

104. Schlüter M, Langenstein BA, Thier W, Schmiegel W-H, Krebber H-J, Kalmar P, Hanrath P: Transesophageal two-dimensional echocardiography in the diagnosis of cor triatriatum in the adult. *J Am Coll Cardiol* 2:1011–1015, 1983.

105. Hanrath P, Schlüter M, Langenstein BA, Polster J, Engel S, Kremer P, Krebber H-J: Detection of ostium secundum atrial septal defects by transoesophageal, cross-sectional echocardiography. *Br Heart J* 49:350–358, 1983.

106. Reifart N, Strohm WD: Detection of atrial septum defects by transesophageal two-dimensional echocardiography with a mechanical sector scanner. In Hanrath P, Bleifeld W, Souquet J (eds): *Cardiovascular Diagnosis by Ultrasound: Transesophageal, Computerized, Contrast, Doppler Echocardiography*. The Hague, Martinus Nijhoff, 1982, pp 247–250.

107. Nellessen U, Daniel WG, Matheis G, Oelert H, Depping K, Lichtlen PR: Impending paradoxical embolism from atrial thrombus: Correct diagnosis by transesophageal echocardiography and prevention by surgery. *J Am Coll Cardiol* 5:1002–1004, 1985.

108. Topol EJ, Biern RO, Reitz BA: Cardiac papillary fibroelastoma and stroke: Echocardiographic diagnosis and guide to excision. *Am J Med* 80:129–132, 1986.

109. Schlüter M, Langenstein BA, Hanrath P, Kremer P, Bleifeld W: Assessment of transesophageal pulsed Doppler echocardiography in the detection of mitral regurgitation. *Circulation* 66:784–789, 1982.

110. Shively B, Cahalan MK, Benefiel D, Schiller N: Intraoperative assessment of mitral valve regurgitation by transesophageal Doppler echocardiography. *J Am Coll Cardiol* 7:228A, 1986.

111. Currie PJ, Schiavone WA, Stewart WJ, Lombardo HP, Burgess LA, Salcedo EE: Evaluation of mitral prosthetic dysfunction with transesophageal color flow Doppler in ambulatory patients (Abstr). *Circulation* 76(Suppl 4):IV39, 1987.

112. De Bruijn NP, Clements FM, Kisslo JA: Intraoperative transesophageal color flow mapping: Initial experience. *Anesth Analg* 66:386–390, 1987.

113. Erbel R, Mohr-Kahaly S, Rohmann S, Schuster S, Drexler M, Wittlich N, Pfeiffer C, Schreiner G, Meyer J: Diagnostic value of transesophageal Doppler echocardiography. *Herz* 12:177–186, 1987.

114. Schlüter M, Kremer P, Hanrath P: Transesophageal 2-D echocardiographic feature of flail mitral leaflet due to ruptured chordae tendineae. *Am Heart J* 108:609–610, 1984.

115. Schlüter M, Langenstein BA, Hanrath P, Kremer P, Bleifeld W: Assessment of transesophageal pulsed Doppler echocardiography in the detection of mitral regurgitation. *Circulation* 66:784–789, 1982.

116. Dahm M, Iversen S, Schmid FX, Drexler M, Erbel R, Oelert H: Intraoperative evaluation of reconstruction of the atrioventricular valves by transesophageal echocardiography. *Thorac Cardiovasc Surg* 35 (Special Issue 2):140–142, 1987.

117. Benefiel DJ, Okuhn SP, Bennett JB, Cahalan MK, Stoney RJ: Intraoperative pediatric transesophageal echocardiography. *J Ultrasound Med*. 5:136, 1986.

118. Goldman ME, Mindich BP: Intraoperative two-dimensional echocardiography: New application of an old technique. *J Am Coll Cardiol* 7:374–382, 1986.

119. Takamoto S, Omoto R: Visualization of thoracic dissecting aortic aneurysm by transesophageal Doppler color flow mapping. *Herz* 12:187–193, 1987.

120. Erbel R, Börner N, Steller D, Brunier J, Thelen M, Pfeiffer C, Mohr-Kahaly S, Iversen S, Oelert H, Meyer J: Detection of aortic dissection by transoesophageal echocardiography. *Br Heart J* 58:45–51, 1987.

121. Erbel R, Mohr-Kahaly S, Rennollet H, Brunier J, Drexler M, Wittlich N, Iversen S, Oelert H, Thelen M, Meyer J: Diagnosis of aortic dissection: The value of transesophageal echocardiography. *Thorac Cardiovasc Surg* 35 (Special Issue 2):126–133, 1987.

122. Engberding R, Bender F, Grosse-Heitmeyer W, Most E, Müller US, Bramann HU, Schneider D: Identification of dissection or aneurysm of the descending thoracic aorta by conventional and transesophageal two-dimensional echocardiography. *Am J Cardiol* 59:717–719, 1987.

123. Kasper W, Hofmann T, Meinertz T, Billmann P, Byrtus M, Lang K, Spillner G, Schlosser V, Just H: Transesophageal echocardiography to detect dissection and aneurysms of the thoracic aorta. *Z Kardiol* 75:609–615, 1986.

124. Engberding R, Bender F, Grosse-Heitmeyer W, Müller US, Schneider D: Diagnosis of thoracic aortic aneurysms by combined transthoracic and

transesophageal 2-echocardiography. *Z Kardiol* 75:225–230, 1986.

125. Börner N, Erbel R, Braun B, Henkel B, Meyer J, Rumpelt J: Diagnosis of aortic dissection by transesophageal echocardiography. *Am J Cardiol* 54:1157–1158, 1984.

126. Hashimoto S, Kumada T, Osakada G, Kubo S, Tamaki S, Yamazato A, Kawai C: Detection of the entry by color Doppler in dissecting aortic aneurysm: Clinical significance of the trans-esophageal color Doppler (Abstr). *Circulation* 76(Suppl 4):IV37, 1987.

127. Mohr-Kahaly S, Rennollet H, Wittlich N, Drexler M, Erbel R: Follow-up of aortic dissection by transesophageal color Doppler echocardiography (Abstr). *Circulation* 76(Suppl 4):IV37, 1987.

128. Geibel A, Hofmann T, Behroz A, Fraedrich G, Schlosser V, Kasper W: Diseases of the descending thoracic aorta—can transesophageal echocardiography add information to conventional echocardiography (Abstr)? *Circulation* 76(Suppl 4):IV37, 1987.

129. Gussenhoven EJ, van Herwerden LA, Roelandt J, Bos E, de Jong N: Detailed analysis of aortic valve endocarditis: Comparison of precordial, esophageal and epicardial two-dimensional echocardiography with surgical findings. *JCU* 14:209–211, 1986.

130. Geibel A, Hofmann T, Behroz A, Birkner H, Meinertz T: Echocardiographic diagnosis of infective endocarditis—additional information by transesophageal echocardiography (Abstr)? *Circulation* 76(Suppl 4):IV38, 1987.

131. Erbel R, Rohmann S, Drexler M, Mohr-Kahaly S, Gerharz CD, Iversen S, Oelert H, Meyer J: Improved diagnostic value of echocardiography in patients with infective endocarditis by transesophageal approach: A prospective study. *Eur Heart J* 9:43–53, 1988.

132. Hanrath P, Schlueter M, Langenstein BA, Polster J, Engel S, Kremer P, Krebber HJ: Detection of ostium secumdum atrial septal defects by transesophageal cross-sectional echocardiography. *Br Heart J* 49:350–358, 1983.

133. Cucchiara RF, Seward JB, Nishimura RA, Nugent M, Faust RJ: Identification of patent foramen ovale during sitting position craniotomy by transesophageal echocardiography with positive airway pressure. *Anesthesiology* 63:107–109, 1985.

134. Kemper AJ, O'Boyle JE, Sharma S: Hydrogen peroxide contrast-enhanced two-dimensional echocardiography: Real-time in vivo delineation of regional myocardial perfusion. *Circulation* 68:603–611, 1983.

135. Smith JS, Feinstein SB, Kapelanski D, Karp RB, Gewertz B, Keamy MF, Segil L, Borow KM, Roizen MF: Intraoperative determination of myocardial perfusion using contrast echocardiography. *Anesthesiology* 65:A27, 1986.

136. Furuya H, Suzuki T, Okumura F, Kishi Y, Uefuji T: Detection of air embolism by transesophageal echocardiography. *Anesthesiology* 58:124–129, 1983.

137. Cucchiara RF, Nugent M, Seward J, Messick JM: Detection of air embolism in upright neurosurgical patients by 2D transesophageal echocardiography (Abstr). *Anesthesiology* 59:A388, 1983.

138. Glenski JA, Cucchiara RF: Transcutaneous O_2 and CO_2 monitoring of neurosurgical patients: Detection of air embolism. *Anesthesiology* 64:546–550, 1986.

139. Glenski JA, Cucchiara RF, Michenfelder JD: Transesophageal echocardiography and transcutaneous O_2 and CO_2 monitoring for detection of venous air embolism. *Anesthesiology* 64:541–545, 1986.

140. Roewer N, Beck H, Kochs E, Kremer P, Schroder E, Schontag H, Jungbluth KH, Schulte-am-Esch J: Detection of venous embolism during intraoperative monitoring by two-dimensional transesophageal echocardiography. *Anasth Intensivther Notfallmed* 20:200–205, 1985.

141. Furuya H, Okumura F: Detection of paradoxical air embolism by transesophageal echocardiography. *Anesthesiology* 60:374–377, 1984.

142. Cucchiara RF, Nugent M, Seward JB, Messick JM: Air embolism in upright neurosurgical patients: Detection and localization by two-dimensional transesophageal echocardiography. *Anesthesiology* 60:353–355, 1984.

143. Oka Y, Inoue T, Hong Y, Sisto DA, Strom JA, Frater RW: Retained intracardiac air: Transesophageal echocardiography for definition of incidence and monitoring removal by improved techniques. *J Thorac Cardiovas Surg* 91 (3):329–338, 1986.

144. Oka Y, Moriwaki KM, Hong Y, Chuculate C, Strom J, Andrews IC, Frater RW: Detection of air emboli in the left heart by M-mode transesophageal echocardiography following cardiopulmonary bypass. *Anesthesiology* 63:109–113, 1985.

145. Topol EJ, Humphrey LS, Borkon AM, Baumgartner WA, Dorsey DL, Reitz BA, Weiss JI: Value of intraoperative left ventricular microbubbles detected by transesophageal two-dimensional echocardiography in predicting neurologic outcome after cardiac operations. *Am J Cardiol* 56:773–775, 1985.

146. Rodigas PC, Meyer FJ, Haasler GB, Dubroff JM, Spotnitz HM: Intraoperative two-dimensional echocardiography: Ejection of microbubbles from the left ventricle after cardiac surgery. *Am J Cardiol* 50:1130–1132, 1982.

22

Echocardiographic and Doppler Assessment of the Fetal Heart

H. Rakowski, M.D.
C. D. Gresser, M.D.
J. Shime, M.D.

INTRODUCTION

Ultrasonic evaluation of the fetus was first described more than 25 years ago. However, the heart, due to its complex structure and rapid motion, has been one of the last fetal organs to be evaluated fully. Improvements in instrument technology and the development of Doppler and color flow imaging have resulted in a remarkable ability to assess fetal cardiac structure and function accurately. These advances have led to a greater use of fetal echocardiography and a better understanding of fetal cardiac function. A normal fetal cardiac study can greatly reassure anxious parents. An abnormal study can alert the perinatologist and pediatric cardiologist to provide optimal care quickly.

FETAL CIRCULATION

The fetal circulation differs from circulation after birth in that the right and left heart work in parallel rather than in series. Since oxygenation does not take place primarily in the lungs, inferior vena caval flow with oxygen-rich blood from the placental circulation and superior vena cava (SVC) flow enter the right atrium (RA). There is streaming of oxygen-rich blood across the foramen ovale into the left atrium (LA), with left ventricular (LV) ejected blood going mainly to the fetal head and upper extremities. Blood ejected from the right ventricle (RV) flows to a lesser degree to the lungs and to a greater degree through the ductus arteriosus to the descending aorta.

TECHNIQUES OF FETAL ECHOCARDIOGRAPHY

Fetal echocardiography can be performed accurately from 16 weeks gestation until term

(1–9), with an initial study being easier technically at 20–24 weeks of age. Initial assessment includes determination of the fetal lie, placental site, biparietal diameter, and a qualitative assessment of amniotic fluid volume. Scanning usually is done with a 5 mHz transducer to optimize structural definition in the small fetal heart. Factors limiting ideal scanning include maternal obesity, polyhydramnios, and a persistent spine-up position of the fetus, resulting in rib shadowing.

Certain views should be attempted in each study. A four-chamber view is best obtained with the beam directed in a cephalic direction through the fetal liver (Fig. 22.1). The left side of the heart can be determined by the position of the interatrial septum, which bows to the left due to the fetal right-to-left shunting. The more apical insertion of the tricuspid valve and the presence of a moderator band identify the RV. Atrial orientation is determined by visualization of the pulmonary veins (LA) and vena caval structures (RA). The four-chamber view is important in quantitating atrial and ventricular size and function, atrioventricular (A-V) valve structure, and the continuity of the atrial and ventricular septum

The parasternal short-axis view is used to determine semilunar valve morphology and great vessel orientation (Fig. 22.2). Parasternal long-axis views and extended views of the aortic arch can define aortoseptal continuity and aortic root integrity and the ductus arteriosus (Fig. 22.3).

Derived M-mode studies are obtained at 100 mm/sec to determine intracardiac dimensions (Fig. 22.4), record valve motion (Fig. 22.5), and help determine the nature of fetal arrhythmias.

431

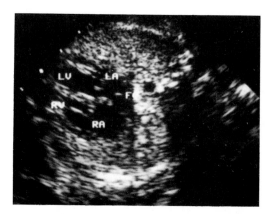

Figure 22.1. A four-chamber view demonstrating the left ventricle (*LV*), right ventricle (*RV*), left atrium (*LA*), and right atrium (*RA*). The interatrial septum can be seen bowing into the left atrium.

QUANTITATIVE ASSESSMENT OF FETAL CARDIAC GROWTH

To assess fetal cardiac growth we studied 75 normal pregnancies at 16–40 weeks gestation (6). Measurements were made from frozen two-dimensional echocardiographic images by using an on-line electronic caliper system. M-mode tracings were not used, since it was often difficult to orient the beam perpendicular to the structure to be measured. We obtained transverse dimension measurements of the left and right atria and the aortic root. The apical four-chamber view was used for all dimensions except the aortic root. The maximal internal transverse dimensions of the left ventricle (LV) and RV were obtained during diastole at the tips of the A-V valves just prior to closure in a plane perpendicular to the ventricular septum. Atrial dimensions were obtained during ventricular systole just after A-V closure, using the widest visible internal diameter in a plane perpendicular to the interatrial septum. The aortic root was measured by the leading edge method at the level of the aortic valves, during valve closure.

Because of the nature of the fetal circulation and elevated pulmonary vascular resistance, there is right heart dominance. This is shown in our study by the RV:LV ratio of 1.16 and the RA:LA ratio of 1.12.

Fetal cardiac structures exhibited a three- to fourfold increase in diameter from 16 to 40 weeks gestation, with a linear increase in size with time (1, 5–7). Growth curves with 95% confidence limits were developed to define normal atrial, ventricular, and aortic root size at different stages of gestation (Figs. 22.6–22.8). A similar relationship existed between chamber size and biparietal diameter (6). These curves can be used to define whether cardiac chambers are normal as well as to assess cardiac growth serially, particularly when cardiac size and function may be affected by hydrops or arrhythmias.

DETECTION OF CONGENITAL HEART DISEASE

Incidence

Major birth defects occur in about 27 of 1000 live births and in about 30% of cases (8/1000) are due to congenital heart disease (10). Although in most instances this outcome cannot be predicted, a

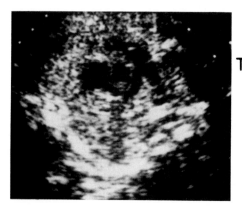
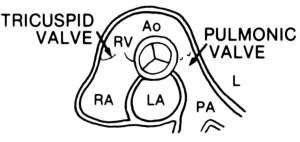

Figure 22.2. *Left panel:* High parasternal short-axis view from a 23-week-old fetus. *Right panel:* Accompanying line diagram. The aorta (*Ao*) and pulmonary artery (*PA*) and its bifurcation can be seen clearly.

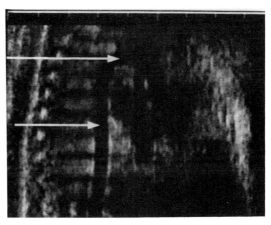

AORTIC ARCH

AORTA

NORMAL

Figure 22.3. In this study taken at 32 weeks gestation, the ascending transverse and descending aorta are clearly visualized.

number of maternal and fetal factors can identify a higher risk.

Identification of High-Risk Groups

Table 22.1 lists the maternal and fetal conditions that help identify a fetus with a higher risk of congenital anomaly. To date, these conditions have been the focus of use of fetal echocardiography as a screening procedure. This risk is increased significantly when a previous child has been affected or when a parent has congenital heart disease. Nora and Nora (11) reviewed eight studies involving 3996 offspring of patients with congenital heart disease. They found the risks of

M-MODE CURSOR

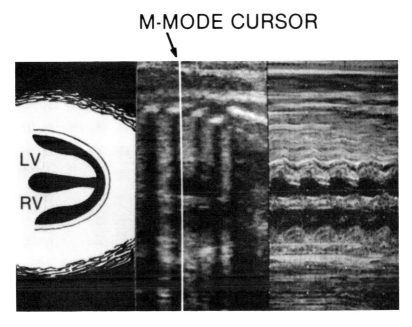

Figure 22.4. A derived M-mode tracing taken at 43 weeks gestation is shown. Measurements are accurate only if the M-mode beam is not tangential to the structure measured.

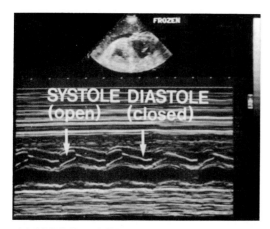

M-MODE NORMAL AORTIC VALVE

Figure 22.5. An M-mode of a normal aortic valve at 38 weeks is shown. Aortic root and left atrial dimensions can be measured as well as the systolic ejection time.

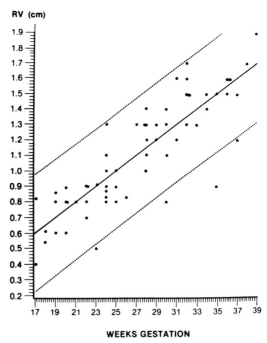

WEEKS GESTATION

Figure 22.7. Maximum right ventricular internal dimension (RV) plotted against gestational age. $n = 63$, $y = 0.50x - 0.25$, $r = 0.857$, $p = 0.0001$.

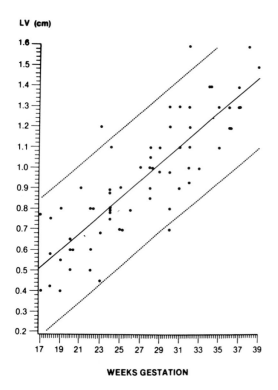

WEEKS GESTATION

Figure 22.6. Maximal left ventricular internal dimension (LV) plotted against gestational age. Dotted lines represent the 95% confidence limits of individual predicted values. $n = 67$, $y = 0.042x - 0.205$, $r = 0.842$, $p = 0.0001$.

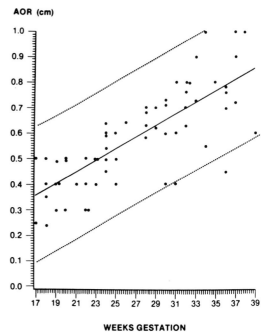

WEEKS GESTATION

Figure 22.8. Maximal aortic root dimension (AOR) plotted against gestational age. $n = 64$, $y = 0.023x - 0.030$, $r = 0.744$, $p = 0.0001$.

Table 22.1. Indications for Fetal Echocardiography

Maternal risk factors
1. Congenital heart disease in parent or previous child
2. Teratogen exposure
3. Collagen vascular disease
4. Hydramnios
5. Uncontrolled maternal diabetes mellitus

Fetal risk factors
1. Extracardiac malformations
2. Abnormal level 1
3. Genetic abnormality
4. Fetal hydrops
5. Intrauterine growth retardation
6. Fetal arrhythmia
7. Abnormal nonstress test

fetal defects were substantially higher if the mother rather than the father was affected, with the risk ratio ranging from a high of 6.39 for aortic stenosis to a low of 1.48 for patent ductus. If the mother was affected, the risk of recurrence was as high as 17.9% for aortic stenosis and as low as 2.6% for tetralogy of Fallot.

Allan et al. (12) studied 1021 mothers referred with a previous history of a child with congenital heart disease. They noted that the overall recurrence rate was 2% if one previous child was affected and 10% if two previous children were affected.

A number of other factors put the fetus at even greater risk of structural abnormality. Allan et al. (13) studied 52 fetuses in which the pregnancy was complicated by nonimmune hydrops. A cardiac etiology was found in 21 of 52 (40%), with structural heart disease in 13 of 21 and tachyarrhythmia in the remaining 8.

Copel et al. (14) demonstrated a 50% incidence of fetal cardiac anomaly when this was suspected on a general obstetrical ultrasound examination and a 26% incidence when an extracardiac anomaly had previously been documented. When a genetic abnormality is identified by amniocentesis, a high risk of cardiac abnormality is present. Conversely, when a fetal anomaly is detected, amniocentesis may identify an associated genetic cause.

Congenital Anomalies Detected

Most forms of congenital heart disease have now been detected in utero, as shown in Table 22.2. This includes atrial septal defect (ASD) (Fig. 22.9); ventricular septal defect (VSD) (Fig 22.10); endocardial cushion defects; valvular lesions (Figure 22.11); conotruncal abnormalities; and lesions incompatible with prolonged life, such as hypoplastic left heart.

The spectrum of abnormalities seen in utero is different from that seen in infancy, since it reflects the inclusion of fetuses with a high rate of death in utero. Kleinman et al. (15) reviewed their center's experience with 72 fetuses that had congenital anomalies detected echocardiographically. They reported a fetal mortality in 57 of 72 cases (79%). In the 15 surviving fetuses, 7 were identified as being dependent on the ductus arteriosus and received prostaglandin E_1 therapy from the time of delivery to surgical palliation. Our experience is quite similar in a smaller series of fetal abnormalities.

ACCURACY OF DIAGNOSIS

The accuracy of a fetal cardiac anomaly detected by echocardiography depends on the pretest likelihood of disease, as well as the sensitivity

Table 22.2. Fetal Cardiac Anomalies Detected in Utero

Septal defects
1. Endocardial cushion defect
2. ASD
3. VSD
4. Premature closure of foramen ovale

Conotruncal abnormalities
1. Tetralogy
2. D-TGA
3. L-TGA
4. Truncus arteriosus
5. Double-outlet RV

Valvular abnormalities
1. Aortic stenosis
2. Pulmonary stenosis
3. Pulmonary atresia
4. Ebstein's anomaly

Aortic abnormalities
1. Coarctation
2. Hypoplastic left heart
3. Subaortic stenosis

Ventricular disproportion
1. Hypoplastic left heart
2. Single ventricle
3. Hypoplastic RV

Malpositions
1. Dextrocardia
2. Splenic syndromes
3. L-Isomerism

Atrial Septal Defect

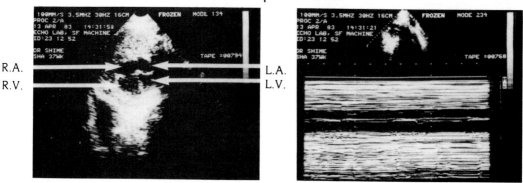

R.A.
R.V.

L.A.
L.V.

4 CHAMBER ENLARGEMENT   PROFOUND BRADYCARDIA H.R.~40/MIN.

Figure 22.9. This study is from a 37-week-old fetus with a dilated cardiomyopathy, an atrial septal defect, and profound sustained bradycardia. Note the dilatation of all four cardiac chambers, the defect in the interatrial septum, and a sustained heart rate (*H.R.*) of 40 beats/min.

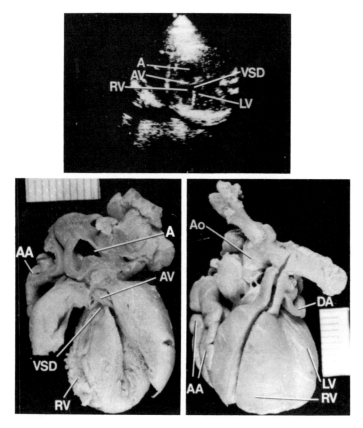

Figure 22.10. A four-chamber view of a fetus with complex congenital heart disease and a VSD is shown. The VSD can be seen as a defect in the four-chamber view with corresponding gross pathologic specimen *below*, showing the site of defect. *A* = Atrium, *A₀* = Aorta, *AA* = Atrial appendage, *AV* = Atrioventricular valve, *DA* = Ductus arteriosus.

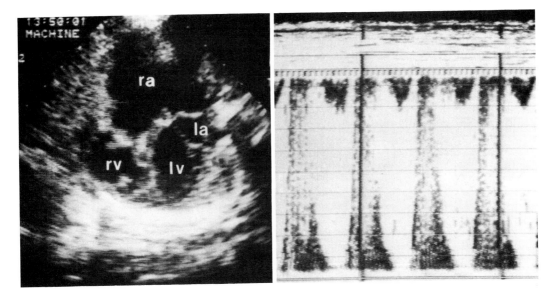

Figure 22.11. *Left panel:* Four-chamber view of a fetus with Ebstein's anomaly of the tricuspid valve. The tricuspid valve can be seen to be displaced apically with a very large right atrial chamber. *rv* = right ventricle, *ra* = right atrium, *la* = left atrium, *lv* = left ventricle. The *right panel* demonstrates high velocity turbulent flow toward the transducer, with the sampling site in the right atrium below the tricuspid valve, indicative of tricuspid regurgitation.

and specificity of echocardiography for a specific lesion. The pretest likelihood of disease can be determined from a genetic assessment as well as previous data presented on the incidence of fetal anomalies in high-risk groups. It is more difficult to define the sensitivity and specificity of fetal echocardiography accurately for all abnormalities separately, since, to date, a large number of fetal abnormalities have not been reported for each condition.

It is reasonable to assume that in an experienced center, the sensitivity of the test will be between 70% and 95%, depending on the lesion examined, and a specificity will be between 80% and 98% (9, 15, 16). Abnormalities most commonly misdiagnosed are small VSDs, aortic coarctation, pulmonary atresia, and occasionally transposition and tetralogy of Fallot.

The importance of pretest likelihood of disease is most critical when screening fetuses at low risk of anomalies is attempted. For example, if the pretest likelihood of disease is 1% and the sensitivity and specificity of the test are 95%, the posttest likelihood of an abnormal study being a true positive is only 16%. However, the likelihood of a negative study truly being negative is 99.99%. If there is a 50% pretest likelihood of disease and only a 90% sensitivity and specificity

of the test, then the positive and negative predictive value of the test is 90%. Thus screening studies for all fetuses generally has not been recommended, and fetal echocardiography has been directed toward assessing high-risk subgroups. Routine obstetric studies should assess cardiac size, and when they are found to be abnormal, a higher level cardiac study should be performed.

INTRACARDIAC MASSES

Isolated cases of intracardiac tumors detected in utero have been reported in the septum (RA), and RV (17, 18). We detected a rhabdomyoma (Fig. 22.12) in a fetus referred for assessment of bradyarrhythmia (17). After birth, the diagnosis of tuberous sclerosis was established.

ASSESSMENT OF VENTRICULAR FUNCTION

Currently it is possible to detect gross abnormalities in ventricular function associated with fetal distress or heart failure (Fig. 12.9). Ventricular dysfunction can be assessed as the percentage of area change of the ventricle from diastole to end-systole. Progressive cardiac enlargement can be documented by plotting ventricular size against time and demonstrating ventricular enlargement that exceeds the 95% confidence limits.

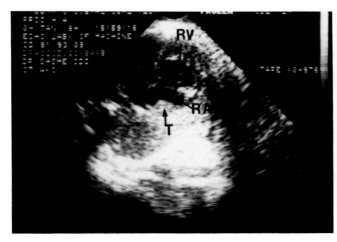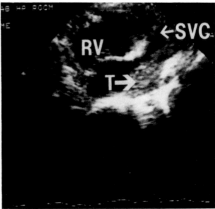

Figure 22.12. This study illustrates a rhabdomyoma at 34 weeks gestation. In the four-chamber view, a 1 cm mass is seen in the right atrium (*left panel*). In the *right panel*, taken shortly after birth, the tumor mass (*t*) can be seen to attach at the site of the junction of the right atrium and superior vena cava (*SVC*).

We have identified two patients with severe ventricular dysfunction, one with four-chamber enlargement and severe global dysfunction (2) and another with severe dysfunction and a large mural thrombus. The latter case at pathologic examination revealed a pattern of global subendocardial infarction with the left ventricle almost filled with mural thrombus. It is not yet clear whether subtle changes in ventricular function can be detected accurately.

ARRHYTHMIAS

A spectrum of fetal arrhythmias has been detected (Table 22.3) (19–24). Some of these arrhythmias have been benign, and others have resulted in heart failure or death.

Bradyarrhythmias

Profound transient bradyarrhythmias are common in the developing fetus. We studied 167 normal pregnancies with normal outcomes and observed transient fetal decelerations in 21% of fetuses between 17 and 25 weeks gestation. This fell to 6.6% after 26 weeks gestation. These episodes are usually transient, lasting 5–30 sec, may be single or multiple, and occasionally are so profound as to constitute transient sinus arrest. It appears likely that this is a physiologic phenomenon with a higher incidence in younger fetuses, reflecting electrical immaturity of the conduction system. Sustained bradyarrhythmias usually indicate serious fetal distress (Fig. 22.9).

Complete heart block is usually associated with serious fetal anomalies or can be seen in association with maternal systemic lupus erythematosus (Fig. 22.13).

Tachyarrhythmias

These arrhythmias are usually supraventricular in origin and, if sustained, usually lead to fetal cardiac enlargement and cardiac failure (19–22). A number of reports have detailed the successful conversion of supraventricular tachycardia with the maternal administration of digoxin alone (Fig. 22.14) or in combination with verapamil, propranolol, or procainamide (19–22). Thus the correct diagnosis and treatment of these tachyarrhythmias may be lifesaving.

Table 22.3. Fetal Arrhythmias

Bradyarrhythmias
1. Transient bradycardia
2. Sustained bradycardia
3. Complete heart block
4. Wandering atrial pacemaker

Tachyarrhythmias
1. Paroxysmal atrial tachycardia
2. Atrial fibrillation
3. Atrial flutter
4. Ventricular tachycardia

Ectopy
1. Atrial premature beats
2. Ventricular premature beats

Complete Heart Block

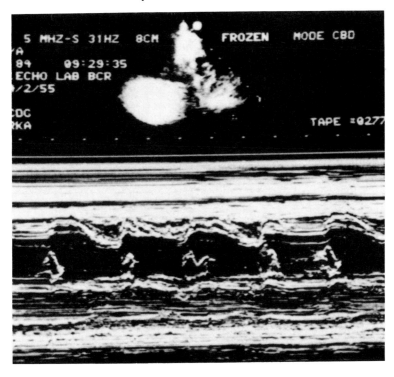

Figure 22.13. Complete heart block. An M-mode tracing taken at the level of the mitral valve demonstrates a regular slow heartbeat, with atrial contraction marching through the tracing with A-V dissociation.

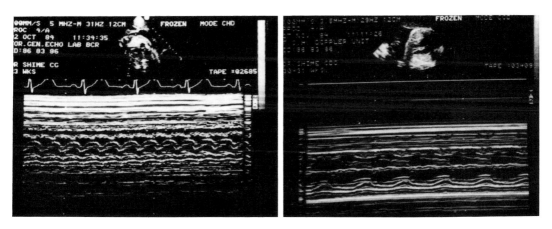

H.R.~300/MIN
REGULAR

H.R.~150/MIN
REGULAR
(MOTHER DIGITALIZED)

Figure 22.14. *Left panel:* M-mode tracing demonstrating a fetal heart rate (*H.R.*) of 300/min. The *right panel* shows reversion to sinus rhythm at 150/min following maternal digitalization.

Ectopy

Ectopy is present in about 2% of normal fetuses (Fig. 22.15) and, in the absence of underlying congenital heart disease, is a benign finding.

Methods of Arrhythmia Detection

A number of methods are available to detect the nature of an arrhythmia. These methods were reviewed recently by Silverman et al. (20). Atrial contraction can be demonstrated by the presence of atrial wall motion as well as the presence of an A wave seen with atrial ventricular valve motion. Ventricular contraction can be detected by the presence of A-V valve closure and semilunar valve opening, as well as the onset of left ventricular wall contraction. Dual M-mode studies can be done or ladder diagrams can be constructed to detect the presence and association between atrial and ventricular contraction. When complete heart block is present, the heart rate is slowed and atrial activity can be shown to be dissociated from ventricular activity (Fig. 22.13).

FETAL DOPPLER ECHOCARDIOGRAPHY

Fetal Doppler studies have been used to provide insights about intracardiac flow in utero. Reed et al. (25) studied 87 fetuses of 17–41 weeks gestation and compared pulmonary artery and aortic outflow diameters, mean and maximal flow velocities, and transvalvular flow. Both outflow tracts increased in size with advancing gestational age, while mean and maximal Doppler flow velocities did not. The pulmonary artery diameter was greater than that of the aorta, while aortic flow velocities were greater than those in the pulmonary artery. The transvalvular PA:AO flow ratio was 1.3:1. Although the accuracy of absolute flow measurements has not been validated, there was a significant increase in flow across the pulmonary artery and aorta with advancing gestational age.

Assessment of diastolic function has revealed a dominance of late diastolic filling of both right and left ventricles, likely due to decreased ventricular compliance (26). Between 17 and 24 weeks gestation, tricuspid and mitral inflow ratios of late flow to early flow (A:E) are 1.56 and 1.55, respectively. Both ratios fall to 1.22 just prior to term. Tricuspid peak atrial filling velocity did not change with advancing gestational age, but peak early velocity (E) increased from 26.3 to 36.5 cm/sec. Mitral inflow early velocity (E) did not change, but peak late velocity (A) decreased from 45.8 to 34.5 cm/sec when fetuses between 17–24 weeks gestation and those close to term were compared. Thus the compliance of the two ventricles appears to differ with advancing fetal age.

Huhta et al. (27) demonstrated the ability and importance of assessing fetal ductal flow. Peak systolic velocities using image-directed pulsed Doppler ranged from 50 to 141 cm/sec (mean:80 cm/sec) and increased with gestational age, al-

Ventricular Premature Beats

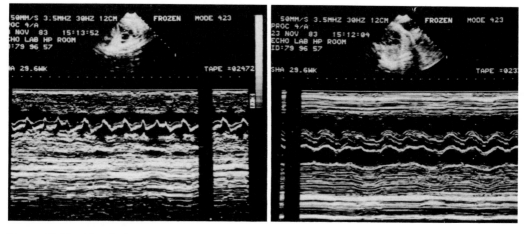

Figure 22.15. Ventricular premature beats occurring in a 29-week-old fetus is shown. An M-mode of mitral valve opening is seen in the *left panel* and an aortic valve opening is seen in the *right panel*. An absence of atrial contraction and a full compensatory pause helped to identify the ventricular origin of the beats.

though there was significant scatter of the data. Diastolic velocities consistently were directed toward the descending aorta and ranged from 6 to 30 cm/sec. Fetal ductal constriction was identified in mothers receiving indomethacin for premature labor, which may have important therapeutic implications.

Valvular regurgitation can be detected in patients with fetal hydrops (28), where it is common, as well as in association with congenital anomalies (28–31). This can be seen in Figure 22.12 in a fetus with Ebstein's anomaly of the tricuspid valve.

Color flow imaging (30, 31) has further improved our ability to recognize and quantitate both valvular regurgitation and intracardiac shunts.

SUMMARY

Fetal echocardiography and Doppler studies have become an essential part of the investigation of the fetus suspected of having underlying heart disease. This permits the rapid and accurate assessment of cardiac size, fetal anomalies, and ventricular function. Doppler studies can assess the degree of valvular regurgitation and intracardiac shunting. Also, our understanding of fetal cardiac physiology and blood flow has been enhanced.

It seems reasonable that all obstetric ultrasound studies should include at least a screening view of the heart. Higher level cardiac studies should be reserved for higher risk groups or suspected arrhythmias. Although the risk of fetal echocardiographic examination is likely very small, the power output of Doppler studies suggest that it should initially be used to assess abnormal fetuses. The risk:benefit ratio appears to be appropriate in this setting.

Since the fetal heart is quite small, a certain level of echocardiographic expertise, understanding of fetal physiology, and congenital heart disease is a prerequisite for those performing fetal cardiac studies.

Although a number of ethical and moral dilemmas regarding termination of pregnancy occasionally may be encountered, these usually are more than offset by the large number of families who can be reassured of having a normal fetus.

REFERENCES

1. Sahn OJ, Lange LW, Allen HD, Goldberg SJ, Anderson C, Giles H, Haber K: Quantitative real time cross-sectional echocardiography in the developing normal fetus and newborn. *Circulation* 62:588–597, 1980.
2. Shime J, Bertrand M, Hagen-Ansert S, Rakowski H: Two-dimensional and M-mode echocardiography in the human fetus. *Am J Obstet Gynecol* 148:679–685, 1984.
3. DeVore GR: The prenatal diagnosis of congenital heart disease: A practical approach for the fetal sonographer. *J Clin Ultrasound* 13:229–245, 1985.
4. Kleinman CS, Donnerstein RL: Ultrasonic assessment of cardiac function in the intact human fetus. *J Am Coll Cardiol* 5:84S–94S, 1985.
5. Wladimiroff JW, Vosters R, Stewart PA: Fetal echocardiography: Basic and clinical considerations. *Ultrasound Med Biol* 10:315–326, 1984.
6. Shime J, Gresser CD, Rakowksi H: Quantitative two-dimensional echocardiographic assessment of fetal cardiac growth. *Am J Obstet Gynecol* 154:543–550, 1986.
7. DeVore GR, Siassi B, Platt LD: Fetal echocardiography V. M-mode measurements of the aortic root and aortic valve in second and third trimester normal human fetuses. *Am J Obstet Gynecol* 152:543–550, 1985.
8. Allan LD, Crawford DC, Anderson RH, Tynan M: Spectrum of congenital heart disease detected echocardiographically in prenatal life. *Br Heart J* 54:523–526, 1985.
9. Presbitero P, Todros T, Pavone G, DeFillipi G: Fetal echocardiography: Diagnosis of congenital cardiomyopathies in a population at risk. *G Ital Cardiol* 15:590–596, 1985.
10. McCallum WD: Fetal cardiac anatomy and vascular dynamics. *Clin Obstet Gynecol* 837–849.
11. Nora JJ, Nora AH: Maternal transmission of congenital heart diseases: New recurrence risk figures and the questions of cytoplasmic inheritance and vulnerability to teratogens. *Am J Cardiol* 59:459–463, 1987.
12. Allan LD, Crawford DC, Chita SK, Anderson RH, Tynan MJ: Familial recurrence of congenital heart disease in a prospective series of mothers referred for fetal echocardiography. *Am J Cardiol* 58:334–337, 1986.
13. Allan LD, Crawford DC, Sheridan R, Chapman MG: Aetiology of non-immune hydrops: The value of echocardiography. *Br J Obstet Gynaecol* 93:223–225, 1986.
14. Copel JA, Pilu G, Kleinman CS: Congenital heart disease and extracardiac anomalies: Associations and indications for fetal echocardiography. *Am J Obstet Gynecol* 154:1121–1132, 1986.
15. Kleinman CS, Donnerstein RL, DeVore GR: Fetal echocardiography for evaluation of in-utero congestive heart failure: A technique for study of non-immune hydrops. *N Engl J Med* 306:568–575, 1982.
16. Wladimiroff JW, Stewart PA, Tonge HM: The role of diagnostic ultrasound in the study of fetal cardiac abnormalities. *Ultrasound Med Biol* 10:457–463, 1984.
17. Gresser CD, Shime J, Rakowski H, Smallhorn JF, Hui A, Berg JJ: Fetal cardiac tumor: A prenatal echocardiographic marker for tuberous sclerosis. *Am J Obstet Gynecol* 3:689–690, 1987.

18. Birnbaum SE, McGahan JP, Janos GG, Meyers M: Fetal tachycardia and intramyocardial tumors. *J Am Coll Cardiol* 6:1358–1361, 1985.

19. Kleinman CS, Donnerstein RL, Jaffe C, DeVore GR, Weinstein EM, Lynch DC, Talner NS, Berkowitz RL, Hobbins JC: Fetal echocardiography: A tool for evaluation of in-utero therapy: Analysis of 71 patients. *Am J Cardiol* 51:237–243, 1983.

20. Silverman NH, Enderlein MA, Stanger P, Teitel DF, Heymann MA, Golbus MS: Recognition of fetal arrhythmias by echocardiography. *J Clin Ultrasound* 13:255–263, 1985.

21. Kleinman CS, Copel JA, Weinstein EM, Santulli TV Jr, Hobbins JC: Treatment of fetal supraventricular tachyarrhythmias. *J Clin Ultrasound* 13:265–273, 1985.

22. Wiggins JW Jr, Bowes W, Clewell W, Manco-Johnson M, Manchester D, Johnson R, Appareti K, Wolfe RR: Echocardiographic diagnosis and intravenous digoxin management of fetal tachyarrhythmias and congestive heart failure. *Am J Dis Child* 140 (3):202–204, 1986.

23. Strasburger FJ, Huhta JC, Carpenter RJ Jr, Gerson A Jr, McNamara DG: Doppler echocardiography in the diagnosis and management of persistent fetal arrhythmias. *J Am Coll Cardiol* 7:1386–1391, 1986.

24. Carpenter RJ Jr, Strasburger JF, Garson A Jr, Smith RT, Deter RL, Engelhardt HT Jr: Fetal ventricular pacing for hydrops secondary to complete atrioventricular block. *J Am Coll Cardiol* 8:1434–1436, 1986.

25. Reed KL, Anderson CF, Shenter L: Fetal pulmonary artery and aorta: Two-dimensional Doppler echocardiography. *Obstet Gynecol* 69:175–178, 1987.

26. Reed KL, Sahn DJ, Scagnelli S, Anderson CF, Shenker L: Doppler echocardiographic studies of diastolic function in the human fetal heart: Changes during gestation. *J Am Coll Cardiol* 8:391–395, 1986.

27. Huhta JC, Moise CJ, Fisher DJ, Sharif DS, Wasserstrum N, Martin C: Detection and quantitation of constriction of the fetal ductus arteriosus by Doppler echocardiography. *Circulation* 75:406–412, 1987.

28. Silverman NH, Kleinman CS, Rudolph AM, Copel JA, Weinstein EM, Enderlein MA, Globus M: Fetal atrioventricular valve insufficiency associated with non-immune hydrops: A two-dimensional echocardiographic and pulsed Doppler ultrasound study. *Circulation* 72:825–832, 1985.

29. Huhta JC, Strasburger JF, Carpenter RJ, Reiter A, Abinader E: Pulsed Doppler fetal echocardiography. *J Clin Ultrasound* 13:247–254, 1985.

30. Maulik D, Nanda NC, Hsiung MC, Youngblood JP: Doppler colour flow mapping of the fetal heart. *Angiology* 37:628–632, 1986.

31. DeVore GR, Hurenstein J, Siassi B, Platt LD: Fetal echocardiography VII. Doppler colour flow mapping: A new technique for the diagnosis of congenital heart disease. *Am J Obstet Gynecol* 156:1054–1064, 1987.

23

Congenital Heart Disease

Samuel B. Ritter, M.D., F.A.C.C.

The severity and manifestations of congenital heart disease may be quite variable; however, the incidence has remained uniform at roughly 1% of all infants. In most cases, it is expressed in neonates, infants, and children as morphologic and anatomic alterations of the heart and great vessels. The prognosis for congenital heart disease has improved dramatically due to improvements in medical and surgical treatment.

Advances in treatment have helped the development of noninvasive imaging and, in turn, have been aided by the new technology. Two-dimensional Doppler flow echocardiography has become more and more widely used preoperatively, intraoperatively, and postoperatively (1).

The instrument we have used for the past 3 years is the Aloka-Corometrics 880, 860, and, currently, 870 scanners. The systems integrate pulsed Doppler with an autocorrelator. This allows visualization of blood flow and its imposition onto an anatomic two-dimensional image. Thus images of intracardiac blood flow can be obtained simultaneously with a two-dimensional display of morphology.

Phased array transducers (2.25 mHz, 3.5 mHz, and 5.0 mHz) continuously sample Doppler shifts throughout the entire two-dimensional echo plane. Sampling occurs on multiple points along the beam line, as well as in multiple beam lines at various levels, from each radial line in the sector plane. In all, 48 transmit-and-receive channels are used.

The ultrasound beam reflected from the heart is separated into two components. One forms the black-and-white B-mode two-dimensional echocardiogram. The other component passes through a comb filter and is transmitted to a quadrature detector. The output from this detector is channeled to an autocorrelator. A digital scan converter then supplies a signal to a color converter, which assigns color according to three basic principles:

1. Direction of flow
2. Velocity of flow
3. Variance of detected frequency shifts

Red is, by convention, assigned to represent visually the flow directed toward the transducer. Flow away from the transducer is rendered in blue. Sixteen shades of intensity (eight red, eight blue) correspond to the velocity of blood flow. The brighter the hue, the faster the velocity. The degree of variance in velocities around the mean velocity (state of turbulence) is displayed in green. This green color, which represents variance of frequency shifts, is superimposed over the red and blue colors, resulting in a "mosaic" color pattern.

Color-coded data may be superimposed over the two-dimensional or M-mode echocardiogram. This is often useful in timing rapidly changing flows at various phases in the cardiac cycle. Various names have been used in an attempt to describe this technique effectively; in this chapter, it will be referred to as Doppler color flow mapping (2–6).

The complexity of congenital cardiac problems and the tomographic nature of two-dimensional echocardiography require that multiple scans of the heart, by various approaches, be performed in a logical, sequential manner. This system, termed the segmental approach, can be applied to both intracardiac and extracardiac anatomy (7, 8).

A study generally begins by defining the abdominal and the atrial situs, goes on to describe atrioventricular connections, and ends with ventriculoarterial connections. Detailed intracardiac

443

analysis is performed by systematically examining the atrial septum, ventricular septum, atrioventricular valves, and semilunar valves. Finally, the extracardiac anatomy is examined, including pulmonary venous systems, systemic venous systems, and the entire aortic arch.

In this segmental analysis, careful identification of details such as systemic venous return will often direct the noninvasive cardiologist to more specific approaches in evaluating cardiac lesions. For instance, in our laboratory we have identified prospectively seven patients with interruption of the inferior vena cava (IVC) with associated azygous or hemiazygous venous continuation of the IVC. Such knowledge obtained prior to cardiac catheterization is invaluable, often saving the patient the undue stress of prolonged invasive procedures.

The two-dimensional echocardiographic study begins with the echo beam parallel to the frontal plane (horizontal cut) at the level of the abdominal aorta. Normally, the abdominal aorta is seen to the patient's left, and the sickle-shaped IVC is seen to the patient's right. The left renal vein is seen to course from the IVC across the midline to the patient's left, running between the posterior abdominal aorta and the more anterior superior mesenteric artery. This defines situs solitus and atrial situs.

Cranial angulation of the echocardiographic beam will follow the infrarenal IVC through its hepatic portion and into the right atrium. Interruption of the IVC above the level of the renal veins will be detected by this approach, as will the appearance of a left-side azygous or hemiazygous structure. The parasagittal/transverse plane will differentiate direct emptying of hepatic vessels into the right atrium from normal IVC drainage. The vertical hemiazygous system will also be seen running parallel to the aorta. Doppler examination of these two structures will demonstrate diagnostic IVC flow patterns in the hemiazygous system with a characteristic Doppler flow tracing in the descending aorta (Fig. 23.1).

CYANOSIS IN THE NEONATE

One must never assume that cyanosis in the newborn is exclusively secondary to malformations of the cardiovascular system. Central nervous system (CNS) problems secondary to intracranial bleeding can result in a cyanotic newborn due to reduced alveolar ventilation. Similarly, cyanosis can be caused by methemoglobinemia. Cyanosis can most certainly also be the result of upper airway obstruction, hyaline membrane disease, pneumonia, or atelectasis. Methemoglobinemia and CNS problems are usually distinguishable clinically, while pulmonary disease can often be determined by history, chest x-ray and response to 100% inspired oxygen. However, persistent pulmonary hypertension in the newborn is often difficult to differentiate from structural cardiovascular abnormalities presenting with similar symptomology. Congenital heart defects can present with right-to-left ductal and atrial shunting, mimicking persistent pulmonary hypertension (9, 10).

Recognizing infants with obstruction to pulmonary venous return, especially total anomalous pulmonary venous drainage below the diaphragm, is most difficult clinically. Echocardiographic images of the heart in the parasternal and apical imaging planes do not reveal gross structural abnormalities. Extracardiac subdiaphragmatic parasagittal imaging best yields the diagnosis. In this approach, the IVC is seen on the right, and the descending aorta is seen on the left. Normally, there is no intermediate vascular channel. In cases of total anomalous venous drainage below the diaphragm, the anomalous pulmonary venous channel is located between these two structures. Confirmation that this is a vertical vascular channel is made by taking a Doppler sample volume in the center of the structure. This shows continuous forward flow toward the transducer in the subxiphoid position (away from the heart), distinctive for pulmonary venous flow (Fig. 23.2).

Experience with this disorder has demonstrated the utility of Doppler color flow mapping (11). Red flow (toward the transducer) is seen in the vertical vascular channel, indicating the direction of flow is caudal. Drainage of the anomalous vein into the intrahepatic portal/vena caval system is also identified, while continuous mosaic turbulent flow in the IVC is noted.

Two-dimensional echocardiography has virtually eliminated the need for cardiac catheterization and its attendant risks in this group of infants (12). The normal stresses of catheterization—injection of contrast material, exposure to radiation, and the cold environment—are exacerbated by the extreme illness of these infants, who are almost always on ventilatory support. Doppler color flow mapping has also proven useful in identifying right-to-left atrial shunts and ductal shunts. This obviates contrast echocardiography, with its

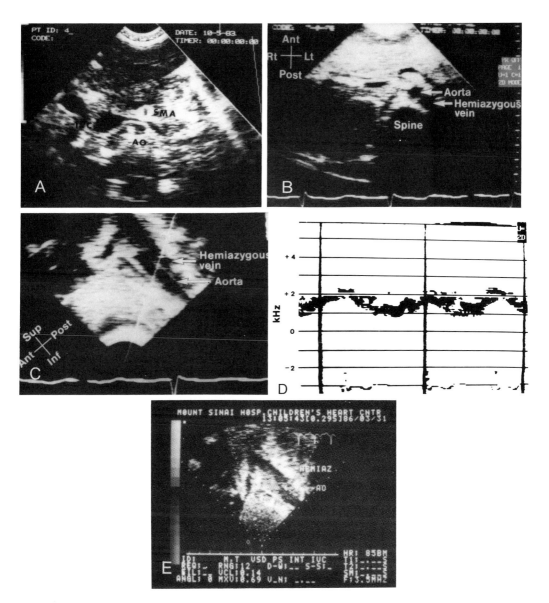

Figure 23.1. *A*, Abdominal horizontal view identifying left-sided aorta (*AO*), right-sided inferior vena cava (*IVC*), and superior mesenteric artery (*SMA*). Note the course of the left renal vein across the midline between the aorta and superior mesenteric artery. *B*, Echocardiographic identification of interruption of the IVC and continuation via a hemiazygous vein to the left of the abdominal aorta. *C*, Subxiphoid transverse view showing a second vertical channel posterior to the abdominal aorta. This is the hemiazygous vein. *D*, A Doppler tracing confirms this as a hemiazygous vein, demonstrating a typical vena caval waveform. *E*, Doppler color flow demonstrating positive (red) flow in the abdominal aorta (toward the transducer) and negative (blue) flow in the hemiazygous vein (*HEMIAZ*) (away from the transducer). See this figure in Color Atlas.

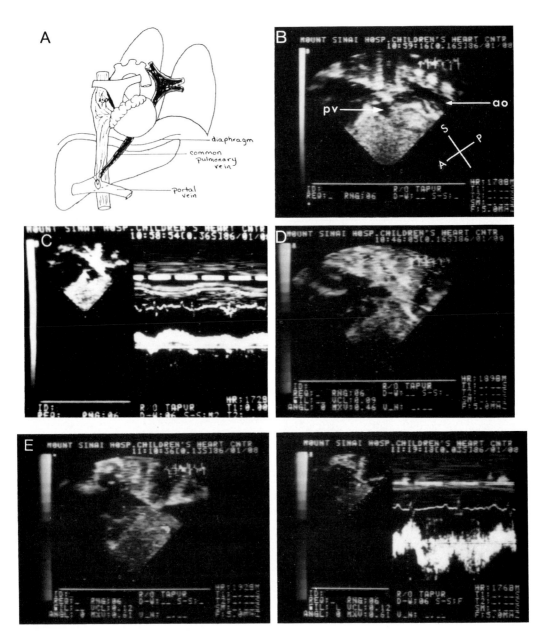

Figure 23.2. *A*, Illustration demonstrating total anomalous pulmonary venous drainage below the diaphragm. The common pulmonary vein is a vertical channel descending infradiaphragmatically and located between the IVC on the *right* and the descending aorta on the *left*. *B*, Two-dimensional echo showing the common pulmonary venous channel (*pv*) (*right*) and the posterior descending aorta (*aO*). *C*, Doppler tracing in the anomalous venous channel. It displays typical positive pulmonary venous waveform, as flow is toward the abdominally placed transducer. *D*, Doppler color flow demonstrates flow toward the transducer (red) in the descending aorta and the anomalous venous channel. *E*, *Left*, Blue flow (toward the right atrium, away from the transducer) in the IVC, located anterior to the anomalous channel. *Right*, Pulsed Doppler flow pattern in this vessel shows typical spectral waveform of IVC flow. See this figure in Color Atlas.

small (but not inconsequential) risk of air embolization.

Other conditions may present as persistent pulmonary hypertension of the newborn. These include hypoplastic left heart syndrome, myopathic left ventricular diseases, left ventricular outflow obstruction, and endocardial fibroelastosis. Differentiation of these structural abnormalities, as well as any others producing cyanosis in the newborn, can be obtained in a similar noninvasive manner.

TRANSPOSITION OF THE GREAT VESSELS

Transposition of the great arteries with an intact ventricular septum is the most common congenital heart lesion causing cyanosis in the neonatal period. In this condition, the right ventricle gives rise to the aorta, and the left ventricle gives rise to the pulmonary artery. Without a large foramen ovale (intracardiac communication) or patent ductus arteriosus (intracardiac communication), the newborn becomes rapidly and progressively cyanotic, acidotic, and shocky. Normal ductal closure occurring in the first 12–24 h almost always causes these infants to present during this time period.

The diagnosis of transposition is best made by subxiphoid imaging, with the echo beam parallel to the horizontal plane of the trunk and angulated cranially toward the left midclavicle. From this position, both left and right ventricular outflow tracts can be identified. Normally, the aorta is seen to arise from the left ventricle posteriorly. The pulmonary artery and its immediate bifurcation into right and left branches is then identified by further cranial angulation anteriorly. In transposition, the main pulmonary artery arises from the posterior ventricle, which assumes a more sickle shape due to the high right ventricular pressure. Anterior angulation reveals the right ventricle giving rise to a nonbranching ascending aorta. Perpendicular subxiphoid views (parasagittal/transverse projection) will identify the ascending aorta arising anteriorly from the right ventricle and continuing to the transverse arch and descending thoracic aorta (13) (Fig. 23.3).

Two dimensional echocardiography has been extremely sensitive and accurate in the prospective diagnosis of transposition of the great vessels. Diagnostic cardiac catheterization is performed rarely; invasive catheter placement is reserved for therapeutic purposes. The lifesaving technique of balloon atrial septostomy augments interatrial blood flow, allowing oxygenated blood from the left atrium to enter the right ventricle and aorta. This procedure has been performed recently under direct imaging by two-dimensional echocardiography, without the use of angiography or irradiation. Determining the size of the subsequent interatrial defect produced by balloon atrial septostomy is important. Assessment of this large flap torn in the interatrial septum may also be made using two-dimensional echocardiography (Fig. 23.4).

PULMONARY/TRICUSPID ATRESIA: HYPOPLASTIC RIGHT HEART SYNDROME

Pulmonary atresia is characterized by lack of continuity between the right ventricle and the main pulmonary artery. Two-dimensional echocardiography can, in a number of views, identify the confluence of the pulmonary arteries and the lack of its connection to the right ventricle. This fibrous discontinuity can best be appreciated in the subxiphoid views (beginning with the four-chamber view and angulating cranially) and the parasternal short-axis views at the level of the great vessels. Pulsed Doppler examination of the main pulmonary artery will reveal no antegrade flow. Doppler color flow mapping will show no flow from the right ventricle into the pulmonary artery. From these views, the size of the right ventricle and the distance between the right ventricular outflow tract and the pulmonary artery can also be evaluated easily.

Planned surgical approaches in the newborn depend heavily on these assessments. A decision

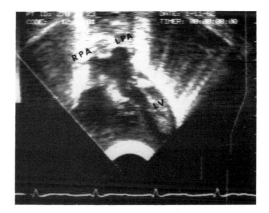

Figure 23.3. Subxiphoid long-axis view (apex down). The sickle-shaped left ventricle (*LV*) gives rise to right (*RPA*) and left (*LPA*) pulmonary arteries.

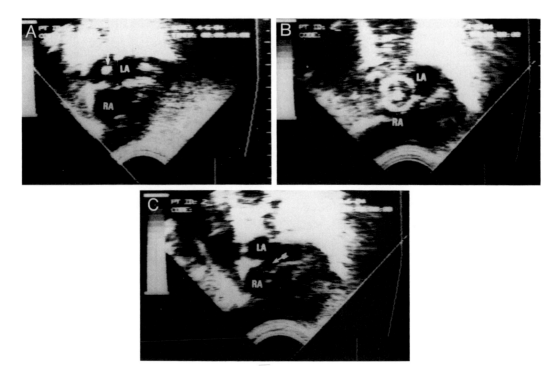

Figure 23.4. Balloon atrial septostomy: subxiphoid four-chamber view (apex down). *A,* Localization of the deflated balloon catheter tip in the left atrium (*LA*) (*arrow*). *RA* = right atrium. *B,* The fully inflated balloon is "jerked" across the interatrial septum. *C,* The resultant large interatrial communication (*arrow*) after septostomy.

can now be made noninvasively depending on whether the newborn has a reasonable size ventricle with a short atretic portion. If the answer is yes, the surgical approach can be valvulotomy; if the answer is no, the approach can be a systemic-to-pulmonary artery shunt.

In tricuspid atresia the thick membranous extension in the region of the tricuspid annulus and absence of a tricuspid valve are seen easily in either the subxiphoid or the apical four-chamber view. The size of the atrial septal defect (ASD) and potential obstruction also are observed, as well as the right-to-left bulging of the septum, implying obstruction to flow. Doppler color flow mapping and pulsed Doppler echocardiography can easily identify the right-to-left atrial shunt and are important in assessing the potential need for balloon septostomy.

Two-dimensional directed M-mode measurement of the pulmonary arteries is also invaluable before and after (as follow-up) systemic-to-pulmonary artery shunts. Anatomic description of the aortic arch (right versus left) and its branching pattern from high parasternal or suprasternal notch

views is essential and can be performed reliably by two-dimensional echocardiography. In our experience, infants with lesions requiring systemic-to-pulmonary artery shunts generally do not re-

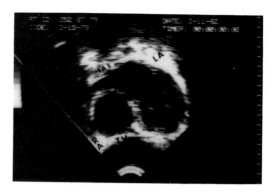

Figure 23.5. Tricuspid atresia: Subxiphoid four-chamber view (apex down). Note the thick *white fibrous band* where the thin tricuspid valve (*TV*) would normally appear. Also note the right-to-left bulging of the interatrial septum (*IAS*). *LA* = left atrium, *RA* = right atrium.

quire cardiac catheterization if the aortic arch and its branches can be delineated noninvasively (Fig. 23.5).

FALLOT'S TETRALOGY

Although Fallot's tetralogy is the most common cyanotic congenital heart disease, it usually does not present symptomatically in the neonatal period. The abnormalities can be demonstrated clearly by two-dimensional echocardiography. The echocardiogram will reveal a large malalignment ventricular septal defect (VSD) with anterodextroposition of the aorta and concomitant infundibular pulmonic stenosis. Parasternal long-axis views will show the VSD and overriding aorta quite well (14).

Pulsed Doppler examination of the VSD will demonstrate the bidirectional shunting across it. Doppler color flow mapping will delineate early left-to-right shunting followed by late systolic right-to-left flow across the VSD. The subxiphoid transverse/parasagittal projection will show the anatomic anomaly clearly. The malalignment VSD with aortic override and anterior leftward displacement of the parietal band in the subpulmonic infundibular area can be demonstrated easily in this view.

Rightward aortic shift, conotruncal hypertrophy, pulmonary artery size, and right ventricular outflow tract are assessed from the subxiphoid view. In this view, the origin of the pulmonary arteries from the right ventricle will differentiate Fallot's tetralogy from truncus arteriosus, since in the latter the pulmonary arteries emanate directly from the trunk (Fig. 23.6).

EBSTEIN'S ANOMALY OF THE TRICUSPID VALVE

Malposition of the tricuspid valve within the right ventricle, distally displaced to the normal tricuspid annulus with atrialization of the right ventricle, often presents in neonates with cyanosis secondary to right-to-left shunting through a dilated foramen ovale. The subxiphoid or apical four-chamber view clearly will demonstrate the caudad displacement of the tricuspid valve.

The tricuspid insufficiency almost always associated with this lesion may be visualized by pulsed Doppler echocardiography or Doppler color flow mapping. The severity of regurgitation is perhaps best delineated by color flow mapping, which gives a more correct spatial orientation of the regurgitant jet than the single-plane pulsed or continuous wave Doppler (Fig. 23.7).

ACYANOTIC CONGENITAL HEART DISEASE: NEONATES

The neonate with pallor and pulselessness who is cold and clammy to the touch, has a gray mottled appearance, and is in severe congestive heart failure is often suffering from low cardiac output secondary to left-sided outflow obstruction. This, in turn, is secondary to critical aortic stenosis, severe coarctation of the aorta, or an interrupted aortic arch.

Because these infants are gravely ill, the noninvasive delineation of the lesions by two-dimensional echocardiography is invaluable. In these neonates, echocardiography often can make cardiac catheterization unnecessary.

Identification of a thickened, doming aortic valve can be made best in the parasternal, apical, or subxiphoid long-axis view. Since left ventricular contractility is poor in critical aortic stenosis, the left ventricular outflow tract gradient is often meaningless. This is because the calculated gradient is decreased falsely by the diminished cardiac output. These infants urgently require valvotomy, and it is our practice to send these infants directly from the echo laboratory to the operating room.

Echocardiography is equally important in evaluating the aortic arch from the high parasternal or suprasternal notch. Discrete coarctation at the juxtaductal level (takeoff of the subclavian artery) can be seen from these views as a distinct narrowing or shelf. Interruption of the arch with continuation, via a ductus arteriosus, can also be seen from this view. Pulsed Doppler echocardiography from the suprasternal notch will show distinct morphologic changes distal to the ductus.

Examination of the abdominal aorta from the subxiphoid parasagittal approach will show similar changes. These changes include decreased upslope and long diastolic runoff, with no return to baseline before the next systolic flow begins. Continuous wave Doppler examination from the suprasternal notch may be useful in calculating the gradient across the area of coarctation. Determination of whether these lesions are associated with a VSD or patent ductus arteriosus can also be made by echocardiography (Fig. 23.8).

Finally, hypoplastic left heart syndrome, with its attendant mitral and aortic atresia, can be identified accurately by two-dimensional imaging. Subxiphoid and apical four-chamber views are perhaps the best imaging windows, although comprehensive scanning using multiple views and

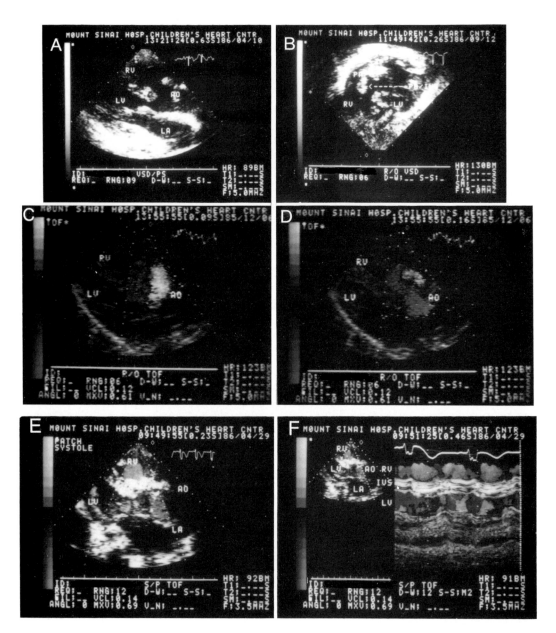

Figure 23.6. *A–F*, Fallot's tetralogy. *A*, Parasternal long-axis projection showing typical malalignment VSD overriding the aorta *(AO)*. *IVS* = intraventricular septum, *LA* = left atrium, *LV* = left ventricle, *RV* = right ventricle. *B*, Subxiphoid transverse section clearly demonstrates the VSD and anterior displacement of the infundibulum or parietal band *(PB)* into the subpulmonic *(PA)* region. *C*, Left-to-right shunt (shown in red) across the malaligned VSD in early systole. *D*, Right-to-left shunt (shown in *blue*) occurring in late systole. *E*, After patch closure of the tetralogy VSD, note echogenic patch. Color flow displays red jet on right ventricular septal surface in systole, indicating patch leak. *F*, Color M-mode confirms this suspicion. Note red color on the right ventricular side of intraventricular septum following the QRS (red flow in diastolic is tricuspid flow). See this figure in Color Atlas.

planes is suggested. In the past, the diagnosis of hypoplastic left heart syndrome was associated with a grave prognosis. Recent advances in surgical technique have improved the odds for these infants. As a consequence, the role of two-dimensional echocardiography has expanded greatly in these cases.

Acyanotic Congenital Heart Lesions

The majority of congenital heart defects are acyanotic, accounting for as much as 80% of congenital heart disease in neonates. Presentation for these lesions can be quite different from cyanotic congenital heart disease, which often results in a critically ill newborn during the neonatal period. Discussion of the noninvasive diagnosis and as-

sessment of these lesions will focus on the integrated and comprehensive approach to imaging. This includes two-dimensional, pulsed wave Doppler, continuous wave Doppler, and color flow Doppler echocardiography.

Ventricular Septal Defect

Although VSDs are true congenital heart lesions and are present in the newborn, symptoms generally do not appear in the neonatal period. These symptoms relate to the increased pulmonary flow secondary to a left-to-right shunt at the level of the defect. The initial lack of symptoms is due to the relationship between pulmonary and systemic vascular resistance and the changes taking place during the first few weeks of life.

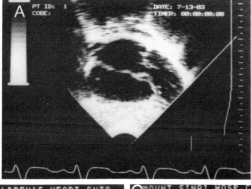

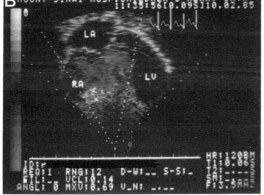
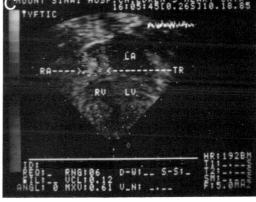

Figure 23.7. Ebstein's anomaly of the tricuspid valve: apical four-chamber view (apex down). *A,* Note the displacement of the tricuspid valve caudad into the right ventricle, well below the mitral valve plane. *B,* Severe tricuspid regurgitation seen as a large blue-colored systolic flow in the right atrium (*RA*). *LA* = left atrium, *LV* = left ventricle. *C,* In comparison to *B,* a small, thin blue-colored regurgitant jet (*TR*) is seen in another patient. *RV* = right ventricle. See this figure in Color Atlas.

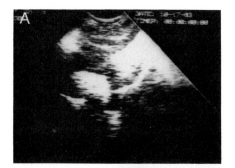

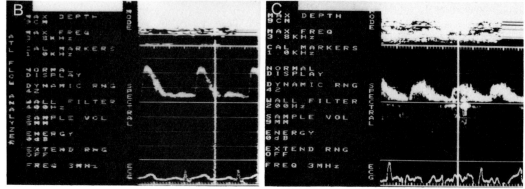

Figure 23.8. Coarctation of the aorta: suprasternal notch view. *A,* A white shelf in the descending aorta, at the level of the left subclavian artery, represents the coarct site. *B,* Normal Doppler spectral waveform in the descending aorta. *C,* Doppler spectral waveform in the descending aorta in coarctation. This is characterized by slow upslope, slow downslope, and contrived runoff flow in diastole.

Identification and differentiation of anatomic types of VSDs can be accomplished easily by two-dimensional echocardiography (15). Although the interventricular septum is a complex curvilinear structure of varied spatial orientation, it can be viewed in its entirety by two-dimensional echocardiography. This allows noninvasive localization of the defect in any position: membranous, endocardial cushion, muscular, or conoventricular.

Subxiphoid parasagittal/transverse imaging is performed with clockwise angulation of the transducer from the junction of the superior and the inferior vena cava to the left. This will display first the membranous and endocardial cushion segments and subsequently the conoventricular/subpulmonic and muscular septum. The subxiphoid four-chamber and apical four-chamber views will also demonstrate the position of these defects. Endocardial cushion portion defects will be seen in these views at the level of the atrioventricular valves. Cranial angulation with the ascending aorta in view will visualize subaortic peri-

membranous VSDs. Continued cranial angulation with the right ventricular outflow tract in view will demonstrate subpulmonic defects.

The parasternal long-axis view often will demonstrate a VSD. However, this view is *most* useful in enabling alignment of a pulsed or continuous wave Doppler beam parallel to flow (left-to-right ventricular flow). This allows estimation of both direction and velocity of the shunt (16, 17).

In cases of dropout of echoes, which can create a false-positive diagnosis of VSD, Doppler echocardiography has greatly aided in differentiating echo dropout from VSD. This sensitivity has been increased by color flow mapping. Doppler echocardiography has aided further in defining flow patterns across a VSD (left-to-right, right-to-left, or bidirectional). Specifically, when the apparent orifice of the VSD is small (septal aneurysm formation with tricuspid septal leaflet apparatus), pulsed Doppler echocardiography can identify a left-to-right shunt in spite of apparent spontaneous closure. The situation of septal aneurysm formation with an apparently small orifice can be quite deceptive; many of these defects have a large flow orifice.

Doppler color flow mapping has aided in identification of these types of shunts (18, 19). Small muscular VSDs, not easily visualized by two-dimensional echocardiography, are identified easily by color flow mapping (20, 21). Often, because of the curvilinear orientation of the interventricular septum, these small VSDs are not detected by pulsed Doppler techniques. Also, multiple VSDs are seen more easily by color flow mapping, especially in the difficult-to-image muscular septum.

Ventricular septal defects characterized by bidirectional shunting (e.g., Fallot's tetralogy, pulmonary hypertension) are visualized easily by two-dimensional echocardiography (22). Flow patterns across the VSD are demonstrated clearly by Doppler color flow mapping techniques. In both cases, early systolic left-to-right shunting is followed by late right-to-left shunting.

In the immediate postoperative period after patch closure of a VSD, regardless of type, it is easy to be confused by residual or altered murmurs. Color flow mapping allows assessment of residual VSD patch leaks.

Compared with other Doppler techniques, color flow mapping does not depend as greatly on the plane of flow being parallel to the Doppler beam. In these cases, however, color flow imaging is best in the parasternal long-axis view. In this orientation, left-to-right or right-to-left transinterventricular septal flows are parallel to the imaging beam.

The natural history of VSDs includes spontaneous diminution in size and often complete closure. Two-dimensional echocardiography is of great value in following these defects over time (Fig. 23.9).

Endocardial Cushion Defects

Two-dimensional echocardiography is often most sensitive and specific for diagnosing endocardial cushion-type VSDs and differentiating complete from partial atrioventricular canals. Ostium primum ASDs with mitral valve abnormalities (cleft) are seen easily on subxiphoid or apical four-chamber views. The cleft mitral valve is demonstrated in either subxiphoid transverse or parasternal short-axis images at the level of the atrioventricular septum and mitral valve. Both apical and subxiphoid four-chamber views clearly show anchoring of the chordae to the crest of the ventricular sep-

tum and identifying criss-crossing of the chordae across the VSD (Fig. 23.10).

Atrial Septal Defect

Two-dimensional echocardiography has been quite useful in imaging ASDs of all types (23–25). Visualization of the complete interatrial septum has been accomplished most successfully from the subxiphoid four-chamber and transverse parasagittal views. The examination begins perpendicular to the frontal plane, parallel to the horizontal axis of the trunk, with the transducer cranially angulated. In this manner, the interatrial septum and right pulmonary vein are identified, along with the mitral and tricuspid annuli. Both the septum primum and the central portion of the interatrial septum (fossa ovalis) are identified in this view. The most superior portion of the interatrial septum, where a sinus venous defect may be present, is best visualized in the parasagittal transverse view at the level of the inferior and superior venae cavae. Due to the great distance from the transducer, echo dropout in the area of the fossa ovalis often can produce a false-positive result. Pulsed Doppler echocardiography has proven to be a reliable tool in discriminating between true and false positives, as well as in determining the presence of a left-to-right shunt at the level of the atrial septal defect (26).

Contrast echocardiography has been used to verify the presence of an ASD. However, Doppler color flow mapping has been used successfully to locate precisely both typical and atypical defects and differentiate between true- and false-positive dropout (27). Quantitative and semiquantitative application of pulsed Doppler echocardiography at the level of the defect has also been reported.

The morphology of the Doppler velocities in the right atrium near the area of a suspected ASD is diagnostic, with a large broad peak occurring during the electrocardiographic QRS complex and a second peak occurring during atrial systole. The second peak is of much lower amplitude and duration than the first. Velocity of flow by pulsed Doppler has correlated well with the Qp:Qs ratio. Planimetry of pulmonary and systemic flow patterns by pulsed Doppler has been validated and correlated with Qp:Qs shunts (28, 29). Quantitative estimation of left-to-right shunt in ASD has been obtained by Doppler color flow mapping (30, 31).

In a number of cases, appearance on two-dimensional echocardiography of a large aneurysm

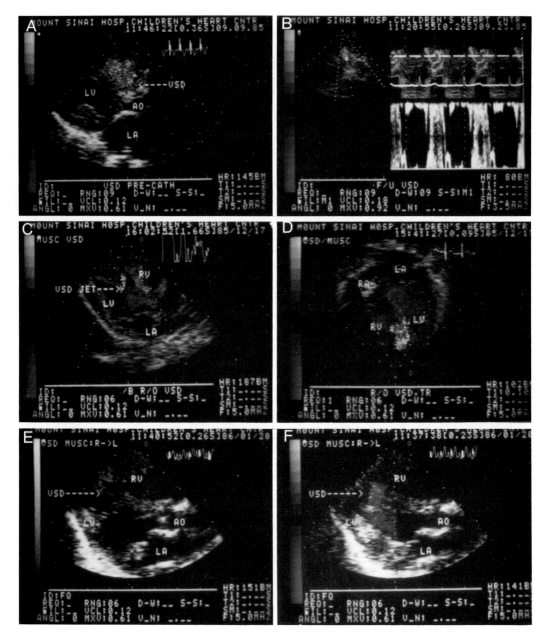

Figure 23.9. *A*, Subaortic, perimembranous type seen in the parasternal long-axis view. Mosaic jet is seen across the VSD from the left (*LV*) to the right ventricle. *AO* = aorta, *LA* = left atrium. *B*, Doppler examination of the mosaic jet in *panel A*. The *lower half* shows a typical pulsed Doppler spectral waveform of high velocity, multifrequency positive flow across the VSD. The *upper half* shows color M-mode of mosaic flow throughout systole. *RV* = right ventricle. *C*, Muscular VSD seen in the parasternal long-axis view. Note the small mosaic jet across the intraventricular septum. *RV* = right ventricle. *D*, Muscular VSD seen in the apical four-chamber view (apex down) and showing the mosaic flow pattern at the level of the VSD. In spite of this view's virtual 90° angle to the septum, the VSD flow is seen easily. *E*, Apicomuscular VSD in a newborn seen from the parasternal long-axis view. Note the moderate-sized VSD deep in the muscular septum. *F*, Right (*RV*)-to-left (*LV*)-shunt at the level of the VSD noted in blue, from the same patient as in *E*. See this figure in Color Atlas.

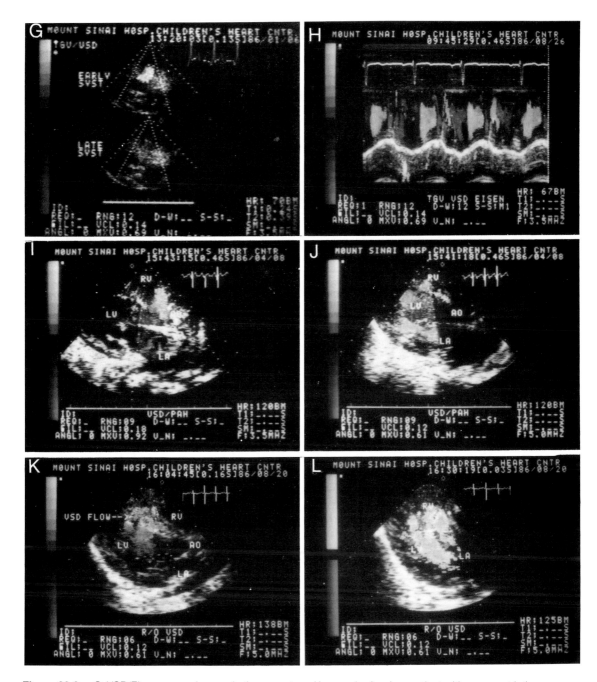

Figure 23.9. *G*, VSD/Eisenmenger's seen in the parasternal long-axis view in a patient with a nonrestrictive VSD and severe pulmonary hypertension. The *upper half* shows early systolic left-to-right flow across the VSD in red. The *lower half* shows late systolic right-to-left flow in blue. *H*, Color M-mode demonstrates quadriphasic trans-VSD flow in Eisenmenger's. Early left-to-right (red) systolic flow and late systolic right-to-left flow (blue), early diastolic left-to-right flow (red) and late diastolic right-to-left flow (blue). *I*, Parasternal long-axis view with color flow clearly demonstrates left-to-right (red) transseptal flow across a perimembranous subaortic defect. *J*, Scanning the septum, we find a small (red) LV-to-RV jet at the lower muscular septum level. *K–M*, Multiple VSDs. *K*, Parasternal long-axis view shows two jets in red across the muscular interventricular septum. *L*, With the velocity indicator off, the two jets are seen more easily (orange). See this figure in Color Atlas.

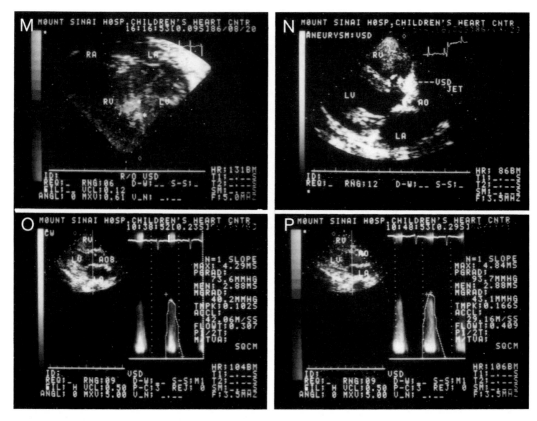

Figure 23.9 *M*, Apical four-chamber view in the same patient. Two muscular VSDs are clearly seen (∗) as displayed by the two transseptal (red) jets. *N–P*, Continuous wave estimation of pulmonary artery pressure in VSD. *N*, Parasternal long-axis shows septal aneurysm across a perimembranous VSD. This often causes the VSD jet to enter the RV eccentrically. *O*, Continuous wave (*CW*) interrogation shows maximal velocity to be 4.29 m/sec across the VSD, calculating a peak gradient of 74 mm Hg by a modified Bernoulli equation. *P*, Color flow-guided continuous wave interrogation of the eccentric trans-VSD jets now gives a peak velocity of 4.8 m/sec, calculating a transseptal pressure drop of 94 mm Hg. In the former case, estimated peak pulmonary artery pressure would have been overestimated by 20 mm Hg. See this figure in Color Atlas.

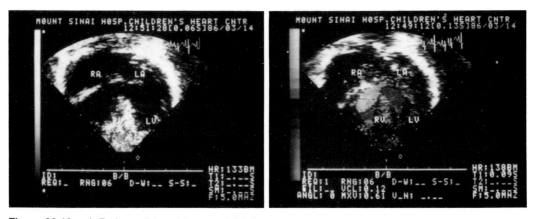

Figure 23.10. *A*, Endocardial cushion-type VSD (apical four-chamber view). Note the VSD located at the level of the atrioventricular valve (posterior). *LA* = left atrium, *LV* = left ventricle, *RA* = right atrium, *RV* = right ventricle. *B*, Color flow in the above case shows red jet across the VSD, from LV to RV. See this figure in Color Atlas.

of the interatrial septum suggested virtual closure of a VSD. The addition of Doppler color flow mapping and color flow guided pulsed Doppler echocardiography demonstrated large left-to-right shunts in spite of the septal aneurysm. These patients underwent surgical closure of the defects (Fig. 23.11).

Patent Ductus Arteriosus

Sahn and Allen (32) were the first to demonstrate direct imaging of the ductus arteriosus. Parasternal short-axis views at the level of the great vessels, with superior angulation, visualized the ductus as a distal continuation of the pulmonary artery extending into the descending aorta. More recent studies by Huhta et al. (33) have demonstrated excellent ductal morphologic imaging in neonates. However, they encountered limitations when two-dimensional echocardiography was used without Doppler echocardiography in determining ductal patency. They concluded that the best method for noninvasive assessment of the ductus arteriosus was combined two-dimensional and Doppler echocardiography. Here again, suprasternal or high left parasternal views were used with an echocardiographic plane directed from the right side of the neck toward the cardiac apex.

In our experience, these two-dimensional echocardiographic views have also been quite successful in identifying the ductus arteriosus, but combined Doppler imaging increases the sensitivity. We have used pulsed Doppler to identify ductal patency, taking the sample volume from the pulmonary artery. We also have examined the aortic arch from both the suprasternal notch and subxiphoid position to identify ductal patency and discriminate other types of systemic-to-pulmonary runoffs. These include aorta-pulmonary window, surgically created systemic-to-pulmonary artery shunts, and coronary arteriovenous fistulas.

Doppler color flow mapping, using the parasternal short-axis view in the main pulmonary artery, gives an excellent color flow pattern in ductal patency (34). This is a characteristic red-orange pattern of left-to-right ductal flow from the aorta to the pulmonary artery along the left superior wall of the main pulmonary artery.

In ductal patency, there is diastolic flow reversal in the descending aorta. By this same principle, pulsed Doppler spectral flow images show color flow reversal. In the subxiphoid parasagittal view there is red systolic flow in the descending aorta (toward the transducer) and blue diastolic flow reversal (flow away from the transducer). This phenomenon may also be viewed from the suprasternal or high parasternal positions (35) (Fig. 23.12).

Pulmonary Artery Hypertension

Pulmonary hypertension associated with a VSD or endocardial cushion defect is a common diagnostic problem in pediatric cardiology. Heretofore, only invasive methods have been available for diagnosis. Recently, pulsed Doppler echocardiography has provided spectral waveform tracing patterns, both qualitative and quantitative, that are diagnostic of pulmonary artery hypertension (36, 37).

In the presence of pulmonary hypertension there is an increase in the slope of acceleration and deceleration, with decreased acceleration time (time to peak flow). We have described changes in the morphology of the pulmonary artery spectral waveform in these patients in response to oxygen administration. These changes are decreased acceleration and deceleration slope with increase in acceleration time and normalization of the spectral waveform trace. Since our first report, we have documented these changes in seven patients with congenital heart lesions and pulmonary hypertension, using simultaneous recording of changes in Qp:Qs and resistance calculations during cardiac catheterization. The usefulness of this Doppler technique is not only in demonstrating pulmonary hypertension, but also in documenting reversibility in response to pulmonary vasodilation with oxygen (Fig. 23.13).

Valvular Lesions

Congenital atrioventricular and semilunar value abnormalities do occur. However, a detailed discussion of the echocardiographic diagnosis of these defects appears elsewhere in this text and will not be repeated here. One exception will be made: the diagnosis of valvular pulmonic stenosis. The advent of pulmonary catheter balloon valvuloplasty has intensified the interest in noninvasive assessment of the severity of pulmonic stenosis.

The use of two-dimensional echocardiography to assess stenotic pulmonary valves is well described. Parasternal short-axis views at the level of the great vessels clearly demonstrate thickened, doming valves. Pulsed Doppler echocardiography can qualitatively identify turbulence of flow distal to the pulmonic valve. At lower velocities of flow, pulsed Doppler can quantify the

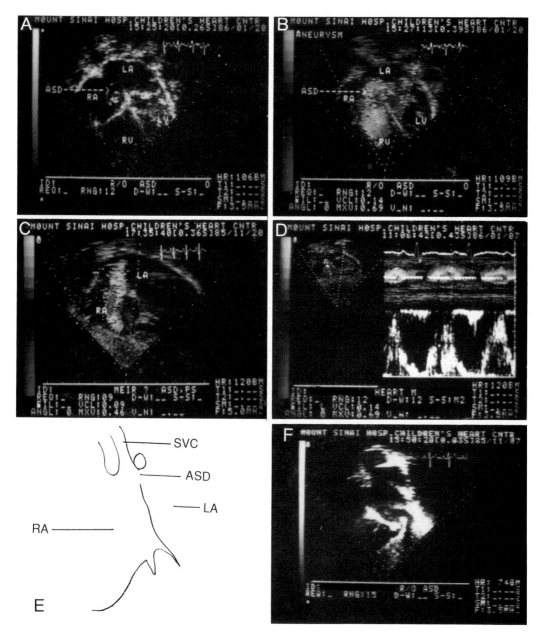

Figure 23.11. ASDs. *A*, A secundum ASD is noted (*arrrow*) in the apical four-chamber view (apex down). The white echogenic area in the right atrium is evidence of aneurysm formation. *RA* = right atrium, *LA* = left atrium, *LV* = left ventricle, *RV* = right ventricle. *B*, In spite of the apparently small orifice seen in *A*, there is moderate-to-large left (*LA*)-to-right (*RA*) shunting. This is seen as the orange color transversing the septum. *C*, Subxiphoid four-chamber view (apex down) in another patient with ASD. The blue center to the large jet (left-to-right shunt) is due to aliasing because of high flow velocity. *D*, The pulsed Doppler sample volume on the right atrial side of the ASD shows a typical spectral waveform pattern (*bottom*). The color M-mode (*upper half*) shows red-colored flow with an aliased blue center. *E*, An illustration of a typical sinus venosus ASD located in the most superior portion of the interatrial septum, just beneath the superior vena cava (*SVC*). Imaging plane is the subxiphoid transverse/parasagittal view. *F*, This plane is best for the two-dimensional echo imaging of this defect. See this figure in Color Atlas.

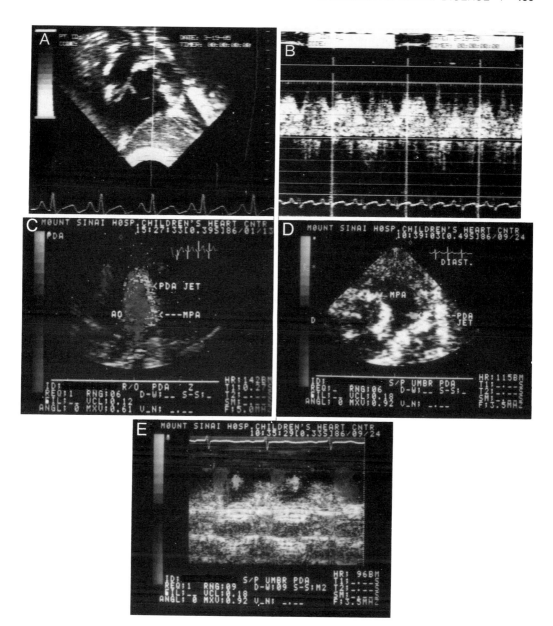

Figure 23.12. Patent ductus arteriosus. *A,* Subxiphoid transverse/parasagittal view showing the entire aortic arch with branch vessels and a large patent ductus arteriosus. The pulsed Doppler sample volume is in this vessel. *B,* Typical Doppler waveform pattern in the open ductus, showing continuous positive flow. *C,* Parasternal short-axis view, main pulmonary artery *(MPA).* Note the mosaic patent ductus arteriosus *(PDA)* jet along the superior left wall of the main pulmonary artery, typically seen on color flow. *AO* = aorta. *D,* Sensitivity of color flow is seen in this example of a child who underwent umbrella closure of a patent ductus arteriosus. Parasternal short-axis view. The echogenic area at the main pulmonary artery bifurcation is the umbrella. Note the thin orange jet entering the pulmonary artery from this umbrella area. It represents residual PDA shunting. *E,* Color M-mode shows blue systolic pulmonary artery blood flow. The small diastolic orange in the main pulmonary area is reflective of the reversed diastolic flow of ductal entry. See this figure in Color Atlas.

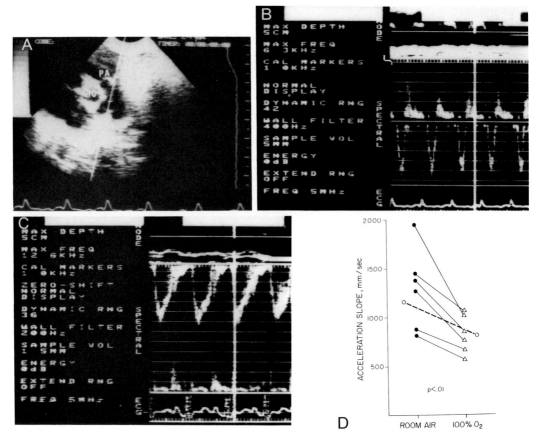

Figure 23.13. Pulmonary hypertension: Doppler study. *A*, Sample volume is seen in the main pulmonary artery (*PA*) distal to the pulmonic valve (parasternal short-axis view). *AO* = aorta. *B*, Doppler spectral waveform in room air in a patient with pulmonary hypertension. Note the rapid acceleration and deceleration and short acceleration time (*AcT* − *time to reach peak flow*). *C*, Changes in waveform in response to 100% inspired oxygen. Note the visibly decreased acceleration and deceleration, as well as increased acceleration time. *D–F*, Graphic representation of our findings on response to oxygen in six infants with pulmonary hypertension and congenital heart lesions. The *Black circles* = room air, *triangles* = 100% oxygen, *open circles connected by dashed lines* = mean values. These studies, performed at the time of cardiac catheterization, reflect catheter-proven differences in pulmonary vascular resistance.

degree of pulmonic stenosis. Where higher velocities of flow are observed, continuous wave Doppler can estimate the peak velocity accurately (38). By calculation using the modified Bernoulli equation, continuous wave Doppler can estimate peak systolic gradient across the valve. Numerous comparison studies of Doppler estimated versus catheterization-measured gradients have shown excellent correlation between the two techniques.

In the past few years many centers have been successful in using balloon dilatation to alleviate outflow obstruction caused by a stenotic pulmonary valve. This has again put a premium on the

accuracy of Doppler as a noninvasive technique used to assess the initial success and subsequent response to valvuloplasty.

In our initial group of 15 patients, Doppler-estimated pulmonic valve gradients were obtained before, immediately after, and in long-term follow-up after balloon valvuloplasty. Comparison of Doppler-derived gradients and catheterization-measured gradients showed a correlation coefficient of 0.98. In these patients, the need for follow-up cardiac catheterization was eliminated (Fig. 23.14).

Measurement of the pulmonary annulus by two-

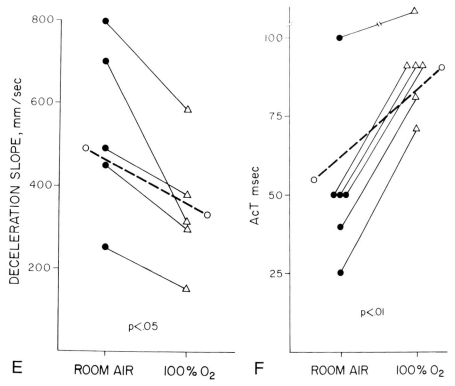

Figure 23.13 *Continued*

dimensional echocardiography has also correlated well with measurements made directly from the angiogram ($r = 0.99$). Correct assessment of the pulmonary annulus is essential in selecting the appropriate balloon diameter for the dilatation.

FETAL ECHOCARDIOGRAPHY
(Also see Chapter 22)

Evaluation of cardiac structure and function in the fetus is a recent advance. Two-dimensional echocardiographic images allow accurate description of fetal cardiac anatomy, and pulsed Doppler can investigate fetal hemodynamics. There is no evidence to suggest routine fetal ultrasound has any adverse effect on the developing human fetus. However, screening for fetal heart disease should be restricted to pregnant women considered to be at higher-than-normal risk (39–41).

Risk factors are classified as fetal, maternal, or familial. Fetal risk factors include intrauterine growth retardation, fetal cardiac arrhythmias, abnormal amniocentesis, or other abnormalities observed by ultrasound. Maternal risk factors include congenital heart disease, alcohol ingestion, polyhydramnios, or diabetes. Familial risk factors

include genetic syndromes or congenital heart disease.

Except for cases where the fetus is in an unfavorable position, echocardiography can provide visualization of fetal cardiac structure. Overall, echocardiography is successful more than 90% of the time. We have found that standard two-dimensional views—including apical four-chamber and parasternal short-axis views at the level of the great vessels—were obtained easily in virtually all cases.

Clear definition of intracardiac anatomy is visualized beginning about 18–20 weeks into gestation. At this time echocardiography can identify the atria, ventricles, atrioventricular valves, concordant great vessel position, and patent foramen ovale. Sequential atrioventricular contraction may be identified on both two-dimensional and M-mode echocardiography. Pulsed Doppler echocardiography can examine flow across the atrioventricular valves and semilunar valves and detect regurgitation if present. Fetal Doppler color flow mapping has been useful in a number of studies in identifying atrioventricular valve regurgitation (42).

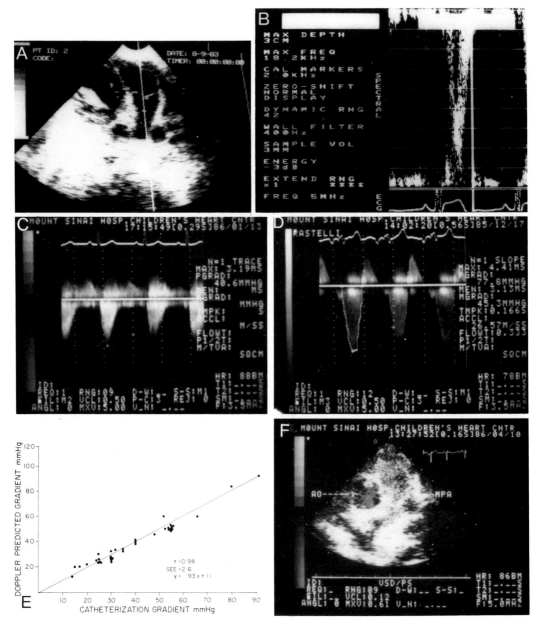

Figure 23.14. Pulmonic stenosis. *A*, Pulsed Doppler sample volume placed distal to the pulmonic valve in the main pulmonary artery (parasternal short-axis view). *B*, Pulsed Doppler spectral waveform showing a turbulent high velocity jet. *C*, Continuous wave Doppler tracing allows accurate calculation of peak flow velocities and gradients in patients with moderate or severe stenosis. *D*, Continuous wave Doppler tracing in the right ventricular outflow tract within a conduit. Note the high peak flow velocity (*4.4 m/sec*) and gradient (*77.8 mm Hg*). *E*, Graphic representation of the correlation between Doppler-estimated and catheterization-measured transpulmonic gradients in patients undergoing balloon valvuloplasty in our institution. *F*, Color flow representation of pulmonic stenosis (parasternal short-axis view). Note that the mosaic color pattern begins proximal to the level of the pulmonic valve, indicating a proximal level of turbulence in the right ventricular outflow tract. This child had infundibular pulmonic stenosis. *AO* = aorta, *MPA* = main pulmonary artery. See this figure in Color Atlas.

We have found Doppler color flow mapping useful in rapidly identifying umbilical arterial and venous flow. In addition, pulsed Doppler has demonstrated its worth in spectral wave pattern analysis of cardiac structures to evaluate the fetoplacental unit. Major structural abnormalities have been detected quite successfully and accurately by this technique in many studies. We have, in this manner, identified prenatally cases of endocardial cushion defect with right-sided predominance, hypoplastic right ventricular syndrome, and hypoplastic left heart syndrome. Continued application in high-risk pregnancies will doubtless allow for increasingly earlier identification of significant lesions. This will allow better planning by the obstetric and pediatric team for medical and psychologic management of the remainder of the pregnancy, delivery, and neonatal period. Normal fetal studies will go far in allaying the fears of parents who have previously had children with severe congenital heart lesions.

SUMMARY

Noninvasive cardiac imaging has greatly enhanced the potential for defining the anatomic and physiologic aspects of cardiac structure and function in infants and children with congenital heart disease. This is largely due to advances in two-dimensional echocardiography; pulsed and continuous wave Doppler in a duplex format; Doppler color flow mapping; and the ability to superimpose blood flow on the two-dimensional echocardiographic image. This technology has resulted in major changes in both diagnostic and therapeutic decisions.

Infants at high risk may no longer need to undergo cardiac catheterization, since accurate anatomic and physiologic assessment is available noninvasively (43). Also, serial follow-up is made easy and risk-free in both surgical and nonsurgical cases. Current intraoperative studies have begun to demonstrate the ability to improve greatly the decision making process even during surgery (44–46). Continued, comprehensive, integrated use of these imaging techniques will continue to add to our understanding of the many facets of congenital heart disease.

REFERENCES

1. Ritter SB: Recent advances in color-Doppler assessment of congenital heart disease. *Echocardiography* 5:457–478, 1988.

2. Omoto R (ed): *Color Atlas of Real Time Two-Dimensional Doppler Echocardiography.* Tokyo, Shindan-To-Chiryo, 1984.

3. DeMaria A (ed): *Two-Dimensional Doppler (Color) Flow Imaging: Principles and Practice.* Echocardiography II, 1985.

4. Namekawa K, Kasai C, Tsukamoto M: Real time blood flow imaging system utilizing autocorrelation techniques. *Ultrasound* 8:203–208, 1982.

5. Namekawa K, Kasai C, Tsukamoto M: Imaging of blood flow using autocorrelation. *Ultrasound Med Biol* 8:138, 1982.

6. Swenson RE, Sahn DJ, Valdes-Cruz LM: Color flow Doppler mapping in congenital heart disease. *Echocardiography* 2:545–549, 1985.

7. Henry WL, DeMaria A, Gramiak R: Report of the American Society of Echocardiography Committee on Nomenclature and Standards in Two-Dimensional Echocardiography. *Circulation* 62:211–217, 1980.

8. Lange LW, Sahn DJ, Allen H: Subxiphoid cross-sectional echocardiography in infants and children with congenital heart disease. *Circulation* 59:513–560.

9. Rice MJ, Seward JB, Hagler DJ: Impact of two-dimensional echocardiography on the management of distressed newborns in whom cardiac disease is suspected. *Am J Cardiol* 51:288–292, 1983.

10. Long WA: Structural cardiovascular abnormalities presenting as persistent pulmonary hypertension of the newborn. In: *Clinics in Perinatology: Symposium on Neonatal Pulmonary Hypertension II.* Philadelphia, WB Saunders, 1984, pp 601–626.

11. Ritter SB, Arnon R, Steinfeld L: Anomalous venous drainage: Identification of Doppler color flow mapping. *Circulation* 1986.

12. Cooper MJ, Teitel DF, Silverman NH: Study of the infradiaphragmatic total anomalous pulmonary venous connection with cross-sectional and pulsed Doppler echocardiography. *Circulation* 70:412–416, 1984.

13. Bierman FZ, Williams RG: Prospective diagnosis of *d*-transposition of the great arteries in neonates by subxiphoid two-dimensional echocardiography. *Circulation* 60:1496–1502, 1979.

14. Sanders SP, Bierman FZ, Williams RG: Conotruncal malformations: Diagnosis in infancy using subxiphoid two-dimensional echocardiography. *Am J Cardiol* 50:1361–1367, 1982.

15. Bierman FZ, Fellows K, Williams RG: Prospective identification of ventricular septal defects in infancy using subxiphoid two-dimensional echocardiography. *Circulation* 62:807–817, 1980.

16. Stevenson JG, Kawabori I, Dooley TK: Diagnosis of ventricular septal defect by pulsed Doppler echocardiography: Sensitivity, specificity, and limitations. *Circulation* 58:322–328, 1978.

17. Marx GR, Allen H, Goldberg SJ: Doppler echocardiographic estimation of systolic pulmonary artery pressure in pediatric patients with interventricular communications. *J Am Coll Cardiol* 6:1132–1137, 1985.

18. Stevenson JG, Kawabori I, Brandestini N: Color coded Doppler visualization of flow within ventricular septal defects: Implications for peak pulmo-

nary artery pressure. *Am J Cardiol* 49:944–949, 1982.

19. Sahn DJ, Swensen RE, Valdes-Cruz LM: Two-dimensional color flow mapping for evaluation of ventricular septal defect shunts: A new diagnostic modality (Abstr). *Circulation* 70:364, 1984.

20. Ritter SB, Kawai D, Rothe WA, Golinko RJ: Doppler color flow mapping in the diagnosis and assessment of ventricular septal defects. *Dynamic Cardiovasc Imag* 1:194–198, 1987.

21. Ritter SB: Color-flow echocardiography: Ventricular septal defect. *Primary Cardiol* 14:27–34, 1988.

22. Kyo S, Omoto R, Takamoto S: Non-invasive analysis of bidirectional multiphasic intracardiac shunts by real time two-dimensional echocardiography (Abstr). *Circulation* 70:365, 1984.

23. Bierman FZ, Williams RG: Subxiphoid two-dimensional imaging of the interatrial septum in infants and neonates with congenital heart disease. *Circulation* 60:80–90, 1979.

24. Shub A, Dimopoulos IN, Seward JB: Sensitivity of two-dimensional echocardiography in the direct visualization of atrial septal defect utilizing the subcostal approach: Experience with 154 patients. *J Am Coll Cardiol* 2:127–135, 1983.

25. Stevenson JG, Kawabori I: Sequential two-dimensional echo/Doppler: Improved noninvasive diagnosis of atrial septal defect (Abstr). *Circulation* 68:110, 1983.

26. Marx GR, Allen HD, Goldberg SJ: Transatrial septal velocity measurement by Doppler echocardiography in atrial septal defect: Correlation with Qp:Qs ratio. *Am J Cardiol* 5:1162–1167, 1985.

27. Sommer RJ, Ritter SB: Color-flow echocardiography: Atrial septal defect. *Primary Cardiol* 15:43–50, 1989.

28. Kitabatake A, Inoue N, Asao M: Noninvasive evaluation of the ratio of pulmonary to systemic flow in atrial septal defect by duplex Doppler echocardiography. *Circulation* 69:73–79, 1984.

29. Valdes-Cruz LM, Horowitz S, Masel E: A pulsed Doppler echocardiographic method for calculating pulmonary and systemic flow in atrial level shunts: Validation studies in animals and initial human experience. *Circulation* 69:80–86, 1984.

30. Kyo S, Omoto R, Takamoto S: Quantitative estimation of intracardiac shunt flow in atrial septal defect by real time two-dimensional color flow Doppler (Abstr). *Circulation* 70:39, 1984.

31. Kyo S, Omoto R, Takamoto S: Clinical significance of color flow mapping real time two-dimensional Doppler echocardiography (2-D Doppler) in congenital heart disease (Abstr). *Circulation* 70:37, 1984.

32. Sahn DJ, Allen HD: Real time cross-sectional echocardiographic imaging of the patent ductus arteriosus in infants and children. *Circulation* 58:343–347, 1978.

33. Huhta JC, Cohn N, Gutgesell HP: Patency of ductus arteriosus in normal neonates: Two-dimensional echocardiography versus Doppler assessment. *J Am Coll Cardiol* 4:P561–564, 1984.

34. Kyo S, Shime H, Omoto R: Evaluation of intracardiac shunt flow in premature infants by color flow mapping real time two-dimensional Doppler echo. *Circulation* 70:456–461, 1984.

35. Ritter SB, Golinko RJ, Cooper RS: Systemic to pulmonary artery anastomoses: Pulsed Doppler evaluation of aortic flow properties (Abstr). *J Utrasound Med* 3:42, 1984.

36. Kitabatake A, Inoue M, Saoa M: Noninvasive evaluation of pulmonary hypertension by a pulsed Doppler technique. *Circulation* 68:302–309, 1983.

37. Ritter SB, Copper RS, Golinko RJ: Noninvasive assessment of pulmonary hypertension, pulmonary vascular reactivity, and intracardiac shunting: Pulsed Doppler application. *J Cardiovasc Ultrasonog* 5:213–221, 1985.

38. Lima CO, Sahn EJ, Valdes-Cruz LM: Noninvasive prediction of transvalvular pressure gradients in patients with pulmonary stenosis by quantitative two-dimensional echocardiographic Doppler studies. *Circulation* 67:866–881, 1983.

39. Kleinman CS, Hobbins JC, Jaffe CC: Echocardiographic studies of the human fetus: Prenatal diagnosis of congenital heart disease and cardiac dysrhythmias. *Pediatrics* 65:1059–1067, 1980.

40. Lange LW, Sahn DJ, Allen HD: Qualitative real time cross-sectional echocardiographic imaging of the human fetus during the second half of pregnancy. *Circulation* 62:799–806, 1980.

41. Silverman N, Golbus MS: Echocardiographic techniques for assessing normal and abnormal fetal cardiac anatomy. *J Am Coll Cardiol* 5:205–210, 1985.

42. DeVore GR, Hornstein J, Siassi B: Doppler color flow mapping: Its use in the prenatal diagnosis of congenital heart disease in the human fetus. *Echocardiography* 2:551–557, 1985.

43. Stark J, Smallhorn J, Huhta J: Surgery for congenital heart defects diagnosed with cross-sectional echocardiography. *Circulation* 68:129–138, 1983.

44. Takamoto S, Kyo S, Adachi H: Intraoperative color flow mapping by real time two-dimensional Doppler echocardiography for evaluation of valvular and congenital heart disease and vascular disease. *J Thorac Cardiovasc Surg* 90:802–812, 1985.

45. Goldman ME, Thys D, Ritter SB: Transesophageal real time Doppler flow imaging: a new method for intraoperative cardiac evaluation (Abstr). *J Am Coll Cardiol* 1, 1986.

46. Hillel Z, Thys D, Ritter SB: Two-dimensional color flow Doppler echocardiography: Intraoperative monitoring of cardiac shunt flows in patients with congenital heart disease. *J Cardiothorac Anesth* 1:42–46, 1987.

24

Echocardiography of Pericardial Diseases

Satyabrata Chatterjee, M.D., Tahir Tak, M.D.,
Shahbudin H. Rahimtoola, M.B.,
P. Anthony N. Chandraratna, M.D.

PERICARDIAL EFFUSION

The noninvasive diagnosis of pericardial effusion was one of the first clinical applications of echocardiography. The pericardial sac normally contains a small amount of fluid and separates the heart from surrounding structures. On the echocardiogram, the anterior wall of the right ventricle adjoins the anterior pericardium and chest wall, and the posterior left ventricle wall is in contact with the posterior pericardium and pleura. Pericardial effusion is relatively echo-free, and a separation between the epicardium and pericardium is seen. It appears anteriorly between echoes from the anterior pericardium and epicardium of the right ventricular wall and posteriorly between the echoes from the left ventricular epicardium and posterior pericardium (1). Typical findings of pericardial effusion on M-mode study are demonstrated in Figure 24.1.

The three echocardiographic hallmarks of pericardial effusion are an echo-free space posterior to the heart, disappearance or marked reduction of the space at the left ventricular-left atrial junction, and the absence of motion of the pericardium (2). Although in many instances the posterior echo-free space stops at the junction of the left ventricle and left atrium, the echo-free space may extend behind the posterior wall of the left atrium into the oblique pericardial sinus in a large pericardial effusion.

The volume of pericardial fluid can be characterized roughly by M-mode echocardiography as mild, moderate, or severe, provided the fluid is not loculated. Horowitz et al. (3) evaluated the efficacy of M-mode echocardiography in estimating the amount of pericardial effusion and described six patterns (Fig. 24.2). In *pattern A*, a single band of echoes representing both the epicardium and pericardium is present, but there is no separation during the cardiac cycle. In *pattern B*, an echo-free space is present between the pericardium and the epicardium during mid to late systole and disappears with early diastole. *Pattern C*, where an echo-free space is present in diastole, represents the transition phase between *patterns B* and *D* and is subdivided into two parts, C_1 and C_2. In C_1, the pericardial movement follows that of the epicardium. In C_2, the pericardial echo is "flat" and shows no movement when compared with that of the epicardium. *Pattern D* is characterized by an echo-free space that persists throughout the cardiac cycle between the posterior epicardium and the flat pericardium. Patients with *pattern D* had more than 50 ml fluid, a larger amount than associated with echocardiographic *patterns A*, *B*, and *C* (4). In *pattern E*, an echo-free space is present between the epicardium and pericardium with parallel motion of these structures. *Pattern E* represents a thickened pericardium.

With large effusions, an echo-free space begins to appear between the anterior pericardium and epicardium of the right ventricular wall (3, 5) (Figure 24.3). As pericardial volume increases, the space for movement of the entire heart within the pericardial sac enlarges. A swinging, twisting motion of the heart around its attachment at the level of the great vessels ensues. The motion is generally posterior during systole and leftward and anterior during diastole. This swinging motion of the heart in the pericardial sac results in the appearance of valvular and wall motion abnormalities in M-mode studies of patients with large pericardial effusions (6–8) (Table 24.1). There may be an illusion of mitral and tricuspid valve

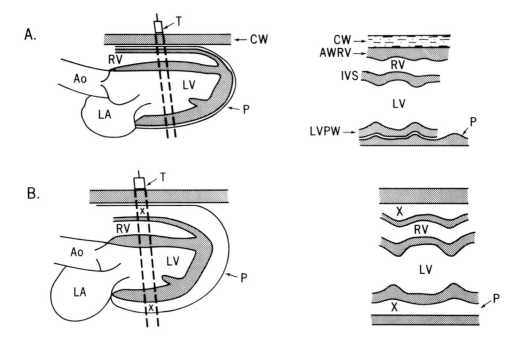

Figure 24.1. Schematic representation of M-mode and two-dimensional echocardiograms. *A*, Normal. *B*, Anterior and posterior pericardial effusion. The echo-free space between the chest wall and anterior right ventricular wall represents a pericardial effusion. The ultrasonic beam is directed through the left ventricular cavity at the same level at which right and left ventricular dimensions are measured. *Ao* = aorta; *AWRV* = anterior wall, right ventricle; *CW* = chest wall; *IVS* = interventricular septum; *LA* = left atrium; *LV* = left ventricle; *LVPW* = left ventricular posterior wall; *P* = pericardium; *RV* = right ventricle; *T* = transducer; *X* = pericardial effusion.

prolapse, systolic anterior motion of the mitral valve (Fig. 24.4), early systolic closure of the aortic valve, midsystolic notching of the pulmonary valve, or paradoxical anterior motion of the interventricular septum. These findings are artifacts only seen on M-mode studies because the chest wall is used as a reference point. With two-dimensional echocardiography, the motion of various intracardiac structures can be compared with one another instead of the chest wall (2, 9).

A major advantage of two-dimensional echocardiography is its ability to assess the distribution of pericardial fluid in pericardial effusion (Table 24.2). Although M-mode echocardiography has better axial resolution, the spatial orientation inherent in two-dimensional echocardiography permits a better estimate of the distribution and amount of fluid (10) (Figure 24.5). This is particularly true with a loculated effusion where M-mode echocardiographic estimation of its size— or even presence—may be grossly in error (10, 11). In some patients, the amount of loculated fluid is small. In others, especially those who have

undergone open-heart surgery, large amounts of loculated fluid may be present and may produce cardiac tamponade. Hence, routine use of two-dimensional echocardiography to detect loculated pericardial fluid is crucial.

ECHOCARDIOGRAPHY DIAGNOSIS OF PERICARDIAL EFFUSION: SENSITIVITY AND SPECIFICITY

As experience increased, many potential pitfalls were recognized in the diagnosis of pericardial effusion by echocardiography. As good as it is, the technique is not 100% sensitive and specific. Pericardial fluid is only relatively echo-free. Increasing gain settings on the echocardiogram may fill the pericardial cavity with echoes and produce false-negative studies. Blood clots in the pericardial sac may cause a false-negative study, since clots are echogenic. In addition, animal studies revealed that when blood is injected into the pericardial sac clots (Fig. 24.6), the effusion becomes more echo-dense (12). Diagnosis of a pericardial clot is especially important. Aspira-

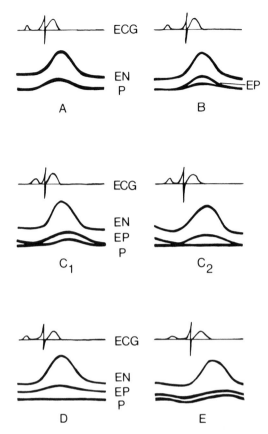

Figure 24.2. Patterns of epicardial and pericardial movement with and without pericardial effusion. (From: Horowitz MS, et al: Sensitivity and specificity of echocardiographic diagnosis of pericardial effusion.)

tion of clots is usually very difficult, and emergent surgery may be indicated if the patient develops hemodynamic embarrassment from the fluid.

False-positive studies for pericardial effusion may be caused by misinterpretation of anatomic structures. A calcified mitral annulus may be identified erroneously as the endocardium, which can result in the posterior left ventricular wall being misinterpreted as pericardial effusion. Direction and location of the M-mode transducer may also influence the echocardiographic appearance of structures (13, 14). Feigenbaum et al. (14) showed that excessive medial transducer angulation may result in misinterpretation of the left ventricular posterior wall as a pericardial effusion. Figure 24.7 illustrates this phenomenon.

A large anterior echo-free space in the absence of a posterior space may be produced by a loc-

ulated pericardial effusion. However, other conditions may produce an identical echocardiographic picture. Figure 24.8 shows an echo-free space between the anterior right ventricle and chest wall. The patient had no evidence of pericardial effusion: the false-positive diagnosis for effusion was probably due to an epicardial fat pad (15, 16). Savage et al. (17) found that the prevalence of epicardial fat mimicking a pericardial effusion was approximately 5%.

The problems of a false-positive diagnosis of pericardial effusion due to epicardial fat is seen both on M-mode and two-dimensional echocardiography. Occasionally, epicardial fat may produce both a posterior and an anterior echo-free space closely mimicking pericardial effusion (17). On two-dimensional echocardiography, fat has a granular appearance. Consequently, an anterior echo-free space with a granular appearance should suggest the possibility of an epicardial fat pad (Fig. 24.8). Other structures reported to present as an echo-free space on M-mode echocardiograms are listed in Table 24.3. These include hernias of the foramen of Morgagni (18), pericardial cysts (19), lymphomas (20), and thrombi interposed between a calcified pericardium and the right ventricular wall in constrictive pericarditis (21).

In the absence of an effusion, a posterior echo-free space may be seen on M-mode examination in patients with an extremely large left atrium that extends inferiorly behind the left ventricle (22) (Fig. 24.9). Massive ascites will produce an anterior echo-free space in the subcostal view that is difficult to distinguish from a large effusion (23). Patients on peritoneal dialysis for renal failure have subdiaphragmatic fluid that can mimic a loculated pericardial effusion. In these patients, the falciform ligament gives the appearance of a linear adhesion (24) (Fig. 24.10A–C). This appearance has been noted only in the subcostal view. Fibrinous pericarditis without effusion and pericardial infiltration by tumor or fibrosis may present as a posterior echo-free space on an M-mode study (25). However, most of these false-positive findings can be diagnosed accurately with two-dimensional echocardiography.

Differentiation between left pleural effusion and pericardial effusion often poses a particularly difficult problem in an M-mode examination. Left-sided pleural effusion presents as a posterior echo-free space on an echocardiogram. An unusually larger posterior echo-free space without evidence of anterior effusion makes the diagnosis of peri-

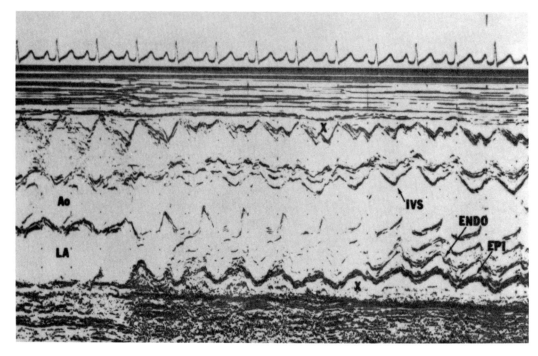

Figure 24.3. M-mode echocardiogram of a patient with anterior and posterior pericardial effusion. (From Chandraratna PAN *Echocardiography* 1:55, 1984.)

cardial effusion unlikely. Furthermore, the space may extend behind the left atrium. When both pericardial and pleural effusion occur together, the key to diagnosis is the presence of pericardial echoes that blend with the posterior left atrial wall on transducer angulation while the pleural space persists (Fig. 24.11). However, pericardial effusions with echo-free spaces posterior to the left atrium have been reported (26, 27), especially in the postsurgical patient (28, 29) and patients with extremely large effusions.

Two-dimensional echocardiography is particularly helpful in differentiating pleural from pericardial effusion. A pericardial effusion is anterior

to the descending aorta, while a pleural effusion is posterior to it (30, 31) (Fig. 24.12).

CARDIAC TAMPONADE

The hemodynamic effects of a pericardial effusion depend in part on the pressure-volume relationship of the pericardium. A small amount of fluid in a noncompliant pericardium may produce severe hemodynamic abnormalities. On the other hand, large amounts of fluid in a compliant pericardium may have no hemodynamic effect. The hemodynamic consequences depend on the amount of fluid, the rapidity with which pericardial fluid accumulates, the pressure-volume relationship of the pericardium, and the compliance of the ventricles. These factors should be borne in mind when assessing the clinical importance of an echocardiographically detected pericardial effusion.

A number of echocardiographic abnormalities have been described in patients with cardiac tamponade (Table 24.4). Excessive cardiac motion, described as "swinging" of the heart in the pericardial sac, is common (32). Phasic respiratory variation in right and left ventricular dimensions has also been described (32, 33). During inspiration, a marked increase of right ventricular di-

Table 24.1. Echocardiographic Artifacts Seen in Large Pericardial Effusions

1. Mitral valve prolapse
2. Tricuspid valve prolapse
3. Systolic anterior motion of the mitral valve
4. Early systolic closure of the aortic valve
5. Midsystolic notching of the pulmonary valve
6. Paradoxical septal motion
7. Attenuated motion of the posterior wall of the aortic root

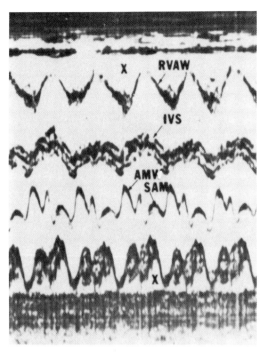

Figure 24.4. M-mode echocardiogram in a patient with pericardial effusion (*X*), illustrating pseudo-systolic anterior motion (*SAM*) of the anterior mitral leaflet (*AMV*). *IVS* = interventricular septum, *RVAW* = right ventricular anterior wall. (From Chandraratna PAN *Echocardiography* 1:55, 1984.)

mension occurs, and there is a corresponding decrease in left ventricular diameter. During expiration, the converse occurs (Fig. 24.13). However, this finding is only an exaggeration of the normal situation. A clear distinction has not been established to separate normal and abnormal findings.

D'Cruz et al. (33) reported a reduced mitral valve anterior diastolic excursion associated with a diminished mitral E–F slope during inspiration, suggesting decreased left ventricular inflow and left ventricular stroke volume. This finding, the echocardiographic correlate of a paradoxical pulse, may also be seen in conditions associated with

Table 24.2. Advantages of Two-Dimensional Echocardiography

A. Better delineation of:
  1. Distribution of fluid
  2. Pericardial cysts
  3. Intrapericardial inclusions
B. Superior imaging of pericardial contrast studies

respiratory distress, such as obstructive lung disease and pulmonary embolism (34). Conversely, patients with tamponade who are unable to produce a sufficient inspiratory effort, who have an atrial septal defect, or who have severe aortic regurgitation will not manifest this echocardiographic sign of cardiac tamponade (35).

Cardiac surgery is an important cause of tamponade, which is associated with sternotomy or thoracotomy. This diminishes the patient's respiratory effort and prevents changes in venous return that result in paradoxical pulse or its echocardiographic correlates. Consequently, these signs are not very sensitive or specific for the diagnosis of tamponade.

More recently, diastolic collapse of the right ventricle and right atrium have been proposed as sensitive indicators of cardiac tamponade. To detect diastolic compression of the right ventricle or right atrium, a slow speed, frame-by-frame playback is necessary. Right ventricular internal dimension is diminished in patients with cardiac tamponade compared with the same measurement after pericardial drainage (36). Right ventricular diastolic collapse, identified by an abnormal posterior motion of the anterior wall of the right ventricle during early to middiastole, was first described by Shina et al. (37) as an early sign of cardiac tamponade (Fig. 24.14). The peak downward motion occurs just before the QRS complex on the electrocardiogram. Following removal of the effusion, anterior right ventricular wall motion becomes normal, and the peak posterior movement occurs at the end of systole.

Cogswell et al. (38) noted that right ventricular diastolic collapse was more sensitive and specific than pulsus paradoxus in detecting increases in intrapericardial pressure during euvolemia and hypervolemia. However, the two tests were equally valuable in hypovolemic states. Figure 24.15 demonstrates diastolic collapse of the right ventricular free wall, best seen in the short-axis view. The collapse occurs in the right ventricular outflow tract, where the free wall is most compressible. Right ventricular diastolic collapse is thought to be a result of an elevated pericardial pressure that exceeds the right ventricular pressure in early diastole (39).

Collapse of the right atrium in diastole is a sensitive sign of pericardial effusion with hemodynamic compromise. During late diastole, there is an abrupt buckling of the free wall of the right and left atria toward the atrial cavity (Fig. 24.16). This collapse continues through a variable portion

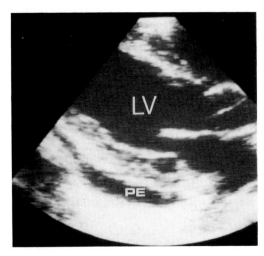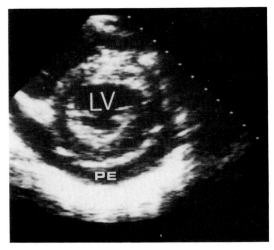

Figure 24.5. Two-dimensional echocardiogram of a patient with a pericardial effusion (*PE*). The parasternal long-axis view is shown on the *left*, and the short axis-view is shown on the *right*. *LV* = left ventricle.

of ventricular systole. Gillam et al. (40) noted this finding to have 100% sensitivity, 82% specificity, and 50% predictive accuracy in the diagnosis of cardiac tamponde. Gillam et al. (40) also suggested that predictive value would be enhanced significantly by considering the duration of right atrial collapse. Consequently, they proposed a right atrial inversion time index, defined as the number of frames demonstrating right atrial inversion divided by the total number of frames per cardiac cycle. An index of 0.34 or more was strongly suggestive of tamponade and improved both the specificity (100%) and predictive value

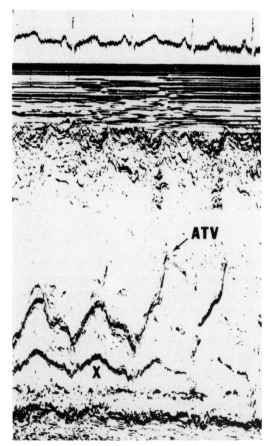

Figure 24.7. M-mode echocardiogram demonstrating how a relatively echo-free space (*X*) can be seen behind the posterior left ventricular wall in a normal subject when the transducer is directed medially. *ATV* = anterior leaflet of the tricuspid valve.

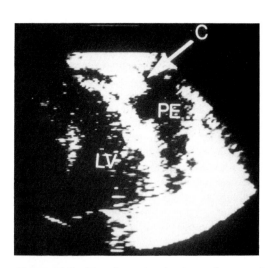

Figure 24.6. Two-dimensional echocardiogram of a patient with a large pericardial clot (*C*). *PE* = pericardial effusion, *LV* = left ventricle.

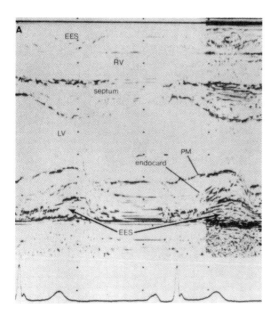

Figure 24.8. M-mode echocardiogram of an epicardial fat pad presenting as an anterior echo-free space. *EES* = extra echo space (representing epicardial fat), *LV* = left ventricle, *PM* = papillary muscle, *RV* = right ventricle, (From Takashi W, et al: *B Heart J* 47:430–8, 1982.)

(100%) of right atrial inversion as a marker of pericardial tamponade without significant loss of sensitivity (94%).

Chamber compression in the presence of a pericardial effusion has improved the ability to diagnose cardiac tamponade (41). Right atrial collapse is probably more sensitive than right ventricular collapse. Kronzon et al. (42) noted that right atrial collapse was a 100% sensitive marker of tamponade, while right ventricular diastolic collapse had a sensitivity of only 78%. Tamponade may occur in the absence of right ventricular or atrial diastolic collapse when there is marked elevation of right heart pressures. For

Table 24.3. Conditions Producing an Anterior Echo-Free Space

1. Epicardial fat pad
2. Hernias of foramen of Morgagni
3. Pericardial cysts
4. Lymphomas and pericardial tumors
5. Calcified mitral annulus
6. Left pleural effusion
7. Left atrial enlargement
8. Thrombi
9. Massive ascites
10. Faulty medial angulation of the transducer

instance, this can occur in patients with severe pulmonary hypertension (43). Using a canine model, Pandian et al. (44) demonstrated that right ventricular diastolic collapse does not appear until baseline cardiac output decreases by more than 20%. Also, they showed that right ventricular diastolic collapse preceded a fall in systemic blood pressure, and chamber collapse preceded the appearance of pulsus paradoxus. Using pulsed Doppler echocardiography in their experimental model, Pandian et al. (44) also noted that gross respiratory phasic variation in pulmonary artery and aortic flow velocity was less than one-half the expiratory aortic flow velocity. Further studies on larger number of patients with tamponade are needed to interpret these echocardiographic findings accurately.

USE OF ECHOCARDIOGRAPHY DURING PERICARDIOCENTESIS

Pericardiocentesis under echocardiographic guidance was first attempted in 1973 using a special M-mode transducer to guide the needle into the pericardial effusion (45). Subsequently, two-dimensional and contrast echocardiographic techniques have been described to identify the location of the tip of the pericardiocentesis needle within the pericardial sac (46–50) (Fig. 24.17; Table 24.5).

The echocardiographic transducer is placed at the cardiac apex while pericardiocentesis is performed from the subcostal position (46, 50). The echocardiogram is recorded continously while the pericardiocentesis needle is being advanced. Negative pressure is maintained during the advance of the needle. Once access to the effusion is achieved, 10–50 cc of fluid are aspirated and discarded, and 5 cc of agitated saline are injected through the needle. The appearance of microbubbles in the pericardial sac confirms the intrapericardiac position of the needle (Fig. 24.18). This technique is particularly useful when there is frank blood in the pericardial sac, and the hematocrit of the pericardial fluid and the patient's blood are similar. Visualization of the pericardial needle by two-dimensional echocardiography is also useful in situations where there is cessation of fluid aspiration after an initially successful tap. A contrast study will determine whether the needle is still intrapericardial. Slight changes of needle position can be made under echocardiographic control and successful pericardiocentesis can be reestablished.

Callahan et al. (48) proposed a different approach to pericardiocentesis, using two-dimen-

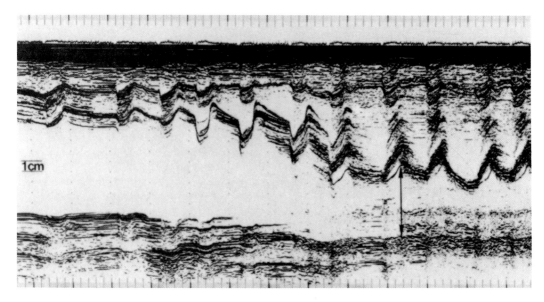

Figure 24.9. M-mode echocardiogram of a patient with massive enlargement of the left atrium. The enlarged left atrium extends inferiorly. This produces an echo-free space behind the left ventricle, mimicking pericardial effusion. (From Engel PJ: *Echocardiography in pericardial disease.* In Folwer NO (ed): *Non-invasive Diagnostic Methods in Cardiology.* Philadelphia, FA Davis, 1983, p 181.

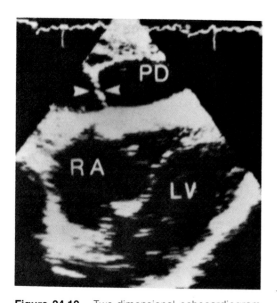

Figure 24.10. Two-dimensional echocardiogram of a patient with subdiaphragmatic fluid mimicking loculated pericardial effusion. *Arrows* point to the falciform ligament. *PD* = peritoneal dialysate; *LV* = left ventricle; *RA* = right atrium. (From Bream R, et al: Subdiaphragmatic fluid mimicking loculated pericardiac effusion on echocardiography. *Am J Cardiol* 54:1288, 1984.)

sional echocardiographic assistance. During the echocardiographic examination, particular note was made of the place on the chest wall closest to the pericardial fluid. An entry tract was then selected for insertion of the pericardiocentesis needle at the point on the chest wall that permits puncture of the pericardial sac without damage to any vital structure. A Teflon-sheathed "intra-cath" needle was then used to complete the pericardiocentesis. In some cases, a large catheter was introduced and connected to a closed drainage system for continous drainage.

CONSTRICTIVE PERICARDITIS

Constrictive pericarditis is associated with characteristic anatomic and physiologic abnormalities (51–55). The typical anatomic abnormality is thickening of the pericardium, with or without pericardial calcification (54). Pericardial thickening produces pericardial motion parallel to the epicardium. On M-mode echocardiography there is an echo-free space between the two structures. If a left pleural effusion is present in addition to a pericardial effusion, the pericardium appears to be sandwiched between the two layers of fluid (Figs. 24.19 and 24.20). In this condition, the actual pericardial thickness can be measured di-

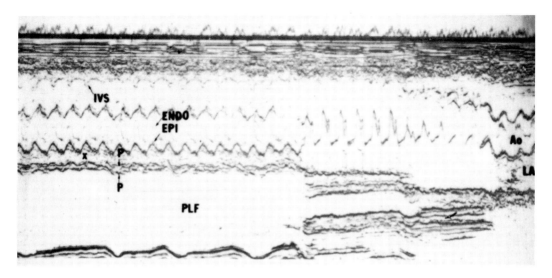

Figure 24.11. M-mode examination of a patient with both pleural effusion (*PLF*) and pericardial effusion (*X*). Transducer angulation causes pericardial echoes to blend with the left atrial posterior wall while the pleural space persists. *Ao* = aorta, *ENDO* = endocardium, *EPI* = epicardium, *IVS* = interventricular septum, *P* = pericardium.

rectly. However, it should be emphasized that evidence of thickened pericardium per se is not sufficient to make a diagnosis of constrictive pericarditis. Pericardial thickening may be present without the hemodynamic findings of constriction.

Rapid early diastolic filling of the ventricles in constrictive pericarditis produces characteristic abnormalities on the echocardiogram. One such abnormality is premature opening of the pulmonic valve (Fig. 24.21). Rapid early diastolic filling may markedly elevate right ventricular early

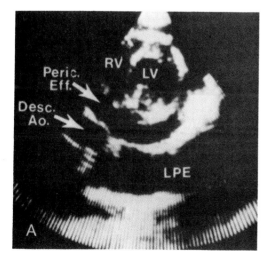

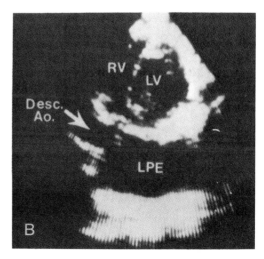

Figure 24.12. Parasternal short-axis views in a patient with both a posterior pericardial (*Peric. Eff.*) and a left pleural effusion. (*LPE*). *A*, The effusions appear as echo-free spaces, both anterior posterior and lateral to the descending thoracic aorta (*Desc Ao*). There is a separation between the descending aorta and left ventricular (*LV*) posterior wall. *RV* = right ventricle. *B*, After pericardiocentesis the anterior echo-free space disappears, but the left pleural effusion remains. (From Haaz WS, et al: Two-dimensional echocardiographic recognition of the descending thoracic aorta: Value indifferentiating pericardial from pleural effusions. *Am J Cardiol* 46:742, 1980.)

Table 24.4. Echocardiographic Abnormalities in Cardiac Tamponade

1. Swinging heart
2. Phasic variation in right ventricular and left ventricular internal diameters
3. Right ventricular compression
4. Notch on epicardial surface of right ventricle in isometric contraction phase
5. Coarse oscillation of left ventricular posterior wall
6. Diastolic indentation of right ventricle
7. Diastolic indentation of right atrium

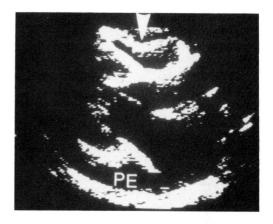

Figure 24.14. Two-dimensional echocardiogram illustrating right ventricular diastolic collapse (*arrow*). *PE* = pericardial effusion.

diastolic pressure, which may exceed the pulmonary artery diastolic pressure and result in premature opening of the pulmonic valve. This finding is not specific for constrictive pericarditis and has also been described in tricuspid regurgitation, pulmonary valve incompetence, ruptured Valsalva's sinus to the right heart, and Löffler's endocarditis (56–58) (Table 24.6).

Another echocardiographic abnormality is rapid posterior motion of the left ventricular posterior wall in early diastole, with little or no posterior motion during rest of diastole. This is caused by the rapid early diastolic filling of the left ventricle.

A similar finding is rapid early diastolic posterior motion of the posterior aortic root wall with little, if any, further posterior motion during the rest of diastole (60, 62) (Fig. 24.22). Rapid early left atrial emptying, in association with rapid early diastolic filling of the left ventricle, causes this

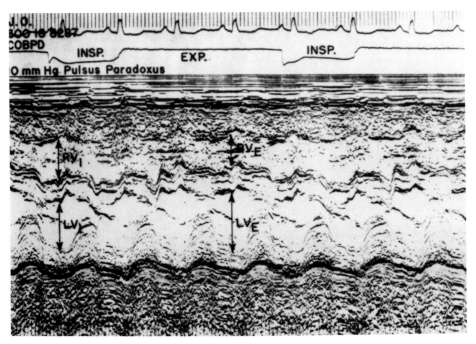

Figure 24.13. M-mode echocardiogram of a patient with cardiac tamponade. The right ventricular size (RV_I) increases during inspiration and decreases during expiration (RV_E). LV_E = left ventricular size in expiration, LV_I = left ventricular size in inspiration. (From Settle Hp, et al: *Circulation* 56:951, 1977.)

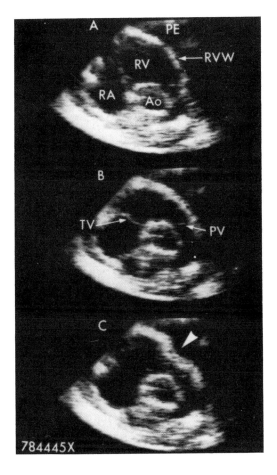

784445X

Figure 24.15. Short-axis view of right ventricular diastolic collapse. Note that the collapse is best seen in the right ventricular outflow tract. *Ao* = aorta, *PE* = pericardial effusion, *PV* = , *RA* = right atrium, *RV* = right ventricle, *RVW* = right ventricular wall. (From Armstrong WF, et al: *Circulation* 65:1491, 1982.)

movement. The normal posterior aortic wall echocardiogram shows an initial posterior motion in diastole, followed by a plateau and then further posterior motion during atrial systole.

A rapid early diastolic E–F slope of the mitral valve has also been noted in patients with constrictive pericarditis (51, 63). However, none of these signs is specific for the diagnosis of constrictive pericarditis. These findings may occur in conditions where there is rapid filling of the left ventricle, such as severe mitral regurgitation.

Interventricular septal motion abnormalities have been described in many cardiac conditions. These include right ventricular volume overload, conduction disturbances, coronary artery disease, and postcardiac surgery. Diastolic septal motion is related primarily to the transseptal pressure gradient (54, 63, 64). Abrupt anterior or posterior motion of the septum in early diastole is characteristic of unusually vigorous ventricular filling. The direction of motion of the septum in early

diastole may depend on a number of factors. These include uneven distribution of fibrosis or calcification in the pericardial sac, timing of mitral and tricuspid opening, relative compliance of the right and left ventricles, and phase of respiration. Candell-Riera and associates (64) studied the interventricular septum in chronic constrictive pericarditis. A brisk, early diastolic anterior movement followed by a rebound toward the left ventricular posterior wall was observed. The beginning of this movement was coincidental with the "pericardial knock", when present. The movement's apex coincided with the "x" descent of the jugular venous pulse. This early diastolic notch in the septum has also been observed in severe aortic and mitral regurgitation, reflecting rapid early diastolic distension of the left ventricle in this disorder. The diastolic notch usually is seen also in patients with restrictive cardiomyopathy (65, 66).

Another recent echocardiographic study reported abnormal notching of the interventricular

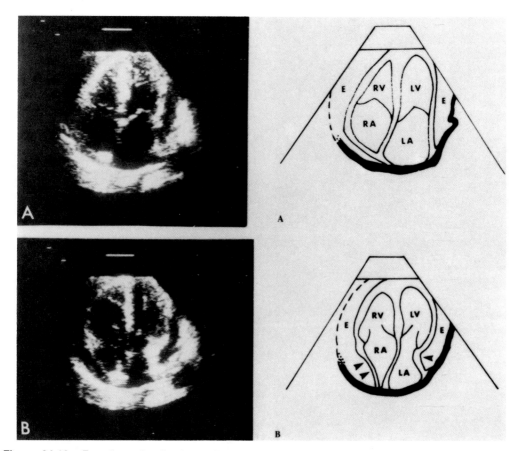

Figure 24.16. Two-dimensional echocardiogram, apical four-chamber view, of a patient with cardiac tamponade. *A,* End-systolic frame. *B,* End-diastolic frame. Note the diastolic compression of both atria. *E* = effusion, *LA* = left atrium, *LV* = left ventricle, *RA* = right atrium, *RV* = right ventricle. (From Kronzon I, et al: Diastolic atrial compression: A sensitive echocardiographic sign of cardiac tamponade. *J Am Coll Cardiol* 2:770, 1983.)

septum (IVS) during atrial systole in patients with constrictive pericarditis (Fig. 24.23) (67). This phenomenon occurred on the M-mode echocardiogram only during sinus rhythm. The onset of the initial posterior ventricular septal motion coincided with the midpoint of the P wave while the nadir of the notch was at the end of the P wave. Subsequent anterior motion of the septum ended before the QRS complex. This atrial systolic notch probably reflects asynchronous filling of the right and left ventricle, resulting from normal atrial asynchrony. Normally the right atrium is activated and contracts before the left atrium.

On real-time two-dimensional echocardiography the pericardium is seen as an immobile, thickened structure (68). A ventricular diastolic filling halt is seen, and transfer of blood from atria to ventricles is accompanied by an increase in motion of the atrioventricular rings. Indentation of the septum into the left heart chambers on inspiration reflects increased right-sided rather than left-sided filling. Increased systemic venous pressure is reflected by a dilated inferior vena cava without respiratory variation (69) (Fig. 24.24). Both atria may be enlarged.

Doppler echocardiography has been used to document pulsus paradoxus. Aortic flow in patients with constrictive pericarditis is decreased dramatically on inspiration. Doppler patterns of mitral inflow demonstrate an early increased diastolic filling velocity followed by a rapid deceleration, leading to a short filling period (69)

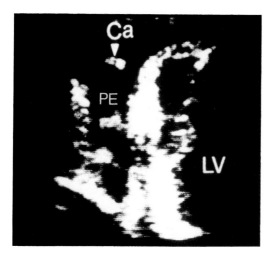

Figure 24.17. Two-dimensional echocardiogram illustrating a pericardial catheter (*Ca*) situated within a large pericardial effusion. (*PE*). *LV* = left ventricle. (From Chandraratna PAN: *Echocardiography* 1:55, 1984.)

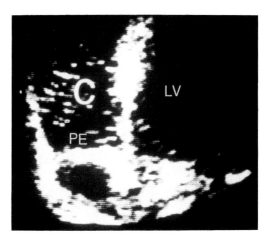

Figure 24.18. Echocardiogram from the same patient as in Figure 24.17, obtained after injection of saline through the catheter. Note the contrast effect (*C*) produced by microbubbles. *LV* = left ventricle, *PE* = pericardial effusion. (From Chandraratna PAN: *Echocardiography* 1:55, 1984.)

(Fig. 24.25). Von Bibra et al. (70) evaluated hepatic venous flow pattern in patients with constrictive pericarditis using pulsed Doppler echocardiography. They described a characteristic W wave pattern similar to the jugular venous pulse in this condition. This was characterized by steep x and y descents with a distinct reflux of the jugular venous pulse at the end of systole and diastole, prior to the A wave.

Thus, multiple echocardiographic signs of constrictive pericarditis exist, none of which is pathognomonic. Echocardiographic evidence of pericardial thickening in association with evidence of rapid early diastolic right and left ventricular filling is highly suggestive of this condition. Accumulation of pericardial fluid in addition to a thickened pericardium has been termed effusive-constrictive pericarditis (71). Following pericar-

diocentesis in patients with effusive-constrictive pericarditis, there is persistence of elevated right and left ventricular end-diastolic pressures.

ABNORMAL INTRAPERICARDIAL ECHOES

Pericardial effusions are usually echo-free. Abnormal echoes within the pericardial sac may be due to pericardial adhesions (Fig. 24.26), peri-

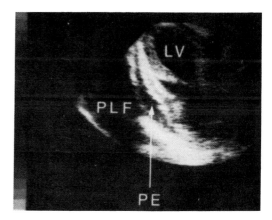

Figure 24.19. Two-dimensional echocardiogram illustrating a small pericardial effusion (*PE*) and a pleural effusion (*PLF*). The pericardium is sandwiched between the pericardial and pleural effusion. *LV* = left ventricle. From Chandraratna PAN: *Echocardiography* 1:55, 1984.)

Table 24.5. Pericardiocentesis Utilizing Echocardiography

1. Place transducer at apex
2. Record echocardiogram continuously
3. Pericardiocentesis via subcostal approach
4. Aspirate and discard 50 cc of fluid
5. Inject 5 ml of saline through exploring needle when fluid is aspirated
6. Cloud of echoes indicates position of needle

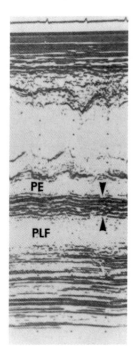

Figure 24.20. M-mode echocardiogram of another patient with pleural (*PLF*) and pericardial (*PE*) effusion. The pericardium (*between arrows*) is thickened. (From Chandraratna PAN, et al: Role of echocardiography in detecting the anatomic and physiologic abnormalities of constrictive pericarditis. *Am J Med Sci* 283:141, 1982.)

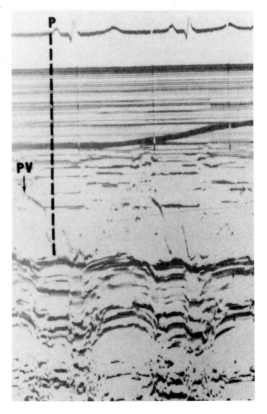

Figure 24.21. M-mode echocardiogram of the pulmonic valve (*PV*) in a patient with constrictive pericarditis, illustrating premature opening of the pulmonic valve (prior to onset of the P wave). The *vertical dotted line* indicates the onset of the ECG P Wave. (From Chandraratna PAN: role of echocardiography in detecting the anatomic and physiologic abnormalities of constrictive pericarditis. *Am J Med Sci* 283:141, 1982.)

cardial metastases (72), intrapericardial clots, or epicardial fat.

Paricardial Adhesions

Dense linear echoes seen on two-dimensional echocardiography that extend from the epicardium to the pericardium probably represent adhesions. Visualization of these adhesions in the pericardial effusion produces a very striking real-time echocardiographic finding. Occasionally, multiple views have to be performed, since adhesions may not be seen on all views (73).

Pericardial Metastases

Manifestations of malignant involvement of the pericardium (Table 24.7) include nodular epicardial tumor deposits, pericardial effusion with or without tamponade, effusive-constrictive pericarditis, and frank constrictive pericarditis (74, 75). Constrictive pericarditis in association with systemic malignancy may result from incasement of the pericardium with tumor or from radiation-

induced pericardial fibrosis. Two-dimensional echocardiography, with or without a Doppler study, is at present unable to differentiate between the two.

Discrete metastatic tumors may be seen on two-dimensional echocardiography as fixed or oscil-

Table 24.6. Conditions Causing Premature Opening of the Pulmonary Valve

1. Constrictive pericarditis
2. Tricuspid regurgitation
3. Pulmonary regurgitation accompanied by atrial septal defect
4. Ruptured Valsalva's sinus to the right atrium
5. Löffler's endocarditis

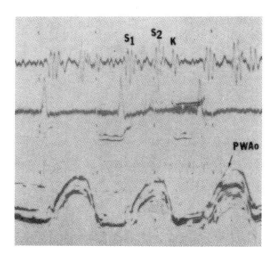

Figure 24.22. An enlargement of the posterior wall of the aortic root (*PWAo*) in a patient with constrictive pericarditis. Note the rapid posterior motion in early diastole with little or no further posterior motion during the rest of diastole. The phonocardiogram shows a pericardial knock (*K*). Chandraratna PAN: Role of echocardiography in detecting the anatomic and physiologic abnormalities of constrictive pericarditis. *Am J Med Sci* 283:141, 1982.)

Echocardiogram In Constrictive Pericarditis

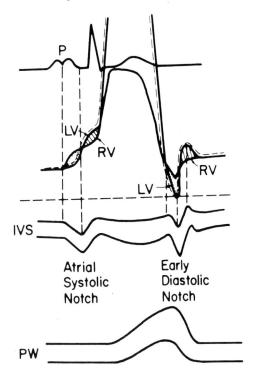

Figure 24.23. Schematic representation of interventricular septal motion in patients with constrictive pericarditis. *IVS* = interventricular septum, *LV* = left ventricle, *P* = P wave, *PW* = posterior left ventricular wall, *RV* = right ventricle. (From Tei C, et al: Atrial systolic notch on the interventricular echogram: An echocardiographic sign of constrictive pericarditis. *J Am Coll Cardiol* 1:907, 1983.)

latory, cauliflower-like, echo-dense masses attached to either the parietal or visceral pericardium (73) (Fig. 24.27). The different patterns seen on echocardiography are: localized nodules (mobile or immobile), diffuse layering of echoes, tumor encasement, and pericardial metastases extending into the myocardium.

The nodular pattern may be mimicked occasionally by a pericardial blood clot. Diffuse layering may, on occasion, be produced by epicardial fat.

Intrapericardial Clots

Pericardial blood clots usually present on the two-dimensional cardiogram as a dense layer of echoes within the pericardium. Occasionally, nodular masses may be seen.

Epicardial Fat

Excessive epicardial fat is an anatomic variant than can simulate a focal pericardial mass or effusion. Conversely, echoes caused by a pathologic mass can be attributed falsely to epicardial fat. Since (CT) distinguishes fat more easily, it may prove superior to echocardiography for this application.

OTHER CONDITIONS

Echocardiography is useful in the diagnosis of pneumomediastinum and pneumopericardium resulting from blunt or penetrating chest trauma (76). The echocardiographic features are.

1. The occurrence of a band of echoes within the cardiac chamber at the anterior cardiac border, beginning in late systole and continuing into early diastole;
2. Total dropout of echoes posterior to this band of echoes causing an "air gap".
3. The cyclic appearance of this "air-gap" sign (Fig. 24.28)

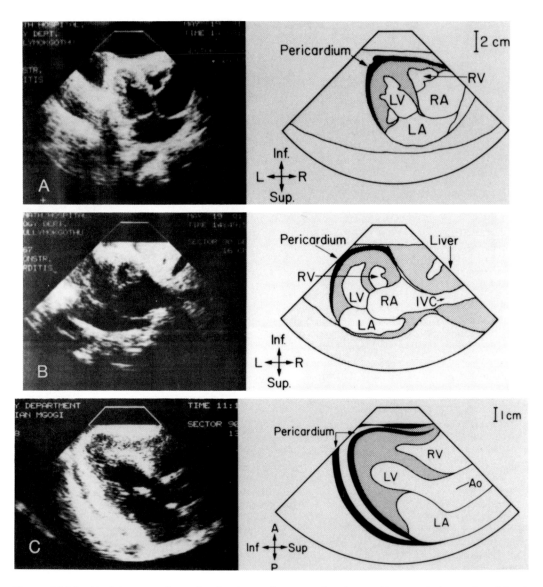

Figure 24.24. Real time two-dimensional echocardiograms of patients with constrictive pericarditis. *A,* Subxiphoid view demonstrating bulging of the interatrial septum into the left atrium. *B,* Subxiphoid view showing a dilated inferior vena cava and right atrium. Both interventricular and interatrial septa deviate to the left. *C,* Parasternal view demonstrating the pericardium as a double echo-dense layer. *A* = anterior, *Ao* = aorto, *inf.* = inferior, *IVC* = inferior vena cava, *L* = left, *LA* = left atrium, *LV* = left ventricle, *R* = right, *RA* = right atrium, *RV* = right ventricle, *Sup.* = superior. (From Lewis BS: *Am J Cardiol* 49:1789, 1982.)

Presumably, air accumulates anteriorly within the mediastinum or pericardium during late systole as ventricular size diminishes. During early diastole, the air is displaced during early diastole by the increasing ventricular volume (Fig. 24.29). The air gap sign can be recorded at the aortic and mitral valve areas. Since air conducts ultrasound poorly, echoes returning from the far field—including intracardiac structures—are severely attenuated and result in an air gap.

Absence of the pericardium, due to either surgical resection or a congential lesion, frequently

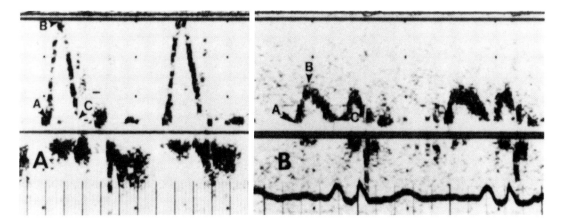

Figure 24.25. Doppler pattern of left ventricular early diastolic filling in a patient with constrictive pericarditis (*A*) compared to a normal control. *B*, Note the higher peak filling velocity (*point B*), rapid deceleration (*slope B-C*), and a shorter early diastolic filling period (*segment A-C*). (From Agatston AS, et al: Diagnosis of constrictive pericarditis by pulsed Doppler echocardiography. *Am J Cardiol* 54:929, 1984.)

causes the heart to expand (77). Posterior left ventricular wall motion may then become hyperkinetic. During ventricular systole, this exaggerated posterior left ventricular wall motion produces anterior displacement (paradoxical motion) of the septum on the M-mode echocardiogram. The heart often shifts to the left, leaving more of the right ventricle visible than is usual on the routine parasternal long-axis view. As a result, an incorrect diagnosis of right ventricular volume overload can be made. Thus, excessive posterior left ventricular wall motion, paradoxical motion of the interventricular septum, and right ventricular dilatation are the three echocardiographic signs of an absent pericardium.

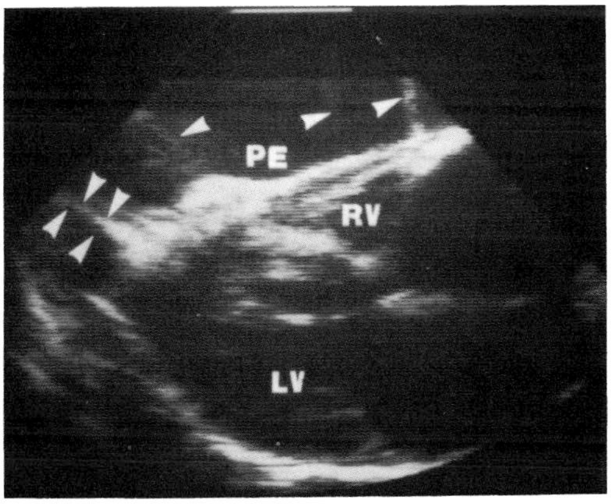

ALTERNATE TECHNIQUES

Although echocardiography has been the primary diagnostic method for pericardial disease, technically adequate echocardiograms are not always possible. Thus, other diagnostic approaches may be required to evaluate a patient with suspected pericardial disease.

Computed Tomography

Computed tomographic (CT) imaging provides an alternative noninvasive means of evaluating pericardial disease. The density differential between the higher density fibrous pericardium and the lower density subepicardial fat allows the pericardium to be clearly delineated by a CT scan. Tomography has been found to be of value in evaluating the congenital absence of the pericardium, pericardial cysts, pericardial effusion, calcific pericarditis, primary and metastatic involvement of the pericardium, and postoperative

Figure 24.26. Echocardiogram showing adhesions within the pericardial effusion (*PE*). *Arrows* point to the adhesions. *LV* = left ventricle, *RV* = right ventricle.

Table 24.7. Manifestations of Malignant Pericardial Involvement

1. Localized nodule
   a. Mobile
   b. Fixed
2. Diffuse layering of echoes
3. Tumor encasement
4. Pericardial metastases extending into myocardium

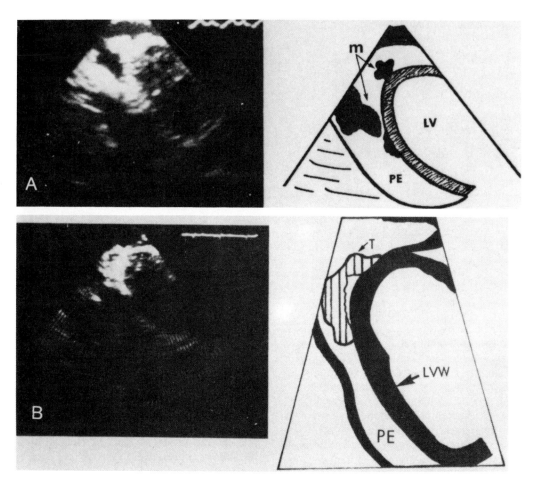

Figure 24.27. *A,* Cross-sectional echocardiogram in the long-axis view of a patient with surgically proved pericardial metastases. Note the abnormal echoes (*m*) that project into the effusion-containing pericardial space (*PE*). These echoes demonstrate a to-and-fro oscillatory motion during the cardiac cycle and represent pericardial metastases. *LV* = left ventricular cavity. *B,* Another example of pericardial metastases (*T*). *LVW* = left ventricular wall.

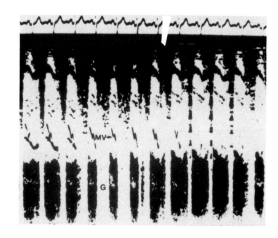

Figure 24.28. The air gap sign recorded at the level of the mitral valve (*MV*). After the onset of the QRS complex and continuing into early diastole, a dense band of echoes obscures the anterior mitral leaflet. An echo-free gap (*G*) is seen posteriorly. (Reprinted with permission from the American College of Cardiology. Reid CL, et al: Echocardiographic detection of pneumomediastinum and pneumopericardium: The air gap signs. *J Am Coll Cardiol* 1:916 1983.)

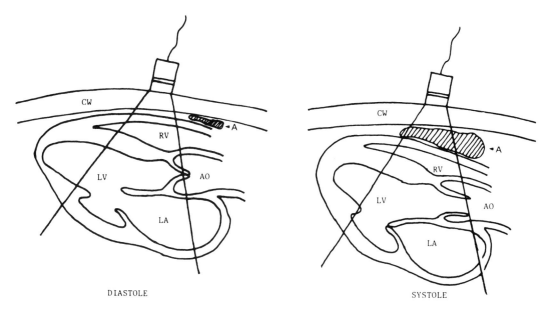

Figure 24.29. Schematic illustrating the air gap sign. Air (*A*) is displaced by the enlarging heart in diastole. In systole it accumulates anteriorly, interfering with the echo beam. *AO* = aorta, *CW* = chest wall, *LA* = left atrium, *LV* = left ventricle, *RV* = right ventricle. (Reprinted with permission from the American College of Cardiology. Reid CL, et al: Echocardiographic detection of pneumomediastinum and pneumapericardium: The air gap sign. *J Am Coll Cardiol* 1:916, 1983.)

changes following pericardiectomy (78). It has been especially helpful in demonstrating pericardial thickening (Fig. 24.30) and neoplastic involvement.

Direct measurement of pericardial thickness by

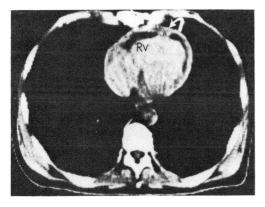

Figure 24.30. CT scan of the heart illustrating the thickened pericardium seen in constrictive pericarditis. Note the adhesions between the right ventricular (*RV*) epicardium and parietal pericardium (*arrow*). (From: Moncada R, et al: Diagnostic role of computed tomography in pericardial heart disease: Congenital defects, thickening, neoplasms and effusions, *Am Heart J* 103:263, 1982.)

CT has shown a sensitivity and specificity of more than 90% in two studies on a small number of patients (78, 79). Isner et al. (79) studied 53 patients prospectively, using both CT of the chest and cardiac ultrasound. A diagnostic-quality CT study was obtained in all 53 patients. However, a technically satisfactory ultrasound examination was not possible in six patients. Of the 47 patients in whom both chest scans and satisfactory ultrasound studies were obtained, CT showed pericardial thickening not seen on ultrasound in 5 patients. Estimated size of pericardial effusion was the same for both CT and ultrasound. Neoplastic pericardial disease was detected by CT scan in 4 of the 53 patients.

Tomography has also been used to differentiate pericardial exudate, large pericardial clots, hemopericardium, and chylous effusion within the pericardial space (78). Tomography complements the role of two-dimensional echocardiography in detecting loculated collections of pericardial fluid (79). Furthermore, since it can facilitate precise catheter placement by angle and depth measurements, drainage of loculated fluid collections might be achieved by CT-guided aspiration (79). Overall, CT provides a sensitive evaluation of the pericardium and quality of pericardial effusion and is a valuable adjunct in patients in whom ultra-sound is technically unsatisfactory.

Nuclear Magnetic Resonance Imaging (MRI)

Another technique used to study the pericardium is MRI. Its advantages include delineation of cardiovascular structures without use of contrast media, lack of ionizing radiation, and the ability to characterize tissues using spin lattice (T1) and transverse (T2) relaxation times (Fig. 24.31). The electrocardiographic-gated technique and the permutation-gated technique allow visualization of variations in the appearance and thickness of the normal pericardial structures during the cardiac cycle. Nonlaminar motion of pericardial fluid caused by motion of the heart in the pericardial sac causes the normal pericardial fluid to have very low intensity on MRI images (Fig. 24.32).

Nonhemorrhagic effusions—especially in patients with uremia, trauma, and tuberculosis—have some regions of medium or high signal intensity within the pericardial sac. This probably represents inflammatory exudate with a high content of fibrinous material that causes considerable shortening of T1. Consequently, the signal intensity is increased. Quantitative MRI estimation of pericardial fluid correlates well with echocardiographic estimations (80).

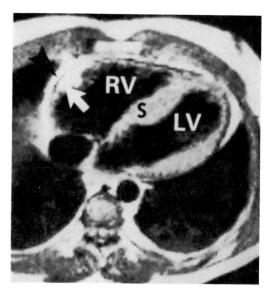

Figure 24.31. Gated magnetic resonance image of the normal pericardium showing it as a 1–2 mm low intensity curvilinear line separating the subepicardial fat (*black arrow*) from mediastinal fat (*white arrow*). *LV* = left ventricle, *RV* = right ventricle, *S* = interventricular septum. (From: Stark DD, et al: Magnetic resonance imaging of the pericardium: Normal and pathological findings. *Radiology* 150:469, 1984.

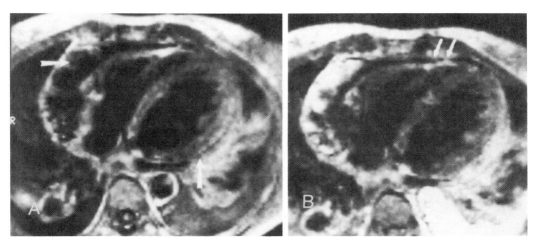

Figure 24.32. Loculated pericardial effusion in a patient with uremia. *A*, Transaxial section through the heart (TE = 28 msec) showing distension of the pericardial space mainly over right atrium and right ventricle. Parts of the effusion show medium signal intensity (*arrows*). *B*, Identical section (TE = 56 msec). There is a relative increase of signal intensity in areas of medium signal intensity on first echo image. Two adhesions are visible between the parietal and visceral pericardium (*arrows*). (From Sechtem U, et al: MRI of the abnormal pericardium. *AJR* 147:245, 1986.)

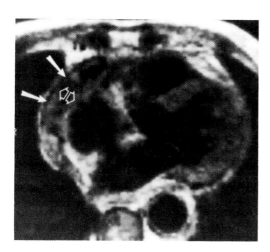

Figure 24.33. Constrictive pericarditis in patient with uremia. On first spin-echo image (TE = 28 msec), a thin, low intensity line representing fibrous parietal pericardium is visible over the right atrium (*closed arrows*). Areas of medium signal intensity (*open arrows*) cover the parietal and visceral pericardium. At surgery, these areas were found to represent dense fibrinous exudate. (From Sechtem U, et al: MRI of the abnormal pericardium. *AJR* 147:245, 1986.

Thickened pericardium is seen on MRI imaging as a 5–7 mm curvilinear line of low signal intensity (81) (Fig. 24.33). Nuclear magnetic resonance imaging also demonstrates differences in signal intensity of the pericardium in patients with thickened pericardium and clinical symptoms of constriction. Pericardial thickening can be excluded by MRI in patients with restrictive cardiomyopathy, enabling differentiation between the two clinical entities (80). However, MRI is not able to differentiate reliably between fibrous and calcified tissue. In these situations, CT remains superior to MRI.

Nuclear magnetic resonance imaging has also been useful in the diagnosis of pericardial cysts, which show the typical magnetic-relaxation characteristics of a fluid-filled lesion. These characteristics are low signal intensity on T1-weighted images and higher signal intensity on T2-weighted images. However, pericardial fat is seen as a homogeneous high intensity signal on T1-weighted images. Electrocardiographic-gated technique with MRI helps in distinguishing pericardial tumors from surrounding noncardiac structures. At present, MRI has not presented any additional in-

formation about the specific pathologic nature of the masses.

Nuclear magnetic resonance imaging can detect a variety of pathologic processes affecting the pericardium. Further studies on larger numbers of patients will determine its potential advantages over existing methods.

REFERENCES

1. Feigenbaum H, Waldhausen JA, Hyde LP: Ultrasound diagnosis of pericardial effusion. *JAMA* 191:711, 1965.
2. Chandraratna PAN, Aronow WS, Lurie M, Murdock K, Milholland H: Role of cross sectional echocardiography in the evaluation of pericardial effusion. *Comprehens Ther* 7:46, 1981.
3. Horowitz MS, Schultz CS, Stimson EB, Harrison DC, Popp RL: Sensitivity and specificity of echocardiographic diagnosis of pericardial effusion. *Circulation* 50:239, 1974.
4. Abbasi AS, Ellis M, Flynn JV: Echocardiographic M-scan technique in the diagnosis of pericardial effusion. *J Clin Ultrasound* 1:300, 1973.
5. Feigenbaum H: Echocardiographic diagnosis of pericardial effusion. *Am J Cardiol* 26:475, 1970.
6. Matsuo H, Matsumoto H, Hamanaka Y, Ohara T, Senda S, Inoue M, Abe H: Rotational excursion of heart in massive pericardial effusion studied by phased array echocardiography. *Br Heart J* 41:513, 1979.
7. Nanda NC, Gramiak R, Gross CM: Echocardiography of cardiac values in pericardial effusion. *Circulation* 54:500, 1976.
8. Martin RP, Rakowski H, French J, Popp RL: Localization of pericardial effusion with wide angle phased array echocardiography. *Am J Cardiol* 42:904, 1978.
9. Windle JR, Felix G, Oinsky WW, Kugler JD: False negative findings in pericardial effusion using M-mode echocardiography. *Pediatr Cardiol* 4:225, 1983.
10. Krozon I, Cohn ML, Winter HE: Cardiac tamponade by loculated pericardial hematoma: Limitations of M-mode echocardiography. *J Am Coll Cardiol* 1:913, 1983.
11. Galve E, Castillo HGD, Evangelista A, Batlle J, Miralda P, Solver JS: Pericardial effusion in the course of myocardial infarction: Incidence, natural history, and clinical relevance. *Circulation* 73:294, 1986.
12. Allen JW, Harrison EC, Camp JC, Borsari A, Turnier E, Law FY: The role of serial echocardiography in the evaluation and differential diagnosis of pericardial disease. *Am Heart J* 93:560, 1977.
13. Feigenbaum, H, Zaky A, Waldhausen JA: Use of ultrasound in the diagnosis of pericardial effusion. *Ann Intern Med* 65:443, 1966.
14. Feigenbaum, H, Zaky A, Waldhausen JA: Use of reflected ultrasound in detecting pericardial effusion. *Am J Cardiol* 19:84, 1967.
15. Rifkin RD, Isner JM, Carter BL, Bankoff MS: Combined postero-anterior subepicardial fat sim-

ulating the echocardiographic diagnosis of pericardial effusion. *J Am Coll Cardiol* 3:1333, 1984.

16. Isner JM, Cartel BL, Roberts WC, Bankoff MS: Subepicardial adipose tissue producing echocardiographic evidence of pericardial effusion. *Am J Cardiol* 51:565, 1983.

17. Savage DD, Garrison RJ, Brand F, Anderson SJ, Castelli WP, Karmel WB, Feinlieb M: Prevalence and correlates of posterior extraechocardiographic spaces in a free living population based sample (the Framingham study). *Am J Cardiol* 51:1207, 1983.

18. Popp RL, Harrison DC: Echocardiography. In Weissler AM (ed): *Noninvasive Cardiology*. New York, Grune & Stratton, 1974, pp 149–226.

19. Feiner JM, Fleming WH, France RH: Echocardiographic identification of a pericardial cyst. *Chest* 68:386, 1975.

20. Tajik AJ: Echocardiography in pericardial effusion. *Am J Med* 63:29, 1977.

21. Klein JJ, Segal BL: Pericardial effusion diagnosed by reflected ultrasound. *Am J Cardiol* 22:57, 1968.

22. Ratshin RA, Smith M, Hood WP: Possible false negative diagnosis of pericardial effusion by echocardiography in presence of large left atrium. *Chest* 65:112, 1974.

23. D'Cruz IA: Echocardiographic simulation of pericardial effusion by ascites. *Chest* 85:93, 1984.

24. Bream R, Campese V, Massry SG, Rahimtoola SH, Chandraratna PAN: Subdiaphragmatic fluid mimicking loculated pericardial effusion on echocardiography. *Am J Cardiol* 54:1388, 1984.

25. Feigenbaum H. *Echocardiography*, ed 4. Philadelphia, Lea & Febiger, 1986, p 548.

26. Martin RP, Rakowski H, French J: Localization of pericardial effusion with wide angle phased array echocardiography. *Am J Cardiol* 42:904, 1978.

27. Greene DA, Kleid JJ, Naidu S: Unusual echocardiographic manifestation of pericardial effusion. *Am J Cardiol* 39:112, 1977.

28. Friedman MJ, Sahn DJ, Haber K: Two-dimensional echocardiography and B-mode ultrasonography for the diagnosis of loculated pericardial effusion. *Circulation* 60:1643, 1979.

29. Teicholz LE: Echocardiography evaluation of pericardial diseases. *Progr Cardiovasc Dis* 21:133, 1978.

30. Haaz WS, Mintz GS, Kotler MN, Parry W, Segal BL: Two-dimensional echocardiographic recognition of the descending thoracic aorta: Value in differentiating pericardial from pleural effusions. *Am J Cardiol* 46:739, 1980.

31. Lewandowski BJ, Jaffer NM, Winsberg F: Relationship between the pericardial and pleural spaces in cross-sectional imaging. *J Clin Ultrasound* 9:271, 1981.

32. Feigenbaum H, Zaky A, Grabhorn L: Cardiac motion in patients with pericardial effusion: A study using ultrasound cardiography. *Circulation* 34:611, 1966.

33. D'Cruz IA, Cohen HC, Prabbu R, Glick G: Diagnosis of cardiac tamponade by echocardiography: Changes in mitral valve motion and ventricular dimensions with special reference to paradoxical pulse. *Circulation* 52:460, 1975.

34. Kronzon I, Winder HE, Weiss EC: Echocardiographic observations of paradoxical pulse without pericardial disease. *Chest* 78:474, 1980.

35. Winer HE, Kronzon K: Absence of paradoxical pulse in patients with cardiac tamponade and atrial septal defects. *Am J Cardiol* 44:378, 1979.

36. Schiller NB, and Botvinick EH: Right ventricular compression as a sign of cardiac tamponade. *Circulation* 56:773, 1977.

37. Shina S, Yaginuma T, Kondo K, Kawai N, Hosoda S: Echocardiographic evaluation of impending cardiac tamponade. *J Cardiogr* 9:555, 1979.

38. Cogswell TL, Bernarth GA, Wann LS, Hoffman RG, Brooks HL, Klopfenstein HS: Effects of intravascular volume state on the value of pulsus paradoxus and right ventricular diastolic collapse in predicting cardiac tamponade *Circulation* 72(5):1076, 1985.

39. Armstrong WF, Helper DJ, Schilt BF, Dillon JC, Feigenbaum H: Diastolic collapse of the right ventricle: Echocardiographic evidence of occult cardiac tamponade. (Abstr). *Am J Cardiol* 42:1010, 1982.

40. Gillam LD, Guyer D, King ME, Marshall J, Weyman AE: Hemodynamic compression of the right atrial free wall, a new highly sensitive echocardiographic sign of cardiac tamponade (Abstr). *Am J Cardiol* 49:1010, 1982.

41. Singh S: Right ventricular and right atrial collapse in patients with cardiac tamponade—A combined echocardiographic and hemodynamic study. *Circulation* 70:966, 1984.

42. Kronzon I, Cohen ML, Winer HE: Diastolic atrial compression: A sensitive echocardiographic sign of cardiac tamponade. *J Am Coll Cardiol*, 2:770, 1983.

43. Singh S, Wann LS, Klopfenstein HS, Hartz A, Brooks HL: Usefulness of right ventricular diastolic collapse in diagnosing cardiac tamponade and comparison to pulsus paradoxus. *Am J Cardiol* 57:652, 1986.

44. Pandian MG, Rifkin RD, Wang SS: Flow velocity paradoxus—a Doppler echocardiographic sign of cardiac tamponade: Exaggerated respiratory variation in pulmonary and aortic blood flow velocities. *Circulation* 70 (Suppl II):381, 1984.

45. Goldberg BB, Pollack HM: Ultrasonically guided pericardiocentesis. *Am J Cardiol* 31:490, 1973.

46. Chandraratna PAN, First J, Langevin E, O'Dell R: Echocardiographic contrast studies during pericardiocentesis. *Ann Intern Med* 87:199, 1977.

47. Chandraratna PAN, Reid CL, Nimalasuriya A, Kawanishi D, Rahimtoola SH: Application of 2-dimensional contrast studies during pericardiocentesis. *Am J Cardiol* 52:1120, 1983.

48. Callahan JA, Seward JB, Tajik AJ, Holmes DR Jr, Smith HC, Reeder GS, Miller FA Jr: Pericardiocentesis assisted by two-dimensional echocardiography. *J Thorac Cardiovasc Surg* 85:877, 1983.

49. Callahan JA, Seward JB, Nishimura RA, Miller FA Jr, Reeder GS, Shub C, Callahan MJ, Schattenberg TT, Tajik AJ: Two-dimensional echocardiographically guided pericardiocentesis: Experience in 117 consecutive patients. *Am J Cardiol* 55:476, 1985.

50. Chandraratna PAN, Reid CL, Kawanishi D, Nimalasuriya A, Rahimtoola SH: Clinical utility of two-dimensional echocardiographic contrast studies during pericardiocentesis. *Circulation* 66:II-91, 1982.

51. Schnittger I, Bowden RE, Abrams J, Popp RL:

Echocardiography: Pericardial thickening and constrictive pericarditis. *Am J Cardiol* 42:388, 1978.

52. Chandraratna PAN, Imaizumi T: Echocardiographic diagnosis of thickened pericardium. *Cardiovasc Med* 3:1279, 1978.

53. Elkayam U, Kotler MN, Segal BY, Parry W: Echocardiographic findings in constrictive pericarditis: A case report. *Isr J Med Sci* 12:1308, 1976.

54. Tavel ME: *Clinical Phonocardiography and External Pulse Recording*, ed 3. Chicago Year Book Medical Publishers, 1978.

55. Voelkel AG, Pietro DA, Folland ED, Fisher ML, Parisi AF: Echocardiographic features of constrictive pericarditis. *Circulation* 58:871, 1978.

56. Wann LS, Weyman AE, Dillon JC, Feigenbaum H: Premature pulmonary valve opening. *Circulation* 55:128, 1977.

57. Weyman AE, Dillon JC, Feigenbaum H, Chang S: Pulmonary valve motion in pulmonary regurgitation. *Br Heart J* 37:1184, 1975.

58. Weyman AE, Dillon JC, Feigenbaum H, Chang S: Premature pulmonic valve opening following sinus of Valsalva aneurysm rupture into the right atrium. *Circulation* 51:556, 1975.

59. Cohen MV, Greenberg MA: Constrictive pericarditis: Early and late complications of cardiac surgery. *Am J Cardiol* 43:657, 1979.

60. Chandraratna PAN, Aronow WS, Imaizumi T: Role of echocardiography in detecting the anatomic and physiologic abnormalities of constrictive pericarditis. *Am J Med Sci* 383:141, 1982.

61. D'Cruz IA, Levinsky R, Anagnostopoulos C, Cohen HC: Echocardiographic diagnosis of partial pericardial constriction of the left ventricle. *Radiology* 127:755, 1978.

62. Strunk BL, Fitzgerald JW, Lipton M: The posterior aortic wall echocardiogram: Its relationship to left atrial volume change. *Circulation* 54:744, 1976.

63. Yamamoto T, Makihata S, Yasutomi H, Tanimoto M, Ando H, Iwasaki T, Yorifuji S, Shimizu Y, Miyamoto T: Echocardiographic and impedance cardiographic manifestations of constrictive pericarditis. *J Cardiogr* 8:719, 1978.

64. Candell-Riera J, Del Castillo G, Permanyer-Miralda G, Soler-Soler J: Echocardiographic features of the interventricular septum in chronic constrictive pericarditis. *Circulation* 57:1154, 1978.

65. Gibson TC, Grossman W, McLaurin LP, Moos S, Craige E: An echocardiographic study of the interventricular system in constrictive pericarditis. *Br Heart J* 38:738, 1976.

66. Acquatella H, Puigbo DA, Folland ED: Sudden early diastolic anterior movement of the septum in endomyocardial fibrosis. *Circulation* 59:847, 1979.

67. Tel C, Child JS, Tanaka H, Shah PM: Atrial systolic notch on the interventricular echogram: An echo-

cardiographic sign of constrictive pericarditis. *J Am Coll Cardiol* 1:907, 1983.

68. Pandian NG, Skorton DJ, Kieso RA, Kerber RE: Diagnosis of constrictive pericarditis by two-dimensional echocardiography: Studies in a new experimental model and in patients. *J Am Coll Cardiol* 4:1164, 1984.

69. Agatson AS, Rao A, Price RJ, Kinney EL: Diagnosis of constrictive pericarditis by pulsed Doppler echocardiography. *Am J Cardiol* 54:929, 1984.

70. Von Bibra H, Jenni R, Sebening H, Blomer H: Diagnosis of constrictive pericarditis by pulsed Doppler echocardiography of the hepatic vein (Abstr). *Proceed X World Cong Cardiol* 4:20, 1986.

71. Hancock BW: Subacute effusive-constrictive pericarditis. *Circulation* 43:183, 1971.

72. Thurber DL, Edwards JE, Achor RW: Secondary malignant tumors of the pericardium. *Circulation* 26:228, 1962.

73. Chandraratna PAN, Aronow WS: Detection of pericardial metastases by cross-sectional echocardiography. *Circulation* 63:197, 1981.

74. Mann T, Brodie BR, Grossman W: Effusive constrictive hemodynamic pattern due to neoplastic involvement of the pericardium. *Am J Cardiol* 41:781, 1978.

75. Kurkijian K, Naber SP, McInerney KP, Caldeira ME, Isner JM, Pandian NG: Echo-pathological correlations from TUFTS: Echocardiographic evaluation of metastatic pericardial disease. *Echocardiography* 3:273, 1986.

76. Reid CL, Chandraratna PAN, Kawanishi D, Bezdek WD, Schatz R, Nanna M, Rahimtoola SH: Echocardiographic detection of pneumomediastinum and pneumopericardium: The air gap sign. *J Am Coll Cardiol* 1:916, 1983.

77. Payvandi MN, Kerber RE: Echocardiography in congenital and acquired absence of pericardium. *Circulation* 53:86, 1976.

78. Moncada R, Baker M, Salinast M, Demas TC, Churchill R, Love L, Reynes C, Hale D, Cardoso M, Pilfarre R, Gunnar RM: Diagnostic role of computed tomography in pericardial heart disease: Congenital defects, thickening, neoplasms and effusions. *Am Heart J* 103:263, 1982.

79. Isner JM, Carter BI, Bankoff MS, Konstam MA, Salem DN: Computed tomography in the diagnosis of pericardial heart disease. *Ann Intern Med* 97:473, 1982.

80. Sechtem U, Tscholakoff D, Higgins CB: MRI of the abnormal pericardium. *AJR* 147:245, 1986.

81. Stark DD, Higgins CB, Lanzer P, Lipton MJ, Schiller M, Crooks LE, Botvinick EB, Kaufman L: Magnetic resonance imaging of the pericardium: Normal and pathological findings. *Radiology* 150:469, 1984.

25

Two-Dimensional Echocardiography in the Detection of Cardiac Masses and Intracardiac Thrombi

John G. Harold, M.D.
Eugenio Carmo, M.D.
Robert Decker, M.D.

Two-dimensional echocardiography is utilized frequently for the clinical assessment and differentiation of cardiac masses. These include tumors, thrombi, vegetations, and foreign bodies. Cardiac tumors may be primary or metastatic; foreign bodies include pacing wires and catheters. This chapter focuses on the identification of cardiac masses by echocardiography.

Primary cardiac tumors are exceedingly rare, with an autopsy incidence of approximately 1 in 10,000. The majority of these tumors are benign, with myxomas being the most frequent type (1, 2). Histologically, benign entities include rhabdomyomas, lipomas, and fibromas. Malignant cardiac tumors are almost all variants of sarcomas. Angiosarcomas are the most frequent, followed by rhabdomyosarcomas, fibrosarcomas, and mesotheliomas. Primary lymphoma of the heart has been recognized, and several other histologic types of malignant tumors have been described in the literature (3).

Metastatic tumors occur 20–40 times more frequently than the primary cardiac tumors and are observed in 10–12% of patients with malignancies. Involvement and distribution are related to the tumor's overall incidence and propensity to spread via direct extension as opposed to vascular or lymphatic channels. The most frequent metastatic tumors involving the heart are lung cancer in men and breast cancer in women. Metastases are also common in esophageal carcinoma, melanoma, leukemia, lymphoma, renal cell carcinoma, and hepatoma. Some patients with acquired immunodeficiency syndrome (AIDS) have been found to have cardiac involvement with Kaposi's sarcoma and lymphoma (4).

Two-dimensional echocardiography has been the most significant advancement in the diagnosis of cardiac masses. Since some primary cardiac tumors may be curable by operation, early diagnosis is essential (5–7). The development of any cardiac symptoms in a patient with known malignancy should prompt an immediate echocardiographic study. Although the prognosis for these patients remains generally poor, effective palliative measures for cardiac problems are frequently available.

BENIGN TUMORS
Myxomas

Myxomas are the most frequent primary cardiac tumor, accounting for approximately 50% of all primary tumors. They occur in all age groups but are most common in adult females. Approximately 75% of cases occur in the left atrium, 20% in the right atrium, and the remainder in either ventricle. Occasionally, myxomas involve more than one cardiac chamber. Left atrial myxomas are usually pedunculated and attached to the fossa ovalis on the interatrial septum by a stalk. Right atrial myxomas are less likely to arise from the atrial septum, and ventricular myxomas tend to arise from the lateral wall. Although the pathologic origin of these tumors has been debated in the past, more recent studies support the argument that these lesions have an endothelial or endocardial origin (8).

Classically, myxomas present with a clinical triad of obstructive, embolic, and constitutional symptoms. Patients with left atrial myxomas may present with symptoms and signs consistent with mitral stenosis. The development of embolic phenomena—particularly to the central nervous system and especially in young patients in sinus rhythm—should prompt echocardiographic evaluation to rule out myxoma or valvular heart disease. Frequently seen constitutional symptoms or laboratory abnormalities in left atrial myxoma include fever, elevated sedimentation rate, hypergammaglobinemia, and anemia (9). The signs and symptoms are proportional to the size of the myxoma. These abnormalities are presumed to be due to production of antibodies or immune complexes stimulated by the myxoma. Cardiac myxomas vary in size and can fill up virtually the left atrium. During systole, the myxoma is contained within the left atrium; in diastole, the myxoma may prolapse into the left ventricle. A large myxoma can obstruct the valve orifice and impede diastolic flow into the ventricle.

The first accounts of echo-diagnosed left atrial myxoma were reported in 1959 (10, 11). Many reports on the echocardiographic manifestations of left atrial myxoma have been published since that time (12–17). The diagnosis of myxoma by M-mode echocardiography may be made difficult or impossible by many factors. For example, if only a few echoes are reflected from the myxoma, the pattern may mimic mitral stenosis (Figs. 25.1 and 25.2). Other factors include a technically inadequate or incomplete study, low gain setting, a small or nonprolapsing myxoma, a normal E–

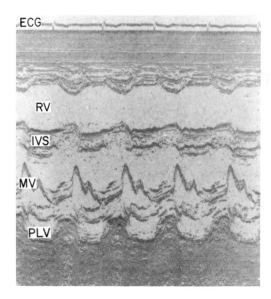

Figure 25.2. M-mode echogram taken 1 month following surgical removal of the left atrial myxoma from the same patient as shown in Figure 25.1. The mitral valve (*MV*) motion is now normal, and the parallel linear echoes have disappeared. *IVS* = interventricular septum, *PLV* = posterior left ventricular wall, *RV* = right ventricle.

F slope, presence of a nonmyxomatous left atrial tumor, a left atrial thrombus, severe mitral valve prolapse, or mitral valve vegetations (18). Pechacek et al. (19) reported on the analysis of 28 patients with a left atrial myxoma and two with a right atrial myxoma. Only 59% of the M-mode echocardiograms in patients with a left atrial myxoma showed the characteristic findings of multiple diastolic echoes within the mitral orifice as well as abnormal systolic echoes within the left atrium (Fig. 25.3). Two-dimensional echocardiography showed the presence of a left atrial mass in all 16 patients who had the procedure. Charuzi et al. (20) proposed a new echocardiographic classification of left atrial myxomas.

The detection of myxomas is best accomplished using several two-dimensional echocardiographic views. Two-dimensional echocardiography is particularly useful in detecting small myxomas (Fig. 25.4). Such small tumors may escape detection by M-mode echocardiography because of an inappropriately low gain setting and a normal E–F slope, as previously mentioned and as seen in Figure 25.5. The parasternal long-axis view is used most frequently because it allows simultaneous

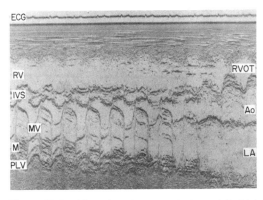

Figure 25.1. M-mode echogram of a large left atrial (*LA*) myxoma (*M*). The myxoma is represented by parallel linear echoes behind the anterior leaflet of the mitral valve (*MV*), rather than the usual cloud of echoes. Confusion with mitral stenosis could have occurred if a two-dimensional echocardiogram had not been performed. *Ao* = aorta, *IVS* = interventricular septum, *PLV* = posterior left ventricular wall, *RV* = right ventricle, *RVOT* = right ventricular outflow tract.

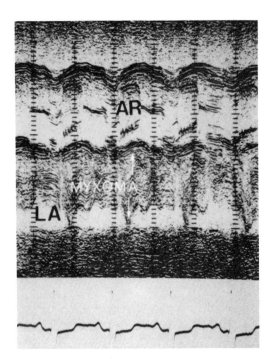

Figure 25.3. M-mode echocardiogram in a patient with a large left atrial myxoma. The myxoma is seen in the left atrium (*LA*) behind the aortic root (*AR*). During systole the myxoma reaches the posterior wall of the left atrium.

visualization of the left ventricle, mitral valve, left atrium, and aorta. Figure 25.6 demonstrates a large, well-circumscribed mass prolapsing into the left ventricle in diastole. An estimate of the size

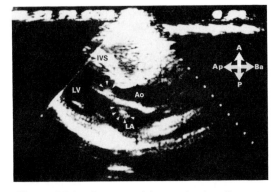

Figure 25.4. Parasternal long-axis view illustrating a thin elongated myxoma (*arrows*) prolapsing into the left ventricle (*LV*) through the mitral orifice during diastole. The myxoma did not interfere with mitral valve function. *A* = anterior, *Ao* = aorta, *Ap* = apex, *IVS* = interventricular septum, *LA* = left atrium, *P* = posterior.

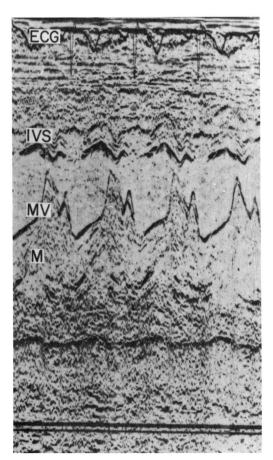

Figure 25.5. M-mode echogram showing a small left atrial myxoma (*M*) from the same patient as shown in Figure 25.4. The motion of the mitral valve (*MV*) is normal. In the last beat on the right, the gain setting was decreased, causing disappearance of most of the echoes from the myxoma. This demonstrates the importance of appropriate gain settings in the diagnosis of left atrial myxoma. *IVS* = interventricular septum.

of this tumor can be made easily from the two-dimensional image, which is the equivalent of the M-mode sweep shown in Figure 25.1. Use of the short-axis view at the aortic level provides visualization of a left atrial myxoma during systole, when the tumor is driven back into the left atrium (Fig. 25.7). No tumor should be seen in the left atrium following surgical resection. As an adjunct to the left parasternal views, apical (Fig. 25.8) and subcostal (Fig. 25.9) views can be utilized. The most suitable is the apical four-chamber view (Fig. 25.10), which provides simultaneous visualization of all four cardiac chambers. In addition

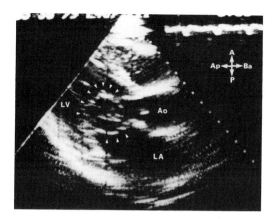

Figure 25.6. Parasternal long-axis view of a large left atrial (*LA*) myxoma (*arrows*) prolapsing into the left ventricle (*LV*) in diastole. The myxoma is seen filling the entire mitral ring. *A* = anterior, *Ao* = aorta, *Ap* = apex; *Ba* = base, *P* = posterior.

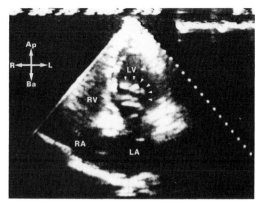

Figure 25.8. Apical four-chamber view demonstrating a large left atrial (*LA*) myxoma (*arrows*) in diastole. The myxoma can be seen extending almost to the apex of the left ventricle (*LV*). *Ap* = apex, *Ba* = base, *L* = left, *R* = right, *RA* = right atrium; *RV* = right ventricle.

to diagnosing left atrial myxoma, a concomitant right atrial myxoma can be eliminated (21, 22).

Two-dimensional echocardiography is significantly more effective than M-mode echocardiography for the detection, localization, and sizing of right atrial masses (23). The visualization of the interatrial septum is important to distinguish between a right atrial myxoma, which is typically attached to the interatrial septum, and tricuspid vegetations, which are attached to the tricuspid

valve (24). Right atrial myxoma also can be visualized using a parasternal short-axis view at the level of the aortic valve and a parasternal long-axis view, which visualizes the right ventricle, right atrium, and tricuspid valve (Fig. 25.11). In the subcostal view, because of the proximity of the transducer, the right atrium can be especially well visualized. In Figure 25.12 a mass is seen in the center of the right atrium. This mass was diagnosed as a right atrial myxoma by M-mode echocardiography. However, the two-dimensional ex-

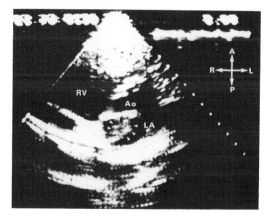

Figure 25.7. Parasternal short-axis view at the level of the aortic root (*Ao*), showing a left atrial (*LA*) myxoma (*arrows*) attached to the interatrial septum. *A* = anterior, *L* = left, *P* = posterior, *R* = right, *RV* = right ventricle.

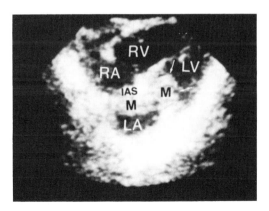

Figure 25.9. Subcostal four-chamber view in a patient with a large left atrial (*LA*) myxoma. The attachment to the interatrial septum (*IAS*) is better seen in this view. The *arrows* show the myxoma (M) prolapsing into the left ventricle (*LV*) during diastole. *RA* = right atrium, *RV* = right ventricle.

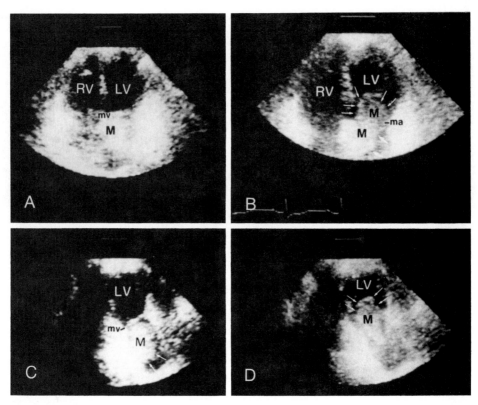

Figure 25.10. Apical view in a patient with a large left atrial myxoma. The four-chamber view is seen at the *top*, and the two-chamber view is seen at the *bottom*. During systole (*A* and *C*), the large myxoma (*M*) fills most of the left atrium from the mitral valve (*mv*) to the posterior wall of the left atrium *LA* (*arrows* on *C*). During diastole (*B* and *D*), the myxoma (*M*) prolapses into the left ventricle (*LV*) passing across the mitral anulus (*ma*). *RV* = right ventricle.

amination demonstrated an attachment to the tricuspid valve rather than to the interatrial septum.

Once the diagnosis of myxoma is made, surgical extirpation is indicated. Routine preoperative angiography need not be performed in uncomplicated cases. Removal of the entire stalk with a rim of normal myocardium is generally adequate, although frequently the interatrial septum is removed and replaced with a patch.

Rhabdomyoma

These benign tumors are the most common primary cardiac tumors of infancy and childhood (25). Eighty-five percent are seen in children younger than 15 years of age. Most of these occur in children less than 1 year old. Cardiac rhabdomyomas are frequently associated with tuberous sclerosis. These lesions are often multiple (in 90% of cases) and are found with equal frequency in both ventricles.

Rhabdomyomas cause symptoms secondary to intracavitary growth, frequently presenting as outflow tract obstructions. Figure 25.13 shows an M-mode echocardiogram suggestive of an intramyocardial tumor. In this case, two-dimensional echocardiography further defined the extent of cardiac involvement. The parasternal long-axis view (Fig. 25.14) and parasternal short-axis view (Fig. 25.15) demonstrate the size and extent of protrusion of the tumor into the right and left ventricles. The subcostal view (Fig. 25.16), which visualized the apex, completed the three-dimensional geometric definition of the tumor. This view demonstrated that the tumor extended all the way to the apex, where it projected into the left ventricular cavity. This information helped differentiate this tumor from asymmetric septal hy-

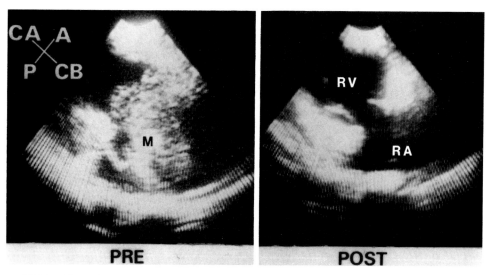

Figure 25.11. Medially angled parasternal long-axis view imaging the right ventricle (*RV*) and right atrium (*RA*). *Left,* From a preoperative (*PRE*) study demonstrating a large right atrial myxoma (*M*). The myxoma is only partially prolapsing into the right ventricle (*RV*). *Right,* Postoperative (*POST*) study demonstrating the complete disappearance of the myxoma. *A* = anterior, *CA* = cardiac apex, *CB* = cardiac base, *P* = posterior.

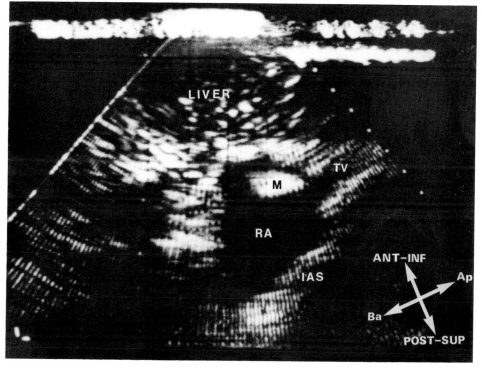

Figure 25.12. Subcostal long-axis view showing an oval mass (*M*) in the right atrium (*RA*) in midsystole. The mass was not attached to the interatrial septum (*IAS*). At surgery, a calcified mass was found to be connected to the septal leaflet of the tricuspid valve (*TV*). *ANT-INF* = anteroinferior, *Ap* = apex, *Ba* = base, *POST-SUP* = posterosuperior.

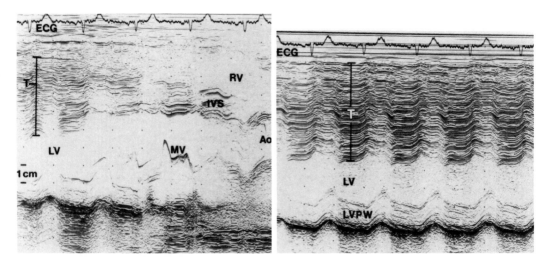

Figure 25.13. This M-mode echogram at the midventricular level (*right*) shows a large intramyocardial tumor (*T, vertical bar*) represented by linear echoes within the interventricular septum (*IVS*), which displays paradoxical motion. In the M-mode sweep (*left*), the mass appears in the midventricular portion of the interventricular septum without encroaching on either the right ventricular (*RV*) or left ventricular (*LV*) outflow tracts. *Ao* = aorta, *LVPW* = left ventricular posterior wall, *MV* = mitral valve.

pertrophy or a diffuse infiltrative cardiomyopathy such as amyloid. The treatment of choice is early, aggressive resection of tumor masses. The untreated patient has a poor prognosis.

Fibroma

These benign tumors are the second most common pediatric cardiac tumor (26). The typical patient is younger than 10 years and presents with a solitary, large ventricular mass. Fibromas usually involve the interventricular septum or the free wall. Patients may present with obstructive symptoms or arrhythmias and have a high risk of sudden death. Aggressive debulking of these tumors has been associated with prolonged asymptomatic survival in some cases.

Other Benign Tumors

Other rarely seen benign tumors include lipomas, hemangiomas, and mesotheliomas. Although rare, mesothelioma is worthy of mention because of its propensity to involve the atrioventricular (A-V) node; hence, presentation with complete heart block is well described (27).

MALIGNANT TUMORS

Most primary malignant tumors of the heart are sarcomas. These tumors are almost always associated with a poor prognosis. However, there are characteristics that allow two-dimensional

echocardiography to distinguish among the various types (28, 29). Angiosarcoma is the most frequently encountered cardiac sarcoma and is seen more often in males. Approximately 80% of angiosarcomas occur in the right atrium. These tumors frequently invade the vena cava, tricuspid valve, and pericardium. Consequently, many patients present with symptoms and signs of right heart failure, pericardial effusion, tamponade, or rapidly progressive vena cava obstruction. The majority of these patients will have metastatic disease at presentation. Patients with rhabdomyosarcoma often present with multiple cardiac lesions. Fibrosarcomas frequently protrude into the ventricular cavity and may cause symptoms of valvular obstruction.

Metastatic Tumors

Metastatic tumors which invade the right atrium can be recognized by M-mode echocardiography as well as by two-dimensional echocardiography. If the mass is large, a parasternal short-axis view is sufficient for diagnosis (Fig. 25.17). If the route of right atrial invasion is via the inferior vena cava, the tumor may be diagnosed best using a subcostal view (Fig. 25.18).

Thrombi

Two-dimensional echocardiography is a useful technique for the detection of intracardiac thrombi.

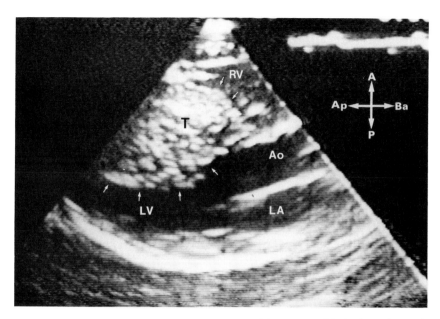

Figure 25.14. Parasternal long-axis view of a large mass of dense, speckled echoes (*arrows*) representing an intramyocardial tumor (*T*) in the same patient as shown in Figure 25.13. The mass replaces the interventricular septum and extends into both the left ventricle (*LV*) and the right ventricle (*RV*). The texture of the echoes in the tumor differs from those of normal myocardium. A = anterior, Ao = aorta, Ap = apex, *Ba* = base, *LA* = left atrium, P = posterior.

The ultrasonic detection of intracardiac thrombi depends on the differences in acoustic properties between the thrombus and the surrounding tissue. Differentiation among intracardiac thrombus, tumor, underlying cavity noise, and adjacent myocardium may be difficult at times (30). Ultrasound tissue characterization techniques may be useful in differentiating thrombi from blood and myocardium.

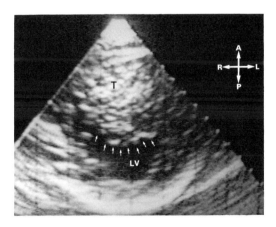

Figure 25.15. Parasternal short-axis view of a large, densely speckled mass of echoes (*arrows*) representing an intramyocardial tumor (*T*) in the same patient as shown in Figures 25.13 and 25.14. The oval tumor is replacing the interventricular septum and protruding into the left ventricular (*LV*) cavity. A = anterior, L = left, P = posterior, R = right.

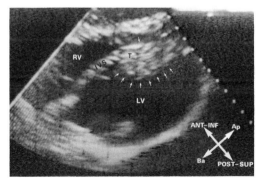

Figure 25.16. Subcostal long-axis view in the same patient as shown in Figures 25.13, 25.14, and 25.15, showing both the right ventricle (*RV*) and left ventricle (*LV*). A mass of dense, speckled echoes (*arrows*) representing the intramyocardial tumor (*T*) is seen in the apical region of the interventricular septum (*IVS*). ANT-INF = anteroinferior, Ap = apex, *ba* = base, *POST-SUP* = posterosuperior.

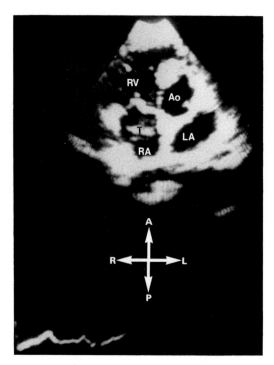

Figure 25.17. Parasternal short-axis view at the aortic root (*Ao*) level. A tumor (*T*) in the center of the right atrium (*RA*) was found to be a metastasis of squamous cell carcinoma of the lung, extending into the right atrium through the inferior vena cava. *A* = anterior, *L* = left, *LA* = left atrium, *P* = posterior, *R* = right, *RV* = right ventricle.

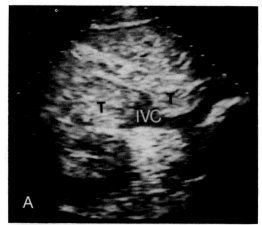

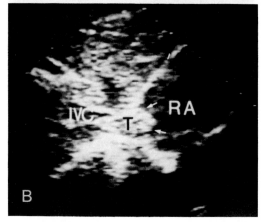

Figure 25.18. *A*, Subcostal view of the inferior vena cava (*IVC*) in a patient with a metastatic tumor (*T*). *B*, The tumor is seen invading the right atrium (*RA*) from the inferior vena cava (*IVC*).

Left atrial thrombi frequently are associated with either rheumatic mitral valve deformities or prosthetic mitral valves. Patients with a large left atrium and paroxysmal atrial fibrillation are at increased risk for embolic complications from left atrial thrombi. Mitral valve prolapse may be associated with valvular thrombi, which may cause embolic strokes. The location, size, and motion of left atrial thrombi are variable. A thrombus fully adherent to the atrial wall, as seen in Figure 25.19, does not have any independent motion. However, thrombi without any firm attachment may show undulation or a jiggling motion during the cardiac cycle. A thrombus attached to the sewing ring of a prosthetic mitral valve will move simultaneously with it. A complete two-dimensional echocardiographic examination is necessary to detect or rule out left atrial thrombi. The parasternal short-axis view is the most reliable echocardiographic window for imaging the left atrial appendage. However, thrombi in the left atrial appendage or mural thrombi adhering to the left atrial wall may be difficult to detect by echocardiography, and a negative study does not rule out their presence. Transesophageal echocardiography is a more sensitive technique in the detection of thrombi in the left atrial appendage (31). Artifact from adjacent cardiac structures may make the diagnosis of intracardiac thrombi difficlt. This is particularly true in patients with prosthetic mitral valves or with extensive mitral annulus calcification. A left atrial thrombus must be differentiated from a myxoma, which may have similar acoustic properties.

Right atrial thrombi occur much less frequently than do left atrial thrombi (32). They are seen

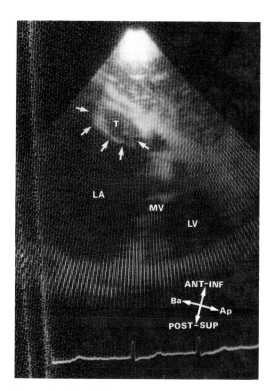

Figure 25.19. Subcostal long-axis view of a patient with severe mitral stenosis. An oval mass (*T*, *arrows*) representing a mural thrombus is seen in the markedly dilated left atrium (*LA*) attached to the interatrial septum. *ANT-INF* = anteroinferior, *Ap* = apex, *Ba* = base, *LV* = left ventricle; *MV* = mitral valve; *POST-SUP* = posterosuperior.

thrombus versus intracavitary tumor or other anatomic structures, such as papillary muscles or chordae tendineae. The presence of an intracavitary mass in a patient with congestive cardiomyopathy or in the left ventricle after a myocardial infarction is most likely a thrombus. Most thrombi are adherent to the left ventricular wall and lack independent motion. However, at times a thrombus is attached loosely to the endocardium, resulting in varying degrees of independent motion.

False-positive diagnosis of a left ventricular thrombus is not uncommon, especially if apical views are utilized. If a high gain setting is required to visualize the left ventricular apex, the presence

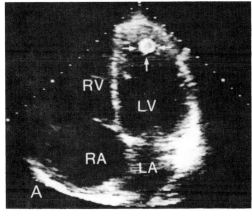

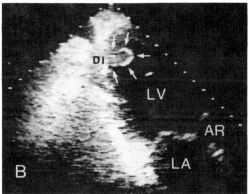

Figure 25.20. Apical view in a patient with a pedunculated thrombus. *A*, The *arrows* show the clear borders of a mass in the apex of the left ventricle (*LV*) when a four-chamber view is obtained. *B*, The two-chamber view shows the attachment of the thrombus to the diaphragmatic surface of the LV apex (*DI*). *AR* = aortic root, *LA* = left atrium, *RA* = right atrium, *RV* = right ventricle.

usually in association with intracardiac catheters, such as indwelling venous catheters or permanent pacemaker electrodes. Inferior vena cava thrombi may be seen in association with certain neoplasms. The most useful view for imaging right atrial thrombi is the subcostal window, which also provides imaging of the inferior vena cava.

Left ventricular thrombi are seen in patients with acute myocardial infarction, left ventricular aneurysms, and congestive cardiomyopathy, with the apex being the most common location (33, 34). Visualization of left ventricular thrombi can be accomplished best using the apical four-chamber and apical long-axis views (Fig. 25.20). Figure 25.21 illustrates a large thrombus filling an apical aneurysm in a patient 2 years after myocardial infarction, which was diagnosed by two-dimensional echocardiography. Attention to anatomy and physiology will facilitate identification of

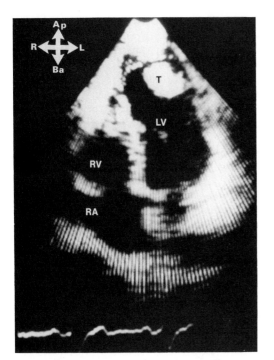

Figure 25.21. Apical four-chamber view demonstrating an apical left ventricular (*LV*) thrombus (*T*). Note that the left ventricular apex is dilated as a result of a myocardial infarction with aneurysm formation. The thrombus was adherent to the left ventricular wall. *Ap* = apex, *Ba* = base, *L* = left, *R* = right, *RA* = right atrium; *RV* = right ventricle.

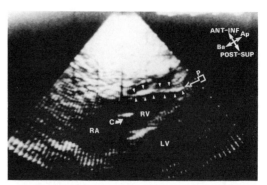

Figure 25.22. Subcostal long-axis view demonstrating a balloon flotation catheter (*C, thick curved arrow*) and a pacing catheter (*P, arrows*) in the right heart. The balloon flotation catheter appears as a short segment at the approximate location of the tricuspid valve. The pacing catheter appears as a long linear echo extending to the right ventricular (*RV*) apex. *ANT-INF* = anteroinferior, *Ap* = apex, *Ba* = base, *LV* = left ventricle, *POST-SUP* = posterosuperior, *RA* = right atrium.

of multiple echoes may be mistaken for an apical thrombus. The best way to increase the efficiency of two-dimensional echocardiography is to visualize the thrombus from at least two different views and through the use of serial studies. Thrombi usually are confined to areas with wall motion abnormalities. Serial studies can assess the regression of thrombi following anticoagulation therapy.

FOREIGN BODIES

In the past, intracardiac foreign bodies were the result of direct cardiac penetration or indirect penetration with migration through the venous system. At present, most foreign bodies visualized by echocardiography are intracardiac catheters, with the majority being balloon flotation or transvenous pacing catheters. Occasionally, foreign bodies are the result of retained catheter fragments.

Echocardiography is recognized as an impor-

tant imaging technique for evaluating intracardiac foreign bodies. Intracardiac catheters are elongated structures with excellent ultrasonic reflective properties. It has been shown that balloon flotation catheters in the right heart can mimic endocardial surfaces, which may give a false impression of pathology when there is none (35).

Similar to balloon flotation catheters, trans-

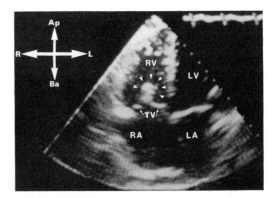

Figure 25.23. In this apical four-chamber view, a thickened mass (*arrowheads*) extends from the tricuspid valve (*TV, small arrows*) into the right ventricle (*RV*). The mass represents a permanent transvenous pacing electrode encapsulated by thick connective tissue. *Ap* = apex, *Ba* = base, *L* = left, *LA* = left atrium, *LV* = left ventricle, *R* = right, *RA* = right atrium.

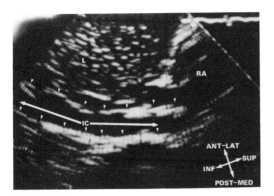

Figure 25.24. Subcostal view showing the right atrium (*RA*) and inferior vena cava (*IC, long arrows*). A loop of retained broken pacing catheter (*arrowheads*) can be seen in the inferior vena cava with edges protruding into the right atrium. *ANT-LAT* = anterolateral; *INF* = inferior, *L* = liver, *POST-MED* = posteromedial, *SUP* = superior.

venous pacing catheters also appear as thick linear structures producing intense echoes which can simulate right heart structures. Motion of the ventricles can be altered because of the abnormal activation sequences created by ventricular pacing. Pacing catheters have been reported to simulate right atrial masses with or without a large loop of the pacemaker electrode in the right atrium. In addition to detecting catheters, two-dimensional echocardiography is an effective tool for evaluating their course within the cardiac cham-

bers. A balloon flotation catheter can be seen crossing the tricuspid valve into the right ventricular outflow tract, while a pacing catheter typically can be followed from the tricuspid valve to the right ventricular apex (Fig. 25.22). Occasionally, a pacing catheter can be followed into the coronary sinus. Furthermore, pacing catheter placement can be aided by the use of echocardiography. Echoes reflected from a permanent catheter that are denser than normal may represent fibrotic growth around the catheter (Fig. 25.23). Occasionally, this complication may involve the tricuspid valve and restrict its motion.

Two-dimensional echocardiography can detect fractured pacing catheters that have migrated out of the superior vena cava and right heart chambers down the inferior vena cava (Fig. 25.24). The subcostal view is the view of choice, as it allows

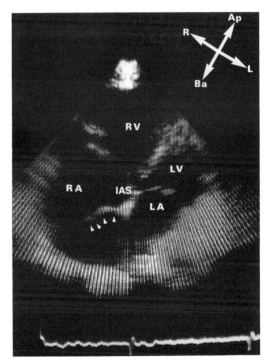

Figure 25.26. Apical four-chamber view taken from a patient with an atrial septal defect. The right atrium (*RA*) and right ventricle (*RV*) are dilated. A curvilinear echo (*arrowheads*) in the right atrium is seen attached to the interatrial septum (*IAS*) and should not be confused with a foreign body. In surgery, this echo was found to be a flap of the interatrial septum attached to the rim of the defect. *Ap* = apex, *Ba* = base, *L* = left, *LA* = left atrium; *LV* = left ventricle.

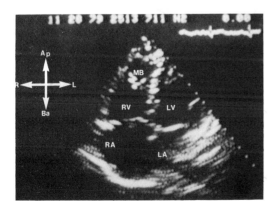

Figure 25.25. Apical four-chamber view demonstrating a prominent moderator band (*MB*) in the right ventricle (*RV*). The fact that it contracted in systole helps distinguish it from a foreign body or mass. *Ap* = apex, *Ba* = base, *L* = left, *LA* = left atrium, *LV* = left ventricle, *R* = right, *RA* = right atrium.

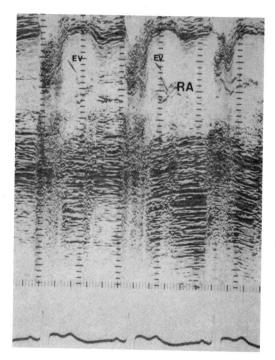

Figure 25.27. M-mode representation of a prominent eustachian valve (*EV*). With the M-mode beam directed through the back of the right atrium (*RA*) from the subcostal approach, the motion of the eustachian valve can be appreciated.

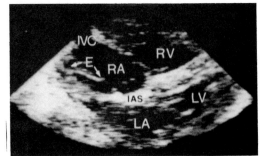

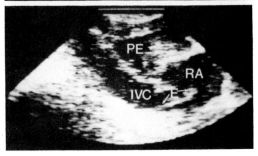

Figure 25.28. Subcostal view of a prominent eustachian valve (*E*). *Top,* A four-chamber view shows the eustachian valve moving inside the right atrium (*RA*) in between the inferior vena cave (*IVC*) and the interatrial septum (*IAS*). *LA* = left atrium, *LV* = left ventricle, *RV* = right ventricle. *Bottom,* Modifying the four-chamber view for better visualization of the inferior vena cava, the attachment of the eustachian valve to the junction of the inferior vena cava to the right atrium can be appreciated. *PE* =

visualization of the inferior vena cava along a substantial length of its course.

Anatomic variations or redundant tissue sometimes may be misinterpreted as masses or foreign bodies (36). A moderator band is a muscle bridge of variable size and location, crossing the right ventricular cavity between the free wall and the interventricular septum. It can be misinterpreted as a mass or thrombus (Fig. 25.25). A flap of the interatrial septum in the case of atrial septal defect may simulate a foreign body (Fig. 25.26). A prominent eustachian valve may be noted in both the M-mode (Fig. 25.27) and the two-dimensional echogram (Fig. 25.28). The subcostal view is the best approach to identify this remnant of the valve over the inferior vena cava and to differentiate it from a possible pathologic condition, such as a vegetation or a thrombus (37). The Chiari network, another congenital remnant in the area of the coronary sinus, also can present as a highly mobile and reflectant echo in the right atrium and may simulate a mass (38). Careful attention to cardiac anatomy, use of multiple echocardio-

graphic views, and clinical correlation are required to minimize these misinterpretations.

SUMMARY

Two-dimensional echocardiography is the diagnostic procedure of choice in the detection of intracardiac masses and foreign bodies. This is due to not only the noninvasive nature of the test but, most importantly, its superior diagnostic capability and ease of image acquisition.

REFERENCES

1. Heath D: Pathology of cardiac tumors. *Am J Cardiol* 21:315–327, 1968.
2. Fyke FE, Seward JB, Edwards WD, Miller FA, Reeder GS, Schattenberg TT, Schub C, Tajik AJ: Primary cardiac tumors: Experience with 30 consecutive patients since the introduction of two-dimensional echocardiography. *J Am Coll Cardiol* 5:1465, 1985.
3. Smith C: Tumors of the heart. *Arch Pathol Lab Med* 110:371–374, 1986.

4. Fink L, Reichek N, St John Sutton MG: Cardiac abnormalities in acquired immune deficiency syndrome. *Am J Cardiol* 54:1161–1163, 1984.

5. Eckstein R, Gossner W, Rienmuller R: Primary malignant fibrous histiocytoma of the left atrium. Surgical and chemotherapeutic management. *Br Heart J* 52:354–357, 1984.

6. Reece IJ, Cooley DA, Frazier OH, Hallman GL, Powers PL, Montero CG: Cardiac tumors. Clinical spectrum and prognosis of lesions other than classical benign myxoma in 20 patients. *J Thorac Cardiovasc Surg* 88:439–446, 1984.

7. Hanson EC, Gill CC, Razavi M, Loop FD: The surgical treatment of atrial myxomas. Clinical experience and late results in 33 patients. *J Thorac Cardiovasc Surg* 89:298–303, 1985.

8. Bulkley BH, Hutchins GM: Atrial myxomas: A fifty year review. *Am Heart J* 97:639–643, 1979.

9. Goodwin JF: Symposium on cardiac tumors. The spectrum of cardiac tumors. *Am J Cardiol* 21:307–314, 1968.

10. Effert S, Domanig E. Diagnostik intraauriculaer tumoren und grosser Thromben mit dem Ultraschall-Ecoverfahren (Diagnosis of intra-auricular tumors and large thrombi with the aid of ultrasonic echocardiography). *Dtsh Med Wschr* 84:6–8, 1959.

11. Edler I, Gustafson A, Karleforst T, Christensson B: Mitral and aortic valve movements recorded by an ultrasonic echo method. *Acta Med Scand* 170:67–82, 1961.

12. Wolfe SB, Popp RL, Feigenbaum H: Diagnosis of atrial tumors by ultrasound. *Circulation* 39:615–622, 1969.

13. Popp RL, Harrison DC: Ultrasound for the diagnosis of atrial tumor. *Ann Intern Med* 71:785–787, 1969.

14. Gustafson A, Edler I, Dahlback O, Kaude J, Person S: Left atrial myxoma diagnosed by ultrasound cardiography. *Angiology* 24:554–562, 1973.

15. Finegan RE, Harrison DC: Diagnosis of left atrial myxoma by echocardiography. *N Engl J Med* 282:1022–1023, 1977.

16. St John Sutton MG, Mercier LA, Guiliani ER, Lie JT: Atrial myxomas: A review of clinical experience in 40 patients. *Mayo Clin Proc* 55:371–376, 1980.

17. Srivastavan TN, Fletcher E: The echocardiogram in left atrial myxoma. *Am J Med* 54:136–139, 1973.

18. Come PC, Riley MF, Markis JE, Malagold M: Limitations of echocardiographic techniques in evaluation of left atrial masses. *Am J Cardiol* 48:947–953, 1981.

19. Pechacek LW, Gonzalez-Camid F, Hall RJ, Garcia E, de Castro CM, Leachman RD, Montiel-Amoroso G: The echocardiographic spectrum of atrial myxoma: A ten-year experience. *Tex Heart Inst J* 13:179–195, 1986.

20. Charuzi Y, Bolger A, Beeder C, Lew AS: A new echocardiographic classification of left atrial myxoma. *Am J Cardiol* 55:614–615, 1985.

21. Fitterer JD, Spicer MJ, Nelson WP: Echocardiographic demonstration of bilateral atrial myxomas. *Chest* 70:282–284, 1976.

22. DeMaria AN, Vismara LA, Miller RR, Neumann A, Mason DT: Unusual echographic manifestations of right and left heart myxomas. *Am J Med* 59:713–720, 1975.

23. Harbold NB, Gau GT: Echocardiographic diagnosis of right atrial myxoma. *Mayo Clin Proc* 48:284–286, 1973.

24. Come PC, Kurland GS, Vine HS: Two-dimensional echocardiography in differentiating right atrial and tricuspid valve mass lesions. *Am J Cardiol* 44:1207–1212.

25. Bass JL, Breningstall GN, Swaiman KF: Echocardiographic incidence of cardiac rhabdomyoma in tuberous sclerosis. *Am J Cardiol* 55:1379–1382, 1985.

26. Feldman PS, Meyer MW. Fibroelastic hamartoma (fibroma) of the heart. *Cancer* 38:314–323, 1976.

27. Nishida K, Kamijima G, Nagayama T: Mesothelioma of the atrioventricular node. *Br Heart J* 53:468–470, 1985.

28. Panella JS, Paige ML, Victor TA, Semerdjian RA, Hueter DC. Angiosarcoma of the heart. Diagnosis by echocardiography. *Chest* 76:221–223, 1979.

29. Duncan WJ, Rowe RD, Freedom RM, Izukawa T, Olley PM: Space-occupying lesions of the myocardium: Role of two-dimensional echocardiography in detection of cardiac tumors in children. *Am Heart J* 104:780–785, 1982.

30. McPherson DD, Knosp BM, Kieso RA, Bean JA, Kerber RE, Skorton DJ, Collins SM: Ultrasound characterization of acoustic properties of intracardiac thrombi: Studies in a new experimental model. *J Am Soc Echo* 4:264–270, 1988.

31. Aschenberg W, Schluter M, Kremer P, Schroder E, Siglow V, Bleifeld W: Transesophageal two-dimensional echocardiography for the dectection of left atrial appendage thrombus. *J Am Coll Cardiol* 7:163–166, 1986.

32. Cameron J, Pohlner PG, Staffor EG, O'Brien MF, Bett JHN, Murphy AL: Right heart thrombus: Recognition and management. *J Am Coll Cardiol* 5:1239–1243, 1985.

33. DeMaria AN, Neumann A, Bommer W, Neumann BS, Grehl L, Weinart L, De Nardo S, Amsterdam EA, Mason DT: Left ventricular thrombi identified by cross-sectional echocardiography. *Ann Intern Med* 90:8–14, 1979.

34. Reeder GS, Tajik AJ, Seward JB: Left ventricular mural thrombus: Two-dimensional echocardiographic diagnosis. *Mayo Clin Proc* 56:82–86, 1981.

35. Charuzi Y, Kraus R, Swan HJC: Echocadiographic interpretation in the presence of Swan-Ganz intracardiac catheters. *Am J Cardiol* 40:989–994, 1977.

36. Keren A, Billingham ME, Popp RL: Echocardiographic recognition and implications of ventricular hypertropic trabeculations and aberrant bands. *Circulation* 70:836–842, 1984.

37. Limacher MC, Gutgesell HP, Vick GW, Cohen MH, Huhta JH: Echocardiographic anatomy of the eustachian valve. *Am J Cardiol* 57:363–365, 1986.

38. Cloez JL, Neimann JL, Chivoret G, Danchin N, Bruntz JF, Godenir JP, Faivre G: Echocardiographic rediscovery of an anatomical structure: The Chiari network. Apropos of 16 cases. *Arch Mal Coeur* 76:1284–1292, 1983.

26

Experimental Advances in Two-Dimensional Echocardiography

Samuel Meerbaum, Ph.D.

INTRODUCTION

The past few years have seen momentous strides in the application of two-dimensional echocardiography (2DE). This is partly as a result of substantial improvement in echo equipment that allows more reliable outlining of blood-muscle interfaces. Consequently, clinical 2DE assessment of cardiac dysfunction and structural abnormalities is now a well-established technique. In addition, new Doppler techniques that significantly supplement 2DE are receiving much current attention.

In spite of these tremendous advances, there appears to be a need for further improvement of 2DE procedures to allow convenient, rapid, and quantitative measurement of the global and regional cardiac geometry and contractile function. Another challenge for experimental 2DE research is to accelerate progress in such new areas as computerized three-dimensional reconstruction, ultrasound characterization of myocardial tissue, and assessment of perfusion.

This chapter focuses on experimental progress in 2DE directed toward quantitation of wall motion, computerization, and enhanced analysis of images; three-dimensional reconstruction; ultrasound tissue characterization; and contrast assessment of myocardial perfusion defects. Sample investigations of cardiac pathophysiology are used to illustrate potential applications.

QUANTITATION OF REGIONAL AND GLOBAL CARDIAC FUNCTION

From an experimental point of view there is little question that 2DE can provide useful measurements of cardiac geometry and function. The concern has been whether such measurements are truly quantitative, as well as how to standardize the method.

Certain imaging problems are common to all noninvasive techniques, while others are specific to 2DE cardiac cross sections and the manner in which quantitative information is derived. Much like nuclear magnetic resonance and fast tomography imaging of the heart, 2DE is used to derive ventricular volumes, ejection fractions, and various indices of global and regional contractile function. It generally is appreciated that results depend on the quality of the cross-sectional images. Although there has been significant improvement in 2DE border delineation, there are frequent limitations on sophisticated analysis. Thus, in certain patient subsets, the yield of sufficiently quantifiable short-axis cross sections may be unsatisfactory. The extent to which the more common apical ventricular images provide quantifiable endocardial edges and wall thickness also can be argued. Finally, there are the bothersome echo "dropouts" that make any standardized quantification procedure difficult to apply.

Most quantitative 2DE procedures were developed from experimental canine short-axis cross-sectional images of the left ventricle. In the closed-chest dog model, which is used for a variety of physiologic and validation studies, image quality recently appears to be quite satisfactory (Fig. 26.1). However, further computer enhancement of the epicardial and endocardial edges is still being developed (2).

An impediment to quantitation is the subjectivity involved in obtaining circular short-axis cross sections presumed to be perpendicular to the long axis of the left ventricle. This assumption generally is true in normal ventricles, permitting

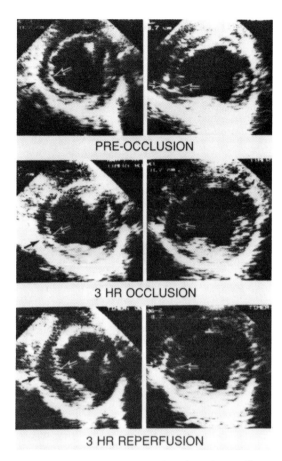

PRE-OCCLUSION

3 HR OCCLUSION

3 HR REPERFUSION

Figure 26.1. Two-dimensional echocardiographic short-axis cross sections at the low papillary muscle level of the left ventricle, taken at the end-diastolic phase in dogs with sudden (*left*) or staged (*right*) reperfusion. *Arrows* indicate epicardial and endocardial interface in the ischemic zone. End-diastolic myocardial wall thickness in the ischemic zone 3 hours after occlusion was slightly decreased in both dogs. Three hours after reperfusion, the ischemic zone wall thickness increased markedly in the dog with sudden reperfusion, whereas the increase in end-diastolic wall thickness was obviously less in the dog with staged reperfusion. (From Yamazaki S, Fujibayashi Y, Rajagopalam RE, Meerbaum S, Corday E: Effects of staged versus sudden reperfusion after acute coronary occlusion in the dog. *J Am Coll Cardiol*, 7:564–572, 1986.) Reprinted with permission from the American College of Cardiology.

quantitative analysis even in the presence of slight sectional obliquity. However, it may not be true in pathologic myocardial states exhibiting significant changes in ventricular shape and/or regional

contractile function. Considering the limits of resolution, a 2DE cross section does not truly represent a discrete transverse plane. Rather, it reflects some average representation of a myocardial "slab." This slab also changes its position along the long axis during systolic contraction. These comments are intended merely to indicate that, while a number of successful experimental validations have been reported, perfect quantitation should not be expected.

FIXED VERSUS FLOATING REFERENCE SYSTEMS

Quantitative regional wall motion analysis presents difficulties for all diagnostic methods that image a three-dimensional body by planar cross sections. One particular problem in studies of the beating heart is its overall intrathoracic displacement, as well as its contractile wall motions. Displacement, which is known to be influenced by respiratory variations, includes long-axis translation and rotation, as well as twisting in transverse planes. Unless these motions are systematically taken into account, a 2DE cross-sectional study often may fail to achieve true quantitation of myocardial segmental function.

Much controversy concerns the use of external versus internal reference systems in quantitative 2DE analysis of changes in segmental area and radial or hemiaxial length from end-diastole to end-systole. The fixed reference system relates all points of an interface, such as the endocardium of the left ventricular short-axis cross section, to an independent X-Y system (3) (Fig. 26.2). The figure demonstrates translation of the cross section due to intrathoracic motion of a normally contracting heart. A fixed reference analysis without appropriate correction would suggest absurd dyskinetic regional motions.

Figure 26.3 demonstrates a floating reference system analysis (3). This approach takes advantage of left ventricular internal landmarks and a derived chamber centroid. This allows superposition of a reference grid system to account for whole heart motion effects. Thus, contractile cardiac wall movements from end-diastole to end-systole can be differentiated. This approach proves adequate for a standardized computer analysis of unselected echo frames in normal or near-uniform contractile motion. However, it does not allow quantitation during significant regional wall motion derangements or major alteration in left ventricular shape. Simple end-diastolic and end-

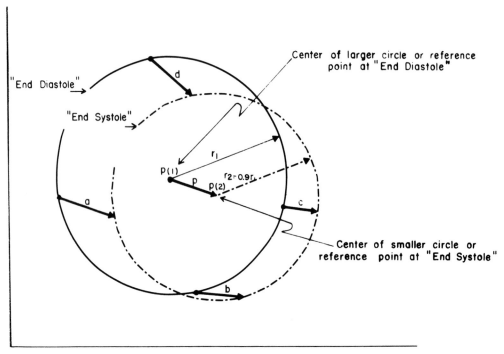

ORIGIN

Figure 26.2. A simple model of ventricular contraction in which there is also translation of the entire ventricle with respect to the laboratory. The radius of the smaller circle is 10% less than that of the larger circle. The center of the circle moves from *P(1)* ("end-diastole") to *P(2)* ("end-systole") in the fixed external coordinate system. The motion of four markers in the fixed system is represented by the vectors $\vec{a}$, $\vec{b}$, $\vec{c}$, and $\vec{d}$. Although the contractile motion for each marker should be equal, the magnitudes of the four vectors are different when measured in the fixed reference system. These differences are attributable to the translation and can be resolved by subtracting the vector *p* from each marker vector. (From Clayton PD, Jeppson GM, Klausner SC: Should a fixed external reference system be used to analyze left ventricular wall motion? *Circulation* 65(7):1518–1521, 1982.) By permission of the American Heart Association.

systolic center superposition may correct for whole heart motions, but unfortunately it also tends to erase information in 2DE cross sections exhibiting pronounced regional contractile abnormalities. This is the dilemma in seeking a quantitative method of wall motion analysis suitable for minimally subjective computerized 2DE image acquisition and analysis. Improved measurement of end-diastolic and end-systolic myocardial wall thickness would help overcome some of these referencing problems.

There appears to be no general consensus about the fixed versus floating reference issue. Depending on the application, either approach has been favored (4). Recent 2DE reports illustrate the usefulness of internal landmarks and standardized subdivision of the ventricle (5). The analytical procedure was generally decided on by the investigators after comparing measurement reproducibility and examining its ability to approximate the expected near-uniform inward wall motions (in areas of normal contraction). Based on such evaluations, quantitative 2DE methods have been described for both apical and short-axis left ventricular cross sections. These have been studied in normal subjects as well as in some patients with coronary artery disease (6).

One experimental investigation attempted to circumvent the problem encountered with floating reference analysis of regional ischemic dysfunction by using an epicardium-derived cross-sectional center (7). Since epicardial motion from end-diastole to end-systole is much less than that of the endocardial border, it was thought that a floating reference system may be suitable even in the presence of regional contractile derange-

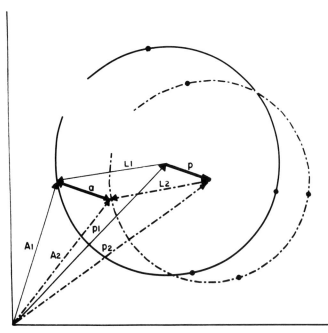

Figure 26.3. The vector approach for measuring marker motion using different reference systems. When measured using the center of the circle as the origin of an internal reference system, the measured marker motion is $\vec{L}_2 - \vec{L}_1$. In the external system the marker motion is equal to the vector difference $\vec{A}_2 - \vec{A}_1$ and is represented by the vector $\vec{a}$. These two measurements give unequal results unless the vector $\vec{p}$ is subtracted from $\vec{a}$. (From Clayton PD, Jeppson GM, Klausner SC: Should a fixed external reference system be used to analyze left ventricular wall motion? *Circulation* 65(7):1518–1521, 1982.) By permission of the American Heart Association.

ments. In this study, the extent of ischemic zones distal to coronary artery occlusions was determined by an independent delineation method using myocardial contrast echocardiography. This provided an important supplemental comparative index to assess the adequacy of several analytical 2DE methods for quantitation of ischemic segments.

The study employed short-axis cross sections of the left ventricle. Floating reference systems used superposition of the end-diastolic and end-systolic centers defined by either the epicardium or endocardium. Compared to fixed referencing, floating reference analysis provided higher interobserver reproducibility of segmental 2DE wall motion analysis. During normal contraction, segment-to-segment variations of the fractional area change contraction index (systolic change in segmental luminal area) were also smallest with floating reference point analysis. Following coronary artery occlusion, sensitivity and specificity for discriminating the independently delineated acutely ischemic regions were highest with the floating reference analysis based on center points computed from the epicardial interface. Endocardially derived center floating point analysis of regional ischemia was not satisfactory. Wall thickness measurements, with the inherent advantage of overcoming the fixed versus floating reference problems, unfortunately exhibited substantial variability in this study.

Another recent study of left ventricular centroids from 2DE images indicated that the center of the area within the endocardial profile is optimal, and should be used in measuring regional myocardial wall motion (1). Further validations of this segmental function analysis will be forthcoming. Standardization of analysis is needed to expand computerized approaches which promise to reduce the current subjectivity (selection of a suitable frame), as well as the tediousness of manual 2DE image measurements.

The clinical importance of these investigations is highlighted in a study looking at segmental evaluation of intraoperative short-axis cross-sectional echocardiograms from 10 patients undergoing cardiopulmonary bypass (8). Using a center of mass floating system of analysis, uniform wall motion was consistent with observed absence of ischemia or perioperative myocardial infarction. On the other hand, standard fixed references showed spurious abnormality of ventricular regional motion. Paradoxical wall motion registered by the time of cardiopulmonary bypass and following sternal closure. In reality, this apparent paradoxical motion was associated with translation of the heart.

IMPROVEMENTS IN QUANTITATIVE ECHOCARDIOGRAPHIC METHODS

Gillam et al presented an intriguing approach to analysis of regional wall motion and delineation of ischemic left ventricular dysfunction (9).

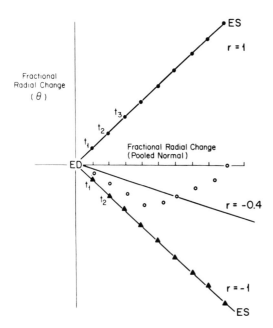

Figure 26.4. Step I of the correlation analysis. Derivation of the correlation coefficients for individual radii. The observed fractional radial change (y axis) at sequential points in systole (t_1, t_2, . . .) is plotted against the pooled normal value at comparable times (x axis). (See text for explanation.) ● = normal ray, ▲ = hypothetical situation in which there is progressive outward rather than inward movement of the endocardial target; ○ = representative ray in the infarcted region of the ventricle. (From Gillam LD, Hogan RD, Foale RA, Franklin TD Jr, Newell JB, Guyer DE, Weyman AE: A comparison of quantitative echocardiographic methods for delineating infarct-induced abnormal wall motion. *Circulation* 70(1):113–122, 1984.) By permission of the American Heart Association.

The usual 2DE analysis examines myocardial wall excursions of end-diastole and end-systole and assumes baseline cross-sectional uniformity of wall motions. Studies suggest significant heterogeneity even in normal states and demonstrate marked regional differences within an ischemic zone (10). The new and apparently superior analytical method for quantitating infarct-induced abnormal motions was validated in short-axis cross sections of the left ventricle. Its essential feature is a correlation procedure that characterizes in detail the entire time course of systolic radial wall motions of each of 36 evenly spaced endocardial targets, in relation to a corresponding course of pooled normal-state wall motions.

Figures 26.4 and 26.5 illustrate the analytical sequence, commencing with endocardial outlines, computation of fractional radial chord changes, and consecutive times in systole; then, designation of the ischemic zone exhibiting abnormal wall motion. A degree of endocardial segment dyskinesis at end-systole actually can be preceded by a peak paradoxical outward motion at an intermediate time during systole. Consequently, the investigators concluded that conventional analysis of overall systolic excursion may fail to detect significant intermediate wall motion abnormalities.

RECENT EXPERIMENTAL APPLICATIONS OF 2DE QUANTITATION

In the experimental laboratory, standardization and computer-assisted 2DE analysis of the left ventricle (primarily short-axis cross sections) allowed significant physiologic applications which yielded important new information. Only a few of these laboratory investigations can be mentioned here, but they illustrate the potential for 2DE assessment of regional cardiac function.

One study measured the changes in percentage from end-diastole to end-systole in total sectional and endocardially bounded segmental luminal area, wall thickness, and circumferential length in 50 dogs and 30 normal humans (10). Detailed 2DE analysis was made possible by satisfactory images in five short-axis cross sections from the base of the left ventricle to the apex. Contraction in a normal ventricle was neither completely uniform nor symmetrical. There was an increase in cardiac contractile function from basal to apical cross sections, most prominently in septal regions of the ventricle (Fig. 26.6).

The significance of this and similar findings is that abnormalities and effects of interventions

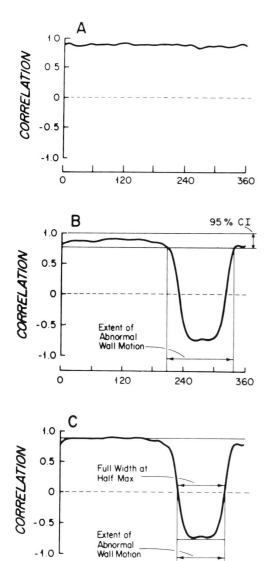

Figure 26.5. Step II of the correlation analysis. Correlation coefficients for individual rays (y axis) plotted against ray location (x axis). (See text for full explanation.) *A*, Control study. *B*, Postinfarct study. The 95% confidence limits of the correlation coefficients of the normal radii (0° to 210°) have been drawn in. Radii for which correlation coefficients fall outside these limits are considered abnormal and used to define the circumferential extent of abnormal wall motion. *C*, Postinfarct study. The full width of the correlation plot at one-half the maximum deflection from baseline was determined. Radii falling within these limits were considered abnormal. (From Gillam LD, Hogan RD, Foale RA, Franklin TD Jr, Newell JB, Guyer DE, Weyman AE: A comparison of quantitative echocardiographic methods for delineating infarct-induced abnormal wall motion. *Circulation* 70(1):113–122, 1984.) By permission of the American Heart Association.

should really be viewed against a background of baseline regional left ventricular contractile heterogeneity. Two further experimental studies, one with atrial pacing at various heart rates and another with nitroglycerin treatment, actually revealed that left ventricular base-to-apex contraction differences in a normal heart were further accentuated during these interventions.

Another series of quantitative 2DE laboratory studies investigated an interventional diagnosis used to characterize coronary artery stenosis or assess acute occlusions (11–13). Dysfunction of ventricular segments during and immediately after atrial pacing was studied in closed-chest dogs at rates up to 210 beats/min (11). Segmental dysfunction was also studied during normal states and with an experimentally induced 70% diameter left anterior descending coronary artery stenosis. Both maximal pacing and immediate postpacing measurements clearly discriminated ischemic from normally perfused myocardial segments in short-axis cross sections of the left ventricle (Fig. 26.7). No significant dysfunction was present in the absence of pacing.

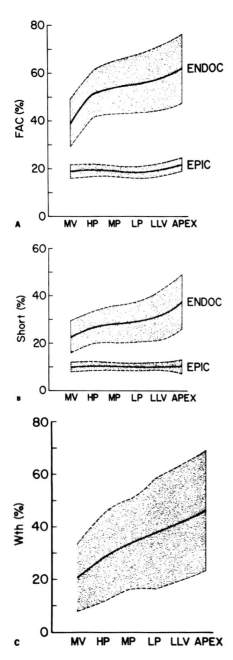

Figure 26.6. Base-to-apex variations of left ventricular sectional function in 50 anesthetized intact dogs. Results are expressed as mean (*solid line*) ± 2 SD (*stippled areas above and below solid line*). *A*, Epicardial (*EPIC*) and endocardial (*ENDOC*) fractional area change (*FAC*). There was a statistically significant difference in *ENDOC FAC* between the various left ventricular short-axis levels, except for *HP* versus *MP*, *MP* versus *LP*, and *LP* versus *LLV*. *B*, *ENDOC* and *EPIC* circumferential fiber shortening (*Short*). *ENDOC SHORT* was significantly different between all levels except for *HP* versus *MP* and *MP* versus *LP*. *C*, Systolic wall thickening (*WTh*), again showing significantly increased contractile function in lower left ventricular sections. All levels were significantly different from each other, except for *LP* vs *LLV*. (From Haendchen RV, Wyatt HL, Maurer G, Zwehl W, Bear M, Meerbaum S, Corday E: Quantitation of regional cardiac function by two-dimensional echocardiography. I. Patterns of contraction in the normal left ventricle. *Circulation* 67(6):1234–1245, 1983.) By permission of the American Heart Association.

To shed light on the use of postextrasystoles or nitroglycerin potentiation to assess myocardial viability during ischemia, quantitative regional 2DE measurements were performed in two other studies (12,13). The extent of myocardial ischemia and necrotic zones was carefully evaluated in left ventricular slices, to establish the degree of damage that significantly diminished or reversed potentiation of regional function. The most impor-

tant observation to come from this study was that when more than 60% of a myocardial wall segment was irreversibly damaged, no significant potentiation of cardiac function could be observed during either postextrasystolic or nitroglycerin intervention.

Recognizing that beat-to-beat measurements are a potentially important feature of 2DE measurement, experimental studies also investigated

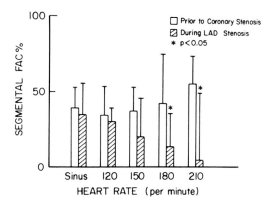

Figure 26.7. Effect of right atrial pacing on anterolateral segment fractional area change percent (*FAC*%) in a low papillary two-dimensional echographic left ventricular cross section, before and during left anterior descending (*LAD*) coronary stenosis (70%). In this segment, supplied by the stenosed coronary artery, fraction area change percent decreased with increasing heart rate, and exhibited a significantly lower value at a heart rate at or above 180 beats/min compared with equivalent measurements before stenosis. *$p < 0.05$ versus prestenosis. (From Kondo S, Meerbaum S, Sakamaki T, Shimoura K, Tei C, Shah PM, Corday E: Diagnosis of coronary stenosis by two-dimensional echographic study of dysfunction of ventricular segments during and immediately after pacing. *J Am Coll Cardiol* 2(4):689–698, 1983.) Reprinted with permission from the American College of Cardiology.

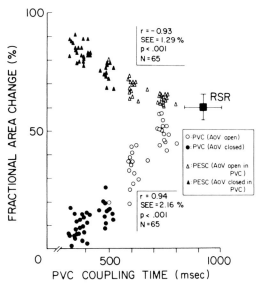

Figure 26.8. Correlation of two-dimensional echocardiographic ventricular contraction coupling intervals with premature ventricular contraction and postextrasystolic contraction fractional area change. This graph indicates a distinct dependence of sectional left ventricular function during the premature ventricular contraction and subsequent postextrasystolic contraction potentiation on the premature ventricular contraction coupling interval. As the latter was progressively reduced, function during premature ventricular contraction, characterized from two-dimensional, echocardiographic, short-axis left ventricular cross sections as systolic fractional area change, decreased successively (correlation coefficient $r = 0.94$). N = number of determinations; p = probability; *SEE* = standard error of the estimate. (From Uchiyama T, Corday E, Meerbaum S, Lang TW, Gueret P, Povjitkov M, Peters T: Characterization of left ventricular mechanical function during arrhythmias with two-dimensional echocardiography: I. Premature ventricular contraction. *Am J Cardiol*, 48:679–689, 1981) with permission.

quantitative assessment of regional cardiac function during arrhythmias (14). Reproducibility studies in dogs indicated that satisfactory measurement could be obtained in short-axis cross sections of the left ventricle. Thus, it proved feasible in the laboratory to characterize regional contractile function during premature ventricular contraction, study function during supraventricular and ventricular paced tachyarrhythmias, and detect the myocardial site of onset of premature ventricular systoles. Figure 26.8 shows the observed relationship between premature ventricular contraction coupling time and 2DE-derived systolic fractional area changes, which were applied to characterize regional contractile function. The pattern observed in dogs in response to direct electrical stimulation featured early systolic contraction with inward wall motion and thickening, followed by paradoxical outward motion and wall thinning in late systole (15). The premature beat contractile derangement was always

maximal at the cardiac site of the stimulus. Thus, 2DE might yet define arrhythmic functional consequences and, in particular, noninvasively establish ectopic foci during arrhythmias.

Global Function Measurements with 2DE

Echocardiography has the potential to acquire several cross-sectional images of the heart rapidly. In the human, it is generally feasible to obtain apical four-chamber and two-chamber cross-sectional views, a high papillary short-axis view, and a parasternal long-axis view of the left ventricle. Improved 2DE equipment, electrocardiogram (ECG) gating, computer-assisted edge delineation, and chamber area measurements have all contributed to enhanced assessment of cardiac chamber volumes and ejection fractions. Yet it is still true that the experienced echocardiographer may have to interpolate any echo dropouts in interfaces observed in gated freeze frames, perhaps noting corresponding local sites in intervening frames or a given cardiac cycle. The myocardial interface seen in apical views seldom represents the exact endocardium, so absolute quantitative assessment of volume should not be expected.

Many 2DE studies have reported on the validity and variability of volume and ejection fraction measurements, both in the human and in the experimental animal. Echocardiographic assessment of changes in chamber areas often are considered quite adequate to derive global indices such as ejection fraction. Both the left and the right ventricle can now be investigated by 2DE, at least in terms of changes in areas or volumes (16).

In the laboratory, several mathematical formulas that use short-axis cross-sectional views and a length measurement have proven helpful for quantitative ventricular analysis. One recent experimental study with potential clinical implications assessed the accuracy of 2DE determination of absolute left ventricular volumes (17). Based upon Simpson's reconstruction from short-axis cross sections, 2DE-derived volumes were compared with direct volume measurements in dogs. This study indicated that the variability of volume measurements became pronounced whenever reconstruction was based on fewer than three short-axis cross sections. However, left ventricular ejection fractions were measured accurately in normal hearts, even when only two short-axis cross sections were available.

Computerization of Two-Dimensional Echocardiography

Although quantitative 2DE measurements have been used for several years in physiologic studies using animal models, the lack of similar quantitation in clinical use has become painfully obvious. This is in spite of the generally acknowledged desirable spatial and real-time features of 2DE. The reasons are myriad. The relative inadequacies of early echo equipment and lack of standard procedures resulted in questionable accuracy of outlined endocardial or epicardial cardiac boundaries. Only recently has image quality been greatly enhanced and border delineation been

improved through appropriate analysis of videotape data. Nonetheless, substantial variability persists and tedious delays are incurred in the manual, subjective tracing of borders and the conventional analysis of 2DE images. Many recognized that the next goal of experimental research must be computerized border recognition along with computer-assisted image data processing, analysis, and display. This objective has not yet been fully achieved, but considerable progress has been made in various laboratories (2, 18–22). Several favorable investigations of computerized 2DE systems portend rapid clinical application.

Basic to the use of computer methods is transformation of the image from an analog to a digital signal. The echo image is subdivided into a large number of tiny spatial elements called pixels. The pixels, characterized by individual gray levels or echo amplitudes, are arranged in a matrix of horizontal rows and vertical columns. Modern 2DE equipment uses digitization and data storage to enhance and display cardiac structure-blood interfaces. Image quality is improved, and effects of echo dropouts are minimized by smoothing and contrast-enhancement algorithms, which facilitate subsequent quantitative analysis of cardiac function.

Fully automated outlining of the endocardium and epicardium has recently been the subject of intensive research. Edge enhancement and 2DE image noise reduction is accomplished by such means as multiple averaging, contrast enhancement, and histogram equalization. The automatic detection of the blood-to-structure interface involves echo gray level thresholding, as well as other mathematical operators, and border detection is also aided by consideration of cardiac wall dynamics.

Among pioneering investigations of computational procedures for 2DE was a study by Dr. E. Garcia in 1980 at the Cedars-Sinai Medical Center in Los Angeles (18). Dr. Garcia first coupled the video output of 2DE units or videotaped echoes to a Nova medical imaging computer. This computer had a 128 K word program, 256 word image memory, 8 megabyte disc storage, and 512×512 pixel video display with 256 gray levels. Images were digitized in a 64×64 matrix and stored on a magnetic disc in real time at 30 frames/sec. This overcame several limitations of then current 2DE. The speed of acquisition was increased greatly over previous methods that digitized only a single still frame at a time. The new system also displayed several different views of the heart simultaneously in a continuous closed-loop fashion, a technique that proved advantageous for comparative assessment of segmental wall motions. Digitization of the echograms and computerized quantitation of ventricular function resulted in significant time and labor savings. This, it was hoped, would avoid the inevitable subjectivity associated with manual processing of 2DE images.

Dr. Garcia next developed computer algorithms. Temporal smoothing of the images replaced the contents of each pixel with a weighted average of itself and a corresponding pixel occurring immediately before and afterward. Spatial smoothing used a weighted average of the pixel and eight surrounding pixels within the same frame. Frame-by-frame automatic edge detection in the 2DE images was assisted by the computer convolving a 3 × 3 Laplacian operator (second derivative) with temporarily and spatially smooth images. A binary image was then created from all the pixels that both exceeded an echo amplitude threshold of the smoothed image and were within a preselected range of the Laplacian images.

The endocardial interface in a typical 2DE cross section was tracked automatically from the binary image by the computer searching from a preselected center in the ventricular chamber until an intensity threshold was encountered at its interface. Once the point on the interface was detected, automatic tracing of the endocardium could proceed all around the ventricle (Fig. 26.9). Following automatic endocardial delineation, the computer program carried out a frame-by-frame quantitation of both global and regional ventricular function. For example, volumes and global ejection fraction were reconstructed from 2DE apical and short-axis cross-sectional views of the left ventricle. Using fixed or floating references and standard subdivision of cross-sectional images into segments, regional wall motions were analyzed frame by frame (18). The system displayed the results in the form of charts, showing alterations in cross-sectional areas of ventricular volumes throughout the cardiac cycle. The percentage of systolic fractional area change or global ejection fractions were displayed and derivatives plotted (Fig. 26.10). Segment-by-segment bar graphs displayed by the computer presented a map of regional contraction and wall thickness.

Since 2DE images obtained in the closed-chest dog preparation were generally excellent, full uti-

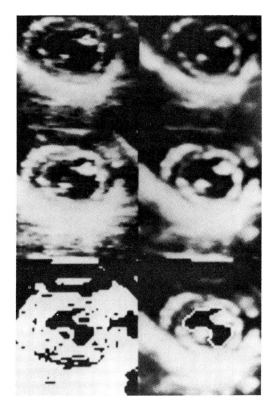

Figure 26.9. Edge detection algorithm implementation in echocardiographic images. *Upper left*, Selected digitized frame of a short-axis cross section at the level of the papillary muscles. *Upper right*, Corresponding frame following space-time smoothing. *Middle*, Images corresponding to those in the upper panels after histogram equalization are shown. Note the decreased dropout in the equalized images. *Lower*, Binary image (*left*) and tracked endocardial outlines (*right*). (From American Society of Echocardiography Subcommittee on Digital Image Processing (Skorton DJ, Collins SM, Garcia E, Geiser EA, Hillard W, Koppes W, Linker D, Schwartz G): Digital signal and image processing in echocardiography. *Progr Cardiol* 110(6):1266–1283, 1985) with permission.

lization of the real-time 2DE computerized system could be demonstrated. A sample application occurred in an experimental study of myocardial ischemia, allowing computerization of measurements previously performed by hand-drawn 2DE methods.

Validation of the Computerized 2DE System

The algorithm explained above was validated in experimental studies against direct measurements in canine left ventricular slabs and also in closed-chest dogs (23). Validation in the latter

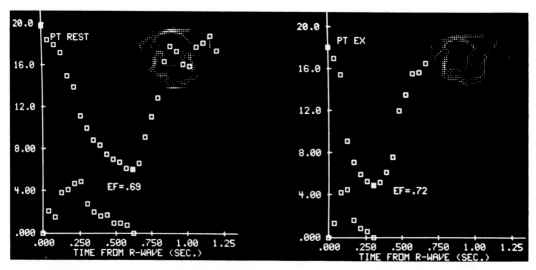

Figure 26.10. 2DE short-axis systolic fractional area change in a normal individual at rest (*PT REST*) and during supine bicycle exercise (*PT EX*). The systolic fractional area change at rest was 0.69 and increased slightly to 0.72 during moderate exercise. Also shown in the *top right corner* of each figure are the superimposed frame-by-frame endocardial delineations in the short-axis 2DE section at the midpapillary level of the left ventricle. (From Garcia E, Gueret P, Bennett M, Corday E, Zwehl W, Meerbaum S, Corday S, Swan HJC, Mermban D: Real time computerization of two-dimensional echocardiography. *Am Heart J* 101(6):783–792, 1981) with permission.

employed contrast cineventriculography which, while not a gold standard, was nevertheless considered to give an acceptable baseline. The computer technique was compared with the conventional hand-drawn 2DE methodology, and interobserver reproducibility was also determined.

An in vitro study was first performed using 10 mm thick canine left ventricular slabs in a water bath. Figure 26.11 compares the computer-processed image with the actual canine slab. Cross-sectional intraluminal areas and segmental areas were computed from directly measured slab dimensions as well as from hand-drawn and computer-processed slab 2DE images. Comparison of intraluminal areas obtained with computerized, hand-drawn, and direct measurements yielded high correlation coefficients (0.95 − 0.96) and satisfactory standard errors. Thus, the computer algorithm was supported by ventricular slab validation of static 2DE images.

Dynamic experimental validations in closed-chest dogs examined automated left ventricular endocardial delineation in characteristic 2DE images and compared the enclosed cross-sectional areas against manually drawn sections. Computer-reconstructed left ventricular volumes were validated with contrast ventriculography. Four or five excellent quality 2DE short-axis cross-sectional images were obtained at different levels of the left ventricle, as well as in one long-axis view. In the conventional manual 2DE method, a dynamic review of endocardial left ventricular wall motion identified the end-diastolic (largest) and end-systolic (smallest) short-axis cross-sectional area. Ventricular length at end-diastole and end-systole were read from 2DE long-axis sections.

Comparison of automatically derived and manually outlined 2DE end-diastolic and end-systolic short-axis cross-sectional areas yielded a high correlation coefficient (0.98 and 0.89) and a small standard error of estimate (Fig. 26.12). Similarly, ventricular volumes correlated well (correlation coefficients: 0.92 and 0.91). Computerized 2DE derivation of end-diastolic and end-systolic left ventricular volumes correlated well with ventriculography. Thus, computerized edge detection of the superior 2DE images obtained in experimental animals allowed accurate analysis of left ventricular cross-sectional areas and volume reconstruction. The prime advantage of the 2DE computer should be its speed and objectivity of analysis.

Relationship of Experimental Validations to Clinical Application

It cannot be stated strongly enough that computerized quantitative analysis of global and re-

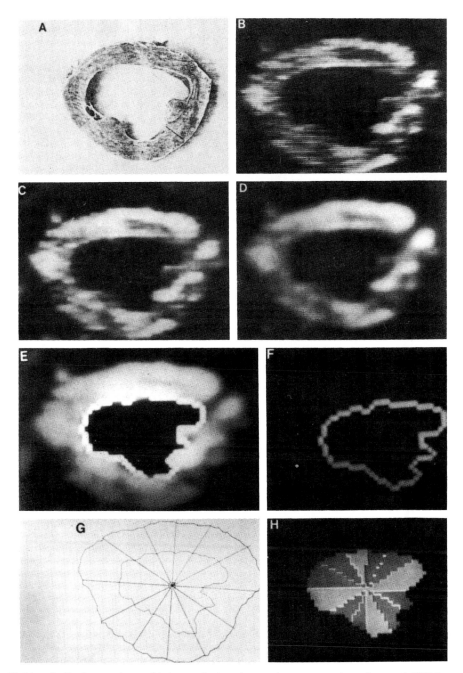

Figure 26.11. *A–D.* Comparison of left ventricular short-axis cross-section slice and 2DE image. *A*, Photocopy of typical canine slab. *B*, Untreated 2DE video image. *C*, Display of computer digitized image. *D*, Display of space-smoothed computer image. (For measurement, all imaging systems were x and y calibrated.) *E*, Computer-processed and space-smoothed 2DE image with automatic endocardial edge outline. *F*, Endocardial edge. *G*, Computer-assisted outline of manually drawn 2DE image (*outer border* represents epicardium; *inner border* represents endocardium), subdivided into 12 segments after locating endocardial center of area, and using midpapillary (3 o'clock reference point) as the intraluminal landmark. *H*, Automatic computer subdivision of cross section into 12 segments with standardized referencing. (From Zwehl W, Levy R, Garcia E, Haendchen RV, Childs W, Corday SR, Meerbaum S, Corday E: Validation of a computerized edge detection algorithm for quantitative two-dimensional echocardiography. *Circulation* 68(5):1127–1135, 1983) by permission of the American Heart Association.

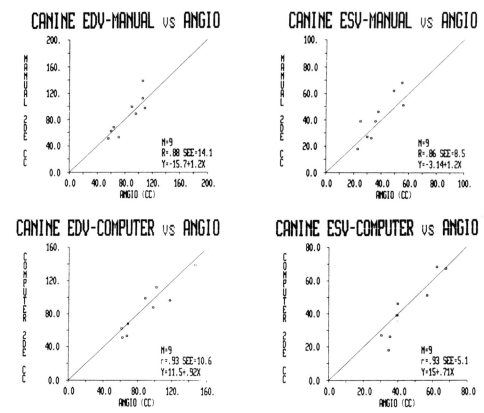

Figure 26.12. Comparison of 2DE-derived reconstructed left ventricular volumes and angiographically determined volumes. Both manually (*upper row*) and computer-derived (*lower row*) 2DE volumes compared favorably with angiographically determined volumes. (From Zwehl W, Levy R, Garcia E, Haendchen R, Childs W, Corday SR, Meerbaum S, Corday E: Validation of a computerized edge detection algorithm for quantitative two-dimensional echocardiography. *Circulation* 68(5):1127–1135, 1983.) By permission of the American Heart Association.

gional cardiac function requires satisfactory 2DE definition of the endocardial and epicardial interfaces. Superior 2DE images obtained in the dog model established the reproducibility and validity of the computerized system. Current clinical 2DE image quality is still variable. Although very good images are obtained in some patients and most healthy volunteers, only a limited number of patients with coronary artery disease are believed suitable for 2DE, real-time, fully automated quantitative computerization. It is still necessary to enhance clinical 2DE images, particularly to minimize echo dropouts and to improve endocardial definition.

An examination of computerized 2DE suggests that automatic edge detection techniques are potentially suitable in the clinical setting (24). Further development of computerized image processing promises wider application, but several problems have yet to be overcome. One relates to less-than-satisfactory epicardial border recognition (a prerequisite for wall thickness quantitation) due to very bright reflections from the strong acoustic impedance mismatch between myocardium and air-filled lungs. Extensive echo dropouts and poor image quality may also interfere with application of computerized techniques.

THREE-DIMENSIONAL ECHOCARDIOGRAPHY

Given the need for reliable and rapid ventricular reconstruction, researchers sought to digitize clearly referenced endocardial and epicardial interfaces in multiple cross sections and utilize computer analysis and display of the reconstructed chamber. This led to the ambitious goal of a computerized dynamic three-dimensional representation of the heart throughout the cardiac cycle. Of most immediate interest was a dynamic display of global and regional wall motion of the left ventricle. An indispensable element for such a three-dimensional echocardiography (3DE) method is a quantifiable spatial location of endocardial and epicardial interfaces in each of the cross sections and satisfactory determination of the spatial relationship.

Investigators have attempted ventricular reconstruction using short-axis and apical 2DE cross sections. This combination helps get the most information from views that, individually, are seldom totally satisfactory (25–29). Apical views present an imperfect view of endocardial and epicardial interfaces, as they are almost parallel to the ultrasonic beam. In the short axis, visualization of the ventricular apex is difficult. Since the most frequent clinical echo viewing of the left ventricle occurs in apical 2DE views, some investigators attempted three-dimensional reconstruction data in several apical sections by simply indexing and incrementally rotating the transducer in 5° to 30° steps (28, 29).

Many investigations have concentrated on transducer spatial registration and systematic localization of digitized 2DE cross sections and segments. An acoustic system devised by Moritz and Shreve (30) locates the transducer position and orientation in space by three orthogonally placed sound sources and three microphone receivers. These authors demonstrated 3DE reconstruction based on short-axis, long-axis, and apical 2DE images. Joskowicz et al. (31) applied laser mirror systems to track transducer motion. Less sophisticated but adequate registration of transducer position and orientation uses simpler and less expensive mechanical systems that involve an articulating arm with a number of degrees of freedom (25–29).

Reconstruction of referenced 2DE cross sections into a 3DE representation involves either hand tracing or digitizing endocardial and epicardial borders. A global 3DE coordinate system is constructed relative to the external axis system of the registration device. The transducer position and orientation for each cross section, along with the digitized positions of the endocardial and epicardial borders, are reviewed to align each of the cross sections within the global X-Y-Z system. After interpolation and contour fitting between cross sections, the ventricular chamber can be reconstructed and its volumes can be readily computed. Dynamic 3DE displays employ available commercial computer-aided visualization methods. Figure 26.13 illustrates an example of what can be expected from a 3DE presentation.

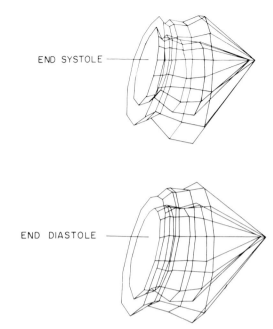

END SYSTOLE

END DIASTOLE

Figure 26.13. End-systolic (*upper*) and end-diastolic (*lower*) 3DE reconstructions from patient RD. These are displayed in a 25° RAO position. (From Geiser EA, Ariet M, Conetta DA, Lupkiewics SM, Christie LG Jr, Conti CR: Dynamic three-dimensional echocardiographic reconstruction of the intact human left ventricle: Technique and initial observations in patients. *Progr Cardiol* 103(6):1056–1065, 1982) with permission.

Chandran et al addressed the important subject of estimating left ventricular volumes in children with congenital heart disease to evaluate their ventricular function (28). A composite 3DE left ventricular reconstruction to measure left ventricular volumes was evaluated in 26 children. Four apical views were used to obtain a "wire cage" model of the left ventricle in three dimensions. Volume estimates were compared with angiographic biplane methods. This study demonstrated that three-dimensional reconstruction can be performed in a clinical setting. One hopes that 3DE assessment of global left ventricular geometry may soon contribute to improved patient management.

ULTRASOUND CHARACTERIZATION OF MYOCARDIAL TISSUE

There is substantial interest in expanding 2DE beyond assessment of anatomy and function. Methods to characterize myocardial tissue by ultrasound have been known for some time. Laboratory studies indicated promise, particularly for detection of myocardial infarction (32–37).

In echocardiography, calcified or scarred myocardial structures are often recognized by significantly increased echo brightness. Myocardial alterations due to cardiomyopathy and amyloidosis are also believed to be distinguishable through conventional or color-enhanced echo. However, such assessment is highly qualitative. One concern is that unstandardized 2DE procedures may present highly variable myocardial images, perhaps simply as a result of changing the equipment's time gain compensation setting. Recently, more sophisticated myocardial texture analysis and analysis of spatial echo patterns have been applied to characterize ischemic or necrotic myocardial tissue.

One approach to characterizing regionally ischemic myocardial tissue is to compare echocardiographic impedance and ultrasound attenuation against normal segments of the heart. Measurement of integrated ultrasound backscatter returning from tissue appears to be a method of choice, since it successfully characterizes regional ischemia after coronary artery occlusion. These studies were performed in the open-chest dog, but recent backscatter techniques correct for the acoustic properties of the chest wall and allow satisfactory characterization of myocardium in intact animal preparations. Figure 26.14 illustrates some of these results.

Of particular interest is research aimed at quantitating patterns of ultrasound reflections by means of radio frequency (RF) data and sophisticated numerical analysis. A sample of the method is shown in Figure 26.15 (37). Digitizing single-echo ultrasound line of sight signals and analyzing amplitude distributions through regional myocardium allow evaluation of infarcted myocardium (38). Unfortunately the RF method cannot be used readily with some 2DE equipment. This method involves huge amounts of data that cannot readily be stored or analyzed with available computers. Consequently, efforts have been aimed at an intermediate quantitative approach to improve image quality. Rather than seeking the basic RF signals, current methods would be improved by acquiring the ultrasound data prior to the 2DE equipment's time gain compensation for attenuation (39). Wide-dynamic-range acquisition and various correction algorithms have been developed to process the original echo.

A new observation relates to phasic differences in cardiac tissue ultrasound parameters (40, 41).

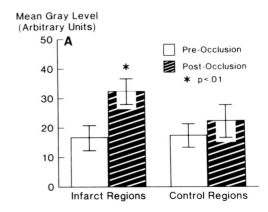

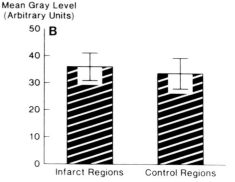

Figure 26.14. Average gray levels in control and infarct regions. *Panel A,* Average gray levels are shown for infarct and control regions before and after coronary artery occlusion. A significant increase in average gray level was found in infarcted regions but not in control regions. *Panel B,* Average gray levels are shown for infarct and control regions within postinfarction images; no statistically significant difference was found. (From Skorton DJ, Melton HE Jr, Pandian NG, Nichols J, Koyanagi S, Marcus ML, Collins SM, Kerber RE: Detection of acute myocardial infarction in closed-chest dogs by analysis of regional two-dimensional echocardiographic gray-level distributions. *Circ Res* 52(1):36–44, 1983.) By permission of the American Heart Association.

Using conventional video images, significantly higher backscatter intensity is noted in normal myocardium in end-diastole than in end-systole. This significant difference diminishes or disappears when the myocardium becomes reversibly ischemic following brief coronary occlusion. It is not yet clear whether analysis based upon these observations will allow characterization of perfusion defects or myocardial blood contact. However, it is likely that current laboratory efforts,

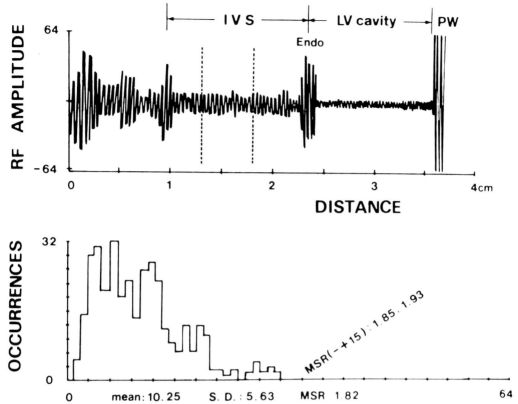

Figure 26.15. *Upper panel*, One sample of unprocessed RF signal displaying amplitude (*RF AMP*) on the y axis and distance on the x axis. The RF signal was obtained from a closed-chest measurement with the cursor cutting slightly obliquely through the septum. A definable window (*dashed vertical lines*) was set in the septum, within the myocardium, for further analysis with use of a histogram of the data. *Endo* = endocardium, *IVS* = interventricular septum, *PW* = posterior wall. *Lower panel*, Histogram constructed with data from 10 samples such as those in the *top panel* and displaying the number of occurrences of a certain amplitude plotted on the y axis and amplitudes on the x axis. The mean amplitude, standard deviation of amplitudes, and MSR are automatically derived by the computer. Gates that were too close to specular interfaces were detected by comparing the MSR values for the selected window with the ones obtained when the window was shifted by a predetermined amount to the left or the right. In this study, the gate was shifted 15 points (1.2 mm) and the corresponding MSR values are displayed in the right in this panel. (From Schnittger I, Vieli A, Heiserman JE, Director BA, Billingham ME, Ellis SG, Kernoff RS, Takamota T, Popp RL: Ultrasonic tissue characterization: detection of acute myocardial ischemia in dogs. *Circulation* 72(1):193–199, 1985.) MSR = mean amplitude/standard deviation of the amplitude. Reproduced with permission of the American Heart Association.

including direct processing or RF ultrasound data, will eventually lead to a quantitative method for 2DE characterization of myocardial tissue.

MYOCARDIAL CONTRAST TWO-DIMENSIONAL ECHOCARDIOGRAPHY

Contrast echocardiography in adult and pediatric patients was introduced by Gramiak and Shah in 1968 (42). In the hands of experienced echocardiographers it has proven to be a useful tool to detect and qualitatively assess valvular or struc-

tural cardiac incompetence. Many studies and case reports have been published (43–45), as well as a comprehensive review of the literature (46). In particular, contrast 2DE evaluation of septal defects or valvular regurgitation has provided extremely useful clinical information. Echocardiographers have employed a number of agents as contrast, ranging from saline to indocyanine green and even to blood itself. In general, the conclusion has been that intravenous, right heart, or even aortic root injections do not pose significant hazards. Yet it is fair to say that there has been only a limited understanding of contrast agent echogenicity effects, beyond observations that some agitational catheter tip cavitation results in gaseous bubbles, which are then responsible for the opacification evident on the echograms during the injection.

The endocardium of the left ventricle may be outlined by intrachamber contrast injection and 2DE. The endocardium of the left ventricle may be outlined by intrachamber contrast injection and 2DE. A sample study was performed using intrachamber contrast injection in 57 consecutive patients (47). Left ventricular ejection fraction calculated on the basis of automatic contour definition by digital subtraction echocardiography demonstrated a better correlation with cineangiographic data than noncontrast 2DE measurement of ejection fraction. In baseline echocardiograms, endocardial definition is deemed imprecise and causes overestimation of the true endocardium. On the other hand, the endocardium is well delineated in contrast echocardiograms. In this particular application, 5.5% oxypolygelatine was used as echo contrast material and injected at a rate of 2–4 ml/sec directly into the left ventricle.

Although 2DE has been extensively applied in studies of mechanical function during myocardial ischemia, a new line of research focuses on detecting perfusion defects and quantitating myocardial blood flow (48). During the past few years many experimental research reports have described investigations of this new technique, including validations and assessment of the method's promise as well as its limitations (49–61).

Echo contrast effects are due to microbubbles created accidentally or formed deliberately in the injectate. Many early studies in the dog used agitated (or sonicated) echo contrast agents. These include saline, Renografin, Renografin-saline mixtures, sorbitol, dextrose hydrogen peroxide and gelatin-encapsulated bubbles. Most initial experimental myocardial contrast echo investigations injected small amounts of the contrast agent either into the aortic root or directly into the coronary arteries supplying the regional myocardium to be investigated (i.e., left ventricular wall). Only a few studies attempted administration intravenously or from the right heart. This was primarily because there was little evidence that quantifiable myocardial opacification could be accomplished with transpulmonary injections.

The sonication technique for preparing my-ocardial echo contrast is attractive because it produces smaller microbubbles. Similar advantages have also been noted with supplemental surfactant additives. The fundamental goal is to allow unhindered contrast passage through the myocardial microcirculation and also to permit sufficient delivery of the agent from the right heart to the left ventricular myocardium. It is necessary to produce extremely small, highly uniform microbubbles (about 3–5 μm) to guarantee absolute safety and still achieve quantitation of myocardial perfusion. Research in this difficult area is being pursued vigorously.

Animal studies of myocardial contrast 2DE demonstrated sufficient reproducibility and validity to justify clinical trials and physiologic studies. Figures 26.16 and 26.17 show early echo observations of regional myocardial opacification during contrast injection into coronary arteries. Many echo contrast agents demonstrated very adequate delineation of underperfused acute ischemic myocardial regions (i.e., risk zones) in canine hearts. These were validated against dye as well as histologic measurements.

Much as with digital angiographic methodologies, computerized procedures were developed for myocardial contrast 2DE. Algorithms were developed to study myocardial contrast dynamics and to compute the degree of regional circulation based on contrast appearance and disappearance (62, 63). Investigators performed detailed studies of errors attributed to ultrasound. These included attenuation, echo contrast microbubble preparation, microbubble injection, and side effects caused by injecting agents of differing viscosity, density, osmolality, and surface tension into the coronary circulation (effects on hyperemic response).

Observations on aortic and pulmonary artery injections of various echo contrast agents (including hydrogen peroxide) have indicated promise. Myocardial contrast 2DE measurements have already been employed successfully in physiologic studies and experimental preparations. Thus, sequential studies of myocardial ischemia following coronary occlusions allow real-time assessment of the underperfused myocardial risk zone. Effects of reperfusion or other interventions also were evaluated. Future evaluations will be aimed at establishing further evidence regarding the safety of the technique and its ultimate potential to quantitate myocardial perfusion.

The prime issue, which is not yet resolved, is whether an optimal echo contrast agent can be

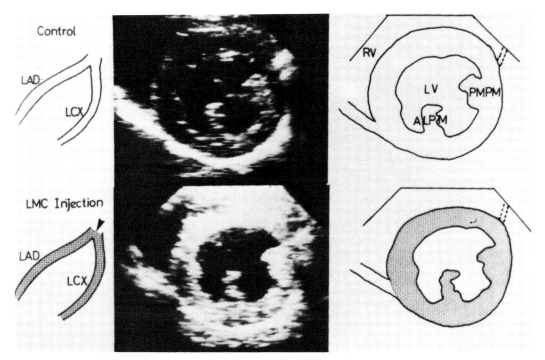

Figure 26.16. Opacification of the myocardium in the short-axis view at the level of high papillary muscle after injection of contrast material into the left main coronary artery (*LMC*) (*arrow*). The entire circumference of the left ventricular myocardium is opacified (*lower panel*). The echolucent area at the junction of the anterior septum and the right ventricle may represent an island of right coronary perfusion. *LAD* = left anterior descending coronary artery, *LCX* = left circumflex coronary artery, *RV* = right ventricle, *LV* = left ventricle, *ALPM* = anterolateral papillary muscle, *PMPM* = posteromedial papillary muscle. (From Tei C, Sakamaki T, Shah PM, Meerbaum S, Shimoura K, Kondo S, Corday E: Myocardial contrast echocardiography: A reproducible technique of myocardial opacification for identifying regional perfusion deficits. *Circulation* 67(3):585–593, 1983.) By permission of the American Heart Association.

produced. This contrast agent would reliably opacify the regional myocardium, delineate perfusion defects, allow quantitation of myocardial perfusion, and be injectable intravenously or from the right heart. Several very promising reports have been published or presented in preliminary form. Several studies reported the feasibility of producing echo contrast agents with a uniform microbubble diameter of about 5 μm. Furthermore, several initial clinical studies during coronary angiography (64, 65), as well as with transpulmonary echo contrast, appear encouraging. Further development of this method are likely to be pursued vigorously, as it may well provide a means for simultaneous determination of contractile function and perfusion.

In spite of all this evidence, more assurance is needed regarding the safety and reliability of echo contrast agents and the accuracy of myocardial measurements. Once developed, many applications can be envisioned, especially during cur-

rently practiced coronary interventions. This promising 2DE contrast method should be developed and related to other new diagnostic approaches for quantitative evaluation of myocardial perfusion defects.

OVERVIEW

Experimental studies in the field of echocardiography are undergoing a change in direction, due to availability of substantially improved 2DE equipment and increasingly extensive clinical investigations. Further major advances in methods and applications are anticipated. The primary goals of experimental 2DE research will probably shift to perfection of newer techniques, such as tissue characterization and myocardial contrast echo, and to validation of quantitative procedures. Validations will be especially important for quantitative analyses, e.g., of segmental contraction and computerized 3DE. To achieve truly useful progress, it is important to maintain an active ex-

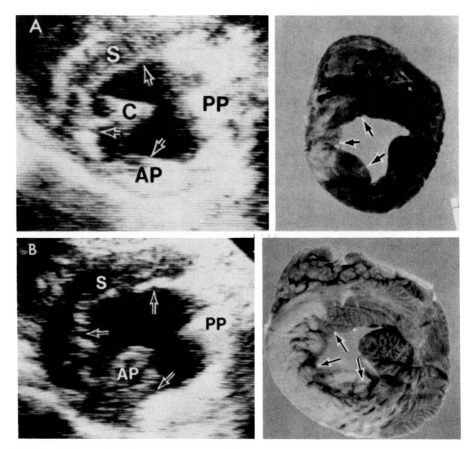

Figure 26.17. *A,* Comparison between contrast echocardiographic images and blue dye-delineated area cross sections in a dog of group A. The echocardiographic contrast medium was injected into the left main coronary artery after left anterior descending coronary artery occlusion. Part of the interventricular septum and left ventricular anterior wall (*arrows*) show a definitive negative contrast area in the *left side panel.* The *right side panel* shows the region free of blue dye in a short-axis slab that corresponds to the section used in the echocardiographic study. *B,* Comparison between contrast echocardiography and the extent of necrosis in a dog of group B. In the *left panel,* a portion of the interventricular septum and a part of the left ventricular anterior wall exhibit negative contrast (*arrows*). The *right panel* shows the necrosis (*arrows*) delineated by triphenyl-tetrazolium-chloride in a slab that corresponded to the left ventricular section used for the contrast echocardiographic study. *c* = catheter. (From Sakamaki T, Tei C, Meerbaum S, Shimoura K, Kondo S, Fishbein MC, Y-Rit J, Shah PM, Corday E: Verification of myocardial contrast two-dimensional echocardiographic assessment of perfusion defects in ischemic myocardium. *J Am Coll Cardiol* 5(1):34–38, 1984.) S = septum. AP = anterior papillary muscle. PP = posterior papillary muscle. Reprinted with permission from the American College of Cardiology. See this figure in the Color Atlas.

change and feedback between the laboratories producing experimental and clinical echocardiographic studies.

REFERENCES

1. Mann DL, Gillam LD, Weyman AE: Cross sectional echocardiographic assessment of regional left ventricular performance and myocardial perfusion. *Progr Cardiovasc Dis* 29:1–52, 1986.

2. Skorton DJ, Collins SM: Digital computer image analysis in echocardiography. *Echocardiography* 1:15, 1984.

3. Clayton TD, Jeppson GM, Klausner SC: Should a fixed external reference system be used to analyze left ventricular wall motion? *Circulation* 67:1518–1521, 1982.

4. Karsh KR, Lamm U, Blanke H, Rentrob K: Comparison of 19 quantitative models for assessment of localized left ventricular wall motion abnormalities. *Clin Cardiol* 3:123, 1980.

5. Grube E, Hansch H, Neumann G, Simon H: Quantitative evaluation of left ventricular wall motion by two-dimensionsl echocardiography (Abstr). *J Am Coll Cardiol* 1:581, 1983.

6. Schnittger I, Fitzgerald PJ, Gordon EP, Alderman EL, Popp RL: Computerized quantitative analysis of left ventricular wall motion by two-dimensional echocardiography. *Circulation* 70:242–254, 1984.

7. Sakamaki T, Lang D, Wong OY, Aosaki N, Kondo S, Shimoura K, Tei C, Meerbaum S, Shah PM, Corday E: Comparative validation of two-dimensional echocardiographic segmental wall motion analysis methods (Abstr). *J Am Coll Cardiol* 1:581, 1983.

8. Durkin M, Lehmann KG, Koprival J, McKenzie WB, Ezekowitz MD, Prokop EK, Barash PG: Center of mass aligorithm spots: Abnormal motion echo that does not mean ischemia. *Cardiovasc News*, p 17, August 1986.

9. Gillam LD, Hogan RD, Foale RA, Franklin TD, Newell JB, Guyer DE, Weyman AE: A comparison of quantitative echocardiography methods for delineation of infarct induced abnormal wall motion. *Circulation* 70:113–122, 1984.

10. Haendchen RV, Wyatt HL, Maurer G, Zwehl W, Bear M, Meerbaum S, Corday E: Quantitation of regional cardiac function by two-dimensional echocardiography: Patterns of contraction in a normal left ventricle. *Circulation* 67:1234–1245, 1983.

11. Kondo S, Meerbaum S, Sakamaki T, Shimoura K, Tei CH, Shah P, Corday E: Diagnosis of coronary stenosis by two-dimensional echocardiographic study of dysfunction of ventricular segments during and immediately after pacing. *J Am Coll Cardiol* 2:689–698, 1983.

12. Sakamaki T, Corday E, Meerbaum S, Torres MAR, Fishbein MC, Rit JY, Aosaki N: Relation between myocardial injury and post-extrasystolic potentiation of regional function measured by two-dimensional echocardiography. *J Am Coll Cardiol* 2:52–62, 1983.

13. Shimoura K, Meerbaum S, Sakamaki T, Kondo S, Fishbein MS, Rit JY, Tei CH, Shah P, Corday E: Relation between functional response to nitroglycerin and extent of myocardial necrosis in dogs: Mapping of the left ventricle by two-dimensional echocardiography. *Am J Cardiol* 52:177–183, 1983.

14. Uchiyama T, Corday E, Meerbaum S, Lang TW, Gueret P, Povzhitkov M, Peter T: Characterization of left ventricular mechanical function during arrhythmias with two-dimensional echocardiography: Premature ventricular contraction. *Am J Cardiol* 48:679–689, 1981.

15. Torres MAR, Corday E, Meerbaum S, Sakamaki T, Peter T, Uchiyama T: Characterization of left ventricular mechanical function during arrhythmias by two-dimensional echocardiography. *J Am Coll Cardiol* 1:819–829, 1983.

16. Foale R, Nihoyannopoulo P, McKenna W, Klienebenne A, Nadazdi A, Rowland E, Smith G: Echocardiographic measurement of the normal adult right ventricle. *Br Heart J* 56:33–44, 1983.

17. Weiss JL, Eaton LW, Kallman Ch, Maugham WL: Accuracy of volume determination by two-dimensional echocardiography: The finding requirements under controlled conditions in the ejecting canine left ventricle. *Circulation* 67:889–896, 1983.

18. Garcia E, Gueret P, Bennett M, Corday E, Zwehl W, Meerbaum S, Swan HJC, Vermon D: Real time computerization of two-dimensional echocardiography. *Am Heart J* 101:783, 1981.

19. Garcia E, Ezekiel A, Levy R, Zwehl W, Ong K, Corday E, Areeda J, Meerbaum S, Corday S: Automated computer enhancement and analysis of left ventricular two-dimensional echocardiograms. Computers in Cardiology, Long Beach, California, IEEE Computer Society, 1982, pp 399–402.

20. Brennecke R, Hahne H, Wessel A, Heintzen PH: Computerized enhancement techniques for echocardiographic sector scans. Computers in Cardiology, Long Beach, California, IEEE Computer Society, 1981, pp 7–11.

21. Skorton DJ, McNary CA, Child JS, Muten FC, Shah PM: Digital image processing of two-dimensional echocardiograms: Identification of the endocardium. *Am J Cardiol* 48:179, 1981.

22. Collins SM, Skorton DJ, Geiser EA, Nichols JA, Connetta DA, Vandian NG, Kerber RE: Computer assisted edge detection in two-dimensional echocardiography: Comparison to anatomic data. *Am J Cardiol* 53:1380, 1984.

23. Zwehl W, Levy R, Garcia E, Haendchen RV, Childs W, Corday SR, Meerbaum S, Corday E: Validation of a computerized edge detection aligorithm for quantitative two-dimensional echocardiography. *Circulation* 68:1127, 1983.

24. Fugii J, Sawada H, Aizawa T, Kato K, Onoe M, Kuno Y: Computer analysis of cross sectional echocardiograms for quantitative evaluation of left ventricular asynergy in myocardial infarction. *Br Heart J* 51:139–148, 1984.

25. Geiser EA, Lupkiewiz SM, Kristy LG, Ariet M, Connetta DA, Conti CR: Framework for three-dimensional time varying reconstruction of the human left ventricle: Sources of error and estimation of their magnitude. *Comput Biomed Res* 13:225, 1980.

26. Ueda K, Kuwaki K, Inoue K: Three-dimensional display and volume determination of the left ventricle by two-dimensional echocardiography (Abstr). *Am J Cardiol* 45:471, 1980.

27. Skorton DJ, Geiser EA: Three-dimensional echocardiography: A geometric reconstruction. In Talano JV, Guardian JM (eds): *Textbook of Two-Dimensional Echocardiography*. New York, Grune & Stratton, 1983, pp 357–369.

28. Chandran KB, Skorton DJ, Attarwalya Y, Orshansky B, Collins SM, Pandian N, Nikraseh PE, Kerber RE: Three-dimensional echocardiographic reconstruction of the intact heart: Calculation of the normal diastolic properties of the canine left ventricle (Abstr). *Circulation* 68:III-4, 1983.

29. Maurer G, Glish A, Nanda NC: Volume determination and three-dimensional reconstruction of echocardiographic images using rotation method (Abstr). *Circulation* 64:IV-206, 1981.

30. Moritz WE, Shreve PL: A microprocessor-based special locating system for use with diagnostic ultrasound. *Proc IEEE* 64:966, 1974.

31. Joskowitz G, Klipcera T, Fachinger O, Probst P,

Mayr H, Kaindel F: Computer supported measurements of 2D echocardiographic images. Computers in Cardiology. Long Beach, California, IEEE Computer Society, 1981, pp 13–17.

32. O'Donnell M, Mimbs JW, Sobel BE, Miller JG: Ultrasonic attenuation in normal and ischemic myocardium: Ultrasonic tissue characterization II. In Linzer M (ed): National Bureau of Standards Special Publication 525, Washington, DC, U.S. Government Printing Office, 1979, pp 63–71.

33. Mimbs JW, O'Donnell M, Miller JG, Sobel BE: Changes in ultrasonic attenuation indicative of early myocardial ischemic injury. *Am J Physiol* 236:H340, 1979.

34. Mimbs JW, Yuhas DE, Miller JD, Weiss AN, Sobel BE: Detection of myocardial infarction in vitro based on altered attenuation of ultrasound. *Circ Res* 41:192, 1977.

35. Skorton DJ, Melton HE Jr, Pandian NG, Nicols J, Koyanagi S, Marcus ML, Collins SM, Kerber RE: Detection of acute myocardial infarction in closed chest dogs by analysis of regional two-dimensional echocardiographic gray level distribution. *Circ Res* 52:36, 1983.

36. Skorton DJ, Collins SM, Nicols J, Pandian NG, Beam JA, Kerber RE: Quantitative texture analysis in two-dimensional echocardiography: Application to diagnosis of experimental contusion. *Circulation* 68:217, 1984.

37. Schnittinger I, Vieli A, Heiseman JE, Director VA, Billingham ME, Ellis SG, Kernoff RS, Takamoto T, Popp RL: Ultrasonic tissue characterization: Detection of acute myocardial infarction in dogs. *Circulation* 72:193–199, 1985.

38. Cohen RD, Motley JG, Miller JG, Kurnick PB, Sobel BE: Detection of ischemic myocardium in vivo through the chest wall by quantitative ultrasonic tissue characterization. *Am J Cardiol* 50:838, 1982.

39. Pincu M, Schwartz G, Corday SR, Fujibayashi Y, Meerbaum S: Attenuation correction in echocardiography. *Ultrason Imag* 8:000–000, 1986.

40. Madaras IE, Barzilia B, Perez JE, Sobel BE, Miller JG: Changes in myocardial backscatter throughout the cardiac cycle. *Ultrason Imag* 5:229–239, 1983.

41. Olshansky B, Collins SM, Skorton DJ: Variation of left ventricular myocardial grey level in two-dimensional echocardiography as a result of cardiac contraction. *Circulation* 70:972, 1984.

42. Gramiak R, Shah PM: Echocardiography of the aortic root. *Invest Radiol* 3:356, 1968.

43. Feigenbaum H, Stowe JM, Lee DA, Nasser WR, Chang S: Identification of ultrasound echoes from the left ventricle by use of intracardiac injections of indocine green. *Circulation* 41:615, 1970.

44. Kerber RE, Kioschos JM, Lauer RM: Use of an ultrasonic contrast method in the diagnosis of valvular regurgitation and intracardiac shunts. *Am J Cardiol* 34:722, 1974.

45. Sahn DJ, Valdez-Cruz LM: Ultrasonic contrast studies for the detection of cardiac shunts. *J Am Coll Cardiol* 3:978, 1984.

46. Meltzer RS, Rollandt J (eds): *Contrast Echocardiography*. The Hague, Martinus Nijhoff, 1982.

47. Grube E, Lampen M, Becher H: Echocontrast-ventriculography: Determination of left ventricular function parameters by digital subtraction echocardiography. *Z Cardiol* 75:650–658, 1986.

48. Corday E, Shah PM, Meerbaum S: Introduction, seminar on contrast two-dimensional echocardiography: Applications and new developments. *J Am Coll Cardiol* 3:1–5, 1984.

49. Armstrong WF, Kinney EL, Mueller TM, Tickner EG, Dillon JC, Feigenbaum H: Assessment of myocardial perfusion abnormalities with contrast enhanced two-dimensional echocardiography. *Circulation* 66:166–173, 1982.

50. Tei C, Sakamaki T, Shah PM, Meerbaum S, Shimoura K, Kondo S, Corday E: Myocardial contrast echocardiography: A reproducible technique of myocardial opacification for identifying regional perfusion defects. *Circulation* 67:585–593, 1983.

51. Kemper A, O'Boyle JE, Sharma S, Cohen CA, Klouer RA, Khuri SF, Pausi AF: Hydrogen peroxide contrast-enhanced two-dimensional echocardiography: Real-time in vivo delineation of regional myocardial perfusion. *Circulation* 68:603–611, 1983.

52. Sakamaki T, Tei C, Meerbaum S, Shimoura K, Kondo S, Fishbein MC, Y-Rit J, Shah PM, Corday E: Verification of myocardial contrast two-dimensional echocardiographic assessment of perfusion defects in ischemic myocardium. *J Am Coll Cardiol* 3:34–38, 1984.

53. Feinstein SB, Ten Cate J, Zwehl W, Oug K, Maurer G, Tei C, Shah PM, Meerbaum S, Corday E: Two-dimensional contrast echocardiography I: In vitro development and quantitative analysis of echo contrast agents. *J Am Coll Cardiol* 3:14–20, 1984.

54. Ten Cate FJ, Drury JK, Meerbaum S, Noordsy, J, Feinstein S, Shah PM, Corday E: Myocardial contrast two-dimensional echocardiography: Experimental examination at different coronary flow levels. *J Am Coll Cardiol* 3:1219–1226, 1984.

55. Feinstein SB, Ong K, Staniloff HM, Fujibayashi Y, Zwehl W, Meerbaum S, Corday E: Myocardial contrast echocardiography: Examination of intracoronary injections, microbubble diameters, and video-intensity decay. *Am J Physiol Imag* 1:12–18, 1986.

56. Kaul S, Pandian NG, Okada RD, Pohost GM, Weyman AE: Contrast echocardiography in acute myocardial ischemia. I: In vivo determination of total left ventricular "area at risk." *J Am Coll Cardiol* 4:1272–1282, 1984.

57. Feinstein SB, Shah PM, Bing RJ, Meerbaum S, Corday E, Chang B, Santillan G, Fujibayashi Y: Microbubble dynamics visualized in the intact capillary circulation. *J Am Coll Cardiol* 4:595–600, 1984.

58. Santoso S, Roelandt J, Mansyoer H, Abdurahman N, Meltzer RS, Hugenholtz PG: Myocardial perfusion imaging in humans by contrast echocardiography using polygelin colloid solution. *J Am Coll Cardiol* 6:612–620, 1985.

59. Gillam LD, Kaul S, Fallon JT, Hedley-White ET, Slater CE, Weyman AE: Functional and pathologic effects of multiple echocardiographic contrast injections on the myocardium, brain and kidney. *J Am Coll Cardiol* 6:687–694, 1985.

60. Keller MW, Feinstein SB, Briller RA, Powsner SM:

Automated production and analysis of echocontrast agents. *J Ultrasound Med* 5:493–498, 1986.

61. Powsner SM, Keller MW, Saniia J, Feinstein SB: Quantitation of echocontrast effects. *Am J Physiol Imag* 1:124–128, 1986.

62. Maurer G, Ong K, Haendchen R, Torres M, Tei C, Wood F, Meerbaum S, Shah P, Corday E: Myocardial contrast two-dimensional echocardiography: Comparison of contrast disappearance rates in normal and underperfused myocardium. *Circulation* 69:418–429, 1984.

63. Schartel M, Fritzsch T, Misalok V: Quantification of myocardial perfusion by contrast echocardiography. *Can J Cardiol* 25:31A, 1986.

64. Moore CA, Smucker ML, Kaul S: Myocardial contrast echocardiography in humans: I. Safety—A comparison with routine coronary arteriography. *J Am Coll Cardiol* 8:1066–1072, 1986.

65. Feinstein SB, Lang RM, Dick C, Neumann A, Al-Sadir J, Chua KG, Carroll J, Feldman T, Borow KM: Contrast echocardiographic perfusion studies in humans. *Am J Cardiol Imag* 1:29–37, 1986.

27

Echocardiographic Changes Related to Space Travel

Michael W. Bungo, M.D.

The United States has put humans into space flight for more than 25 years. In this unique environment, the effects of gravity are negligible. However, humans have developed an efficient set of cardiovascular regulating mechanisms to maintain blood pressure and flow in spite of the hydrostatic forces applied by gravity (1).

Before the first journey into space there were dire predictions that the cardiovascular system might be unable to adjust to this absence of gravity. Since the zero-gravity environment of space cannot be duplicated on Earth for any longer than a fraction of a minute, there was no experience on which to base recommendations. Data were generated in ground-based bedrest tests and short journeys into space using animal subjects. In 1961, only a few months after an historic orbital flight by a Soviet cosmonaut, the first United States astronaut ventured into space.

The goal of placing a human into near space created complex engineering requirements. Coupled with the existing medical technology and small capacity of the spacecraft, this resulted in minimal cardiovascular monitoring. For a simple monitoring device to be acceptable, it had to provide little interference, use no space capsule power, and occupy virtually no room. As flight experience was gained without obvious deleterious clinical effects, the argument for additional testing or examination of astronaut crew members found little support within the National Aeronautics and Space Administration (NASA).

Cardiovascular studies in the early United States space program (Mercury, Gemini, and Apollo) were largely limited to inflight electrocardiographic monitoring and pre- and postflight testing of orthostatic intolerance. This latter response

had been noted as the most obvious consequence of exposure to zero gravity (2, 3).

The theory employed to explain the observation of orthostatic intolerance stated that during exposure to zero gravity, the hydrostatic forces (which normally have the greatest influence on the venous system) are removed. This negates the natural pooling effect of blood in the lower extremities, allowing increased venous return to the central cardiovascular system. The increased central volume subsequently is sensed as volume overload, and reflex mechanisms are initiated to return central blood volume to "normal." Prime among theoretical mechanisms at the time was an initiation of the Gauer-Henry reflex, which states that atrial stretch receptors cause inhibition of antidiuretic hormone and therefore a resultant renal diuresis (4). More current theories invoke atrial naturetic factor as an important mechanism (5).

These explanations were advanced in response to observations made during the early ventures of humans into space. It was noted that the legs became smaller in circumference during space flight, resulting in a bird-like appearance. The facies also became puffy with distended veins and congested mucous membranes. Plasma volume was decreased after flight. Although crew members experienced no limitations in flight, after return to Earth a loss of orthostatic tolerance was observed (6). This behavior, consistent with relative intravascular volume depletion, conformed to the above theories. Again, because of the severe technical and political limitations placed on NASA, dedicated inorbit data collection in an expanded and comprehensive program was delayed until the Skylab series of the early 1970s.

The Skylab orbital workshop provided the first in-depth medical investigations in flight. In this more opportune setting a large volume of cardiovascular data were collected. However, the open literature contains little statistical analysis of grouped samples, reporting anecdotal individual findings instead. As a result, our knowledge consists of a series of case reports severely hampered by questions of controlled environment and "mean ± error" presentation (7).

During the Skylab flights, circulatory parameters were measured during the application of stresses such as bicycle ergometry and lower body negative pressure (LBNP). As part of the final Skylab mission, pre- and postflight M-mode echocardiograms were performed on the three crew members. These demonstrated that cardiac mass, stroke volume, and left ventricular end-diastolic volume were decreased postflight and the decrements persisted for more than a week after landing (8).

Between 1982 and 1985 NASA launched a number of space shuttle missions. From these missions, pre- and postflight (but not inflight) two-dimensional echocardiograms were obtained on 30 individuals at selected intervals. Flight durations ranged from 120 to 168 hr. The following parameters were examined: resting heart rate, blood pressure (systolic, diastolic, and mean), left ventricular (LV) dimensions and volumes (end-systole and end-diastole), stroke volume, cardiac output, left atrial and right ventricular dimensions, LV posterior wall and interventricular septal wall thickness, LV fractional shortening, ejection fraction, velocity of circumferential fiber shortening, and LV mass. When appropriate, values were normalized for body surface area and presented as indices. The data acquisition schedule was not uniform, since studies had to be obtained at times that would have the least impact on the astronauts' other activities. However, the postflight data were divided into two groups: those echocardiograms obtained immediately postflight (within hours of landing) and those obtained approximately 1 week after landing (range of 5–11 days).

In 13 crew members, these data were obtained both immediately postflight and 1 week later. Most postflight measurements were not statistically different from the preflight values, as there were wide variations in the measured results, further complicated by the added errors compiled when calculations (such as LV mass) were performed.

Nevertheless, there were clear differences ($p <$ 0.01) in several areas. Heart rate was 24% higher immediately postflight and 1 week later was still 8% higher than preflight. LV diastolic index was decreased by 16% immediately postflight. One week later, LV diastolic index was not significantly different from preflight, although there appeared to be a tendency toward a slight increase over preflight values. On landing day, measurements of systolic volume, stroke volume, and cardiac index could not be clearly distinguished from preweightlessness values. However, 1 week later, cardiac index and stroke volume index were elevated 29% and 17%, respectively. Total peripheral resistance, estimated from the cardiac output and blood pressure measurements, was unchanged immediately postflight but was decreased by 15% a week later (9). The decrease in left ventricular diastolic volume index (LVDVI) tended to be greater the larger the preflight heart size. Figure 27.2 illustrates preflight LVDVI, plotted on the abscissa, compared against the postflight change in heart size, plotted on the ordinate (10).

While these investigations were being performed, the French space agency became involved in a joint experiment with the Soviet Union's space program. In June 1982, the Soviet space lab Salyut VII took off with a custom-built echocardiographic instrument on board. Data on the peripheral vasculature were also obtained, as this equipment was capable of continuous wave Doppler examination. Unfortunately, as was the case in earlier United States programs, data were only obtained from one individual. The most significant achievement of this experiment was that, for the first time, inflight echocardiographic data were recorded. Postflight decrease in left ventricular diastolic volume (LVDV) and increase in heart rate were similar to other reported studies. However, LVDV was elevated early in the flight before the subsequent drop, while heart rate remained increased during the entire period of weightlessness. No changes in any parameters of cardiac contractile function could be implied (11).

In April 1985, the United States space shuttle program carried a commercial two-dimensional echocardiographic sector scanner into low Earth orbit for more detailed human examinations (Fig. 27.1). Studies were obtained on four individuals several days before the flight, on each day except day 4 of the 7-day mission, within 2 hr of landing, 1 day postflight, and 4 days postflight. For the

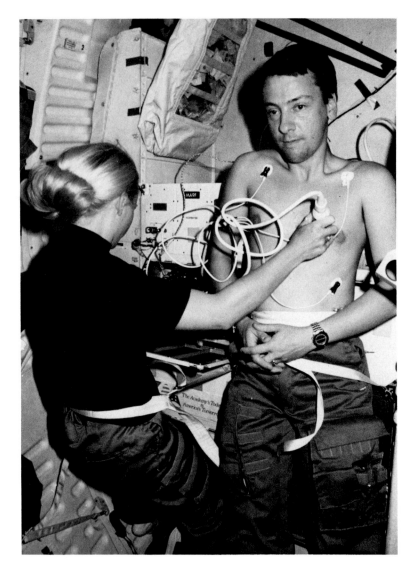

Figure 27.1. Echocardiographic study being performed during space flight. There is no up or down in space, so the apparent "standing" posture is artifactual. Note the strap restraints required to prevent the subjects from floating away. The heart shifts somewhat medially and cephalid during weightlessness.

first time in the United States program, actual inflight data were available for comparison with the pre- and postflight data. Also, there were enough subjects to at least show inflight hemodynamic trends, even if statistical analysis was difficult.

The parameters evaluated were similar to those used in previous studies. Right ventricular dimension was found to be decreased by 35% throughout weightlessness, returning to baseline postflight (Fig. 27.3). LVDVI, when compared to preflight values, was increased by 20% on the first day of flight but decreased by 15% thereafter. Stroke volume changes were similar to those for LVDVI. Mean blood pressure and heart rate were both increased by 20% during weightlessness (Fig. 27.4). Increases in both diastolic and systolic pressure contributed to the rise in mean pressure. After an 85% rise in cardiac index the first day, values returned to preflight levels for the duration of the mission. However, cardiac index was elevated again by 59% during the post-

LVDVI AND SPACE FLIGHT
(PERCENT CHANGE)

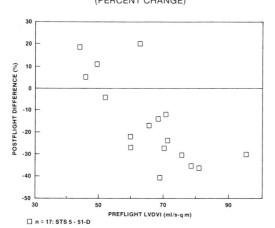

□ n = 17: STS 5 - 51-D

Figure 27.2. Change in left ventricular diastolic volume index (*LVDVI*) versus preflight left ventricular size. The larger the preflight heart size, the greater the loss in left ventricular volume.

flight recovery period (Fig. 27.5). Trends toward elevation in cardiovascular work and total peripheral resistance were noted throughout the flight (Figs. 27.6 and 27.7). Recovery from weightlessness appeared to require at least a week of reexposure to Earth's gravity (12).

Considering the limited number of observa-

RIGHT VENTRICULAR DIMENSION
DURING SPACE FLIGHT

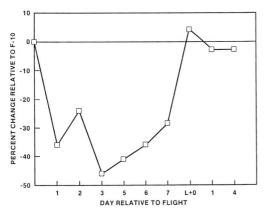

Figure 27.3. Change in right ventricular dimension during space flight. The *zero line* represents the preflight value; the day of space flight is represented on the abscissa, with L + 0 indicating landing day (2 hr after flight) and subsequently 1 and 4 days after landing. *F-10* represents the baseline data obtained 10 days prior to launch.

AFE - 51-D

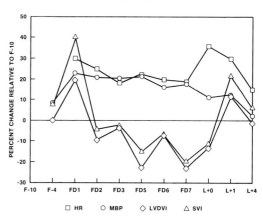

□ HR   ○ MBP   ◇ LVDVI   △ SVI

Figure 27.4. Composite of heart rate (*HR*), mean blood pressure (*MBP*), left ventricular diastolic volume index (*LVDVI*), and stroke volume index (*SVI*) as these parameters change during space flight. See the legend to Figure 27.3 for explanation of axis labeling.

tions, it is difficult to imply that these are absolute changes in the central hemodynamics of the human cardiovascular system that can be expected as gravitational force is withdrawn. However, these studies have produced several important and encouraging points. First, the limited inflight data compare well with the larger body of data obtained pre- and postflight, at times where there is overlap in the time of measurement. Second,

CARDIAC INDEX
DURING SPACE FLIGHT

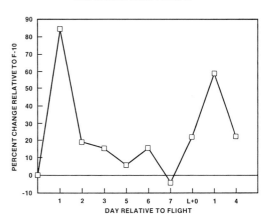

Figure 27.5. Change in cardiac index during space flight. Volumes are expressed as a percent change similar to Figure 27.3.

CARDIOVASCULAR WORK
DURING SPACE FLIGHT

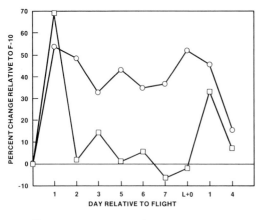

□ LV STROKE WORK　　○ RATE-PRESS. PRODUCT

Figure 27.6. Changes in cardiovascular work during space flight, expressed both as left ventricular (*LV*) stroke work and the rate pressure product. Axis labeling is as noted in the legend to Figure 27.3.

data obtained during bedrest studies in large numbers of volunteers show similar trends (13). Third, inflight values conform to theoretical predictions of headward fluid shifts and subsequent vascular adaptation and fluid redistribution.

When changes observed in LVDVI, heart rate, and other parameters are compared with preflight standing (rather than supine) values, many sta-

VASCULAR RESISTANCE (TPR)
DURING SPACE FLIGHT

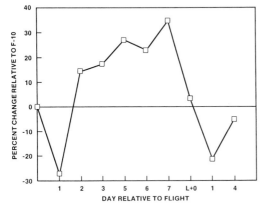

Figure 27.7. Changes in total peripheral resistance (TPR) from preflight as a function of time in weightlessness See the legend to Figure 27.3 for description of axis labeling.

tistical differences disappear (Charles JB, Bungo MW: unpublished data, NASA-Johnson Space Center, Houston, Texas). This observation may imply that the cardiovascular system is resetting to preferred parameters, those that exist during most of the life cycle of the human organism (in the upright posture). Additional investigation will be necessary to define the absolute magnitude and mechanisms of these adaptive changes, as well as the consequences of prolonged or repeated exposure to conditions of altered gravity.

Echocardiography is an ideal tool for these future investigations. Equipment is becoming more sophisticated, more compact, and more reliable. The technique is noninvasive and with negligible risk, justifying its use in human volunteers. The amount of data obtained in a single investigative study, by either direct measurement or subsequent calculation, makes the technique cost effective. Finally, the accuracy of the procedure allows conclusions to be reached after a smaller number of observations than with most other approaches.

The role of medicine in the exploration of space faces many challenges (14). Currently, the United States flight program plans more extensive investigations as part of the routine health program for astronauts, in collaboration with domestic universities and foreign governments (15).

REFERENCES

1. Sandler H: Effects of bedrest and weightlessness on the heart. In Boure GH (ed): *Heart and Heart-Like Organs*. New York Academic Press, 1980, vol 2, pp 435–524.
2. Berry CA, Coons DO, Catterson AD, Kelly GF: Man's responses to long duration space flights in the Gemini spacecraft. In: Gemini Midprogram Conference, NASA SP-121. Washington, DC, National Aeronautics and Space Administration, 1966, pp 253–263.
3. Hoffler GW, Johnson RL: Apollo flight crew cardiovascular evaluations. In: *Biomedical Results of Apollo*, NASA SP-368). Washington, DC, National Aeronautics and Space Administration, 1975, pp 227–264.
4. Gauer OH, Henry JP, Behn C: The regulation of extracellular fluid volume. *Ann Rev Physiol* 32:547–595, 1970.
5. Needleman P, Greenwald JE; Atriopeptin: A cardiac hormone intimately involved in fluid, electrolyte, and blood pressure homeostasis. *N Engl J Med* 314:828–834, 1986.
6. Bungo MW, Johnson PC Jr: Cardiovascular examinations and observations of deconditioning during the space shuttle orbital flight test program. *Aviat Space Environ Med* 54:1001–1004, 1983.
7. Johnston RS, Dietlein LF (eds): Section V, Car-

diovascular and metabolic function. In: *Biomedical Results from Skylab*, NASA SP-377). Washington, DC, National Aeronautics and Space Administration, 1977, pp 284–405.

8. Henry WL, Epstein SE, Griffith LH, Goldstein RE, Redwood DR: Effects of prolonged spaceflight on cardiac function and dimensions. In: *Biomedical Results from Skylab*, NASA SP-377). Washington, DC, National Aeronautics and Space Administration, 1977, pp 366–371.

9. Bungo MW, Goldwater DJ, Popp RL, Sandler H: Echocardiographic examination of space shuttle crewmembers. *J Appl Physiol* 62:278–283, 1987.

10. Charles JB, Bungo MW: Post-space flight changes in resting cardiovascular parameters are associated with preflight left ventricular volume (Abstr). *Aviat Space Environ Med* 57:493, 1986.

11. Pottier JM, Patat F, Arbeille P, Pourcelot L: Car-

diovascular system and microgravity simulation and inflight results. *Acta Astronaut* 13:47–51, 1986.

12. Bungo MW, Charles JB, Riddle J, Roesch J, Wolf DA, Seddon MR: Echocardiographic investigation of the hemodynamics of weightlessness. *J Am Coll Cardiol* 7:192A, 1986.

13. Sandler H, Goldwater DJ, Bungo MW, Popp RL: Changes in cardiovascular function: Weightlessness and ground-based studies. *NATO Advisory Group for Aerospace Research and Development*, Conference proceedings No. 377. 1985, pp 6-1–6-9.

14. Hillman AL: After the Challenger. *N Engl J Med* 315:1196–1200, 1986.

15. Charles JB, Bungo MW: Cardiovascular research in space: Considerations for the design of the human research facility of the United States space station. *Aviat Space Environ Med* 57:1000–1005, 1986.

28

Echocardiographic Techniques in the Dog and Cat

Robert H. Lusk, Jr., D.V.M.
Stephen J. Ettinger, D.V.M.

INTRODUCTION

Ultrasonography, the technique of soft tissue imaging using pulsed high frequency sound waves, represents one of the most dramatic advances in the clinical practice of veterinary medicine. Introduced to human clinical medicine in the 1970s, it has been used in animals primarily for medical research and only recently for clinical purposes. A number of well-designed studies in dogs and cats have established its use for qualitative and quantitative assessment of cardiac function (2, 4, 7, 9, 12, 16, 18, 22).

Echocardiography permits safe, noninvasive evaluation of a minimally restrained animal. In high-risk situations, echocardiography can be safely used to measure heart size and provide real-time tomographic images. Occasionally, with the addition of Doppler, echocardiography is used to evaluate the physiologic status of the heart. This is extremely important in the critically ill veterinary patient, since the clinician cannot reason with the patient.

Echocardiographic studies of cardiac structure, function, and hemodynamics give the clinician and researcher an excellent tool to measure progression of a disease or response to treatment. Accurate diagnosis requires reliable, repeatable echocardiographic measurements (24). We believe that the use of ultrasonography in veterinary cardiology provides accurate and repeatable assessment of both cardiac anatomy and function.

Two echocardiographic techniques are now available. M-mode echocardiography employs a narrow beam, "ice pick" view of the heart. Visualization of the heart requires the beam to be directed manually at different cardiac structures. The result is an anatomically unfamiliar and somewhat difficult-to-read image. However, the rapid sampling rate permits characterization of more subtle abnormalities of motion, especially of the mitral and aortic valves. Two-dimensional real-time echo (2DE), also referred to as sector scanning, is created by a fan-shaped ultrasound beam that is directed through different cardiac planes. This allows the viewer to see an anatomically familiar two-dimensional tomographic image (22). Noninvasively, the clinician is informed of the cardiac spatial anatomy and function. In 2DE the heart is seen beating, and the size and shape of intra- and extracardiac structures are seen. Both symmetric and asymmetric enlargement are recognizable, soft tissue can be distinguished from fluid, and neoplasms and vegetations can be visualized. The motion of the heart relative to the surrounding extracardiac structures may be recognized and quantitated.

We use echocardiography principally for evaluating patients with suspected cardiac disease, identifying unexplained cardiomegaly interpreted from electrocardiography or thoracic radiography, and evaluating patients with unexplained or questionable heart murmurs. Echocardiography provides a useful anatomic description of the cardiac disorder, a semiquantitative functional description of the disorder, and it may identify progression of cardiac malfunction. Left ventricular function is quantifiable without the need for invasive studies.

Dogs with known mitral valvular insufficiency are evaluated to determine chordae integrity, the extent of the valvular damage, and left atrial size. Congestive cardiomyopathy of dogs and left ventricular function quantitated by shortening fraction may be determined specifically by echocardiographic examination. In the feline species, the

530

exam is used to differentiate clinically between congestive and hypertrophic myocardial disease, something that cannot otherwise be done non-invasively. Ultrasound studies permit the repeated measurement of cardiac indices in animals with systemic hypertension and hyperthyroidism.

Pericardial effusion, pericardial masses, cardiac tumors (left ventricle, left atrium, right atrium or heart base), and penetrating foreign bodies are identified readily by 2DE (23). Pleural effusions, pleural, lung, and mediastinal masses, and diaphragmatic hernias are identified regularly. This often permits a rapid diagnosis to be made in otherwise difficult clinical circumstances. Ultrasound is also extremely useful in the diagnosis of congenital cardiac diseases, since specific anatomic descriptions provide the fundamental details for the diagnosis. Right-to-left shunting lesions are identifiable when agitated saline bubbles or indocyanine green dye is used to elucidate anatomic defects (1).

In humans, dogs, and cats, the left heart is easier to image than the right. This is due to difficulty in adjusting near-field echoes and the right heart's proximity to the transducer. Right-sided structures are best imaged when there is fluid between them and the transducer (16).

Investigators have found that 2DE planes are highly reproducible in the dog. Most indices of left ventricular function are independent of body weight in dogs, but Jacobs and Knight (9) suggested that variations in weight influence other indices that may, in turn, affect left ventricular function in the cat. Dimensions as measured from the standard left- and right-sided windows are nearly identical.

In the short time since the introduction of 2DE in veterinary medicine, the technique has been shown to permit repeatable assessment of cardiac anatomy. 2DE images from the cat are similar qualitatively to those from dogs and humans, but there are problems in the cat relating to the small size of the heart, narrow intercostal spaces, and rapid heart rate (4).

THE ECHOCARDIOGRAM OF THE NORMAL DOG AND CAT

Good quality images may be obtained in most dogs and cats with traditional cardiac ultrasonographic techniques and equipment. Images are usually better in the presence of cardiomegaly, the result of a larger "echo window." However, images acceptable for measurement may be obtained in normal animals also. Dogs rarely are

anesthetized or sedated for the procedure, but often it is not as easy to work with cats. It is important to note that sedation does affect cardiac indices. In most situations, special handling, modified positions (Figs. 28.1–28.4), a good caring technician, and a quiet environment will produce good echoes. However, these techniques may be difficult to perform in cats, obese animals, animals with thoracic deformities, or those with severe respiratory distress.

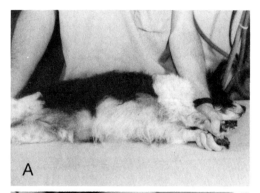

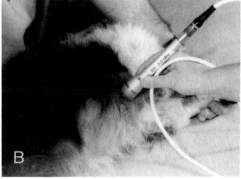

Figure 28.1. *A*, Normal dog in the left lateral position being imaged from the right parasternal position. Imaging is facilitated by extending the right forelimb cranially. *B*, The hair over the thorax is clipped, and liberal amounts of water-soluble coupling gel are used. Chemical restraint rarely is required in the dog but may be used in the cat. The transducer is placed along the area of the third to seventh intercostal space, usually from 1–8 cm dorsolateral to the midline (sternum). Longitudinal and cross-sectional views are usually obtained in the fourth or fifth intercostal space. The beam is swept from the cardiac apex to the base to obtain three imaging planes. These include the left ventricle, mitral valve-aortic root, and left atrial regions. The short-axis plane is used to obtain the best image of the papillary muscles, chordae tendineae, mitral valve, and the aortic Valsalva's sinuses.

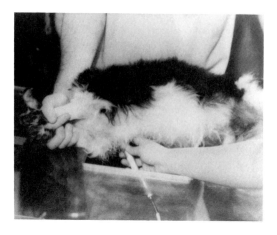

Figure 28.2. The heart is imaged with the transducer placed on the thoracic wall from below, using a Plexiglas table with holes cut out for the transducer placement. This gives better images from the right side because of the cardiac notch in the right lung. This increases cardiac contact with the right thoracic wall, thus providing a larger cardiac window.

Initially, imaging was performed in the traditional positions used in humans. However, good echo windows were not obtainable routinely, and images were often quite variable. Over the past few years many studies in dogs and cats have

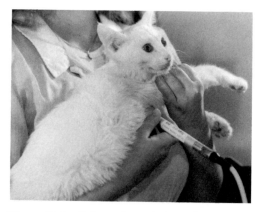

Figure 28.3. Feline echo technique. Although the normal recording position is preferred, some cats do not permit such positioning. However, they may allow the technician to hold them upright while placing the transducer against the thoracic wall in the usual left and right parasternal positions. This often is accomplished in the cat without sedation. The overall image quality in the cat is poorer than in dogs. Technical difficulties arise from near-field transducer artifacts, limitation of near-field settings, and poor resolution of septal echoes. Use of 7.5 MHz transducers improves endocardial resolution to the detriment of subjective appreciation of cardiac motion. In small dogs and cats, occasionally, a water-filled balloon is held next to the thoracic wall to act as a distancer to improve the depth required for good imaging.

identified the best positions for M-mode or two-dimensional echocardiography. Cardiac images obtained from the thoracic inlet and the cranial abdomen are usually unacceptable. The two favored windows are the right and left parasternal (apical) locations.

The veterinary community has adopted the image planes identified by Thomas (22) in his comprehensive report and study of the echo-tomographic anatomy of the dog. The same imaging planes are also applicable to the cat (4). In a more recent article on quantitative 2DE in the dog, O'Grady et al. (16) identified the following image planes obtained in the dog:

1. Right parasternal long-axis view, optimized for the
   a. Left ventricular apex and mitral valve
   b. Left ventricular apex, left ventricular outflow tract, aortic valve, and proximal ascending aorta
   c. Left atrium
   d. Interventricular septum, left ventricular outflow tract, aortic valve, mitral valve, and left ventricular posterior wall (a plane between *c* above and *e* below)
   e. Aortic annulus, visualization of aortic cusps, and the Valsalva's sinuses
2. Right parasternal short-axis view, optimized for the
   a. Left ventricular, high papillary muscle level
   b. Chordae tendineae of the left ventricle
   c. Aortic root and valve
3. Left parasternal apical long-axis view, optimized for the
   a. Left ventricle, mitral valve, and left atrium
   b. Left ventricle, left atrium, right ventricle, and right atrium (four-chamber view)

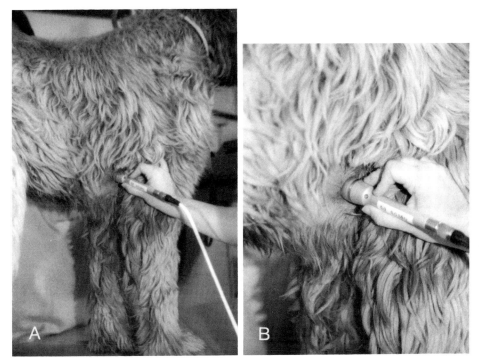

Figure 28.4. Giant dog echocardiography. *A*, Giant breeds of dogs are often difficult to position when they are critically ill, especially with pulmonary edema. Due to severe respiratory distress the dog cannot be held down comfortably, and the rapid, deep thoracic excursions preclude obtaining a reasonable recording. Often, echoes are made with the dog in a standing position instead. *B*, The transducer position is right parasternal.

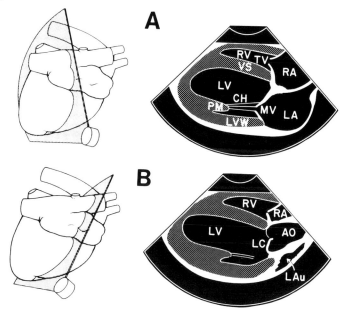

Figure 28.5. Diagram of long-axis views—right parasternal position. The diagrams represent a view of a dog's heart being transected by the fan-shaped transducer beam. To the right of the cardiac diagram are the echo-tomographic images of the planes shown. *A*, Long-axis four-chamber view of the heart. *B*, Long-axis view of the heart with emphasis on the left ventricular outflow region. The heart cannot be viewed in one single image to show the left atrium (*LA*), left ventricle (*LV*), mitral valve (*MV*), chordae tendineae (*CH*), left auricle (*LAu*), ventricular septum (*VS*), left cusp of the aortic valve (*LC*), aorta (*AO*), right atrium (*RA*), tricuspid valve (*TV*), right ventricle (*RV*), papillary muscle (*PM*), and left ventricular wall (*LVW*). (From Thomas WP: Two-dimensional real-time echocardiography in the dog. *Vet Radiol* 25:50−64, 1984.)

4. Left parasternal long-axis view, optimized for the
   a. Left ventricular outflow tract, aortic valve, and ascending aorta
   b. Right ventricular inflow tract and tricuspid valve
   c. Right ventricular outflow tract, pulmonary valve, and pulmonary artery
5. Left parasternal short-axis view, optimized for the
   a. Right ventricular inflow tract, and short-axis view of the aorta at the level of the aortic cusps

Echocardiography in the dog is generally possible to a depth of 20 cm, using standard unaltered equipment. Transducer frequencies vary from 2.5 to 7.5 MHz in the dog and 5.0 to 7.5 mHz in the cat.

In lateral recumbent positions the animal lies on its right or left side. Although not required, we obtain better echo quality when the hair is clipped over the parasternal region. A water-soluble coupling gel is applied to remove air space and improve sound transmission. Electrocardiographic leads with alligator clips are positioned just below the level of the stifles and olecranon. The electrocardiogram (ECG) is monitored primarily for timing purposes. The cardiac window may be found by moving the transducer and imaging in the intercostal spaces. Depending on the size of the patient, the window is 1 to 7 cm dor-

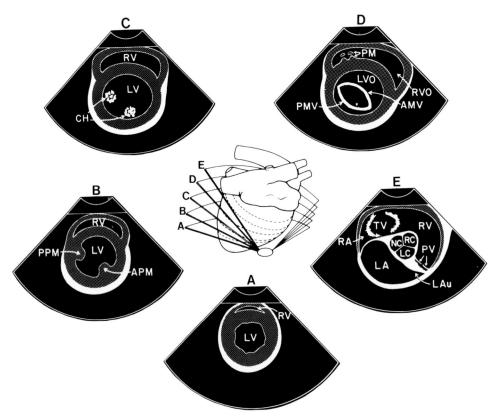

Figure 28.6. Diagram of short-axis views—right parasternal position. The *center diagram* illustrates the transducer beam location used to obtain the images shown in A–E. A, Apical level. B, Papillary level. C, Chordal level. D, Mitral valve level in diastole. E, Aortic valve level in diastole. *LVO* = left ventricular outflow tract, *PMV* = posterior mitral valve cusp, *RVO* = right ventricular outflow tract, *AMV* = septal (anterior) mitral valve cusp, *PPM* = posteromedial papillary muscle, *APM* = anterolateral papillary muscle, *PV* = pulmonary valve, *NC* = noncoronary or septal cusp of the aortic valve. Definitions of other abbreviations are the same as those in Figure 28.5. (From Thomas WP: Two-dimensional real-time echocardiography in the dog. *Vet Radiol* 25:50–64, 1984.)

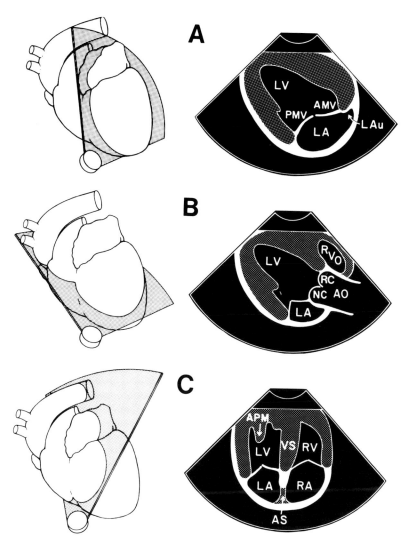

Figure 28.7. The echo beam is at the left caudal parasternal (intercostal) position but is not a true left ventricular apex view. The pictures show the heart diagram and the position of the echo beam as well as the corresponding echo-tomographic images. *A,* The long-axis two-chamber view of both the left atrium and left ventricle. *B,* Long-axis view of the left ventricular outflow tract region. *C,* Four-chamber view. *AS* = atrial septum, *RC* = right coronary aortic cusp. Definitions of other abbreviations are found in the legends to Figures 28.5 and 28.6. (From Thomas WP: Two-dimensional real-time echocardiography in the dog. *Vet Radiol* 25:50–64, 1984.)

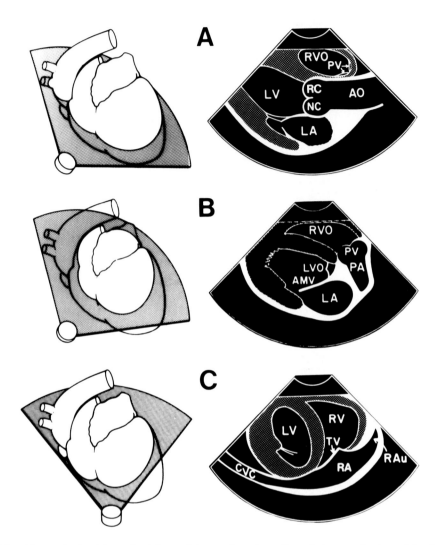

Figure 28.8. Views obtained from the left cranial parasternal position. *A*, Long-axis view of the left ventricular outflow tract. *B*, Long-axis view of the right ventricular outflow tract. *C*, Oblique view of the heart with a long-axis view of the right atrium and caudal vena cava. (The transducer is shown in the caudal position, but Thomas reported this view to be present in either cranial or caudal locations.) *CVC* = caudal vena cava, *PA* = pulmonary artery, *RAu* = right auricle. Definitions of other abbreviations are found in the legends to Figures 28.5–28.7. (From Thomas WP: Two-dimensional real-time echocardiography in the dog. *Vet Radiol* 25:50–64, 1984.)

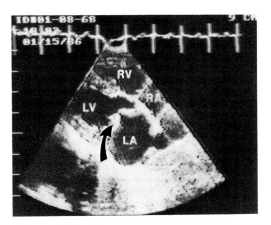

Figure 28.9. Right parasternal long-axis view of the left ventricle (*LV*) and the mitral valve. This four-chamber view shows the position of the left atrium (*LA*), left ventricle, right atrium (*RA*), and right ventricle (*RV*). The semilunar valves (*arrow*) are seen between the atria and ventricles.

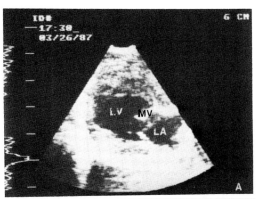

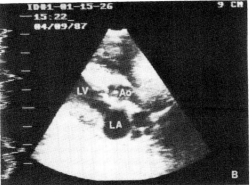

Figure 28.11. Right parasternal long-axis view of the left atrial cavity. *A*, The left ventricular cavity (*LV*) and partially opened mitral valve (*MV*) are viewed with the transducer turned to allow full visualization of the left atrial cavity (*LA*). *B*, Moving the transducer slightly allows comparison of size between the left atrium (*LA*) and the aortic outflow tract (*Ao*). Normally, there is almost a 1:1 size ratio in both the dog and cat.

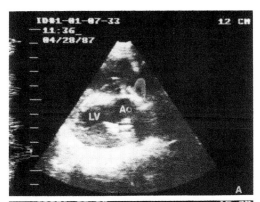

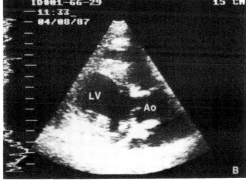

Figure 28.10. Right parasternal long-axis view. *A*, The left ventricular (*LV*) and aortic outflow region (*Ao*) at the level of the aortic valve. The cavity is seen in full dimension. The aortic leaflets are observed in the open position, and the aorta is fully distended.

solateral to the sternum, usually near the costochondral junction. The image is found in the region of the third to seventh intercostal space. Acoustic gain and gray scale are set to optimize images for both epicardial and endocardial surfaces. The anteroposterior terminology in the human is analogous to ventral-dorsal in the dog and cat.

Imaging the recumbent patient from the underside often provides a better image of the heart, since it is closer to the thoracic wall. Air space resulting from interposed lung tissue also is diminished. This approach, useful in humans also, uses a stand or table (we use a Plexiglas table) with several small holes cut out (Fig. 28.2). This allows placement of the patient in a comfortable

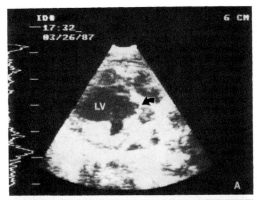

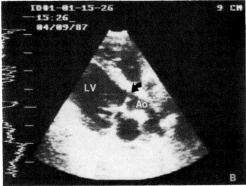

Figure 28.12. Right parasternal long-axis view of aortic valve region. The left ventricular cavity and outflow tract (*LV*), aortic valve leaflets (*arrow*), and the aortic root (*Ao*) are visualized in both figures.

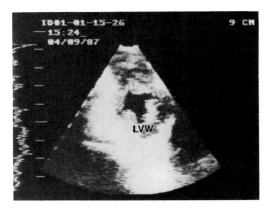

Figure 28.14. Right parasternal cross-sectional view. The left ventricular cavity and the thick left ventricular wall (*LVW*) are seen in systole.

lying position with ready access to the cardiac window. The echocardiographer then saturates the thoracic wall with coupling gel and examines the heart from below.

Transducer orientations in the right and left parasternal positions are demonstrated in Figures 28.5–28.19. The methods of obtaining long-axis and cross-sectional images in the dog and cat are similar to those used in humans. A detailed description of the technique along with anatomic correlations in the dog were published by Thomas (22). Images in the cat are acceptable with either 5 or 7.5 MHz transducers, but the quality of the image is often not as good as in the dog (4).

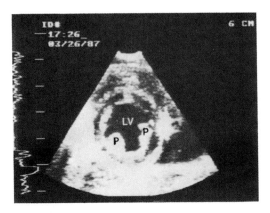

Figure 28.13. Right parasternal cross-sectional view. At the level corresponding to that shown in Figure 28.6*B*, the left ventricular cavity (*LV*) is seen in diastole at the level of the papillary muscles (*P*). The right ventricular cavity is above the left ventricular cavity.

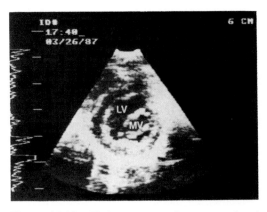

Figure 28.15. Right parasternal cross-sectional view at the mitral valve—diastole. The left ventricular cavity (*LV*) and the mitral valve (*MV*) leaflets are visualized. At this level, the leaflets have a fish-mouth appearance.

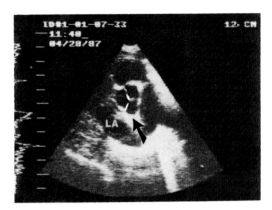

Figure 28.16. Right parasternal cross-sectional view at the level of the aortic root (*arrow*). The valve leaflets at this level give the characteristic appearance of the "Mercedes" logo. The left atrial (*LA*) cavity is below and to the left of the aortic root in this image (see Fig. 28.6*E*).

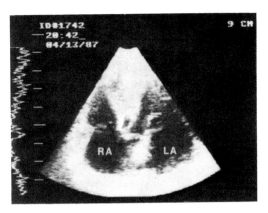

Figure 28.18. Left parasternal apical long-axis (four-chamber) view. This view optimizes the appearance of the right (*RA*) and left (*LA*) atria for measurement. The aorta is poorly seen on cross section between the four chambers of the heart at the level of the intercavitary septa.

Although voluntary expiration is the preferred phase of respiration for recording the echocardiogram in humans, the influence of the respiratory cycle in small animal echoes has not been studied adequately.

MEASURING THE CANINE AND FELINE ECHOCARDIOGRAM

Most echocardiographers recommend that M-mode measurements be performed in accordance with the American Society of Echocardiography (17). This has been adhered to generally in veterinary medicine. However, some recent studies used slightly varying analytic methods to determine these values (9).

M-mode tracings and two-dimensional images of most dogs and cats are quite reproducible. These recordings usually are better taken from the right side. In cats, views are taken occasionally in positions other than lateral recumbency due to restraint problems. Occasionally, the sternal position is used in cats.

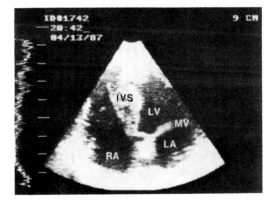

Figure 28.17. Left parasternal apical long-axis view. The mitral valve (*MV*) septal leaflet is seen well in the four-chamber view of the heart. *IVS* = interventricular septum, *LA* = left atrium, *LV* = left ventricle, *RA* = right atrium.

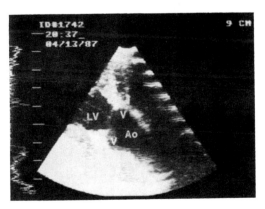

Figure 28.19. Left parasternal long-axis view. The left ventricular outflow tract, aortic valves, and Valsalva's sinuses (*V*) are seen in this view. *Ao* = aorta, *LV* = left ventricle.

For 2DE the error is usually less than 10% in repeat measurements on the same animal (4, 16). Body weight must be regarded critically in most linear measurements in dogs. Use of a mean population ± the standard deviation in cats was suggested by Pipers and Hamlin (18). Jacobs and Knight (9) examined 41 healthy normal cats and reported a significant correlation of measurements to body weight as well as a significant inverse relationship among heart rate and body weight, circumferential fiber shortening, and many right ventricular, left ventricular, and left atrial measurements. They concluded both body weight and heart rate influence echo measurements in the cat, and changes in one cardiac dimension may significantly affect other measurements.

A significant correlation has been demonstrated between long- and short-axis image plane measurements in both the dog and the cat. Human images should be obtained at the end of the respiratory period (17). However, no attempts have been made in veterinary medicine to identify the significance of varying measurements throughout the respiratory cycle. Most quantitative measurements described have been performed using the echoanalyzer activated on the screen from previously recorded video images.

In dogs with left atrial enlargement associated with mitral regurgitation, both electrocardiographic and echocardiographic enlargement are present. Radiographic indications of left atrial enlargement is not always supported by 2DE. This is thought to be due to overreading of the radiographic study. Left ventricular hypertrophy determined electrocardiographically could not be correlated with either radiographic or echocardiographic enlargement ratios. The left atrium-to-aorta echo ratio of 0.99 (range: 0.8–1.20) is very sensitive for the early recognition of left atrial enlargement (13).

Several studies in the dog, with both M-mode and 2DE used, related echo dimensions to body surface area. These studies demonstrated a linear relationship between increasing body size and increasing heart size. Correlations exist for all cardiac chamber dimensions, wall thicknesses, and amplitudes of motion studies (3, 12, 16). In these studies there were no differences between male and female subjects, and all dimensions from the left and right parasternal positions were nearly identical. However, internal measurements from M-mode studies are not interchangeable with those from 2DE unless an M-mode cursor is employed

(16). Nomograms for weight-related measurements in dogs were given by Boon et al. (3).

Left ventricular function, mitral valve motion velocities, and dimension ratios were not correlated to body surface area in any of the studies by Boon et al. (3). This was true of echoes in any size dog. Fractional shortening of the left ventricle was 39% ± 6%. Early in the study of echocardiography Dennis et al. (5) demonstrated a good correlation between the ejection fraction slope determined by transcutaneous echocardiography and that determined by esophageal echocardiography. However, a recent study by Fox (7) reported that no canine or feline studies correlated body surface area or weight to indices of ventricular performance.

M-mode echo was demonstrated to be a sensitive technique for documenting right ventricular dilation in heartworm-infected dogs. This correlated well with radiographic impressions of right ventricular enlargement. The ECG was not as specific as either radiographic or echocardiographic measurements (11).

Wingfield et al. (25) showed that there was abnormal mitral valve motion during diastole in all dogs with atrial fibrillation. Also, there was no evidence of atrial contraction. Left ventricular, interventricular septum, and posterior left ventricular wall contractility were decreased, suggesting congestive cardiomyopathy. Observed pulse deficits were explained by the lack of systolic or diastolic motion in the mitral and aortic valve leaflets in association with some of the QRS complexes.

Mass is constant throughout the cardiac cycle, unlike wall thickness and cavity volume. A study by Shiller et al. (21) showed that left ventricular weight at postmortem was very close to that determined through echocardiography. Wall thickness alone does not provide full information regarding left ventricular mass. In pericardial effusion, left ventricular wall thickness appears increased, yet the measurement is still normal. Conversely, in congestive cardiomyopathy, left ventricular hypertrophy may be severe but is masked by obligatory thinning of the left ventricular wall. Gooding et al. (8), in a study of ten clinically normal English cocker spaniel dogs, reported that left ventricular weight determined by M-mode images correlated significantly with autopsy determined weights.

M-mode and 2DE have detected changes in left ventricular wall thickness in experimentally induced renal hypertension. Both dogs and cats are afflicted with naturally occurring systemic hypertension and may benefit from ultrasound measurements and hypertension studies (15, 19).

Left ventricular volume is best determined by 2DE rather than by M-mode echo. Sector scanning provides accurate in vitro estimates of the canine left ventricle. The optimal sector scan views for left ventricular volume estimation are those providing maximal dimensional information and making the fewest assumptions about left ventricular geometry (20, 21).

There is close agreement between reported and reviewed echo values in cats (4, 7, 9, 18). Although 2DE is often performed, results are limited by resolution and near-field distortions. Cats often have 3 mm size walls; an error of 0.5 mm combined with a resolution error of 1 or 2 mm can cause serious measurement problems. Still, consistent and repeatable studies have demonstrated similar results for both M-mode and 2DE measurements.

Lower fractional shortening results observed in cats are attributed to the use of tranquilizers. Jacobs and Knight (10) studied left ventricular internal diameter, shortening fraction percentage, and the velocity of circumferential fiber shortening. These measurements were significantly decreased from baseline values after usual dosages of ketamine (3–5 mg/kg intramuscularly) were given to healthy cats: shortening fraction dropped from 49.90% to 40.60%. DeMadron et al. (4) suggested left atrial 2DE measurements in the cat are more accurate than those determined by M-mode. This may be because a true right-cranial to left-caudal measurement of the left atrium is made instead of the cranial left atrium or left auricle.

The cardiac dimensions of the normal cat vary over only a small range. Thus, some studies have not correlated body surface area with cardiac measurements. Clearly, from the work of Jacobs and Knight (9) and others, this consideration may require a revision in our method of analysis.

In a study by DeMadron et al. (4), aortic annulus and ventricular wall thickness were related to weight, while left ventricular and left atrial internal diameters were not. In this study, posterior wall thickness and fractional shortening determined by M-mode were closer to short-axis 2DE studies. M-mode results tended to be higher than those produced by 2DE. Long-axis measurements were more likely to give better results

when measuring the interventricular septum, left ventricular internal diameter, posterior left ventricular wall thickness, left atrial internal diameter, and aortic root size.

Feline hyperthyroidism is associated with a high incidence of echocardiographic abnormalities. Bond et al. (2) reported on 30 cats with this disease and noted left ventricular hypertrophy, aortic root and left atrial enlargement, and an increased shortening fraction (49.72%) when compared to a similar series of normal cats (41.0%). After cats were made euthyroid, either medically or surgically, the echocardiogram showed a decrease in left atrial size but not a consistent decrease in left ventricular wall thickness (14).

Normal M-mode and 2DE measurements (Tables 28.1–28.5) are available for the dog and the cat. The data for these tables have been taken from studies published by several authors during the past 3 years.

ACKNOWLEDGMENTS

This chapter was supported by the Berkeley Veterinary Research Foundation, Inc.

We wish to acknowledge the technical support of Mara Gottesman, B.S., A.H.T. in developing the technique and in the production of some of the echo studies used in this report. Drs. David Knight, David Sisson, and William Thomas provided helpful commentary in their reviews of this paper.

REFERENCES

1. Bonagura JD, Pipers FS: Diagnosis of cardiac lesions by contrast echocardiography. *J Am Vet Med Assoc* 182:396–401, 1983.
2. Bond BR, Fox PR, Peterson ME: Echocardiographic evaluation of 30 cats with hyperthyroidism. *Proc ACVIM* 39, 1983.
3. Boon J, Wingfield WE, Miller CW: Echocardiographic indices in the normal dog. *Vet Radiol* 24:214–221, 1983.
4. DeMadron E, Bonagura JD, Herring DS: Two-dimensional echocardiography in the normal cat. *Vet Radiol* 26:149–158, 1985.
5. Dennis MO, Nealeigh RC, Pyle RL, et al: Echocardiographic assessment of normal and abnormal valvular function in beagle dogs. *Am J Vet Res* 39:1591–1598, 1978.
6. Felner JM, Blumenstein BA, Schland RC, et al: Sources of variability in echocardiographic measurements. *Am J Cardiol* 45:995–999, 1980.
7. Fox P: Echocardiographic reference values in healthy cats sedated with ketamine HCl. *Am J Vet Res* 46:1479, 1985.
8. Gooding JP, Robinson WF, Mews GC: Echocardiographic assessment of left ventricular dimen-

sions in clinically normal English cocker spaniels. *Am J Vet Res* 47:296–302, 1986.

9. Jacobs G, Knight DH: M-mode echocardiographic measurements in nonanesthetized healthy cats: Effects of body weight, heart rate, and other variables. *Am J Vet Res* 46:1705–1711, 1985.

10. Jacobs G, Knight D: Change in M-mode echocardiographic values in cats given ketamine. *Am J Vet Res* 46:1712–1713, 1985.

11. Lombard CW, Ackerman N: Right heart enlargement in heartworm-infected dogs. *Vet Radiol* 25:210–217, 1984.

12. Lombard CW: Normal values of the canine M-mode echocardiogram. *Am J Vet Res* 45:2015–2018, 1984.

13. Lombard CW, Spencer CP: Correlation of radiographic, echocardiographic and electrocardiographic signs of left heart enlargement in dogs with mitral regurgitation. *Vet Radiol* 26:89–97, 1985.

14. Moise NS, Dietze AE: Echocardiographic, electrocardiographic and radiographic detection of cardiomegaly in hyperthyroid cats. *Am J Vet Res* 47:1487–1494, 1986.

15. Morioka S, Simon G: Echocardiographic evidence for early left ventricular hypertrophy in dogs with renal hypertension. *Am J Cardiol* 49:1892, 1982.

16. O'Grady MR, Bonagura JD, Powers JD, Herring DS: Quantitative cross-sectional echocardiography in the normal dog. *Vet Radiol* 27:34–49, 1986.

17. O'Rourke RA, Hanrath P, Henry WN, et al: Report of the Joint International Society and Federation of Cardiology/World Health Organization task force on recommendations for standardization of measurements from M-mode echocardiograms. *Circulation* 69:854A–857A, 1984.

18. Pipers FS, Hamlin RL: Clinical use of echocardiography in the domestic cat. *J Am Vet Med Assoc* 176:57–61, 1980.

19. Salcedo EE, Gockowski K, Tarazi RC: Left ventricular mass and wall thickness in hypertension. *Am J Cardiol* 44:939, 1979.

20. Schapira JN, Kohn MS, Beaver WL, Popp RL: In vitro quantitation of canine left ventricular volume by phased-array sector scan. *Cardiology* 67:1–11, 1981.

21. Schiller NB, Skioldebrand CG, Schiller EJ, et al: Canine left ventricular mass estimation by two-dimensional echocardiography. *Circulation* 68:210–216, 1983.

22. Thomas WP: Two-dimensional, real-time echocardiography in the dog. *Vet Radiol* 25:50–64, 1984.

23. Thomas WP, Sisson D, Bauer TG, Reed JR: Detection of cardiac masses in dogs by two-dimensional echocardiography. *Vet Radiol* 1984;25:65–72, 1984.

24. Wallerson DC, Devereux RB: Reproducibility of quantitative echocardiography. *Echocardiography* 3:219–235, 1986.

25. Wingfield WE, Boon J, Miller CW: Echocardiographic assessment of mitral valve motion, cardiac structures, and ventricular function in dogs with atrial fibrillation. *J Am Vet Med Assoc* 181:46–49, 1982.

Table 28.1. M-Mode Echocardiographic Measurements and Body Weight[a] Correlations in 40 Dogs[b]

Dimension (units)	Measurements		Correlation with Body Weight (r^2)	Significant Diff of Slope from Zero (P)
	Mean ± SD	Range		
LVIDd	39 ± 8	19–55	0.785	<0.0001
LVIDs	24 ± 6	9–36	0.729	<0.0001
RVIDd[a]	11 ± 3	5–17	0.440	<0.0001
ST	9 ± 2	5–13	0.445	<0.0001
LVWT	9 ± 2	7–14	0.689	<0.0001
LVW exc	10 ± 3	5–17	0.320	<0.0005
AOd	23 ± 4	13–29	0.748	<0.0001
AO exc	8 ± 2	3–13	0.496	<0.0001
LAs	22 ± 5	14–32	0.622	<0.0001
MV exc	14 ± 3	8–22	0.569	<0.0001
S exc	5 ± 2	2–9	0.125	<0.05
D (%)	39 ± 6	30–53	0.099	NS
LA/AO	0.99 ± 0.1	0.7–1.3	0.0006	NS
D–E slope (mm/sec)	403 ± 116	190–670	0.224	<0.005
E–F slope (mm/sec)	138 ± 51	60–255	0.033	NS
Heart rate (beats/min)	99 ± 19	60–145		

[a]Body weight (mean ± SD) = 24 ± 10 kg (range: 5–44 kg).
[b]Data are from Lombard CW: Normal values of the canine M-mode echocardiogram. *Am J Vet Res* 45:2015–2018, 1984.

Table 28.2. Two-Dimensional Echocardiographic Pooled Data for 17 Normal Dogs[a,b]

Parameter	Mean	SD	Minimum Value	Maximum Value
LV Length 1-D (mm)	61.04	10.97	35.60	76.40
LV Length 1-S (mm)	49.32	10.11	28.40	62.20
LV Length 2-D (mm)	60.45	10.73	35.20	75.40
LV Length 2-S (mm)	48.44	9.76	27.40	59.00
LV Length 3-D (mm)	58.16	10.82	31.40	75.60
LV Length 3-S (mm)	44.86	8.38	25.20	61.00
LA Right-Left LAx(RP) (mm)	32.24	5.65	21.40	47.80
LA Base-Apex LAx(RP) (mm)	27.92	4.99	17.80	38.20
LA Area LAx(RP) (cm^2)	9.75	3.14	3.68	16.92
IVS LAx-D(mm)	6.91	1.65	5.00	10.00
LV Dimension LAx-D (mm)	33.92	5.54	23.80	46.80
LVFW LAx-D (mm)	7.88	2.16	4.20	11.20
IVS LAx-S (mm)	10.08	2.43	6.60	14.80
LV Dimension LAx-S (mm)	24.64	4.79	17.80	37.00
LVFW LAx-S (mm)	10.85	2.25	6.40	14.20
Aorta-Annulus (RP) (mm)	13.71	2.22	8.40	18.80
Aorta-Sinuses (RP) (mm)	19.27	3.41	10.20	24.60
LV Area 1-Internal (cm^2)	9.17	2.67	4.90	15.02
LV Area 1-External (cm^2)	22.85	7.67	10.92	38.26
IVS Sax-D (mm)	8.26	1.97	5.60	12.00
LV Dimension Sax-D (mm)	34.55	5.60	24.20	46.00
LVFW Sax-D (mm)	8.01	2.32	4.40	11.00
IVS Sax-S (mm)	10.19	2.15	7.40	15.20
LV Dimension Sax-S (mm)	25.89	4.44	17.00	34.80
LVFW Sax-S (mm)	10.33	2.77	6.20	16.20
Mitral Area SAx (cm^2)	3.69	1.42	1.70	7.42
LV Area 2 (cm^2)	8.02	2.78	3.96	15.00
Aorta Area SAx(RP) (cm^2)	2.68	0.87	0.70	4.30
LV Length-D (LPA) (mm)	51.74	10.42	29.20	74.40
LV Length-S(LPA) (mm)	39.68	8.89	23.20	59.00
LA Base-Apex (LPA) (mm)	25.33	5.52	12.60	34.80
LA Medical-Lateral (LPA) (mm)	31.04	7.79	18.20	50.80
LA Area (LPA) (cm^2)	8.44	3.31	2.66	16.62
Aorta-Annulus (LP) (mm)	14.71	2.50	11.40	18.80
Aorta-Sinuses (LP) (mm)	20.76	2.92	16.40	26.60
Aorta-Ascending (LP) (mm)	14.42	2.19	11.40	17.80
Aorta Area (LP) (cm^2)	2.82	0.97	0.72	4.86
Weight-pounds	40.82	15.23	10.00	64.00
Weight-kilograms	18.52	6.91	4.54	29.03
Body Surface Area (m^2)	0.69	0.18	0.27	0.94
FS LAx (nu)	0.28	0.04	0.21	0.34
FS SAx (nu)	0.25	0.05	0.17	0.34
Stroke Volume 1 LAx (ml)	25.46	11.40	7.84	52.15
Stroke Volume 2 LAx (ml)	15.78	6.37	4.69	27.38
Stroke Volume 3 LAx (ml)	26.20	8.72	10.30	43.34
Stroke Volume 1 SAx (ml)	24.45	13.55	9.31	54.91
Stroke Volume 2 SAx (ml)	14.98	9.02	5.47	31.84
Stroke Volume 3 SAx (ml)	25.64	11.00	12.23	46.97
EF 1 LAx (nu)	0.61	0.06	0.50	0.71
EF 2 LAx (nu)	0.45	0.08	0.30	0.59
EF 3 LAx (nu)	0.54	0.06	0.42	0.64
EF 1 SAx (nu)	0.57	0.08	0.42	0.70
EF 2 SAx (nu)	0.39	0.12	0.19	0.58
EF 3 SAx (nu)	0.50	0.08	0.37	0.64
LA:Aorta (RP)	2.37	0.27	1.96	2.91
% thickening IVS LAx	0.50	0.23	0.22	0.92
% thickening IVS SAx	0.26	0.11	0.07	0.44

(*continued*)

Table 28.2. *(continued)*

Parameter	Mean	SD	Minimum Value	Maximum Value
% thickening LVFW LAx	0.41	0.15	0.15	0.73
% thickening LVFW SAx	0.31	0.12	0.09	0.52
IVS:LVFW LAx	0.91	0.17	0.60	1.30
IVS:LVFW SAx	1.07	0.20	0.75	1.45
Mitral Area SAx:LV Area 2	0.46	0.04	0.38	0.52

[a]Linear dimensions are reported in millimeters (mm), area dimensions in square centimeters (cm²), slopes in millimeters per sec (mm/sec), intervals in seconds (sec), and volumes in milliliters (ml). A number of parameters have no units (nu). LV = left ventricle; D = diastole; S = systole; RP = right parasternal position; LA = left atrium; IVS = interventricular septum; LVFW = left ventricular free wall; LAx = long-axis view; SAx = short-axis view; LP = left parasternal position; LPA = left parasternal apical position; FS = fractional shortening; EF = ejection fraction; LA:Aorta (RP) = left atrial dimension right-left LAx to aortic dimension at annulus; LV Length 1 = LV length per Figure 28.2 (line B); LV Length 2 = LV length per Figure 28.2 (line A); LV Length 3 = LV length per Figure 28.1; LV Area 1 = measured at LV papillary level; LV Area 2 = measured at LV mitral level; Stroke Volume 1, EF 1 = using cube formula; Stroke Volume 2, EF 2 = using Mashiro's formula; Stroke Volume 3, EF 3 = using Teichholz's formula.
[b]Data are from O'Grady MR, et al: Quantitative cross-sectional echocardiography in the normal dog. *Vet Radiol* 27:34–49, 1986.

Table 28.3. Values for Quantitative 2DE in the Cat[a]

Parameter	Awake (n = 7)		Sedated (n = 6)		Pooled (n = 13)		Correlation with Body Weight (r)	P Value
AOR SIN	9.0	(1.18)	10.3	(0.95)	9.6	(1.24)	0.39	NS
LA	12.1	(1.01)	12.0	(0.51)	12.1	(0.92)	0.37	NS
AOR ANN	7.5	(0.75)	8.1	(0.53)	7.7	(0.74)	0.52	<0.01
AOR AREA	0.7	(0.16)	0.8	(0.07)	0.7	(0.15)	0.62	<0.05
IVSD SAX	3.6	(0.60)	5.0	(0.46)	3.9	(0.83)	0.70	<0.001
IVSS SAX	5.6	(0.67)	6.9	(0.42)	5.9	(0.82)	0.67	<0.001
LVIDD SAX	13.7	(1.49)	12.9	(0.58)	13.5	(1.38)	0.10	NS
LVIDS SAX	8.2	(1.58)	9.0	(0.72)	8.4	(1.46)	0.06	NS
LVWD SAX	3.2	(0.44)	4.6	(0.36)	3.5	(0.71)	0.64	<0.05
LVWS SAX	5.2	(0.70)	6.4	(0.56)	5.5	(0.83)	0.84	<0.001
IVSD LAX	3.4	(0.51)	4.0	(0.31)	3.6	(0.52)	0.50	<0.01
IVSS LAX	5.6	(0.51)	6.4	(0.29)	5.8	(0.58)	0.65	<0.01
LVIDD LAX	12.6	(1.16)	12.7	(0.34)	12.6	(1.04)	0.09	NS
LVIDS LAX	7.7	(1.59)	8.8	(0.72)	8.0	(1.49)	0.23	NS
LVWD LAX	3.6	(0.50)	4.0	(0.28)	3.7	(0.49)	0.60	<0.001
LVWS LAX	6.0	(0.55)	6.5	(0.40)	6.1	(0.55)	0.37	NS
WEIGHT (KG)	3.2	(0.64)	5.0	(1.02)	3.6	(1.05)	1.00	
FS$_1$ SAX	0.40	(0.08)	0.30	(0.05)	0.38	(0.09)	0.06	NS
FS$_2$ LAX	0.39	(0.10)	0.31	(0.07)	0.37	(0.10)	0.23	NS
LA-MM	11.0	(0.82)	10.8	(1.30)	10.9	(1.00)	0.39	NS
AO-MM	7.9	(0.38)	8.6	(0.89)	8.2	(0.72)	0.85	<0.001
IVS-D-MM	3.7	(0.49)	4.8	(0.45)	4.2	(0.72)	0.71	<0.01
IVS-S-MM	6.4	(0.53)	7.7	(0.45)	7.0	(0.81)	0.80	<0.001
LVID-D-MM	13.6	(1.27)	13.1	(0.74)	13.4	(1.07)	0.00	NS
LVID-S-MM	8.6	(0.98)	8.4	(0.55)	8.5	(0.80)	0.05	NS
LVW-D-MM	3.6	(0.53)	4.5	(0.50)	4.0	(0.69)	0.62	<0.05
LVW-S-MM	5.6	(0.53)	6.8	(0.45)	6.1	(0.79)	0.83	<0.001
FS$_3$-MM	0.37	(0.06)	0.36	(0.03)	0.36	(0.05)	0.06	NS
HR	188.6	(30)	205	(29.5)	196.1	(29.9)		

[a]Data are from DeMadron E, et al: Two-dimensional echocardiography in the normal cat. *Vet Radiol* 26:149–158, 1985.

Table 28.4. Feline M-Mode Echocardiographic Data Population Means, SD, and Estimated Acceptable Limits on 21 Variables for 30 Randomly Selected Healthy Cats[a]

Variable	Mean	SD
BW (kg)	4.11	1.05
HR (beats/min)	194.00	23.25
STS (cm)	0.58	0.06
STD (cm)	0.31	0.04
LVID$_s$ (cm)	0.80	0.14
LVIDd (cm)	1.59	0.19
PWS (cm)	0.68	0.07
PWD (cm)	0.33	0.06
LA (cm)	1.23	0.14
AO (cm)	0.95	0.11
LA/AO	1.30	0.17
LVET (s)	0.14	0.02
SF (%)	49.80	5.27
Vcf (cm/s)	3.65	0.63
EPSS (cm)	0.02	0.09
RVID$_s$ (cm)	0.33	0.17
RVID$_d$ (cm)	0.60	0.15
RWS (cm)	0.33	0.04
DESLP (mm/s)	232.70	77.38
EFSLP (mm/s)	87.23	25.99
DEXC (mm)	3.87	0.48

[a]Data are from Jacobs G, Knight DH: M-mode echocardiographic measurements in nonanesthetized healthy cats: Effects of body weight, heart rate, and other variables. *Am J. Vet Res* 46:1705–1711, 1985.

Table 28.5. M-Mode Eachocardiographic Mensurals of 30 Healthy Cats Lightly Sedated with Ketamine Hydrochloride[a]

Value	X	SD	Range	Coefficient of Variation
Ao EDD (cm)	0.94	0.11	0.71–1.15	11.73
LA (cm)	1.03	0.14	0.72–1.33	13.20
LA/Ao	1.10	0.18	1.07–1.73	16.47
LVEDD (cm)	1.40	0.13	0.49–1.16	9.52
LVESD (cm)	0.81	0.16		19.57
LVCW (cm)	0.35	0.05	0.21–0.45	14.85
IVS (cm)	0.36	0.08	0.22–0.49	21.04
IVS/LVCW	1.03	0.18	0.69–1.42	17.85
RV (cm)	0.50	0.21	0.12–0.75	46.56
PEP (s)	0.044	0.009	0.024–0.058	21.81
LVET$_1$	0.118	0.118	0.093–0.176	15.26
LVET$_2$	0.116	0.011	0.100–0.132	9.14
PEP/LVET	0.379	0.077	0.228–0.513	20.37
% D	42.72	8.05	30.00–60.00	18.85
Vcf$_1$ (s-1)	3.68	0.87	2.27–5.17	23.74
Vcf$_2$ (s-1)	3.50	0.84	2.44–5.00	23.94
HR (bpm)	245.3	35.60	160.00–300.00	14.51
Age (yr)	3.36	3.15	0.58–15.00	—
Weight (kg)	3.88	1.17	2.05–6.80	30.22
BSA (m^2)	0.23	0.05	0.15–0.34	20.16

[a]Data from Fox P: Echocardiographic reference values in healthy cats studied with ketamine HCl. *Am J Vet Res* 46:1479, 1985.

SELECTED CLINICAL EXAMPLES

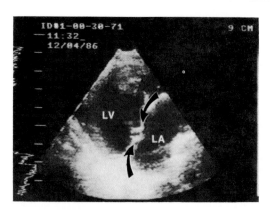

Figure 28.20. Mitral valvular fibrosis. The *black arrows* indicate thickened mitral valve leaflets in this dog. The closed valves are insufficient, and there is a space between the tips of the shriveled and thickened valve leaflets, resulting in mitral regurgitation and a dilated left atrium (*LA*). *LV* = left ventricle.

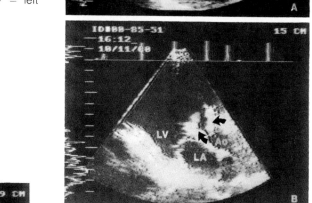

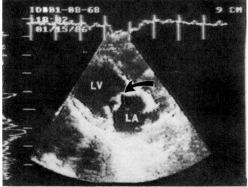

Figure 28.21. Flail mitral valve. In dogs with chronic valvular fibrosis, the septal leaflet (*arrow*) of the mitral valve is usually thicker than the posterior leaflet. The septal leaflet is flailed and protrudes into the left atrium during systole. *LA* = left atrium, *LV* = left ventricle.

Figure 28.22. Valvular vegetations and insufficiency. *A*, The septal leaflet (*arrow*) of the mitral valve is thickened and insufficient in mitral valvular bacterial endocarditis. Fever, cough, and heart failure are presenting clinical signs. *B*, The entire aortic valve is thickened, disfigured, and insufficient (*arrows*) in aortic valve vegetative endocarditis. The dog presents with a waterhammer pulse and signs of heart failure. *Ao* = aorta, *LA* = left atrium, *LV* = left ventricle.

SELECTED CLINICAL EXAMPLES (cont.)

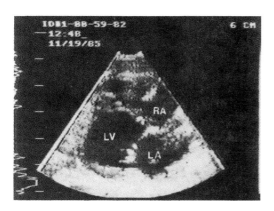

Figure 28.23. Mitral valve annular disease. This dog has chronic fibrosis of the mitral leaflets. There is thickening of the leaflets and also generalized left ventricular dilation, resulting in annular dilation and further insufficiency of the valve, resulting in dilation of the left atrium (*LA*). *LV* = left ventricle, *RA* = right atrium.

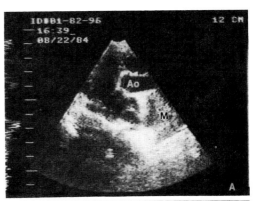

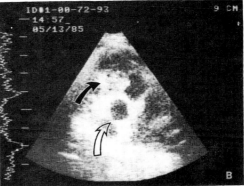

Figure 28.25. *A*, The mass (*M*) in this dog with an aortic body or heart base tumor lies physically above and around the aorta (*Ao*) in the right parasternal position. *B*, In another dog on cross-sectional view the mass (*black arrow*) lies physically below the aorta (*open arrow*).

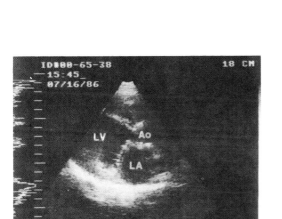

Figure 28.24. Subvalvular aortic stenosis—congenital. Dogs with this lesion are difficult to differentiate from those with valvular disease. The echocardiogram demonstrates narrowing of the sub-aortic region with post-stenotic dilation of the aorta beyond the stenosis.

SELECTED CLINICAL EXAMPLES (cont.)

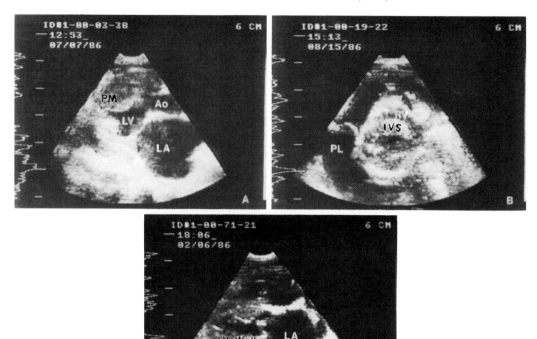

Figure 28.26. Hypertrophic cardiomyopathy. *A,* The papillary muscles (*PM*) are thickened and reduce the size of the left ventricular cavity (*LV*) and the aorta (*Ao*) in this cat. There is marked dilation of the left atrium (*LA*) as a result of disease. *B,* Pleural effusion (*PL*) and thickening of the interventricular septum (*IVS*) are observed on the cross-sectional view of this cat.

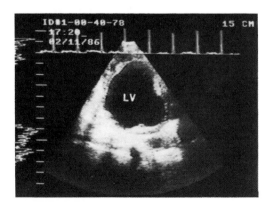

Figure 28.27. Massive dilation of the left ventricular cavity is typical of congestive cardiomyopathy in giant breeds of dogs. Shortening fractions in these dogs are decreased markedly.

SELECTED CLINICAL EXAMPLES (cont.)

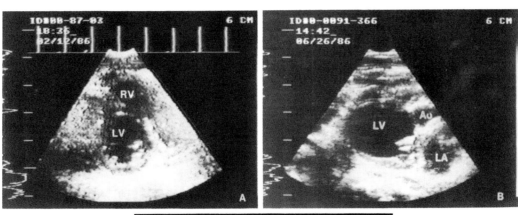

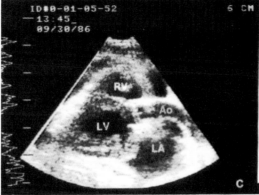

Figure 28.28. *A*, Dilation of both left ventricular (*LV*) and right ventricular (*RV*) cavities seen on a cross-sectional view typifies congestive cardiomyopathy in the cat. *B* and *C*, In this right parasternal view, generalized dilation of all cardiac chambers as well as the aortic arch is seen.

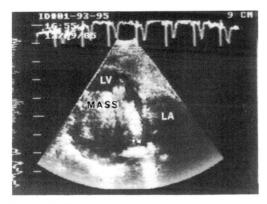

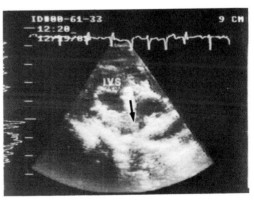

Figure 28.29. A mass invading the left ventricular muscle in this dog was determined to be a leiomyosarcoma. The mass is obliterating the ventricular cavity (*LV*) due to its continued growth and pressure on the heart. *LA* = left atrium.

Figure 28.30. Following an accidental shooting, this dog presented with a slow heart rate and syncope. An air pellet was found lodged in the interventricular septum (*IVS*), and the tractor beam from the pellet is seen (*arrow*). The rythm was a stable right bundle-branch block. Surgical removal was not required, and the dog has continued to thrive posttrauma.

SELECTED CLINICAL EXAMPLES (cont.)

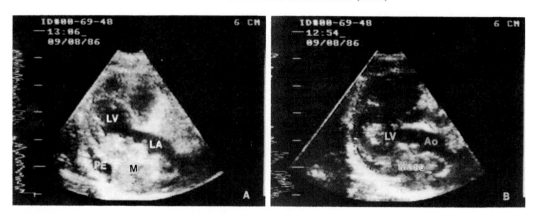

Figure 28.31. *A* and *B*, Views of a cat with signs of heart failure demonstrate a mass obstructing the left atrium (*LA*) and left ventricle (*LV*). Pericardial fluid (*PE*) is present. The mass (*M*) was histologically a carcinoid tumor. *Ao* = aorta.

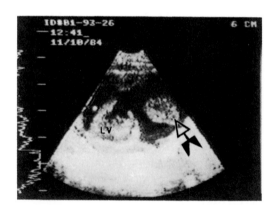

Figure 28.32. Cats with cardiomyopathy occasionally present with large ball thrombi in the left atrium (*arrow*) as noted in this view. These masses are particularly dangerous because embolic phenomena usually develop during the course of the disease. *LV* = left ventricle.

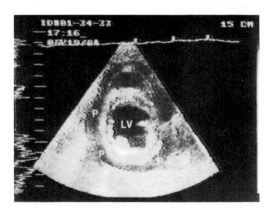

Figure 28.33. Benign pericardial effusion in the dog is one of the causes of effusion in middle- to older-aged dogs. The fluid (*PE*) usually is a port wine color and must be differentiated from hemangiomas affecting the heart. *LV* = left ventricle.

SELECTED CLINICAL EXAMPLES (cont.)

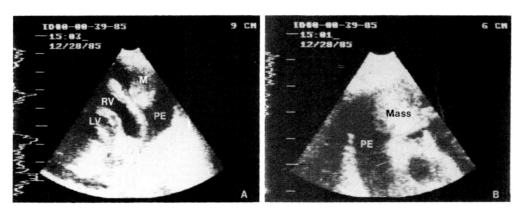

Figure 28.34. Right atrial neoplasm. *A,* Left (*LV*) and right ventricular (*RV*) cavities are shown surrounded by pericardial effusion (*PE*). Within the pericardial sac and extending from the right atrium is a pedunculated tumor (*M*). *B,* On closer view, the mass is a mixed hyper-hypoechoic structure. On cut section it is a dense tissue mass with blood-filled cystic areas. The histopathology showed a malignant hemangiosarcoma of the right atrium, a fairly common neoplasm of the right atrium, spleen, and liver.

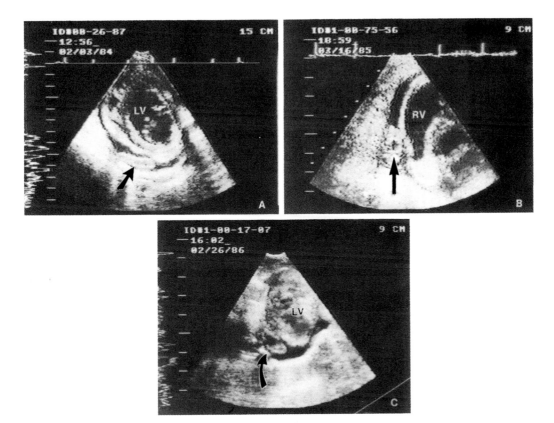

Figure 28.35. Pericardial tumor. Adenocarcinoma of the pericardial space is less frequent in the dog than either hemangioma or benign pericardial effusion. A discrete nodule (*arrow*) in the pericardial space is beside the left ventricle (*LV*) (*A*) and the right ventricle (*RV*) (*B*) in two dogs.

SELECTED CLINICAL EXAMPLES (cont.)

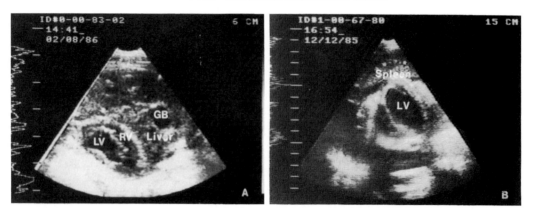

Figure 28.36. Congenital diaphragmatic pericardial-peritoneal hernia in a cat (*A*) and dog (*B*). In the cat, the liver and gallbladder (*GB*) are seen resting against the right ventricular wall (*RV*). The dog's window demonstrates the spleen within the pericardial sac lying against the left ventricular wall (*LV*).

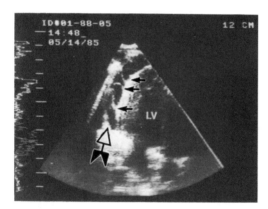

Figure 28.37. Pericarditis with fibrin strands in a chimpanzee. This primate presented with pericardial effusion, which was drained and treated. She returned several months later with a recurrence of the problem, this time with fibrin strands within the pericardial space (*arrows*). The condition eventually cleared without surgery and was thought to be a viral pericarditis.

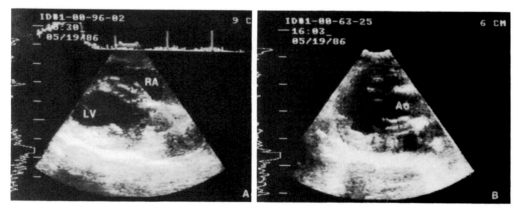

Figure 28.38. *A* and *B*, Patent ductus arteriosus in a dog. This condition is usually not seen but rather is diagnosed on the basis of clinical, radiographic, and electrocardiographic signs. The echocardiogram rarely shows the ductus but does reveal a dilated left ventricle (*LV*) with good contractility and a widely dilated aortic arch (*Ao*) far out of proportion to the normal size of the aorta. *RA* = right atrium.

SELECTED CLINICAL EXAMPLES (cont.)

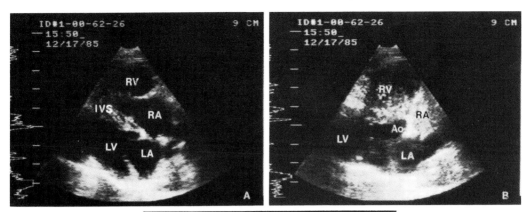

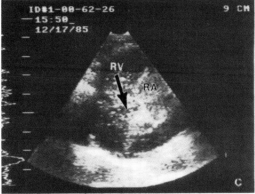

Figure 28.39. Fallot's tetralogy in a young dog with signs of exercise intolerance and cyanosis. There was a right ventricular hypertrophic pattern on the ECG and a thick right ventricle (*RV*) with undercirculation radiographically. The ultrasound examination showed a thick interventricular septum (*IVS*) and a thickened right ventricular wall (*A*). When bubbles of Renografin (Squibb) and saline were injected into the right atrium (*RA*) in *B*, the right atrium and right ventricle immediately opacified. *C*, The dye crossed the IVS into the LV cavity (*arrow*). Ao = aorta, *LA* = left atrium, *LV* = left ventricle.

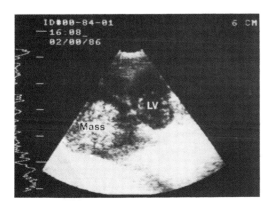

Figure 28.40. Cranial mediastinal mass in a cat. The thickened homogeneous mass cranial to the heart was seen both on radiographic and ultrasound examination of the thorax. The mass was a solid, dense lesion that, on aspiration, revealed abnormal lymphocytes diagnostic of lymphosarcoma. Treatment is often successful for a brief period in reducing the size of the tumor. *LV* = left ventricle.

29

Doppler Echocardiography in Small Animals

David H. Knight, D.V.M.

Doppler echocardiography with spectral frequency analysis has become available only recently in veterinary medicine. For the time being, Doppler expertise in the veterinary field will be limited primarily to university-based, veterinary teaching hospitals, where its valuable clinical, teaching, and research applications can be developed.

The potential of cardiac Doppler to provide an efficient way to perform a hemodynamic assessment in animals represents a major clinical advance for veterinary cardiologists. Although important, this kind of information often was not available in the past because the time commitment, potential risks to the patient and expense of cardiac catherization could not be justified. The utility of performing noninvasive, nonstressful, hemodynamic measurements by cardiac Doppler is similar both for small domestic animals and for humans. In fact, it appears that much of the human experience is transferable to animals.

Experiments in dogs have validated many clinical applications, including calculation of volume flow (1–6), pressure gradients (7–9), ventricular performance (10–12), and detection of valve regurgitation (13). However, with few exceptions (1, 9), these studies have been performed in open-chest dogs. Consequently, at this early stage of veterinary application, reference values for Doppler measurements in normal, intact animals have not been published, although data is being compiled independently by several investigators. For now, human reference values for blood flow velocity through valve orifices appear to be good approximations (14), but may be lower than actual values in dogs and cats. If reference values for species such as the dog are to be useful, adjustments for the large, breed differences in body size will have to be made. Despite the pressing need, this information is likely to be accumulated slowly because technically satisfactory examinations are much more difficult to obtain from animals with normal-sized hearts. For this reason and because of the importance of aligning the Doppler beam with the direction of blood flow, most experimental animal work has been done through an open chest.

TECHNICAL CONSIDERATIONS

Transducers

Examination of small domestic animals can be likened to human pediatric practice. Even grossly enlarged cat hearts can be imaged at a depth of 4–8 cm, and the hearts of all but the giant breed dogs can be imaged within 16 cm. Sample volume placement actually is considerably closer to the transducer, even when interrogating from the left apex. Consequently, the physiologic range of blood flow velocities in cats and most dogs is usually within the capabilities of 5–3.5 MHz pulse wave transducers. For dogs weighing over 50 kg, measurement of flow velocity in the physiologic range may require lower frequency Doppler transducers. Dense fur between the chest wall and the transducer does not appreciably affect signal quality so long as the area is saturated with ultrasound couplant. Rib spaces, particularly in cats, are narrow. Therefore, it is an advantage to have transducers with small contact surfaces, and it may be necessary to apply firm pressure.

Restraint and Patient Positioning

With few exceptions, dogs and cats can be immobilized adequately in lateral recumbency by an experienced holder without resorting to the use of chemical restraint. Since the Doppler examination usually is performed from both sides of the chest, it is necessary to reposition patients during the course of a study. In animals with enlarged hearts or pleural effusion, the acoustic window along both right and left parasternal borders is ample, and quality signals can be obtained with the transducers directed from the upper, exposed side. However, in some normal animals, more lung is interposed between the chest wall and the heart, degrading the quality of the examination. In these instances, better results may be obtained by directing the transducer from the underside through a cutout in the top of the examination table. In general, this approach has been more useful in improving image quality than in optimizing Doppler signals.

Windows of Interrogation

Due to the relatively deep, narrow chest conformation of dogs and cats, the cardiac apex tends to lie directly behind the sternum rather than to the left, as in the human. Nevertheless, the most readily accessible acoustic windows for Doppler interrogation are similar to those used for humans. The right parasternal and left apical views provide the best access. As in humans, the right ventricular outflow tract and main pulmonary artery can be visualized from the short-axis, right parasternal projection. The angle between the Doppler beam and the pulmonary trunk is usually much less than 20°. By slightly elevating the sector plane, the left branch of the pulmonary artery is brought into view, and the pulsed Doppler sample volume can be placed in the vicinity of the pulmonary orifice of a patent ductus arteriosus. At the level of the cross section through the aortic root, the interatrial septum is in a good position to be visualized and probed with the Doppler beam.

In the right parasternal long-axis view, both the atrial septum and ventricular septum lie nearly perpendicular to the echo beam. Consequently, this is an excellent view to visualize septal defects and position the Doppler beam to detect the presence of shunts. Both atrioventricular valves can be visualized from this position, but the Doppler beam cannot be aligned satisfactorily to measure peak blood velocity through the orifices of these valves accurately. However, this view still can be very useful for detecting regurgitant jets behind both valves. By directing the transducer slightly craniad of the right parasternal four-chamber projection, the left ventricular outflow tract and

ascending aorta are intersected. Because the angle of interrogation can be quite wide, flow velocity measurements in these locations ordinarily are not attempted from this approach.

From the left apical view, the Doppler beam can be pointed directly into the orifice of the mitral and aortic valves and at a shallow angle through the tricuspid valve. This is the most satisfactory approach to these three valves and the left ventricular outflow tract. Because the Doppler beam in the left apical four-chamber view is parallel to the atrial and ventricular septa, alignment with the flow velocity vector of an atrial or a ventricular septal defect is poor. By moving the transducer craniad along the left sternal border, it may be possible to visualize the right ventricular outflow tract and main pulmonary artery. For Doppler examinations, generally this has not provided better access to these locations than the right parasternal short-axis approach, when cardiac anatomy is normal. However, in some dogs with severely hypertrophied right ventricles, the heart becomes rotated in such a way that the right ventricular outflow tract can be interrogated more effectively from the anterior left parasternal approach.

Neither the subcostal nor suprasternal approaches seem to work well in unanesthetized dogs and cats. The high-domed, deeply recessed diaphragm greatly increases the distance between the heart and the transducer in the subcostal position. Furthermore, animals tend to resist maneuvers with the transducer at these positions.

In dogs, it is possible to measure velocity in the ascending aorta from the thoracic inlet. This is facilitated by using an angulated, nonimaging, continuous wave transducer. However, in our experience, this approach is much more difficult and usually yields lower peak flow velocities than measurements made at the aortic valve from the left apex. The limitations of the suprasternal approach in animals are similar to those encountered in humans (6).

Clinical Applications

The range of applications for Doppler echocardiography in animals parallels that in humans, but clinical experience is limited at present. The ability to determine the pressure gradient accurately across a discrete, subaortic stenosis in dogs with a hereditary form of this condition has been demonstrated (9). To date, this is the only published report documenting the clinical utility of Doppler echocardiography in a naturally occurring cardiac disease of animals. However, this successful demonstration is only one example of many practical uses that are now being evaluated.

Stenosis of the pulmonary valve, sometimes accompanied by hypertrophic narrowing of the right ventricular outflow tract, is one of the most common cardiac anomalies in dogs. As with subaortic stenosis, cardiac Doppler has been useful in assessing severity of the obstruction. Although a

functional diagnosis usually can be made, it may be impossible to calculate a valid pressure gradient in some severe cases (Fig. 29.1). This is because cardiac chamber enlargement often repositions the right ventricular outflow tract, making it less accessible to Doppler interrogation.

Doppler ultrasound has proved to be a very sensitive method for identifying valve incompetence. Chronic valvular disease (endocardiosis)

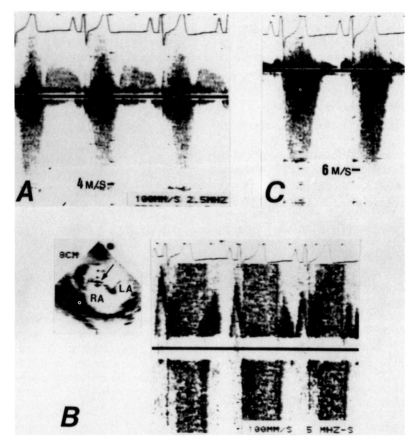

Figure 29.1. Recordings from a 4-month-old, 17 lb, mixed breed dog with congenital stenosis and regurgitation of the pulmonary valve and tricuspid regurgitation secondary to right ventricular enlargement. *A*, From the right parasternal border, a recording in the continuous wave Doppler mode shows high systolic flow velocity in the region of the right ventricular outflow tract and pulmonary artery. The indistinct border and bidirectional quality of the signal indicate that the beam does not pass through the stenotic jet at a satisfactory angle. However, from this location, a weak signal of pulmonary regurgitation was seen. No diastolic murmur was audible. *B*, A pulsed Doppler recording from the left apex, with the sample volume (*arrow*), immediately behind the tricuspid valve, documented regurgitant flow with aliasing. The right ventricular inflow velocity following atrial systole was higher than in early diastole, consistent with diminished diastolic ventricular compliance. *C*, From the same transducer location, a tricuspid regurgitant peak flow velocity of 5.6 m/sec was recorded in the continuous mode. The calculated gradient of 125 mm/ Hg gives a better indication of the severity of this dog's outflow tract obstruction than could be determined from the Doppler recording at the obstruction (*A*). Timing markers at 200 msec intervals, 8 cm scanning depth. *RA* = right atrium, *LA* = left atrium.

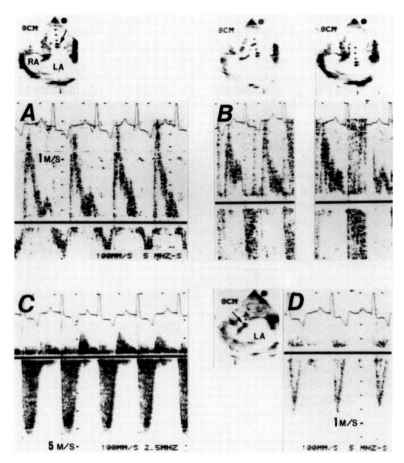

Figure 29.2. Chronic mitral valve endocardiosis with regurgitation in a 10 lb, 10-year-old male miniature poodle. *A*, From the left apex, the sample volume was positioned at the tip of the open mitral valve. The early left ventricular peak inflow velocity was high (1.6 m/sec), consistent with elevated filling pressure and a compliant ventricle. A small A-wave was present during filling cycles greater than 400 msec but became superimposed upon the early passive inflow at higher heart rates. Mitral stenosis is not a feature of this disease. The signal below the zero baseline was caused by systolic flow in the left ventricular outflow tract. *B*, Regurgitant flow was detected with the sample volume placed at the mitral orifice and could be tracked into the atrium for a considerable distance. *C*, In a continuous wave recording from the left apex, the signal from the peak regurgitant flow velocity (4.4 m/sec) was weak. The velocity may have been underestimated because of Doppler beam orientation. Low arterial blood pressure and elevated left atrial pressure may also have contributed to the low peak flow velocity. Although this dog's valvular incompetence was severe, the velocity profile of the regurgitant jet did not indicate a high, pressure V wave in the left atrium, probably because the volume of the atrium was large relative to the regurgitant volume. *D*, Aortic flow velocity measured with the sample volume (*arrow*) at the valve. Peak flow velocity (80 cm/sec) was in the low range of normal. At this heart rate, the left ventricular ejection time (95 msec) was greatly reduced. This dog's low stroke output is consistent with its severe degree of mitral regurgitation. Timing markers at 200 msec intervals, 8 cm scanning depth. *RA* = right atrium, *LA* = left atrium.

causing mitral regurgitation is the major acquired cardiac disease in dogs. A large proportion of dogs with mitral valve disease also have some involvement of the tricuspid valve. The murmur of mitral regurgitation projects to both left and right precordia, making it difficult to determine by auscultation if the tricuspid valve is also incompetent.

Pulse wave Doppler with imaging has been a useful way for separate identification of right and left atrioventricular (A-V) regurgitation. Most cases of tricuspid regurgitation caused by endocardiosis of the valve or cardiac dilatation appear to be functionally minor, since the regurgitant jet can only be found immediately behind the valve. On the other hand, the regurgitant jet caused by mitral endocardiosis ordinarily can be tracked at much greater distances into the left atrium (Fig. 29.2). The major component of the mitral jet usually is directed toward the posterior wall of the left atrium. Although mitral regurgitation is localized readily with the broad beam of the continuous wave transducer, alignment with the peak flow velocity vector can be difficult, accounting for the fact that velocities of 3.5–4.5 m/sec are commonly recorded and probably underestimate the true A-V pressure differential (Fig. 29.2). A clinically useful approximation of right ventricular systolic pressure can be obtained in cases with tricuspid regurgitation by measuring peak regurgitant flow velocity (Fig. 29.1).

The sensitivity of Doppler ultrasound also has made it possible to detect subclinical incompetence of all four cardiac valves. In dogs with idiopathic dilated cardiomyopathy, murmurs are frequently inaudible, despite modest degrees of mitral regurgitation. Similarly, nearly every consequential case of either subaortic or pulmonic valvular stenosis is accompanied by a small degree of regurgitation from the corresponding valve (Fig. 29.1).

Small membranous ventricular septal defects with left-to-right shunting frequently can be identified by cardiac Doppler when visualization by two-dimensional echocardiography is ambiguous. Most cases of atrial septal defect with left-to-right shunting in dogs are benign and therefore are often either unsuspected or unconfirmed. Now, with the aid of combined two-dimensional imaging and Doppler echocardiography, this defect is being recognized more often.

One application of Doppler ultrasound that may be particularly useful in the clinical evaluation of animals is the noninvasive assessment of acute, cardiac responses to drug therapy. The close correspondence between the aortic flow velocity integral and stroke volume on a beat-to-beat basis has been documented in open-chest dogs (10). The clinical utility of using the flow velocity integral to monitor acute changes in relative stroke volume has been demonstrated in humans (15).

In the clinical setting, objective and quantitative evaluation of cardiovascular responses in unanesthetized animals is handicapped by the difficulty of obtaining essential measurements that require either invasive procedures or a greater degree of patient cooperation than can be achieved. However, Doppler studies are still feasible in unanesthetized animals and are particularly suited to serial observations. Use of the aortic flow velocity integral has worked well for assessing the acute effects of sodium nitroprusside, captopril, and milrinone in dogs. Changes in stroke output can be determined in dogs with congestive heart failure and either mitral regurgitation or primary dilated cardiomyopathy. The aortic flow velocity curve is also a more convenient and dependable way to obtain systolic time intervals than is either the M-mode measurement of aortic valve motion or the classical phonocardiogram-arterial pressure pulse method.

REFERENCES

1. Darsee JR, Mikolich JR, Walter PF, Schlant RC: Transcutaneous method of measuring Doppler cardiac output: I. *Am J Cardiol* 46:607–612, 1980.
2. Fisher DC, Sahn DJ, Friedman MJ, Larson D, Valdes-Cruz LM, Horowitz S, Goldberg SJ, Allen HD: The effect of variations on pulsed Doppler sampling site on calculation of cardiac output: An experimental study in open-chest dogs. *Circulation* 67:370–376, 1983.
3. Meijboom EJ, Valdes-Cruz LM, Horowitz S, Sahn DJ, Larson DF, Young KA, Lima CO, Goldberg SJ, Allen HD: A two-dimensional Doppler echocardiographic method for calculation of pulmonary and systemic blood flow in a canine model with a variable-sized left-to-right extracardiac shunt. *Circulation* 68:437–445, 1983.
4. Valdes-Cruz LM, Horowitz S, Mesel E, Sahn DJ, Fisher DC, Larson D: A pulsed Doppler echocardiographic method for calculating pulmonary and systemic blood flow in atrial level shunts: Validation studies in animals and initial human experience. *Circulation* 69:80–86, 1984.
5. Meijboom EJ, Horowitz S, Valdes-Cruz LM, Sahn DJ, Larson DF, Lima CO: A Doppler echocardiographic method for calculating volume flow across the tricuspid valve: Correlative laboratory and clinical studies. *Circulation* 71:551–556, 1985.
6. Stewart WJ, Jiang L, Mich R, Pandian N, Guerrero JL, Weyman AE: Variable effects of changes in flow rate through the aortic, pulmonary and mitral valves on valve area and flow velocity: Impact on quantitative Doppler flow calculations. *J Am Coll Cardiol* 6:653–662, 1985.
7. Valdes-Cruz LM, Horowitz S, Sahn DJ, Larson D, Lima CO, Mesel E: Validation of a Doppler echocardiographic method for calculating severity of discrete stenotic obstructions in a canine preparation with a pulmonary arterial band. *Circulation* 69:1177–1181, 1984.
8. Smith MD, Dawson PL, Elion JL, Booth DC, Handshoe R, Kwan OL, Earle GF, DeMaria AN:

Correlation of continuous wave Doppler velocities with cardiac catheterization gradients: An experimental model of aortic stenosis. *J Am Coll Cardiol* 6:1306–1314, 1985.

9. Valdes-Cruz LM, Jones M, Scagnelli S, Sahn DJ, Tomizuka FM, Pierce JE: Prediction of gradients in fibrous subaortic stenosis by continuous wave two-dimensional Doppler echocardiography: Animal studies. *J Am Coll Cardiol* 5:1363–1367, 1985.

10. Steingart RM, Meller J, Barovick J, Patterson R, Herman MV, Teichholz LE: Pulsed Doppler echocardiographic measurement of beat-to-beat changes in stroke volume in dogs. *Circulation* 62:542–548, 1980.

11. Wallmeyer K, Wann LS, Sagar KB, Kalbfleisch J, Klopfenstein HS: The influence of preload and heart rate on Doppler echocardiographic indexes of left

ventricular performance: Comparison with invasive indexes in an experimental preparation. *Circulation* 74:181–186, 1986.

12. Colacousis JS, Huntsman LL, Cuneri PW: Estimation of stroke volume changes by ultrasonic Doppler. *Circulation* 56:914–917, 1977.

13. Waggoner AD, Quinones MA, Young JB, Brandon TA, Shah AA, Verani MS, Miller RR: Pulsed Doppler echocardiographic detection of right-sided valve regurgitation. *Am J Cardiol* 47:279–286, 1981.

14. Hatle L, Angelsen B: *Doppler Ultrasound in Cardiology*, 2nd ed. Philadelphia, Lea & Febiger, 1985.

15. Elkayam U, Gardin JM, Berkley R, Hughes CA, Henry WL: The use of Doppler flow velocity measurement to assess the hemodynamic response to vasodilators in patients with heart failure. *Circulation* 67:377–382, 1983.

30

Biologic Effects of Diagnostic Ultrasound

Frank G. Shellock, Ph.D.

INTRODUCTION

The widespread use of ultrasound in diagnostic medicine is a testament to its perceived safety, especially compared to imaging techniques that require ionizing radiation. Although there has never been any report of adverse effects caused by the clinical application of ultrasound (2, 20, 26, 30, 37, 39, 40, 43), the data concerning biologic effects are not sufficient to assume absolute safety.

Potential health hazards associated with ultrasound are currently receiving much attention from the United States Food and Drug Administration (FDA) (22), professional groups, and manufacturers of ultrasound equipment. This interest is largely due to the fact that new ultrasound devices tend to have higher energy outputs and ultimately will require regulatory labeling.

This chapter describes what is presently known about the mechanisms underlying the biologic effects of diagnostic ultrasound. The specific intent is to examine clinically relevant research so the reader may appreciate the essential risks. Measurement of acoustic energy, recommended exposure levels, and safety considerations are also discussed.

MEASUREMENT OF ACOUSTIC ENERGY

To understand the potential of ultrasound for producing biologic effects, it is essential to have a basic knowledge of how to determine exposure parameters or "dosage." There are a number of methods for measuring the energy output of ultrasound equipment (30, 38). However, not one of the methods is universally accepted. Similarly, there are a variety of terms used to express exposure to ultrasound. The following discussion of acoustic power output levels, however, is limited to the four terms most commonly used in reference to biologic effects: spatial peak-temporal average (SPTA) intensity, spatial average-temporal average (SATA) intensity, spatial peak-pulse average (SPPA) intensity, and maximum intensity (I_m) (30, 33, 38).

The ultrasound dose is a function of the duration of exposure and peak concentration of acoustic power within a specific area. Exposure time depends on the mode of operation of the ultrasound equipment. Continuous wave systems deposit more energy than pulsed wave devices, since the former emit constant sound waves, while the latter intermittently produce sound waves for only a few cycles (Fig. 30.1).

The acoustic power (amount of energy per unit time) produced by a particular instrument is expressed in watts or milliwatts (mW). One watt equals 1 J/sec, and 1 J equals 0.239 cal. SPTA intensity is a common and more precise term for quantitatively expressing acoustic power. This is calculated by determining the maximum value of intensity occurring in an ultrasound beam averaged over the pulse repetition period (for pulsed ultrasound) (30, 33, 38). SPTA intensity is considered an important exposure parameter for biologic effects studies. This is because it essentially characterizes the changes associated with thermal mechanisms (30, 33, 37–39).

An exposure parameter of ultrasound that is determined easily and used frequently by manufacturers to specify the intensity of pulsed ultrasound instruments is SATA intensity. Simply put, SATA intensity is obtained by measuring the average power output of an ultrasound beam and then dividing that by the surface area of the transducer (30, 33, 38).

An additional indication of the ultrasound dos-

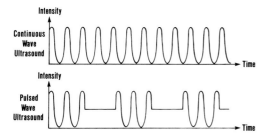

Figure 30.1 Graph of intensity versus time, comparing continuous wave and pulsed wave ultrasound.

age is SPPA intensity, defined as the maximum acoustic intensity in space averaged as it exists during each pulse. SPPA intensity is thought to correspond to nonthermal biologic effects of ultrasound (30, 33, 37–39).

The final exposure parameter routinely used to describe power output involves a measurement of the spatial peak intensity averaged over the longest one-half cycle of pulse. This is called I_m (30, 33, 38). As in all the previous designations of acoustic power levels, I_m is expressed as either watts per meter squared or milliwatts per centimeter squared. Table 30.1 lists typical ranges of acoustic power for commercial ultrasound equipment.

MECHANISMS OF BIOLOGIC EFFECTS

Absorption of ultrasonic energy by tissues in living systems may result in significant functional and structural changes if the exposure is at a sufficient level or threshold (4, 6, 9, 10, 14, 21, 23, 27–30, 32). Certain mechanisms correlate with these biologic alterations and are considered to be the primary sources of potential tissue damage due to irradiation by ultrasound. Understanding the causes of the biologic effects of ultrasound is important to anticipate and study conditions under which significant changes can occur.

Mechanisms responsible for biologic effects of ultrasound are usually classified as being related to either thermal or athermal causes. In general, thermal effects of ultrasound are those that produce biologic changes at similar temperatures, as would occur by heating through other means. Athermal effects are not directly attributable to changes in temperature and are produced by either mechanical forces or cavitation (15, 18, 19, 30, 31, 41). Under appropriate conditions, both thermal and athermal effects can occur simultaneously.

Thermal Mechanisms

As ultrasound propagates through tissue, absorbed energy is continually converted to heat. Tissue temperature may increase significantly. The elevation in temperature depends on a number of factors, including ultrasonic frequency, mean intensity, total time of irradiation, and thermal characteristics of the tissue (16, 17, 20, 30).

Most researchers believe the main cause of ultrasound-associated tissue damage is a direct result of thermally induced changes, especially since an increase in temperature appears to potentiate mechanical and cavitation mechanisms of biologic effects (30, 31).

With respect to tissue heating during diagnostic ultrasound, it is extremely unlikely for an appreciable amount of heat to be generated with pulsed wave systems at the frequencies and time exposures currently employed. However, at least one in vivo study has demonstrated that continuous wave Doppler flowmeters used for diagnosis are capable of producing significant changes in surface temperature when operated at maximum power output levels (17). This currently is undergoing further investigation because of the obvious safety implications.

Mechanical Effects

Because ultrasound is a physical entity, it stands to reason that mechanical effects—changes re-

Table 30.1. Typical Ranges of Acoustic Power Output for Commercial Ultrasound Equipment[a]

	SPTA (mW/cm^2)	SATA[a] (mW/cm^2)	SPPA (W/cm^2)
Static pulse-echo scanner	10–200	0.4–20	0.5–280
Automatic sector scanners	45–200	2.7–60	25–100
Sequenced linear arrays	0.1–12	0.06–10	25–100
Continuous wave Doppler	0.6–80	0.2–20	—
Pulsed Doppler	350–700	80–180	1–12

[a]Values obtained from the American Institute of Ultrasound in Medicine and the National Electrical Manufacturer's Association.
[b]Measured at transducer face.

lated to physical disturbances—will occur under certain conditions. Specific mechanical effects described in association with sonation of biologic systems include development of radiation pressure, radiation force, acoustic torque, and acoustic streaming (18, 30, 31, 37).

Acoustic streaming is due to nonlinearities in the ultrasonic field, which may be due to either radiation pressure absorption or cavitation. Velocity gradients can be caused by acoustic streaming, which can produce permeability changes in cell membranes and alter intracellular organization (43).

For a more comprehensive explanation of mechanical effects, see the report by the National Council on Radiation Protection and Measurements (30). The presence of one or more of these mechanical effects of ultrasound may partially explain the significant changes that can be produced by athermal mechanisms.

Cavitation

The term cavitation describes the development and subsequent responses of cavities in acoustically affected media. It is another mechanism whereby the application of ultrasound may cause serious adverse effects. This complex phenomenon is associated with the cyclically varying pressure that occurs in relation to sound wave transmission (13, 18, 30).

Two primary types of cavity or bubble behavior have been identified. Most biologic tissues contain air or other gases. At the negative phase of the transmitted ultrasound wave, gas from tissue can be drawn into a bubble which is then compressed during the positive phase. If the bubble grows to a resonant size and pulsates without collapsing or "oscillates," it is referred to as *stable cavitation*. The hydrodynamic forces surrounding the oscillating bubble are believed to cause biologic effects (18, 19, 30, 31).

At relatively high ultrasound intensities, bubbles that continually collapse and reform—called *transient cavitation*—can occur. These cavities oscillate in an unstable fashion and collapse within one or two pressure cycles. As the cavities collapse, powerful shock waves which are believed to be extremely destructive are generated within the medium. Transient cavitation may result in the violent implosion of bubbles, producing temperatures as high as 2000° Kelvin (30). Free radicals, which have been demonstrated to cause serious biologic effects (30), can also develop in association with transient cavitation.

Most studies on acoustic cavitation have employed in vitro models (13, 15, 18, 19). Only recently has there been in vivo evidence that cavitation can take place in mammalian tissue (41). However, this appears to require ultrasound intensities used clinically for physical therapy and not for diagnostic ultrasound (41). Further studies are needed to determine the threshold for the development of cavitation and its ultimate biologic consequences.

RECOMMENDED SAFE EXPOSURE LEVELS

At present, there is considerable controversy surrounding the manner in which acoustic power output of diagnostic ultrasound equipment is measured and reported (22, 38, 39). Over the years, new developments in assessing power levels have resulted in a lack of standardization by those involved in the regulation and manufacture of ultrasound devices. Of course, at the forefront of this controversy is what the recommended safe exposure levels should be.

In the United States there are two federal laws that set safety standards for diagnostic ultrasound. In 1968, the Radiation Control for Health and Safety Act required ultrasound equipment manufacturers to provide the FDA with data concerning the acoustic power output of all new products. In 1976, the Medical Device Amendments were enacted under the Food, Drug and Cosmetics Act. This made it mandatory for manufacturers to submit advance notification to the FDA of plans to market a new device. In this notification the manufacturer must include information on power output levels so that the FDA can determine whether or not exposures exceed the maximum output of devices used prior to 1976.

A primary goal of this legislation was to allow for a maximum amount of diagnostically relevant information at a minimum of ultrasound exposure for the patient. It is anticipated that future safety guidelines for ultrasound equipment with high acoustic output levels will require records of exposure dosages, especially for examinations involving the fetus.

The American Institute of Ultrasound in Medicine (AIUM) has stated that no independently confirmed significant biologic effect has been observed in mammalian tissue at a threshold level at or below an SPTA of 100 mW/cm² (2). The AIUM considers this to be a general guideline and acknowledges the indicated energy level is only one aspect of diagnostic ultrasound that must be considered in regard to biologic effects.

Although the vast majority of ultrasound devices operate below 100 mW/cm^2, a number of the newer Doppler systems exceed this recommended exposure level (22). Therefore, additional research is necessary to evaluate potential risks associated with the use of this equipment in comparison to the important diagnostic information it provides for patients.

POTENTIAL BIOLOGIC EFFECTS OF ULTRASOUND DURING PREGNANCY

Ultrasound has provided diagnostic information vital to the management of the pregnant patient as well as the fetus (26). One of the reasons for the predominant use of ultrasound for examinations during pregnancy (as well as the use of Doppler ultrasound for monitoring fetal heart rate) is that only minimal risks are believed to be involved with this diagnostic procedure.

It is important to note that cells undergoing division, as is the case in the developing fetus, are more susceptible to damage from a variety of physical agents, including ultrasound (3, 5, 6, 26, 29, 30, 35). Certain laboratory studies have also implied that exposure to ultrasound during pregnancy may not be entirely innocuous and could result in subsequent risk of congenital anomalies, developmental problems, childhood cancer, and other harmful effects (24, 28, 29, 35, 44, 45). These observations provide the impetus for the continual search for adverse effects when diagnostic ultrasound is used in pregnant patients.

The few investigations that suggest ultrasound can cause irreversible damage to the embryo and fetus tended to use exposures greatly exceeding levels commonly encountered in diagnostic applications. In instances when teratologic effects were identified, it was usually at ultrasonic energies capable of producing substantial tissue heating, and the association between hyperthermia and teratogenesis is well known (26, 32).

To date, epidemiologic investigations have indicated the lack of deleterious effects on the fetus with respect to immediate or later occurrence of harmful abnormalities or pathologic conditions (1, 7, 11, 26, 36, 47). Irrespective of available evidence, a cautionary and judicious approach to the use of ultrasound during pregnancy is still warranted. Additional studies are required to establish definitively the safety of diagnostic ultrasound in pregnancy.

According to the National Institutes of Health (NIH) Consensus Development Conference on the Use of Diagnostic Ultrasound Imaging during Pregnancy (34), ultrasound examination of pregnant women should be used only for a specific medical indication and not for routine screening. Furthermore, ultrasonic examinations should not be performed solely to satisfy the family's desire to view the fetus, determine its sex, or obtain a picture of the fetus. Similarly, visualization of the fetus for educational or commercial demonstrations of no clinical benefit to the patient should be discouraged (34).

Some new echocardiographic Doppler instruments have power output levels greatly exceeding the equipment of the past. This has prompted the FDA to reassess the need for more comprehensive data regarding the clinical efficacy of these instruments from a health risk-benefit perspective. Obviously, it is unwise to believe that diagnostic ultrasound will be safe for examination of the fetus under all conditions.

POTENTIAL BIOLOGIC EFFECTS OF ULTRASOUND DURING CARDIAC IMAGING

Cardiac imaging applications of diagnostic ultrasound are not considered to be associated with significant thermal or athermal changes because of the comparatively low exposure levels required for the examination of the heart. Most of the acoustic energy used during echocardiography is absorbed and attenuated by the skin and muscle of the chest wall. This is believed to provide a wide margin of safety, even during the use of continuous wave Doppler instruments, which expose the patient to higher average intensities than does pulsed ultrasound (30).

Echocardiography may indirectly produce harmful effects when various contrast agents (i.e., indocyanine green dye, saline, autologous blood, and dextrose solution) are used. These agents typically scatter the sound beam, producing strong echoes that enhance image quality.

For the most part, only short-term neurologic deficits or other minor side effects have been observed in relation to the use of ultrasonic contrast agents (8, 46). However, a recent case report has demonstrated that significant neurologic changes, presumably from microbubble air embolism, can occur in patients with suspected right-to-left shunts (25). Therefore, contrast echocardiography should be used with particular caution in this patient group.

Of additional concern is the possibility that microbubble contrast agents may provide a source for cavitation effects (46). In vitro studies have demonstrated that gas bubbles can promote platelet aggregation, even at low acoustic output levels generated by diagnostic equipment (46). This subject clearly merits further investigation.

CONCLUSION

According to the vast literature on biologic effects of ultrasound, it appears as though there are no deleterious effects associated with the clinical application of this imaging technique. In support of the scientific studies is the fact that a substantial number of patients have been examined over the years by ultrasound without any serious side effects.

As newly developed ultrasound systems appear with higher acoustic energy outputs, additional research will be necessary to evaluate the potential health hazards associated with the application of this equipment. Clinicians must take a responsible role in their use of diagnostic ultrasound and be cognizant of the exposures that they are subjecting patients to in order to maintain the outstanding safety record of this imaging technique.

REFERENCES

1. Abdulla U, Dewhurst CJ, Campbell C, Talbert D, Lucas M, Mullarkey M: Effect of diagnostic ultrasound on maternal and fetal chromosomes. *Lancet* 2:829–831, 1971.
2. AIUM Committee Report, Bioeffects Committee: Statement on mammalian in vitro ultrasonic biological effects. *Reflections* 4:311–314, 1978.
3. Akamatsu N: Ultrasound irradiation effects on preimplantation embryos. *Acta Obstet Gynaecol Jap* 33:969–378, 1981.
4. Anderson DW, Barrett JT: Depression of phagocytosis by ultrasound. *Ultrasound Med Biol* 7:267–273, 1981.
5. Au WW, Obergoenner N, Goldenthal KL, Corry P, Willingham V: Sister-chromatid exchanges in mouse embryos after exposure to ultrasound in utero. *Mutat Res* 103:315–320, 1982.
6. Barnett SB, Bonin A, Mitchell G, Mehr-Homji KM, Baker RSU: An investigation of the mutagenic potential of pulsed ultrasound. *Br J Radiol* 55:501–504, 1982.
7. Bernstine, RL: Safety studies with ultrasonic Doppler technique: A clinical follow-up of patients and tissue culture study. *Obstet Gynecol* 34:707–709, 1969.
8. Bonmer W, et al.: Report of the Contrast Committee, American Society of Echocardiography. *ASE Communicator* 8:1, 1982.
9. Buckton KE, Baker NV: An investigation into possible chromosome damaging effects of ultrasound on human blood cells. *Br J Radiol* 45:340–342, 1972.
10. Carstensen EL, Law WK, McKay ND, Muir TG: Demonstration of nonlinear acoustical effects at biomedical frequencies and intensities. *Ultrasound Med Biol* 6:359–368, 1980.
11. Cartwright RA, McKinney PA, Hopton PA, Birch JM, Hartley AL, Mann Jr, Waterhouse JA, Johnston HE, Draper GJ, Stiller C: Ultrasound examinations in pregnancy and childhood cancer. *Lancet* 3:999–1000, 1984.
12. Ciaravino V, Bulfert A, Miller MW, Jacobson-Kram D, Morgan WF: Diagnostic ultrasound and sister chromatid exchanges: Failure to reproduce positive findings. *Science* 227:1349–1351, 1985.
13. Ciaravino V, Flynn HG, Miller MW: Pulsed enhancement of acoustic cavitation: A postulated model. *Ultrasound Med Biol* 7:159–166, 1981.
14. Coakley WT, Slade JS, Braeman JM: Examination of lymphocytes for chromosome aberrations after ultrasonic examination. *Br J Radiol* 45:328–332, 1972.
15. Doulah MS: Mechanism of disintegration of biological cells in ultrasonic cavitation. *Biotechnol Bioeng* 19:649–660, 1980.
16. Fahim MS, Fahim Z, Der R, Hall DG, Harmen J: Heat in male contraception (hot water 60°C, infrared, microwave and ultrasound). *Contraception* 11:549–562, 1975.
17. Filipcznski L: Measurement of the temperature increases generated in soft tissue by ultrasonic diagnostic Doppler equipment. *Ultrasound Med Biol* 4:151–155, 1978.
18. Flynn HG: Physics of acoustic cavitation in liquids. In Mason WP (ed): *Physical Acoustics*. New York, Academic Press, 1964, vol 1B, pp. 57–172.
19. Flynn J: Generation of transient cavities in liquids by microsecond ultrasound. *J Acoust Soc Am* 72:1926, 1982.
20. Fry FJ: Biological effects of ultrasound—A review. *Proc IEEE* 67:604–619, 1979.
21. Glick D, Nolen HW, Edmonds PD: Blood, chemical and hematological effects of ultrasonic irradiation of mice. *Ultrasound Med Biol* 7:87–90, 1981.
22. Hess TP: FDA wants users warned against high-intensity ultrasound of fetuses. *Diagn Imag* 77–85, December 1986.
23. Hill CR: Ultrasonic exposure thresholds for changes in cells and tissues. *J Acoust Soc Am* 52:667–672, 1972.
24. Kinnier M, Wilson LM, Waterhouse JAH: Obstetric ultrasound and childhood malignancies. *Lancet* 3:997–999, 1984.
25. Lee F, Ginzton L: A central nervous system complication of contrast echocardiography. *J Clin Ultrasound* 11:292–294, 1983.
26. Lele PP: Safety and potential hazards in the current applications of ultrasound in obstetrics and gynecology. *Ultrasound Med Biol* 5:307–320, 1979.
27. Loch EG, Fischer AB, Kuwert E: Effect of diagnostic and therapeutic ultrasonics on normal and malignant human cells in vitro. *Am J Obstet Gynecol* 110:457–460, 1971.
28. Macintosh IJC, Davey DA: Relationships between intensity of ultrasound and induction of chromosome aberration. *Br J Radiol* 45:320–327, 1972.
29. Mole R: Possible hazards of imaging and Doppler ultrasound in obstetrics. *Birth* 13:29–38, 1986.
30. National Council on Radiation Protection and Measurements. *Biological Effects of Ultrasound: Mechanisms and Clinical Implications*. NCRP Report No 74, 1983.
31. Nyborg WL: *Physical Mechanisms for Biological*

Effects of Ultrasound, HEW Publication FDA 78-8062. Washington, D.C., US Government Printing Office, 1977.

32. Poswillo D, Nunnerley H, Sopher D, Keith J: Hyperthermia as a teratogenic agent. *Ann R Coll Surg* 55:171–174, 1974.

33. Repacholi MH, Benwell DA: *Essentials of Medical Ultrasound.* Clifton, NJ, Humana Press, 1982.

34. Shearer MH: Revelations: A summary and analysis of the NIH Consensus Development Conference on Ultrasound Imaging and Pregnancy. *Birth* 11:23–36, 1984.

35. Shoji R, Momma E, Shimizu T: Influence of low intensity ultrasound irradiation on prenatal development of two inbred mouse strains. *Teratology* 12:227–232, 1975.

36. Stark CR, Orleans M, Haverkamp AD, Murphy J: Short and long-term risks after exposure to diagnostic ultrasound in utero. *Obstet Gynecol* 63:194–200, 1984.

37. Stewart HD, Stewart HF, Moore RM, Garry J: Compilation of reported biological effects data and ultrasound exposure levels. *J Clin Ultrasound* 13:167–186, 1985.

38. Stewart HF: Output levels from commercial diagnostic ultrasound equipment. *Ultrasound Med* (Suppl) 2:39–48, 1983.

39. Stewart HF, Moore RM: Development of health risk evaluation data for diagnostic ultrasound: A historical perspective. *J Clin Ultrasound* 12:493–500, 1984.

40. Stewart HF, Stratmeyer ME: *An Overview of Ultrasound: Theory, Measurement, Medical Applications and Biological Effects*, HHS Publication FDA 82-8190. Washington, DC, US Government Printing Office, 1982.

41. Ter Haar G, Daniels S: Evidence for ultrasonically induced cavitation in vivo. *Phys Med Biol* 26:1145–1149, 1981.

42. Watts PL, Hall AJ, Fleming JE: Ultrasound and chromosome damage. *Br J Radiol* 45:335–339, 1972.

43. Wells PNT: The possibility of harmful biological effects in ultrasonic diagnosis. In Reneman RS (ed): *Cardiovascular Applications of Ultrasound.* New York, Elsevier, 1973, pp. 1–17.

44. Wenger RD, Meyenburg M: Investigation into possible genetic effects of diagnostic ultrasound. *Ultrasound Med Biol* (Suppl) 2:49–53, 1983.

45. Wenger RD, Obe Meyenburg M: Has diagnostic ultrasound mutagenic effects? *Human Genet* 56:95–98, 1980.

46. Williams AR: Effects of ultrasound on blood and the circulation. In Nyborg WL, Ziskin MC (eds): *Biological Effects of Ultrasound.* New York, Churchill Livingstone, 1985, pp. 49–66.

47. Wilson JMK, Waterhouse JAH: Obstetric ultrasound and childhood malignancies. *Lancet* 2:997–998, 1984.

31

Training of the Echocardiographer

Jay S. Simonson, M.D.

INTRODUCTION

For a physician to consider himself qualified to perform and interpret echocardiograms, special training and extensive experience are required. The necessity for prolonged training requirements is well understood in other cardiology subspecialties such as angioplasty, pacemaker implantation, or electrophysiology. In echocardiography, time and experience are every bit as necessary as with these other modalities.

A request for an echocardiogram must be considered as a consultation. Another physician is asking for an examination for specific cardiac abnormalities to answer specific clinical questions. This requires the physician-echocardiographer not only to be able to acquire images and interpret them, but also to be able to understand the significance of these findings within the context of the clinical problem.

The term *echocardiography* as used in this chapter includes M-mode, two-dimensional, pulsed wave Doppler, color Doppler, and contrast echocardiography. These are all interrelated procedures and use of several of these modalities is often required in a given patient. Indeed, the decision of when to use a particular modality is one of the cornerstones of echocardiography training. Physicians responsible for echocardiographic studies should be thoroughly familiar with all modalities.

The noninvasive and nonharmful nature of echocardiography, combined with the user friendliness of current equipment, has created an important potential problem. Decreasing costs have made equipment acquisition feasible for the majority of physician practices. Consequently, it is now possible for physicians to perform studies and yet, intentionally or unintentionally, not know how to interpret them. Echocardiography is a

procedure in which it is more difficult to acquire interpretative skills than the skills of use.

The optimal training for a physician to perform and interpret echocardiograms competently and accurately is defined in terms of the training required to provide the best patient care. These requirements change rapidly, since increasing use and sophistication have raised steadily the standard of training. What was minimal knowledge several years ago may now be considered inadequate. The ability to interpret echocardiograms today requires extensive training and exposure to images from a wide variety of cardiac disorders. The rapid changes in this field require carefully planned continuing education to maintain expertise.

PHYSICIAN TRAINING IN IMAGE ACQUISITION

The ease with which echocardiographic images can be correlated with anatomy has given rise to the current trend of introducing the basics of echocardiography to medical students and residents. Ideally, physicians in training will enter subsequent formal training in echocardiography with prior exposure to the field. However, this exposure is intended only to enhance formal training and not shorten it.

Echocardiography is an extremely operator-dependent procedure. Consequently, it is not enough only to be able to interpret the echocardiogram. Physicians who interpret studies must also have the technical skill to obtain high quality images. The physician must be able to judge the data's quality and reliability. The ability to judge continuous data as they are imaged and to recognize the audible Doppler characteristics of various cardiac lesions requires a physician experienced at performing studies alone. Although the majority of studies are done by technicians, often the physician must perform part of the examination to exclude alternative diagnoses or obtain subtle data.

It is also important to know when another echocardiographer has not obtained a complete study, especially since echocardiography's strength is its ability to recognize unsuspected or clinically inapparent abnormalities. The physician-echocardiographer must be able to direct and assist the technician during difficult studies and be able to recognize artifact and discard erroneous or misleading information. The major pitfalls of echocardiography are (a) the risk of introducing confounding artifacts and (b) failing to record data of diagnostic importance. By obtaining experience with image acquisition the physician can learn the appearance and many manifestations of artifact.

Echocardiographers must know the limitations and strengths of both the technique and their own abilities. Much of the potential usefulness of the procedure requires an extensive knowledge of what images can be obtained with persistent image acquisition. Mediocrity must not be tolerated.

QUANTITATIVE ECHOCARDIOGRAPHY

Increased technical sophistication has resulted in quantitative techniques that have strengthened and increased enthusiasm for echocardiography. It is now possible to provide immediate quantitative anatomic and physiologic information that can be compared with that from normal people or tracked in a given patient over time to detect changes. The physician-echocardiographer must now be able to provide quantitative and semi-quantitative data regarding chamber sizes, wall motion, ejection fraction, wall thickness, Doppler gradients, and valve area estimates. A training program should include instruction in quantitative techniques, as well as the power and pitfalls of these measurements.

TRAINING ENVIRONMENT

Instructor

Training should be done under the supervision of an established and experienced physician-echocardiographer who has reached at least level three of expertise as defined by the American Society of Echocardiography (ASE) (see section on levels of training). Ideally, training should include exposure to several sonographers with a wide variety of experience.

Equipment

The training facility must have modern, well-functioning equipment that can give clear M-mode, two-dimensional, pulsed wave, and continuous wave Doppler echocardiographic images. This can be achieved using single units with all these capabilities or several units that provide them in combination. Currently, color Doppler capabilities may be considered optional. However, given the many advances in this field and the increasing clinical use of this modality, training site availability of color Doppler must be considered highly desirable.

Location and Facilities

Training should be done at a facility that performs at least 1000 studies per year. These studies should include patients of all ages and both sexes with a wide variety of acquired and congenital heart disease. Optimally, this facility would perform studies on patients from many clinical settings: inpatient services, outpatient clinics, the emergency department, the coronary care unit, critical care units (including cardiac surgery patients), and the catheterization and angiography laboratory. Clinical correlation with other diagnostic modalities, such as auscultation, electrocardiography, pulmonary pressure measurement, and angiography, is also helpful to confirm observations and hone skills.

Classes of Physician-Echocardiographers in Training

The widespread use of echocardiography in a clinical setting has a relatively short history. However, its rapid development has led to its application in the majority of medical populations in this country over the past 10 years. This growth has led to the development of two groups of physician-echocardiographers: (a) cardiology fellows currently in training programs and (b) cardiologists who have completed fellowship training and learn this technique postfellowship.

The Bethesda Conference on Adult Cardiology Training has recognized the existence of these two separate categories of physicians performing echocardiography. Although differences between the two groups were recognized, it was thought that requirements for expertise should remain almost identical.

One difference between these groups is that physicians out of formal training programs may have more clinical experience than fellows in formal training. Also, time constraints of a busy practice make meeting formal requirements much more difficult. Although the value of clinical experience is unquestioned, most believe that this insight and time constraint do not preclude the need for substantially equivalent training requirements for both groups. Due to the time constraints on a cardiologist postfellowship, it may be necessary for that individual to spread training out over a longer period of time.

CONTENT OF TRAINING

Basic Physical Principles

Understanding the physical principles and instrumentation of ultrasonography must be a basic ingredient in training at all levels of expertise. An increased appreciation of the physics involved will greatly improve understanding of the technique and its potential. Instruction in cardiac anatomy, physiology, and pathophysiology is crucial to the understanding of echocardiography. When the operator knows what to look for, subtle details may be imaged.

Steps in Learning Echocardiography

Initial exposure should be focused primarily on M-mode and two-dimensional echocardiography. These form the cornerstone of echocardiography and a good working knowledge is required prior to the introduction of Doppler techniques. Typically, 3–6 weeks of experience will prepare physicians to add Doppler examination to their studies. Likewise, a fundamental knowledge of pulsed wave and continuous wave Doppler is required prior to the use of color flow Doppler. Even though some argue that color flow may be simpler in its technical application, lack of prerequisite Doppler knowledge will considerably limit the successful use of color flow techniques.

Although initial learning may occur in a stepwise approach, advanced learning requires the use of multiple modalities in a given patient. After 2 or 3 months of training the physician should be able to use all modalities in combination, as clinically indicated in a given patient.

Levels of Training

The 17th Bethesda Conference on Adult Cardiology Training and the ASE have made official guideline recommendations for the training of physicians responsible for the performance and interpretation of echocardiographic examinations (1, 2). Since echocardiography plays such a fundamental clinical role in cardiology, it is thought that all cardiologists need to be well trained in this discipline. However, these groups recognize the needs of cardiologists for varying involvement and have recommended three levels of training in echocardiography, corresponding to three levels of expertise.

The first level of expertise is that which each trainee must achieve. This requires 3 months of training with at least 80% of that time devoted to echocardiography. During this time the trainee should perform and/or interpret more than 150 echocardiographic imaging procedures and 75 Doppler examinations under the supervision of the director of the laboratory. This level does not qualify an individual to perform or interpret echocardiograms independently.

The second level of training in echocardiography provides the basic knowledge and experience necessary to perform and/or interpret examinations independently in the clinical setting. An additional 3 months of experience (6 months total) performing and interpreting a minimum of 150 echocardiographic imaging and 150 Doppler studies are recommended to reach the second level of competence. During this period the trainee should have no other primary responsibilities.

The third level of expertise enables the individual to administer and direct an echocardiography laboratory. Training requires an additional 6 months (total of 1 year) devoted primarily to echocardiography. During this period a minimum of 450 additional echocardiographic studies should be performed and/or interpreted by the trainee "in a patient population in which a broad spectrum of adult congenital and acquired heart disease is present."

The number and type of procedures suggested for each level of training are summarized in Figure 31.1. It must be stressed that these numbers refer both to the number of procedures actually performed by the physician and to the number interpreted in a didactic fashion. A balance between these interrelated functions must be reached by each trainee on an individual basis.

Developing a minimum number of procedures and a length of time in specific training to declare competence is admittedly arbitrary. The rate at which a given physician trainee becomes skilled in performing and interpreting echocardiographic studies depends on several factors. Previous training, clinical experience, technical abilities, knowledge of cardiology, the type of patients examined, and the teaching abilities of the techni-

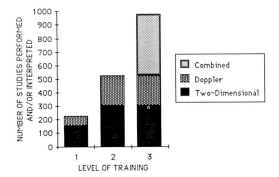

Figure 31.1. The number and types of studies recommended by the ASE for each level of physician echocardiographer training. Level 1 requires 3 months of training and will not qualify an individual to perform or interpret echocardiograms independently. Level 2 requires an additional 3 months of experience and qualifies an individual to perform and interpret examinations independently in a clinical setting. Level 3 requires 12 months of training and enables the individual to administer and direct an echocardiography laboratory.

cians and the physician-supervisor may all influence the time needed to acquire expertise.

As in all of medicine, exposure to a breadth of disorders is as important—or more important—than exposure to sheer volume of patients. In the majority of centers doing large volumes of patients, variety naturally occurs. Thus the guidelines outlining a minimum number of procedures to be performed are reasonable. It is important to note that these numbers refer both to the number of procedures actually performed by the physician and the number interpreted in a didactic fashion to achieve the necessary balance.

The final determination of competency for a physician-echocardiographer must rest with the director of the cardiology training program. At present, formal testing of echocardiography skills is minimal. The cardiovascular diseases subspecialty board offered by the American Board of Internal Medicine requires only a level one competence to understand and correctly answer the questions relating to echocardiography. However, subspecialty certification in echocardiography is currently being considered and will undoubtedly occur in the future.

CONTINUING EDUCATION

Technology changes rapidly, and trained echocardiographers will require continuing education lectures to keep abreast of developments.

The physician-echocardiographer must read current peer review journals. The quality and completeness of studies in these journals should be compared with their own. Studies that are difficult to interpret should be reviewed with colleagues in the field to teach and help one another.

Many formal courses lasting less than 1 week are available and can be an excellent way to acquire specific skills and keep abreast of current developments. However, these courses do not eliminate the need for more prolonged hands-on experience to develop technical echocardiographic expertise. These courses can only supplement—not replace—the formal training outlined in the three-level system.

PEDIATRIC ECHOCARDIOGRAPHY TRAINING

The suggested requirements for physician training in pediatric echocardiography made by the ASE are akin to those for the adult echocardiographer, although the official number of studies is slightly less (3). The pediatric cardiologist must spend a similar amount of time exposed to a large number of pediatric patients. In this training program, understanding congenital heart disease assumes more importance. Exposure to a large percentage of patients under the age of 1 year will facilitate this. Fetal echocardiography is considered a separate skill and requires additional training.

REFERENCES

1. Pearlman AS, Gardin JM, Martin RP, Parisi AF, Popp RL, Quinones MA, Stevenson JG: Guidelines for optimal physician training in echocardiography: Recommendations of the American Society of Echocardiography Committee for Physician Training in Echocardiography. *Am J Cardiol* 60:158–163, 1987.
2. Demaria AN, Crawford MH, Feigenbaum H, Popp RL, Tajik AJ: Task Force IV: Training in echocardiography. 17th Bethesda Conference: Adult cardiology training. *J Am Coll Cardiol* 7:1207–1208, 1986.
3. Meyer RA, Hagler D, Huhta J, Smallhorn J, Snider R, Williams R: Guidelines for physician training in pediatric echocardiography: Recommendations of the Society of Pediatric Echocardiography Committee on Physician Training. *Am J Cardiol* 60:164–165, 1987.
4. Filly K, Hagen-Ansert S, Hagen A, Carney D, Kisslo J, Christie L, Korfhagen J: *Report of the American Society of Echocardiography Committee on Education and Training of the Echocardiographer (Cardiac Sonographer)*. American Society of Echocardiography, August 1982.

32

Peripheral Vascular Duplex Imaging

David Cossman, M.D.
Robert Carroll, M.D.
Jean Ellison, R.V.T.

VENOUS IMAGING

Noninvasive techniques have long been sought to diagnose deep venous thrombosis of the upper and lower extremities. In part, this search has been due to the vagaries of clinical presentation which make accurate diagnosis by clinical signs and symptoms so difficult (1). Most of us were impressed by the low sensitivity of the Homan's sign even as we were learning it in medical school.

Another impetus involves morbid and sometimes lethal complications of inadequately diagnosed and treated thrombophlebitis. Pulmonary emboli, sometimes fatal, may occur without overt signs of deep venous thrombosis.

Also, dye venography of the upper and lower extremities is not always possible. Even when feasible, it is painful and expensive. This makes the technique unacceptable for screening or following patients with known or suspected deep venous thrombosis. Radionuclide ^{125}I-fibrinogen is a sensitive test, but has a low specificity (2, 3). Another disadvantage of this test is its reliance upon human fibrinogen, which carries the risk of AIDS and other diseases common to pooled human blood products.

Duplex scanning of carotid arteries has largely displaced qualitative physiologic studies. Similarly, venous imaging is emerging as the single most important noninvasive study in the diagnosis of venous diseases of the upper and lower extremities. This is due to the reproducibility, accuracy, and cost effectiveness of the technique (4–6). Real-time B-mode venous ultrasound permits direct visualization of the femoral, popliteal, tibial, subclavian, axillary, and antecubital veins. This provides anatomic information not available through traditional physiologic techniques, such as impedance plethysmography and audible interpretation of the continuous wave Doppler signal.

In our laboratory, all venous examinations are performed with a commercially available duplex scanner. A 7.5 MHz probe is used on the femoral, popliteal, and tibial veins. These veins are assessed for patency, valvular incompetence, and intraluminal thrombosis. To promote venous filling while examining the veins in the lower extremities, the patient is placed supine in a slight reversed Trendelenburg position. In this position, the femoral, posterior tibial, and saphenous veins are imaged.

Patients are then placed in a left lateral decubitus position for examination of the distal superficial femoral and popliteal veins. Doppler signals are used to confirm the anatomic findings by evaluating spontaneity, augmentation, and phasicity. Examination of the veins in the upper extremities (jugular, subclavian, axillary, and antecubital) is done using a 7.5 MHz probe with the patient in a supine Trendelenburg position. Although the innominate vein may be seen, it is not well imaged because of depth.

Criteria for interpretation have been described by Sullivan et al. (6). These values have been corroborated by more than 4000 venous examinations performed in our laboratory at Cedars-Sinai Medical Center in Los Angeles. The major diagnostic criteria are absence of intraluminal thrombus, compressibility of the vein by the probe, changes in vein diameter with quiet respiration and the Valsalva maneuver, and visualization of blood flow and venous valve motion.

Absence of Intraluminal Thrombus

The ability of high resolution B-mode ultrasound to visualize a thrombus in the lumen of a vein has been demonstrated repeatedly. The echogenicity of these clots is the subject of some disagreement (7, 8). However, in our experience, recent thrombus is less echogenic than chronic

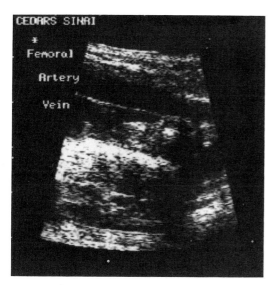

Figure 32.1. Thrombus tip in the femoral vein.

thrombus. Clot retraction, migration of cellular components, and deposition of blood-borne solutes probably result in increased echogenicity of recent thrombi as they age. Since a thrombus may be invisible in its early stages, absence of a detectable clot does not rule out the presence of deep venous thrombosis. When a clot is detected, it tends to distend the involved venous segment (Fig. 32.1), may be free-floating within the lumen of the vein, and is more easily compressible by the examining probe head. Old and new thrombi may coexist and may be difficult to differentiate.

Compressibility of the Vein

Veins of the lower extremities, especially the femoral and popliteal veins, are compressed easily by moderate transducer pressure during the venous examination (Fig. 32.2). In both the longitudinal and transverse planes, vein walls will coapt with mild pressure unless the vein is filled with clot or the wall is rigid secondary to chronic deep venous thrombosis. The femoral vein is dilated but sometimes difficult to compress in iliac thrombosis or external compression or with elevated central venous pressures. No thrombus is seen and patency may be verified by venous Doppler or observation of normal valve function in real time.

Respiration-Induced Changes in Vein Diameter

Changes in the diameter of patent common femoral veins have been studied by Effeney et al. (9). The Valsalva maneuver produced increases in vein diameter of 50–200% with a quick return to the normal resting state. A damped response was associated with proximal iliofemoral thrombosis or acute and chronic femoral vein thrombosis. There was an 8% false-positive rate associated with gross congestive heart failure. No false-negative examinations occurred.

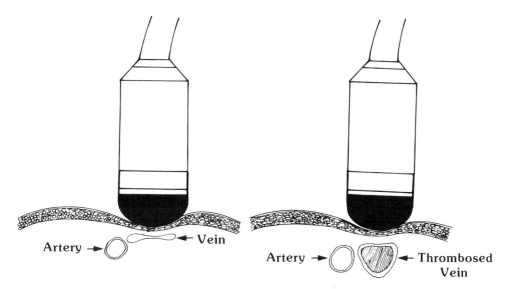

Figure 32.2. Probe compression technique. *Left*, Compressibility compatible with normal vein. *Right*, Noncompressibility compatible with thrombus.

Visualization of Blood Flow and Valve Motion

Venous valves frequently are visualized (Fig. 32.3). Their motion in response to distal compression or the Valsalva maneuver provides confirmation of patency. Blood flow is often echogenic secondary to red blood cell rouleau formation.

Using these four criteria, venous imaging has a sensitivity of 97% and a specificity of 90% (4, 9). In our experience, a false-negative examinations usually are caused by small thrombi in the calf detected by venography and missed on ultrasonic imaging. Peroneal vein thrombosis has consistently been the most difficult to detect. There is considerable evidence in the literature that calf vein thrombosis poses little or no risk of pulmonary emboli and therefore does not require heparinization (10, 11). We have also been concerned about overtreatment (i.e., hospitalization, heparin, and Coumadin) in patients with isolated calf vein thrombi. Consequently, we recommend follow-up examinations 3–5 days after the initial study in patients with strongly suspicious clinical presentations and negative examinations or in patients with positive examinations confined only to the tibial veins. Anticoagulation is recommended in this latter group if a follow-up examination shows propagation of the thrombus into the larger popliteal veins. Serial examinations are also helpful in assessing the efficacy of anticoagulation. In concert with continuous wave venous Doppler and impedance plethysmography, these

studies can identify recanalization and collateralization of major veins.

Physiologic venous studies cannot discriminate between deep venous thrombosis and extrinsic compression of major veins by masses or hematoma. Venous ultrasound is useful in diagnosing venous compression by aneurysm, Baker's cyst, lymph nodes, tumors, and hematoma. The distinction between extrinsic compression and deep venous thrombosis is especially crucial when hematoma, calf tenderness, and swelling masquerade as thrombophlebitis, since anticoagulation obviously is contraindicated when bleeding is present.

Upper extremity venous thrombosis appears to be increasingly common. This is because of the ever-increasing number of foreign objects being inserted into the jugular and subclavian veins. Swan-Ganz catheters, peritoneal jugular shunts, pacemaker wires, dialysis catheters, and hyperalimentation and antibiotic catheters are left in place for long periods of time with an inevitable risk of thrombosis of the great veins. The incidence of pulmonary emboli secondary to upper extremity venous thrombosis is estimated to be as high as 12%. However, controversy remains regarding treatment and the incidence of long-term complications of pain and swelling (12, 13).

The lower extremity criteria for patency also are applied to the axillary, subclavian, and brachial veins. The subclavian vein is difficult to compress because of the clavicle. However, satisfactory imaging may be obtained by placing a 7.5 MHz probe above or below the clavicle. Continuous wave Doppler is then used to evaluate spontaneity, phasicity, and augmentation with distal compression to improve diagnostic accuracy.

MAPPING SAPHENOUS AND ARM VEINS FOR BYPASS SURGERY

The preoperative assessment of saphenous, basilic, and cephalic veins for suitability in bypass surgery is an important contribution of venous imaging to the clinical practice of vascular and cardiac surgery. Preoperative assessment of these veins allows the surgeon to avoid unnecessary, time-consuming, and potentially harmful exploration of an inadequate vein. If the saphenous vein is absent, the basilic and cephalic veins of the arms are mapped and marked preoperatively if they are suitable for use.

The patient is placed in a reverse Trendelenburg position in order to distend the saphenous vein for examination. The course of the vein and

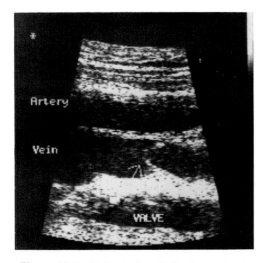

Figure 32.3. Valve leaflets in the femoral vein.

its branches are marked on the skin. The diameter of the vein in the high thigh, distal thigh, calf, and ankle are recorded. The diameter of the saphenous vein is usually at least 1.0–1.5 mm greater when distended at the time of surgery than when measured preoperatively. In our experience, veins smaller than 2.5 mm preoperatively are inadequate at the time of surgical exploration. Others have used any vein measured preoperatively that is greater than 2.0 mm (14).

By marking the course of the saphenous vein along the inner aspect of the thigh and calf, unnecessary skin flaps made by misplaced incisions are avoided. This results in a lower incidence of wound necrosis and infection as well as an increased efficiency in harvesting the veins. Also, when veins are to be used for in situ nonreversed femoral-popliteal bypass grafts, large side branches may be marked preoperatively. In this way, strategically placed incisions may be made along the course of the veins without exploring the entire length.

After implantation of saphenous or cephalic veins for femoral-popliteal bypass grafts, duplex scanning of the grafts is performed at 6-month intervals to detect stenoses that precede graft occlusion. Special attention is paid to valve sites and vein-to-vein anastomoses, as well as to proximal and distal anastomoses. Areas of increased turbulence and high velocities indicate stenoses that may be repaired easily prior to graft thrombosis. During the past 2 years, color flow duplex scanning has greatly facilitated the imaging of implanted grafts. Color flow scanners produce color-coded images of blood flow that correspond to the spectrum of velocities at specific locations within an artery or vein. Points of stenosis may be rapidly identified by color changes indicating increased blood flow velocity and turbulence. Color changes themselves are qualitative markers of areas of stenosis but serve to focus the technologist's attention to points of interest where quantitative Doppler shift or velocity measurements may be obtained.

COMMON FEMORAL ARTERY PSEUDOANEURYSMS

Duplex scanning of the common femoral artery has gained wider application following this vessel's use as the point of access for peripheral and coronary balloon or laser angioplasty and atherectomy. Pseudoaneurysms of the common femoral artery are detected easily, especially with color flow Doppler (Fig. 32.4). Diagnostic criteria

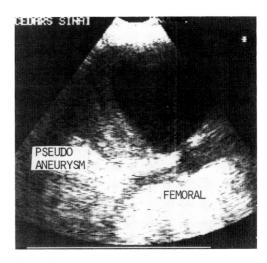

Figure 32.4. Large pseudoaneurysm with laminated clot overlying the femoral artery.

include demonstration of a pulsatile cystic mass and arterial blood flow in the needle track from the common femoral artery to the pseudoaneurysm. The location of this tract is greatly facilitated by color flow duplex scanning. Early detection of pseudoaneurysms by duplex scanning can help avoid late complications, such as thrombosis, rupture, or compression of the femoral nerve. The incidence of pseudoaneurysm was previously estimated at 0.1% by clinical examination and subsequent angiography. With today's wider application of duplex scanning, the incidence appears to be five times greater than originally estimated, perhaps reflecting the complexity of endovascular procedures and the size of the sheaths required.

DUPLEX SCANNING OF THE CAROTID ARTERIES

Duplex scanning is a reliable, reproducible, and noninvasive method of examining the extracranial carotid arteries. Combined real-time B-mode ultrasonic imaging and Doppler spectrum analysis provide accurate information about the morphology of plaques at the carotid bifurcation and the degree of stenosis present. To a lesser degree, they also provide information on plaque ulceration and hemorrhage. Tortuosity, kinking, intimal dissection, and aneurysms can also be diagnosed noninvasively. Carotid artery surgery is being performed increasingly without contrast arteriography, long considered the gold standard in evaluating the carotid bifurcation (15–17).

The duplex scan is used to evaluate patients with asymptomatic cervical bruits, transient ischemic attacks, amaurosis fugax, past history of strokes, status after carotid endarterectomy, and nonlateralizing neurologic symptoms. In patients with cervical bruits it is important to remember that not all patients with bruits have significant carotid stenosis. Conversely, not all patients with severe stenosis have bruits (18–20). Noncritical bifurcation lesions may be followed at regular intervals to detect changes in morphology or degree of stenosis. This is of considerable clinical importance, since these changes are associated with new transient ischemic attacks or completed strokes unheralded by premonitory warnings (21). Plaque morphology is also a significant factor in managing the asymptomatic patient with carotid arteriosclerosis. Plaque hemorrhage and ulceration more frequently are associated with transient ischemic attacks and strokes, because of intimal disruption and embolization of debris, than are comparable stenotic lesions of fibrofatty composition or inert calcification (22, 23).

In the B-mode examination, longitudinal and sagittal views of the common, internal, and external carotid arteries are obtained. An attempt is then made not only to estimate the percentage of stenosis but also to characterize the histology of the plaque. Hemorrhagic and ulcerative plaques are more likely to cause transient ischemic attacks and strokes than are smooth plaques of comparable size.

Without accompanying spectral analysis, percentage of stenosis is difficult to estimate with B-mode imaging alone. Underestimation of the percentage of stenosis is caused often by soft asymmetrical plaques. Also, calcification of the near wall causes "shadowing" that obscures visualization of the far wall. Conversely, percentage of stenosis can be overestimated as a result of artifacts and viewing asymmetric plaques in only one plane. Therefore, we rely on B-mode imaging to estimate percentage of stenosis only in 50% diameter reduction or less.

Although degree of stenosis is difficult to assess with B-mode imaging alone, this technique is extremely useful in determining the histologic nature of the plaque. This is especially true in asymptomatic patients with less than severe stenosis. Bright echogenic plaques are calcified, whereas echolucent areas are composed of either thrombus or lipid (Fig. 32.5). Plaques can be either simple or complex, depending on whether their composition is homogeneous or heterogeneous.

Surface characteristics of plaques are also important. Even with the high resolution scanner's definition of 1.0–2.0 mm, small ulcerations are difficult to identify. Although Johnson et al. (24) and O'Donnell et al. (25) claimed to have detected ulcerations within plaques with extremely high accuracy, most investigators believe that small ulcers are missed easily with current commercially available equipment (26). The specificity in detecting large ulcerations is between 70% and 80%, but the large number of false-negative examinations make B-mode imaging, by itself, unreliable in detecting plaque ulcers.

The B-mode examination is helpful in managing patients with asymptomatic carotid stenosis. Fibrofatty plaques, which are homogeneous and smooth, demonstrate a more benign natural history than calcified plaques with lipid deposition and subintimal hemorrhage (27). Calcified plaques tend to disrupt with the disgorgement of particulate emboli, producing either transient ischemic attacks or strokes. In the future, B-mode imaging may be of considerable value in settling the debate over which patients with asymptomatic carotid stenosis are surgical candidates.

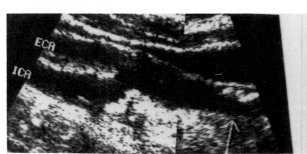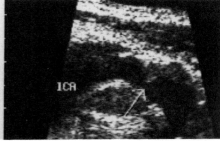

Figure 32.5. *Left,* Carotid bifurcation with irregular plaquing. *Right,* Internal carotid artery with soft irregular plaquing. *ECA* = external carotid artery, *ICA* = internal carotid artery.

DOPPLER SPECTRUM ANALYSIS OF THE CAROTID ARTERIES

Limitations of B-mode imaging require the addition of Doppler spectrum analysis to assess accurately the severity of arteriosclerotic occlusive disease in the extracranial carotid and vertebral arteries. Spectrum analysis is particularly valuable in quantifying stenotic lesions with more than 50% vessel diameter reduction. Interpretation of the audible Doppler signal by the technologist performing the study is as important as the spectrum analysis, since high grade stenoses have characteristic acoustic qualities recognizable by the experienced sonographer.

Modern black and white duplex scanning equipment possesses on-line, fast Fourier transform (FFT) frequency spectrum analysis capabilities. This evaluates the Doppler shift signal for frequency, velocity, and turbulence. Blood flow across a given point also can be calculated once the velocity and vessel diameter are known. Either continuous wave Doppler or range-gated pulsed Doppler systems are available. The latter system is preferable, since signal shifts from a single point in the Doppler beam may be sampled. This discrete sample volume has the advantage of identifying the vessel from which the signal is being obtained. This largely eliminates confusion between the internal and external carotid arteries. The one disadvantage of the pulsed Doppler system is its insensitivity to high frequency Doppler shifts, resulting in aliasing or simultaneous display of the Doppler spectrum above and below the display baseline. However, aliasing becomes a diagnostic criterion for high grade stenosis.

Recently, color flow duplex systems have become available. Color flow Doppler systems utilize pulse Doppler emanating from a multigate transducer that allows for simultaneous multiple line sampling (a "packet"). Unlike the black and white signal analyzer that uses FFT to display all reflected velocities, the color Doppler system utilizes autocorrelation of reflected signal strengths compared to stored signals, and mean velocities are displayed in colors that vary in intensity or hue. By performing over a quarter million calculations/sec, the true color display gives the appearance of blood flow. The mosaic of color changes at stenotic areas corresponds to spectral broadening in black and white systems.

After complete ultrasonic imaging of the carotid artery, the technologist obtains Doppler shift signals from the common, internal, and external carotid arteries. In the absence of disease, these arteries have characteristic spectral patterns determined by the runoff bed into which each vessel empties. The brain is a low resistance organ resulting in a Doppler spectrum for the internal carotid artery characterized by a sloped systolic upslope, low peak frequency, and continuous forward flow during diastole. The higher resistance runoff bed of the external carotid artery results in a sharp systolic upstroke, a more discrete dichrotic notch, and little forward flow in diastole. As would be expected, the signal from the common carotid artery is a combination of the signal from the internal and external carotid arteries (Fig. 32.6).

Alterations in the normal Doppler spectrum characterize disease states in the carotid arteries. Changes in peak frequency, velocity, and "spectral broadening" vary with percentage of stenosis in the involved arteries (Fig. 32.7). Since flow characteristics differ proximal to the plaque, dis-

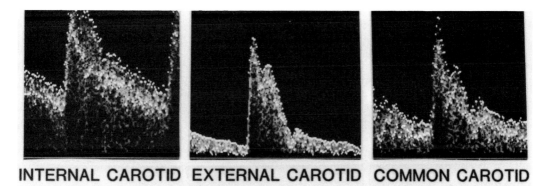

INTERNAL CAROTID   EXTERNAL CAROTID   COMMON CAROTID

Figure 32.6. Typical Doppler spectrums from internal, external, and common carotid arteries.

DOPPLER SPECTRAL ANALYSIS

DIAMETER STENOSIS	DOPPLER SPECTRAL WAVEFORM ANALYSIS

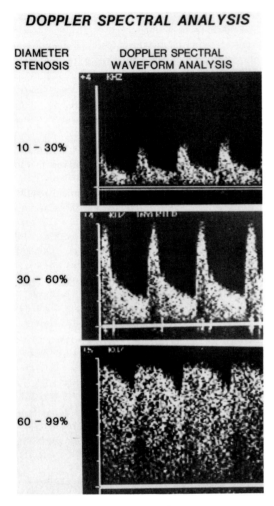

10 – 30%

30 – 60%

60 – 99%

Figure 32.7. Representative Doppler spectrums with varying degrees of disease, using a 3.5 MHz pulsed Doppler.

tal to the plaque, and within the plaque, the technologist must obtain sample signals from several locations within each vessel. Significant diagnostic errors can occur if these signals are not obtained. With color Doppler, the "jet" of blood moving through a stenosis may rapidly be identified by a color change, allowing the technologist to find the tightest area of stenosis without a lengthy search.

Within the stenotic area of an artery, frequency or velocity is increased as defined by Poiseuille's law. Laminar flow usually is maintained, and little spectral broadening is evident. Turbulent flow occurs distal to the plaque, producing lower frequency Doppler signals and a disorganized Dopp-

ler waveform. Bidirectional flow may also be observed, especially if the stenosis is severe. The audible Doppler signal is high pitched and whistling within the area of stenosis and fluttering or bubbling beyond the stenotic zone.

Quantifying the magnitude of stenosis involves measuring maximal systolic velocity within the stenotic zone. Velocities greater than 100 cm/sec correlate with stenoses of greater than 50% (28). Peak systolic velocities increase until a residual lumen of 1.0–1.5 mm is reached, at which point velocities decrease (29). An accurate diagnosis depends more on spectral broadening than on peak velocity. Because of the abrupt decrease in flow velocity in highly stenotic lesions, velocity ratios have been developed that estimate luminal narrowing. These ratios compare maximal velocities from within the stenotic zone with velocities in the more normal distal artery (30). Normally, the internal carotid artery to common carotid artery maximum velocity ratio is less than 0.8. Ratios greater than 1.5 are diagnostic of diameter reductions of more than 50% and area reductions of more than 80% (31). Of perhaps more use is the observation that within the stenotic area of an artery, peaked diastolic velocities increase. The lower the ratio between the systolic and diastolic peak velocities, the greater the luminal narrowing (32).

Spectral broadening is an important diagnostic criterion of luminal narrowing, particularly within critical stenoses that retard rather than accelerate blood flow. If a particular point in a normal artery is analyzed, laminar flow causes most red blood cells within the sample volume to move at the same speed. In gray scale spectrum analysis, the slower velocity will be depicted as white and the faster velocities will be depicted as dark. A waveform or curve is thereby generated corresponding with the cardiac cycle. If all or most of the cells produce the same Doppler shift, the area beneath the curve will be black. As increasing stenoses create turbulence, a wider spectrum of Doppler shifts or velocities will occur at a single point, leading to "filling in" of space beneath the Doppler waveform. A smooth outer envelope will be lost, since laminar flow has been replaced by disorganized flow. Lesser degrees of stenoses produce spectral broadening in the downslope of systole. As the stenotic lesion becomes tighter and diastolic velocities increase, spectral broadening is evident throughout the cardiac cycle. Quantification of spectral broadening is difficult, but "filling in" of the diastolic and systolic window are generally associated with stenoses of more than 75% (32, 33).

The diagnosis of internal carotid artery occlusion is a critical part of duplex examination. A false-positive test will deny a patient with a tight stenosis but patent artery the opportunity to have a carotid endarterectomy. A false-negative test may lead to unnecessary angiography. Since a tight stenosis may reduce blood flow to a trickle, many vascular surgeons believe that any patient with internal carotid artery occlusion by duplex scan should undergo confirmatory angiography so as not to overlook a potentially surgically correctable lesion.

The diagnosis of total occlusion is made by the absence of detectable Doppler noise from within the lumen of an artery. It is important then to be able to differentiate between the internal and external carotid artery; however, confusion between the two can occur. Normally, at the carotid bifurcation, the larger internal carotid artery lies posterior and lateral to the external carotid artery, which has several branches. Variations exist, particularly in disease states, and ultrasonic identification of the two vessels is unreliable. When the internal carotid artery is totally occluded, the Doppler waveform of the external carotid artery may resemble that of the internal carotid artery. This is particularly true if the internal carotid artery has large collateral branches to the cerebral vascular bed. This may result in a mistaken impression that the single patent vessel is the internal carotid artery rather than the external carotid artery. Although it is rarely the case in the nonoperated carotid artery, postoperative occlusions of the external carotid artery have been observed with patency of the internal carotid artery. This is because the endarterectomy of the external carotid artery is blind and frequently unsatisfactory. With occlusion of the internal carotid artery, the ipsilateral common carotid artery waveform should demonstrate no flow in the latter third of the cardiac cycle. This is because the low resistance bed has been eliminated. Increased or compensatory flow frequently can be demonstrated in the contralateral internal carotid artery, but this phenomenon is highly variable. To confirm that the technologist is sampling from the external carotid artery, the ipsilateral temporal artery is rapidly and repeatedly compressed, and the corresponding oscillation is observed in the signal display.

Table 32.1 is a compilation of clinical results from leading investigators using duplex scanning to evaluate carotid bifurcation disease. As experience is gained with Doppler ultrasonography and spectrum analysis, greater accuracy has been achieved. Several authors have now reported performing carotid endarterectomy without prior angiography (15–17).

We currently have experience with 136 patients who have undergone carotid endarterectomy without angiography. Operative findings have correlated with the results of the duplex scan in each case. However, one patient with a 99% stenosis diagnosed by duplex scanning had a patent but unreconstructable internal carotid artery due to stenosis distal to the area examined by the duplex scan. It is not known whether an angiogram would have altered the surgical approach in this patient. Further experience needs to be gained before carotid endarterectomy without angiography can be recommended in all cases.

REFERENCES

1. Barnes RW, Wu KK, Hoak JC: The fallibility of the clinical diagnosis of venous thrombosis. *J Am Med Assoc* 234:605–607, 1975.
2. Kakkar VU: The diagnosis of deep vein thrombosis using I125 fibrinogen test. *Arch Surg* 104:152–159, 1977.

Table 32.1. Concordance Duplex Scanning versus Angiography

Angiography	Duplex results (% diameter reduction)						Total
	Normal	1–15%	16–49%	50–79%	80–99%	100%	
Normal	47	9					56
1–15%	4	49	8				61
16–49%		14	62	4			80
50–79%		1	7	56	8		72
80–99%				5	22	1	28
100%					1	38	39
Total	51	73	77	65	31	39	336

3. Moser KM, Brach BB, Dolan DF: Clinically suspected deep venous thrombosis of the lower extremities: A comparison of venography, impedance plethysmography and radiolabeled fibrinogen. *J Am Med Assoc* 237:2195–2198, 1977.
4. Raghavendra BN, Rosen RJ, Cam S, Riles T, Horti S: Deep venous thrombosis: Detection by high resolution real time ultrasonography. *Radiology* 152:789–793, 1984.
5. Barnes BW: Ultrasound techniques for evaluation of lower extremity venous disease. In Zweibel WJ (ed): *Introduction to Vascular Ultrasonography*, 2nd ed. New York, Grune & Stratton, 1982, pp 273–288.
6. Sullivan ED, Peter DJ, Crawley JJ: Real time B-mode venous ultrasound. *J Vasc Surg* 1:465–470, 1984.
7. Peter DJ, Flanagan LD, Crawley JJ: Analysis of blood clot echogenicity. *J Clin Ultrasound* 14:111–116, 1986.
8. Coehlo JCU, Sigel B, Ryan JC: B-mode sonography of blood clots. *J Clin Ultrasound* 10:323–327, 1982.
9. Effeney DJ, Friedman MB, Gooding GAW: Iliofemoral venous thrombosis: Real time ultrasound diagnosis, normal criteria, and clinical applications. *Radiology* 150(3):787–792, 1984.
10. Lundh B, Fagher B: The clinical picture of deep vein thrombosis correlated to the frequency of pulmonary embolus. *Acta Med Scand* 210:353–356, 1981.
11. Switt S: Venous thrombosis and pulmonary embolism. *Am J Med* 33:703–704, 1962.
12. Demeter SL, Pritchard JS, Piedad OH, Cordasco EM, Taheri S: Upper extremity thrombosis: Etiology and prognosis. *Angiology* 3(11):P734–755, 1982.
13. Prescott SM, Tikoff G: Deep venous thrombosis of the upper extremity: A reappraisal. *Circulation* 59(a):350–355, 1979.
14. Salles-Cunha S, Andros G, Harris R, Dulawa L, Oblath R: Preoperative noninvasive assessment of arm veins to be used as bypass grafts in the lower extremities. *J Vasc Surg* 3(5):813–816, 1986.
15. Goodson SF, Flanigan P, Bishara RA, Schuler JJ, Kikta MJ, Meyer JP: Can carotid duplex scanning supplant arteriography in patients with focal carotid territory symptoms? *J Vasc Surg* 5:554–557, 1987.
16. Thomas GI, Jones TW, Starney LS, Mankas DR, Spencer MP: Carotid endarterectomy after ultrasonic examination without angiography. *Am J Surg* 151:616–619, 1986.
17. Orlow JR, Dean M, Johnson JM, et al: Carotid surgery without angiography. *Am J Surg* 148:217–220, 1984.
18. David TE, Humphries AW, Young JR, Bevan EG: A correlation of neck bruits and arterosclerotic arteries. *Arch Surg* 107:729, 1973.
19. Riles TS, Lieberman A, Kopelman J, Imparato AM: Symptoms stenosis and bruits. *Arch Surg* 116:218–220, 1981.
20. Ziegler DK, Zileli T, Dick A, Sebaugh JL: Correlations of bruits over the carotid artery with angiographically demonstrated lesions. *Neurology* 21:860–865, 1971.
21. Roederer GO, Langlois YE, Strandess DE: The natural history of carotid arterial disease in asymptomatic patients with bruits. *Stroke* 15:605–613, 1984.
22. Lusby RJ, Ferrell LD, Ehrenfeld WK: Carotid plaque hemorrhage. *Arch Surg* 117:1479–1487, 1982.
23. Moore WE, Hill AD: Importance of emboli from carotid bifurcation in pathogenesis of cerebral ischemia attacks. *Arch Surg* 101:708–715, 1970.
24. Johnson JM, Ansel AL, Morgan S, DeCesare D: Ultrasonic screening for evaluation and follow-up of carotid artery ulceration. A new basis for assessing risk. *Am J Surg* 144(6):614–618, 1982.
25. O'Donnell TF, Erdoes L, Mackey WC, et al: Comparison of B-mode ultrasound imaging and arteriography with pathogenic findings at carotid endarterectomy. *Arch Surg* 120:443–449, 1985.
26. Zweibel WJ: B-mode Duplex carotid sonography. In Zweibel WJ (ed): *Introduction to Vascular Ultrasonography*, 2nd ed. New York, Grune & Stratton, 1982, pp 139–170.
27. Imparato AM, Riles TS, Mintzer R, Baumanson FG: The importance of hemorrhage in the relationship between gross morphology characteristics and cerebral symptoms in 376 carotid artery plaques. *Ann Surg* 197:195–203, 1983.
28. Garth KE, Carroll BA, Summer EG, et al: Duplex ultrasound scanning of the carotid arteries with velocity spectrum analysis. *Radiology* 147:823–827, 1982.
29. Zweibel WJ, Zagzebski JA, Crummy AB, et al: Correlation of peak Doppler frequency with lumen narrowing in carotid stenosis. *Stroke* 3:386–391, 1982.
30. Spencer MP, Reid JM: Quantification of carotid stenosis with continuous wave Doppler ultrasound. *Stroke* 3:326–330, 1979.
31. Blackshear WM, Phillips DJ, Chikos PM, et al: Carotid artery velocity patterns in normal and stenotic vessels. *Stroke* 1:67–71, 1980.
32. Barnes RW, Rittgers SE, Putney WW: Real time Doppler spectrum analysis. *Arch Surg* 117:52–57, 1982.
33. Keagy BA, Pharr WF, Thomas D, et al: A quantitative method for the evaluation of spectral analysis patterns in carotid artery stenosis. *Ultrasound Med Biol* 6:625–630, 1982.

APPENDIX A

CLINICAL CASE STUDIES USING DOPPLER ECHOCARDIOGRAPHY

CASE STUDY 1*,†

MITRAL PROSTHETIC DYSFUNCTION-ASSOCIATED AORTIC VALVE DISEASE (FIG. A.1)

History

Forty-four year old, white male who underwent mitral valve replacement (Starr-Edwards prosthesis) in September of 1974 for rheumatic mitral valve disease. At that time, he had mild aortic insufficiency. The patient did well until the early to mid 1980's when he noted a gradual onset of fatigue, dyspnea on exertion and intermittent atrial fibrillation. In 1983 he developed fevered chills, but no obvious organisms were found on performing blood cultures. The patient was referred for further evaluation for increasing fatigue, DOE, orthopnea, and chest pain.

Physical Examination

A slender, white male in no acute distress; blood pressure 138/64, pulse 64 and irregularly irregular. No significant neck vein distention. Cardiac exam revealed crisp prosthetic valve sounds. There was a II/VI systolic ejection murmur at the base, radiating to the carotids. There was a III/VI diastolic decrescendo murmur at the base. There was a III/VI holosystolic murmur at the apex.

EKG

Atrial fibrillation with prominent voltage of LVH.

X-Ray

Showed moderately significant cardiomegaly.

Echo/Doppler

The two-dimensional echo showed marked left atrial enlargement, with the Starr-Edwards valve apparently being well seated. There were some faint extra echos near the apex of the cage with numerous micro bubbles seen in the left ventricular cavity. There were multiple dense echos in the region of the aortic valvular structures. The cardiac Doppler (see representative samples) revealed the patient to have 2–3+ mitral regurgitation with a mitral valve area of 1.3–1.6 cm². There was a 1+ aortic insufficiency with moderate aortic stenosis.

Disposition

Due to cardiac Doppler findings the patient will be scheduled for cardiac catheterization with most likely valvular replacement to follow.

CASE STUDY 2‡

MEMBRANOUS VENTRICULAR SEPTAL DEFECT (FIG. A.2)

History

A 20 year old, college student who had been followed by a pediatric cardiologist for a presumed membranous VSD. His EKGs and chest X-rays in the past have been normal. No echocardiogram had been performed. The patient presented with a 2 week history of vertigo-like symptoms and was referred from student health for evaluation.

Physical Examination

The patient is a well-developed young male with no acute distress. Blood pressure is 130/60 with his pulse being 54 and regular. There was

*Copied, with permission, from Johnson & Johnson, Ultrasound 1986, IREX Cardiology Group.
†Courtesy of Randolph P. Martin, M.D., F.A.C.C., Noninvasive Diagnostics-Consultative Cardiology, Charlottesville, Virginia.

‡Courtesy of Randolph P. Martin, M.D., F.A.C.C., Noninvasive Diagnostics-Consultative Cardiology, Charlottesville, Virginia.

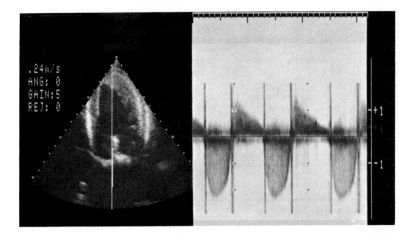

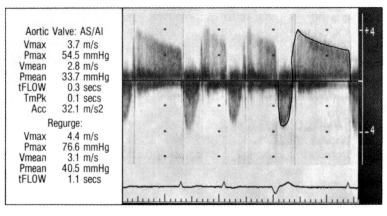

Aortic Valve: AS/AI	
Vmax	3.7 m/s
Pmax	54.5 mmHg
Vmean	2.8 m/s
Pmean	33.7 mmHg
tFLOW	0.3 secs
TmPk	0.1 secs
Acc	32.1 m/s2
Regurge:	
Vmax	4.4 m/s
Pmax	76.6 mmHg
Vmean	3.1 m/s
Pmean	40.5 mmHg
tFLOW	1.1 secs

Figure A.1. Case Study 1.

no neck vein distention. His precordium was quiet. The first and second heart sounds were normal with the pulmonic component of the second sound being normal and moving normally. There was a IV/VI harsh systolic murmur heard at the base with radiation across the entire precordium. There were no diastolic sounds heard.

EKG

Shows prominent voltage with sinus arrhythmias.

X-Ray

Was within normal limits.

Echo/Doppler

Echcardiogram showed normal cardiac chamber size. There was a very small membranous VSD seen with a small septal aneurysm. Sampling with the pulse and continuous wave Doppler reveals a high velocity jet at the mouth of the VSD (in the RV outflow tract). Pulmonic flow velocity was not increased and equalled the aortic flow velocity. There was pulmonic insufficiency recorded by the Doppler, a common Doppler finding. There were no Doppler findings suggestive of pulmonary hypertension.

Disposition

While the patients symptoms were thought to be secondary to inner ear disturbances, a Holter monitor and exercise tests were performed, both of which were normal. The patient has been encouraged to have SBE prophylaxis prior to dental procedures.

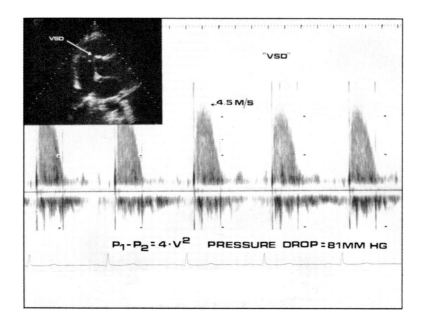

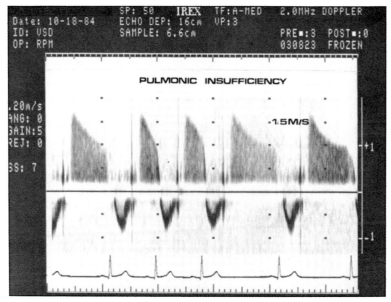

Figure A.2. Case Study 2.

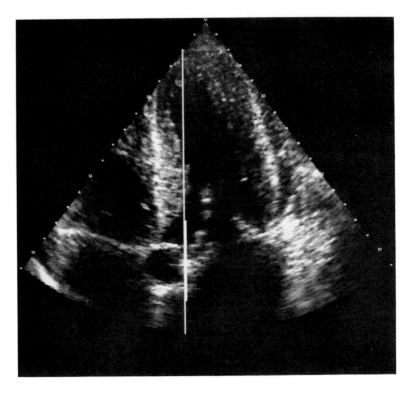

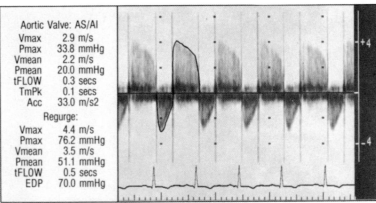

Figure A.3. Case Study 3.

CASE STUDY 3§

AORTIC VALVE DISEASE—QUESTION OF SEVERITY (FIG. A.3)

History

Sixty-one year old, white male with a complaint of leg fatigue and dyspnea on exertion of increas-

§Courtesy of Randolph P. Martin, M.D., F.A.C.C., Noninvasive Diagnostics-Consultative Cardiology, Charlottesville, Virginia.

ing nature over the past two years. The patient has been followed for chronic glomerulonephritis for approximately 24 years, but has recently needed dialysis. There has been no significant history of PND or edema.

Physical Examination

Shows an alert, white male in no acute distress. Blood pressure is 160/62 with the pulse being 70 and regular. There was no neck vein distention. Cardiac exam revealed a normal first and second heart sound. There was a II/VI systolic murmur heard at the base, which radiated to the carotids. There was a II/VI diastolic decrescendo murmur heart at the base.

EKG

Shows left ventricular hypertrophy.

X-Ray

Shows borderline cardiomegaly with a prominent aorta.

Echo/Doppler

There is left ventricular hypertrophy with mild left ventricular enlargement. There are multiple dense echos in the region of the aortic valve, but one of the leaflets shows good excursion. The cardiac Doppler does detect moderate (2+) aortic insufficiency with no significant aortic gradient. The peak gradient measured by Doppler (in the setting T + AI) was 36 mm of mercury.

Disposition

Based upon the echo-Doppler findings, a further invasive workup is not planned at this time.

CASE STUDY 4‖

RHEUMATIC HEART DISEASE WITH MITRAL STENOSIS, MITRAL INSUFFICIENCY AND TRICUSPID REGURGITATION (FIG. A.4)

History

Eighty year old, white male who first presented with cardiac problems in 1981. At that time, while hospitalized for acute dyspnea, he sustained a right cerebral hemispheric stroke. Cardiac workup at that time (noninvasive) revealed rheumatic mitral valve disease. Over the past 2–3 years, the patient had 2–3 pillow orthopnea with 1–2+ ankle edema but no increase in abdominal girth. The patient has complained of a decrease in exercise capacity and prominent dyspnea on exertion.

Physical Examination

Shows an alert, white male appearing younger than his stated age. His blood pressure is 128/72 with his pulse being 64 and irregularly irregular. Cardiovascular exam reveals slight neck vein dis-

tention with his precordium showing an RV heave. The patient had an accentuated first heart sound with a normal second heart sound. There was an opening snap heard .09 seconds after A_2. There was a II/VI blowing systolic murmur at the left sternal border, which radiated toward the upper right quadrant. There were no diastolic rumbles heard. There was minimal hepatomegly.

EKG

Revealed atrial fibrillation with prominent precordial voltage and digitalis effect.

X-Ray

Revealed marked cardiomegaly with evidence of left atrial and right ventricular enlargement.

Echo/Doppler

Two-dimensional echo and Doppler revealed rheumatic mitral valve disease with the two-dimensional echo giving a mitral valve area of 1.4 cm². The cardiac Doppler showed a mitral valve area of 1.3 cm² with a mean gradient of 9.5 mm Hg. The Doppler also revealed mild to moderate mitral regurgitation. There is moderate tricuspid regurgitation with peak RV systolic pressures calculated at 44.2 mm Hg. Left ventricular function was mildly to moderately depressed.

Disposition

The patient will be considered for cardiac catheterization, although in light of the right ventricular size and mild to moderate RV hypertension his operative risks are increased.

CASE STUDY 5¶

RHEUMATIC MITRAL STENOSIS AND INSUFFICIENCY STATUS POSTCOMMISSUROTOMY (FIG. A.5)

History

A 29 year old woman who had scarlet fever as a child. In May of 1981 she underwent cardiac catheterization and commissurotomy for significant mitral stenosis with mild mitral regurgitation. Her postoperative course was complicated by postpericardiotomy syndrome. For the past two years she has had intermittent episodes of pericarditis or pleuritis. Recently, after one of the

---

‖Courtesy of Randolph P. Martin, M.D., F.A.C.C., Noninvasive Diagnostics-Consultative Cardiology, Charlottesville, Virginia.

¶Courtesy of Randolph P. Martin, M.D., F.A.C.C., Noninvasive Diagnostics-Consultative Cardiology, Charlottesville, Virginia.

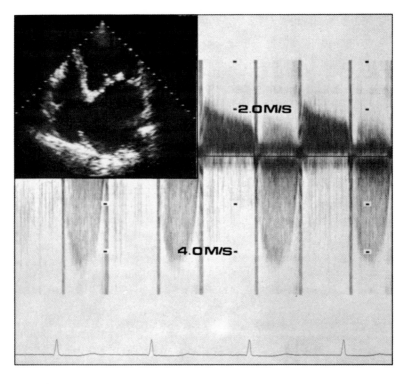

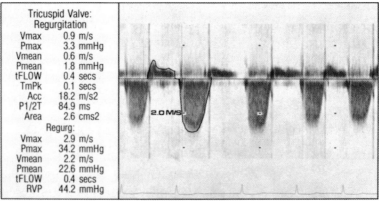

Tricuspid Valve:	
Regurgitation	
Vmax	0.9 m/s
Pmax	3.3 mmHg
Vmean	0.6 m/s
Pmean	1.8 mmHg
tFLOW	0.4 secs
TmPk	0.1 secs
Acc	18.2 m/s2
P1/2T	84.9 ms
Area	2.6 cms2
Regurg:	
Vmax	2.9 m/s
Pmax	34.2 mmHg
Vmean	2.2 m/s
Pmean	22.6 mmHg
tFLOW	0.4 secs
RVP	44.2 mmHg

Figure A.4. Case Study 4.

episodes of presumed pleuritis, a lung scan was performed which showed the possibility of a small pulmonary embolus. The patient has, over the past one year, noted a gradual decrease in her exercise capacity, but denies any significant orthopnea. The patient was sent in for noninvasive evaluation.

Physical Examination

Shows an alert, white female and no acute distress. Her blood pressure was 130/80 with her pulse being 68 and regular. Her lungs were clear. There was no neck vein distention. Cardiovascular exam revealed an accentuated first heart sound with a normal second heart sound. There was a II/VI holosystolic murmur heard maximally at the apex and radiating to the axilla. There was an opening snap heard .09 seconds after A_2. There was a II/VI diastolic rumble heard with a presystolic accentuation. Additionally, there was a question of I/VI faint diastolic decrescendo murmur heard at the base.

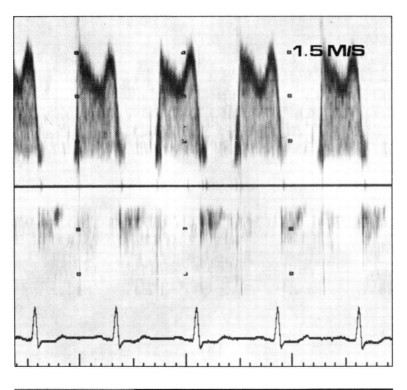

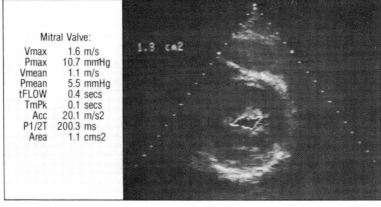

Mitral Valve:
Vmax	1.6 m/s
Pmax	10.7 mmHg
Vmean	1.1 m/s
Pmean	5.5 mmHg
tFLOW	0.4 secs
TmPk	0.1 secs
Acc	20.1 m/s2
P1/2T	200.3 ms
Area	1.1 cms2

Figure A.5. Case Study 5.

EKG

Within normal limits.

X-Ray

Mild left atrial and left ventricle prominence.

Echo/Doppler

The two-dimensional echo and Doppler shows a rheumatic mitral valve disease with the left ventricle being at the upper limits of normal for size, with a mild decrease in its overall function. There is good pliability of the anterior leaflet of the mitral valve. The two-dimensional echo shows a mitral valve area of 1.3 cm². The cardiac Doppler calculates a mitral valve area of 1.2 cm² with a mean gradient of 6 mm of mercury at rest. There is a mild mitral regurgitation. Additionally there is a 1+ aortic insufficiency with no significant findings of RV hypertension.

Disposition

It is felt that the patient's symptoms are secondary to some restenosis of the mitral valve orifice, and she will be followed closely.

CASE STUDY 6*

FOLLOW-UP OF COMMISSUROTOMY FOR MITRAL STENOSIS

D.K.

The patient is a 42 year old white female who underwent a mitral valve commissurotomy in 1964. She has not seen a physician in 20 years. From a cardiovascular standpoint, symptomatically, she is in NYHA Class II.

The physical examination showed sinus rhythm, a normal first heart sound, a normal second heart sound, an opening snap with $A_2 - OS = 0.06$ seconds, a grade 3/6 apical diastolic rumble with presystolic accentuation, and a grade 2/6 systolic ejection murmur at the lower left sternal border.

The two-dimensional echocardiogram showed a thickened, restricted mitral valve characteristic of rheumatic mitral stenosis; the mitral valve area was 1.3 cm^2. The left ventricle was normal sized and had normal wall motion. The left atrium was enlarged; the derived M-mode left atrial dimension was 5.0 cm.

The Doppler cardiac ultrasound study showed a mean gradient of 6 mm Hg and mild mitral insufficiency. As a result, the planned repeat cardiac catheterization has been deferred, and she is being followed clinically.

CASE STUDY 7†

NORMAL MITRAL VALVE PROSTHESIS WITH SEVERE PULMONARY HYPERTENSION

W.P.

The patient is a 59 year old, white male who underwent surgery for severe mitral stenosis with severe pulmonary hypertension, severe right coronary artery disease, and mild to moderate aortic insufficiency. In August 1983 a 31 mm St. Jude

*Courtesy of Gary S. Mintz, M.D., F.A.C.C., Director of Cardiology Ultrasound Laboratory, Likoff Cardiovascular Institute, Hahnemann University Hospital.
†Courtesy of Gary S. Mintz, M.D., F.A.C.C., Director of Cardiology Ultrasound Laboratory, Likoff Cardiovascular Institute, Hahnemann University Hospital.

mitral valve prosthesis was implanted and a saphenous vein bypass graft was anastomosed to the distal right coronary artery. Prior to discharge, phonoechocardiographic study showed normal disc motions, normal left ventricular size, significant right ventricular enlargement (3.4 cm), significant left atrial enlargement (6.0 cm), and a normal A_2-mitral prosthesis opening interval of 0.07 seconds. First-pass radionuclide angiography showed a left ventricular ejection fraction of 0.51 and a right ventricular ejection fraction of 0.22.

Seven months later he was readmitted with progressive shortness of breath, paroxysmal nocturnal dyspnea, and peripheral edema. The physical examination showed an acutely ill, cyanotic patient. There was sinus rhythm with episodes of atrial fibrillation and flutter. Prosthetic valve sounds were normal; there was a closing click, but no opening click. There was a grade 3/6 holosystolic murmur at the lower left sternal border and apex.

Initial laboratory studies showed that anticoagulation was not within therapeutic range; the prothrombin time was 12.6 seconds with a control of 11.6 seconds. The arterial blood gas showed a pH of 7.25, PCO_2 of 63 mm Hg and a PO_2 of 52 mm Hg on 100% FIO_2. A phonoechocardiographic study still showed normal disc motion, but the A_2-mitral prosthesis opening interval had shortened from 0.07 seconds to 0.02 seconds. Left atrial size (6.0 cm) and radionuclide left ventricular and right ventricular ejection fractions (0.05 and 0.02, respectively) were unchanged, but right ventricular size had increased (3.4 cm to 4.9 cm).

The Doppler ultrasound study showed a mean mitral prosthetic valve gradient of 3.6 mm Hg, mild mitral insufficiency, and moderate tricuspid insufficiency. Cardiac catheterization confirmed normal prosthetic function except for mild mitral insufficiency. There was a persistent severe pulmonary hypertension (pulmonary artery pressure measured 90/40).

CASE STUDY 8‡

EARLY ENDOCARDITIS INVOLVING A TISSUE MITRAL VALVE PROSTHESIS

R.P.

The patient is a 63 year old, white female with rheumatic mitral valve disease who underwent

‡Courtesy of Gary S. Mintz, M.D., F.A.C.C., Director of Cardiology Ultrasound Laboratory, Likoff Cardiovascular Institute, Hahnemann University Hospital.

valve replacement with an Ionescu-Shiley tissue prosthesis. Her postoperative course was complicated by mediastinitis and *Staphylococcus aureus* septicemia. She was treated with mediastinal drainage and antibiotics. However, she became dyspenic, and despite medical therapy for congestive heart failure, her respiratory distress worsened.

The physical examination showed normal first and second heart sounds and a grade 2/6 systolic murmur along the left sternal border.

The two-dimensional echocardiogram study showed a vegetation attached to one of the leaflets of the tissue valve prosthesis.

The Doppler cardiac ultrasound study detected significant mitral insufficiency with an eccentric regurgitant jet in the left atrium. On the basis of this information, without preoperative cardiac catheterization, she underwent replacement of the infected prosthesis. A St. Jude mitral valve was implanted. This time her postoperative course was uncomplicated, and, at discharge, she was asymptomatic.

CASE STUDY 9§

AORTIC STENOSIS
G.R.

The patient is a 63 year old, white male who began to complain of dyspnea on exertion 4 years ago. At that time cardiac catheterization showed mild aortic stenosis, mild aortic insufficiency, and normal coronary arteries. For the past 2 months he has been having increasing exertional dyspnea; symptomatically he is in the NYHA Class III.

The physical examination showed a normal carotid pulse, an irregular heart rhythm, a third heart sound, and a grade 3/6 systolic murmur loudest at the lower left sternal border and apex.

First-pass radionuclide angiography showed a left ventricular ejection fraction of 0.18. Two-dimensional echocardiography showed a thickened and restricted aortic valve, marked left atrial enlargement, and marked left ventricular enlargement with severe diffuse hypokinesis.

Doppler cardiac ultrasound detected an aortic valve gradient of 64 mm Hg and mild aortic insufficiency.

Despite the poor ventricular function, the Dop-

pler study prompted cardiac catheterization which confirmed the presence of critical aortic stenosis, the calculated valve area 0.6 cm². He underwent aortic valve replacement with a St. Jude prosthesis. There were no postoperative complications. His functional status significantly improved.

CASE STUDY 10*

ATRIAL SEPTAL DEFECT
N.K.

The patient is a 24 year old, white female who went to her physician complaining of dyspnea on exertion.

The physical examination showed normal vital signs and pulses. There was a normal first pulse heart sound, a widely split second heart sound, and a grade 2/6 systolic ejection murmur localized to the mid-left sternal border.

The electrocardiogram showed an incomplete right bundle branch block.

The two-dimensional echocardiogram showed an atrial septal defect of the ostium secundum type, right ventricular and pulmonary artery enlargement, and abnormal interventricular septal motion, but no other cardiac anomalies.

Doppler cardiac ultrasound detected a left to right shunt across the interatrial septum. There were no other shunts, valvular gradients, valvular insufficiency, or evidence of pulmonary hypertension. As a result of the above information, without having cardiac catheterization, she underwent surgery; a "silver-dollar-sized" atrial septal defect was successfully patched.

CASE STUDY 11†

PULMONIC STENOSIS
J.D.

The patient is a 2 year old, white female who was referred for evaluation at the age of 5 months with a heart murmur. The physical examination showed a normally developing child (25th percentile in weight, 50th percentile in height). There

§Courtesy of Gary S. Mintz, M.D., F.A.C.C., Director of Cardiology Ultrasound Laboratory, Likoff Cardiovascular Institute, Hahnemann University Hospital.

*Courtesy of Gary S. Mintz, M.D., F.A.C.C., Director of Cardiology Ultrasound Laboratory, Likoff Cardiovascular Institute, Hahnemann University Hospital.
†Courtesy of Gary S. Mintz, M.D., F.A.C.C., Director of Cardiology Ultrasound Laboratory, Likoff Cardiovascular Institute, Hahnemann University Hospital.

was a harsh grade 3/6 systolic ejection murmur, loudest at the upper sternal border, a pulmonic ejection sound, and a soft pulmonic component of the second heart sound which was widely split. The electrocardiogram showed severe right ventricular hypertrophy. A cardiac catheterization showed moderate pulmonic stenosis with a peak gradient of 60 mm Hg.

During the past 18 months she has been active and gaining weight, but has had frequent upper respiratory tract infections. The physical examination was unchanged. Prior to consideration for cardiac catheterization, she was referred for ultrasound study.

A two-dimensional echocardiogram showed a thickened and restricted pulmonic valve.

Doppler ultrasound showed a peak gradient of 64 mm Hg. Because the pulmonic valve gradient (Doppler gradient now compared to the catheterization gradient 18 months ago) has not changed, cardiac catheterization has been postponed. She is being followed medically.

CASE STUDY 12‡

RECOARCTATION OF THE AORTA
M.L.M.

The patient is a 26 year old, white female who at 19 years of age underwent resection of a coarc-

---

‡Courtesy of Gary S. Mintz, M.D., F.A.C.C., Director of Cardiology Ultrasound Laboratory, Likoff Cardiovascular Institute, Hahnemann University Hospital.

tation of the aorta. Because she now wants to become pregnant, she was referred for cardiac evaluation.

The physical examination showed a blood pressure of 150/74. Compared to the carotid and radial pulses, the femoral and pedal pulses were diminished. The left ventricular impulse and the first and second heart sounds were normal. There was an ejection sound along the left sternal border and a grade 3/6 systolic ejection murmur that was audible diffusely over the precordium and also over her back between her shoulder blades.

Except for radiographic evidence of a previous thoracotomy, her chest X-ray was normal. Her electrocardiogram was normal. The two-dimensional echocardiogram showed a dilating ascending aorta and aortic arch. The descending thoracic aorta was distorted and appeared narrowed just distal to the left subclavian artery.

Doppler cardiac ultrasound measured a pressure gradient of 64 mm Hg through this narrowed segment. As a result, the patient underwent cardiac catheterization which confirmed the severity of the gradient. The patient is scheduled for surgery to repair the coarctation, whether residual or recurrent.

APPENDIX B
CLINICAL CASE STUDIES USING COLOR FLOW DOPPLER

CASE STUDY 1*,†

RHEUMATIC HEART DISEASE WITH MITRAL, AORTIC TRICUSPID AND PULMONIC INSUFFICIENCY (FIG. B.1)

History

This 67 year old, white male was being evaluated for chronic rheumatic heart disease. He had a known history of rheumatic fever as a child and had been followed for mitral stenosis and insufficiency since the early 1960's. He initially underwent cardiac catheterization in 1976 when he was found to have mild aortic stenosis, severe mitral regurgitation and mild mitral stenosis. He had mild left ventricular dysfunction at that time. The patient was clinically well until a symptomatic deterioration occurred in 1980. Repeat cardiac catheterization revealed mild aortic stenosis and regurgitation, moderate mitral regurgation with unquantitated mitral stenosis, and new pulmonary hypertension with tricuspid regurgitation. The patient declined surgical repair of his valve disease, and has been managed medically.

The patient was hospitalized in 1985 with the new onset of hepatomegaly and ascites.

Physical Examination

The patient was in moderate distress. His peripheral pulses were reduced. His lungs were clear. His point of maximal impulse revealed a diffuse lift. His first heart sound was soft, and his second heart sound was absent at the aortic area. No gallops were present. Grade 2/6 systolic ejection

---

*Copied, with permission, from Johnson & Johnson, Ultrasound 1986, IREX Cardiology Group.
†Courtesy of Arthur J. Labovitz, M.D., F.A.C.C., and George A. Williams, M.D., F.A.C.C., Associate Professors of Medicine, St. Louis University School of Medicine, St. Louis, MO.

murmur was present at the right upper sternal border, and a lower pitched holosystolic murmur was present at the left lower sternal border. A grade 2/6 diastolic rumble with presystolic accentuation was present at the apex. No opening snap was audible. The liver was enlarged to 22 cm and pulsatile.

2-D Echo

Routine echocardiography revealed marked left atrial enlargement, a heavily calcified aortic and mitral valve, an anatomic mitral valve orifice of 0.9 cm^2, and marked right ventricular enlargement with right ventricular volume overload pattern. The left ventricular function was relatively normal with left ventricular hypertrophy.

Echo/Doppler

There was mitral stenosis, with a calculated area of 0.9 cm^2, and mitral insufficiency, which was not quantitatable by flow mapping. The aortic valve gradient calculated was 64 mm Hg, and mild aortic insufficiency was present. Moderate to severe tricuspid insufficiency was present with a calculated tricuspid valve gradient of 16. The tricuspid valve pressure half-time was consistent with a valve area of 1.1 cm^2.

Color Flow Mapping

Real-time color flow mapping in this patient provided additional information. The jet of mitral insufficiency was visualized to the mid-left atrium, and confirmed the presence of continuing moderate mitral insufficiency. The aortic insufficiency was seen to be mild. Pulmonic insufficiency was also present. Flow mapping also documented the presence of severe tricuspid regurgitation, and a narrowed diastolic flow jet through the tricuspid valve provided evidence of previously unsuspected tricuspid stenosis and helped to explain the patient's present symptoms.

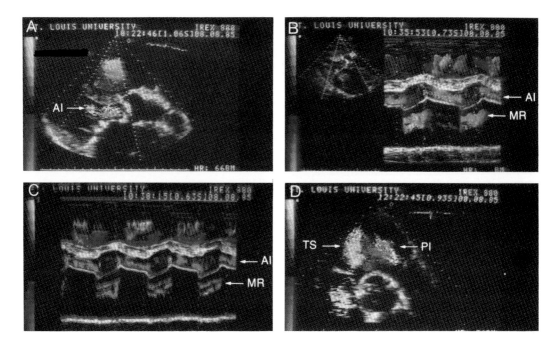

Figure B.1. *A*, Parasternal long axis view. Mosaic pattern, representing the turbulent flow of aortic insufficiency, is demonstrated in the left ventricular outflow tract. *B*, Color flow 2-D and M-mode demonstrating aortic insufficiency in the left ventricular outflow tract and mitral regurgitation in the left atrium. *C*, Color flow M-mode demonstrating aortic insufficiency in the left ventricular outflow tract and mitral regurgitation in the left atrium. Color M-mode aids in the timing of cardiac events and allows for quick identification of multiple lesions. *D*, Short axis parasternal view at the aortic level. Color flow mapping demonstrates tricuspid stenosis as a red jet toward the transducer and pulmonic insufficiency as a mosaic pattern also toward the transducer. Both of these lesions occur at the same time in the cardiac cycle. CFM allows for rapid identification of both lesions. See this figure in the Color Atlas.

CASE STUDY 2‡

VENTRICULAR SEPTAL DEFECT AND MITRAL REGURGITATION (FIG. B.2)

History

Four month old infant referred for a murmur and failure to thrive. She was the 6 lb. 10 oz. product of a full-term uncomplicated pregnancy. The neonatal period was unremarkable. Beginning at 2½ months of age, the mother noted more rapid breathing and difficulty in feeding. After 2 ounces, she began to sweat and breathe more rapidly. She was referred for cardiac evaluation.

‡Courtesy of Samuel B. Ritter, M.D., F.A.A.P., F.A.C.C., Director, Noninvasive Cardiology, Childrens Heart Center, Mount Sinai Hospital of New York, NY.

Physical Examination

The infant was an acyanotic black female in mild respiratory distress; heart rate was 130/minute, respiratory rate 45/minute with mild intercostal and subcostal retractions. Pulses were equal in upper and lower extremities. There was a thrill over the left midsternal border to palpation. The first heart sound was normal, and the second heart sound physiologically split with respiration. A grade IV/VI harsh holosystolic murmur was auscultated best at the left mid-to-lower sternal border, radiating to the base and apex. A II/VI short, low-pitch diastolic rumble was appreciated apically.

EKG

Normal sinus rhythm, normal axis for age, with evidence of biventricular enlargement.

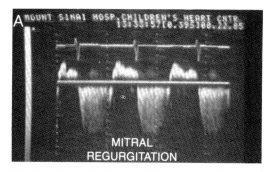 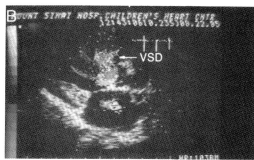
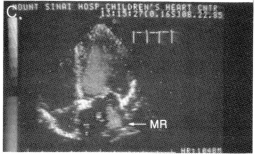 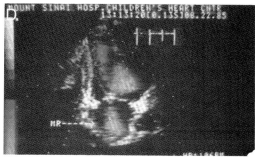

Figure B.2. *A,* Continuous wave Dopper is used to confirm the CFM diagnosis of mitral regurgitation. MR is displayed below the baseline in systole, and mitral inflow is seen above the baseline in diastole. *B,* Parasternal long axis view. This example of a ventricular septal defect clearly demonstrates blood flow from the left ventricular outflow tract to the right ventricle. *C,* Four-chamber apical view. Mitral regurgitation is seen in the left atrium. Note the eccentricity of the regurgitant jet. *D,* A modified apical two-chamber view was obtained to optimize the color flow pattern. Moderate mitral regurgitation is visualized in the left atrium. This lesion was not detected by clinical auscultation or pulsed Doppler. See this figure in Color Atlas.

X-Ray

Cardiomegaly with prominent pulmonary vasculature.

Impression

Ventricular septal defect causing congestive heart failure.

2-D Echo

(Initial study performed on noncolor mechanical scanner.)

The two-dimensional echo showed normal situs, ventricular looping, and great vessel position. There was biventricular enlargement and marked left atrial dilation. A subaortic, perimembranous ventricular septal defect was identified, moderate in size.

Doppler/Echo

Pulsed Doppler examination revealed harsh, turbulent left-to-right flow across the VSD; there

was no evidence of ductal patency with the sample volume in either the aorta or pulmonary artery. Atrioventricular valve flow was normal.

Color Flow Mapping

Follow-up noninvasive studies were performed with a color flow mapping system. Ventricular septal defect shunting was clearly demonstrated. Surprisingly, 2+ mitral insufficiency was seen on color flow mapping, with a discrete jet ascending along the left atrial lateral wall. Placement of a pulsed Doppler sample volume within the color coded regurgitant jet as well as CW interrogation along the lateral left atrial wall confirmed the finding.

Importance

Neither clinical evaluation by auscultation nor pulsed Doppler without color flow suggested mitral regurgitation. Anatomically, the valve is normal.

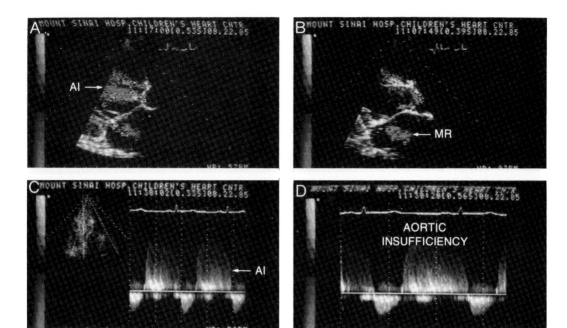

Figure B.3. *A*, Parasternal long axis view. A mosaic pattern, representing turbulence, is demonstrated in the left ventricular outflow tract during diastole, which is consistent with aortic insufficiency. A mosaic jet of mitral regurgitation can also be seen in the left atrium. *B*, A parasternal long axis view demonstrating the mosaic pattern of mitral regurgitation in the left atrium. *C*, Four-chamber apical view. A continuous wave Doppler beam is easily placed through the characteristic mosaic pattern of aortic regurgitation for the spectral analysis tracing. *D*, This spectral tracing was recorded at an increased sweep speed to increase the accuracy of derived calculations. Aortic insufficiency is represented as flow above the baseline during diastole. See this figure in Color Atlas.

Disposition

As a result of the color flow mapping examination cardiac catheterization was deferred. The patient will continue to be followed noninvasively for possible future surgical intervention. The infant continues on digoxin and diuretic.

CASE STUDY 3§

RHEUMATIC MITRAL AND AORTIC INSUFFICIENCY (FIG. B.3)

History

Twenty year old female with history of rheumatic fever at age 6. Asymptomatic during childhood. Over the past two years, she developed progressive dyspnea on exertion.

§Courtesy of Samuel B. Ritter, M.D., F.A.A.P., F.A.C.C., Director, Noninvasive Cardiology, Childrens Heart Center, Mount Sinai Hospital of New York, NY.

Physical Examination

The patient was a slender white female in no acute distress. Her blood pressure was 130/60. Cardiac examination reveals a left ventricular lift with prominent laterally displaced PMI. Heart sounds were normal. A grade 3/6 blowing systolic murmur at the third left intercostal space and a grade 3/6 diastolic blowing murmur were auscultated.

EKG

Left atrial and left ventricular enlargement.

X-Ray

Cardiomegaly with left atrial and left ventricular dilitation.

2-D Echo

The two-dimensional echo revealed moderately enlarged left atrium and dilated left ventricle.

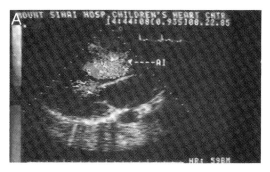
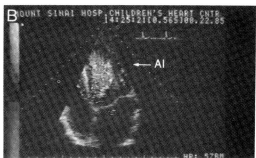
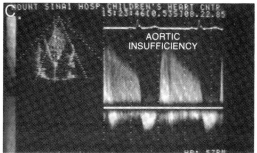
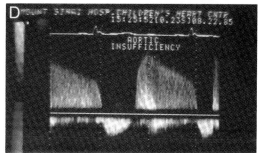

Figure B.4. *A*, Parasternal long axis view. The mosaic pattern of turbulent blood flow is easily visualized in the left ventricular outflow tract diagnostic of aortic insufficiency. *B*, Four-chamber apical view. The mosaic pattern of turbulent blood flow is easily located and visualized in the left ventricular outflow tract, consistent with aortic insufficiency. This confirms our diagnosis of AI obtained from the parasternal long axis view. *C*, Continuous wave Doppler can be placed in the AI jet (which is easily visualized by a mosaic flow pattern) for rapid confirmation and quantitation. *D*, Spectral analysis tracing is recorded at increased speed to allow for more accurate quantitative measurements. See this figure in Color Atlas.

Color Flow Mapping

Color flow displayed significant aortic and mitral regurgitation. Both appeared to be hemodynamically severe. Doppler (CW) confirmed these above findings.

Disposition

Cardiac catheterization has been deferred as a result of this color flow mapping study. This patient will continue to be followed noninvasively for eventual double valve replacement.

CASE STUDY 4‖

RHEUMATIC AORTIC INSUFFICIENCY (FIG. B.4)

History

Eighteen year old with a history of rheumatic fever in early childhood. Followed for a number

‖Courtesy of Samuel B. Ritter, M.D., F.A.A.P., F.A.C.C., Director, Noninvasive Cardiology, Childrens Heart Center, Mount Sinai Hospital of New York, NY.

of years with a diagnosis of aortic insufficiency and mitral regurgitation. Until recently, she has been asymptomatic. Over the past year, mild dyspnea on exertion has developed.

Physical Examination

The patient is a well-developed young female in no distress. The pulse was 75 and regular; blood pressure was 13/65. Cardiac examination revealed a left ventricular lift palpated with PMI laterally displaced. Heart sounds were normal. A grade 2–3/6 high-pitch blowing diastolic murmur was heard best at the third–fourth left intercostal space on the left. A second blowing murmur was heard in systole at the apex, and a low-pitch diastolic rumble was auscultated at the same place.

EKG

Sinus rhythm with left atrial and left ventricular enlargement.

X-Ray

Moderate cardiomegaly, left atrial and left ventricular enlargement.

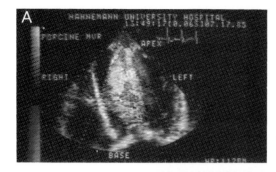
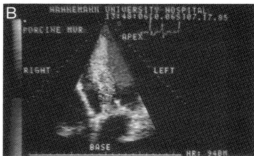
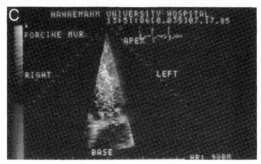

Figure B.5. *A–C*, Apical four-chamber view. A mosaic pattern, representing turbulent blood flow, is easily visualized in the left ventricular inflow tract of this heart with a Hancock heterograft. See this figure in Color Atlas.

2-D Echo

Echocardiogram showed left ventricular dilatation with good contractility. No intracardiac defects were noted. The aortic valve opened well.

Color Flow Mapping

Color flow revealed moderate to severe aortic regurgitation, seen best in the parasternal long axis view.

Disposition

As a result of this color flow mapping study, cardiac catheterization has been deferred. This patient will continue to be followed noninvasively for eventual aortic valve surgery.

CASE STUDY 5¶

PROSTHETIC MITRAL VALVE (FIG. B.5)

History

A 68 year old male presented with both rheumatic and coronary heart disease. In 1980, he

¶Courtesy of Gary S. Mintz, M.D., F.A.C.C., Associate Professor of Medicine, Associate Professor of Radiology, The Likoff Cardiovascular Institute of Hahnemann University, Philadelphia, PA.

underwent triple coronary artery bypass graft surgery. Three years later, two of the grafts were occluded and there was progression of aortic and mitral valve disease. At that time, he underwent double coronary artery bypass graft surgery and aortic and mitral valve replacement with Hancock heterografts. He was better symptomatically until the last 6 months when progressive heart failure necessitated frequent hospitalization several times during the month before he was transferred to Hahnemann University Hospital.

Physical Examination

On admission, his heart rate was 110/min and regular, his blood pressure was 80/60, and his respiratory rate 30/min. There was marked jugular venous distention and hepatomegaly and rales over the lower half of his lung fields. Cardiac exam showed a diffuse and displaced cardiac apex, loud third and fourth heart sounds, and a grade 3/6 holosystolic murmur audible between the lower left sternal border and the apex.

EKG

The electrocardiogram showed sinus tachycardia and a left bundle branch block. The chest X-ray showed marked cardiomegaly and pulmonary edema.

Current Medication

At this time, his medications consist of Lasix, digoxin, captopril, dobutamine, dopamine, aspirin and Persantine.

2-D Echo

Two-dimensional echocardiographic study showed marked four-chamber enlargement and severe left ventricular dysfunction. The leaflets of neither heterograft were seen clearly.

Doppler Echo

Doppler ultrasound study showed normal antegrade flow velocities and (probably) trivial aortic insufficiency. However, because of the size of the left ventricle, it was difficult to interrogate the mitral prosthesis for valvular insufficiency.

Color Flow Mapping

Color flow showed no prosthetic mitral valve insufficiency and detected moderate tricuspid insufficiency.

Disposition

With the possibility of prosthesis malfunction excluded, he was treated with and responded to experimental inotropic drugs. He was discharged showing significant symptomatic improvement.

APPENDIX C
CARDIAC DOPPLER CALCULATIONS

Joan C. Main, R.C.P.T., R.C.T.

THE DOPPLER EQUATION

Cardiac Doppler data are generally reported as velocity expressed in either meters or centimeters per second (Fig. C.1). Each system has its own calibration standards which are indicated on the screen and the hard copy.

On some instruments, Doppler shift is displayed in kilohertz (see Table C.1). Consequently, blood flow velocity must be calculated manually using the following equation:

$$V = \frac{F_d \times C}{2\,F_o \times \cos O} \qquad \text{Eq. C.1}$$

where V = blood flow velocity, F_d = Doppler shift from display, C = velocity of sound through tissue, F_o = transmit frequency, cos = cosine, and O = angle of blood flow to the ultrasound beam.

For example, if we use a 2.0 MHz transmit frequency and the angle of blood to the ultrasound beam is 45°, the cosine of this angle is 0.70.

The velocity of sound through tissue is 1540 m/sec. The observed Doppler shift is 4.6 kHz.

Therefore, the blood flow velocity is:

$$V = \frac{(4.6)\,(1540)}{2\,(2)\,(0.70)}$$

and

$$V = 1.8 \text{ m/sec.}$$

OBTAINING THE PRESSURE GRADIENT (FIG. C.2)

Transvalvular gradients can be obtained within the heart using either pulsed or continuous wave Doppler. However, pulsed wave Doppler can be used to record peak velocity only if velocities do not exceed the Nyquist limit of the instrument (Table C.2).

Many common conditions militate against the use of pulsed Doppler. Valvular obstructions usually produce accelerated forward flow velocities.

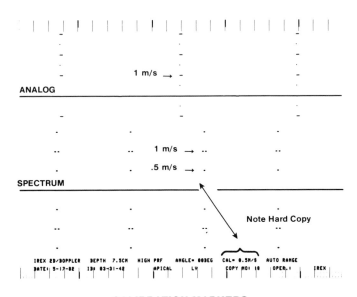

Figure C.1. An example of calibration markers. The scale settings vary with each system. When the spectrum is on the *CAL*, notation on the bottom of the strip chart recorder refers to the spectrum calibration.

CALIBRATION MARKERS

Table C.1. Conversion Table (kHz to m/sec; m/sec to kHz)

Probe Frequency (MHz)	Angle of Sound Beam			
	0	10	20	30
2.0	2.56/0.39	2.53/0.40	2.41/0.42	2.22/0.45
2.25	2.88/0.35	2.84/0.35	2.71/0.37	2.5/0.40
2.50	3.21/0.31	3.16/0.32	3.01/0.33	2.78/0.36
3.0	3.85/0.26	3.79/0.26	3.61/0.28	3.33/0.30
3.5	4.49/0.22	4.42/0.23	4.22/0.24	3.89/0.26
5.0	6.41/0.16	6.31/0.16	6.02/0.17	5.55/0.18
7.5	7.69/0.13	9.47/0.11	9.04/0.11	8.33/0.12
10	12.8/0.08	12.6/0.08	12.0/0.08	11.1/0.09
cos	1	0.98	0.94	0.87

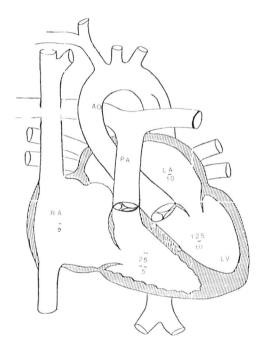

Figure C.2. An illustration of intracardiac chamber pressures. In normal flow, the pulmonary artery (*PA*) has the same systolic pressure as the right ventricle. Similarly, aortic (*AO*) systolic pressure normally is equal to left ventricular (*LV*) systolic pressure. *LA* = left atrium, *RA* = right atrium.

Regurgitant flows have a high velocity opposite to normal flow. To resolve these peak velocities, continuous wave Doppler must be used.

Velocity is related directly to the pressure drop across an orifice or obstruction. It is expressed by the formula in Figure C.3, where P is the pressure proximal (*1*) and distal (*2*) to the obstruction and V is the proximal (*1*) and distal (*2*) velocity. Viscous resistance in the blood is represented as R, and the mass density of blood is given by $\rho = 1.06 + 10^3$ kg/m³ (*4*).

Calculating the pressure drop across a valve uses a simplified Bernoulli's equation:

$$P_1 - P_2 = \overset{\downarrow}{4}\, V_m^2 \qquad \text{Eq. C.2}$$

where V_m is the maximum velocity found, $P_1 - P_2$ is the pressure drop, and *4* is the blood density constant.

In aortic stenosis, the peak velocity in systole

$$\underbrace{P_1 - P_2}_{} = \underbrace{\frac{1}{2}\rho\,(v_2^2 - v_1^2)}_{\text{CONVECTIVE ACCELERATION}} + \underbrace{\rho\int_1^2 \frac{d\bar{v}}{dt}\,d\bar{s}}_{\text{FLOW ACCELERATION}} + \underbrace{R\,(\bar{v})}_{\text{VISCOUS FRICTION}}$$

Figure C.3. Bernoulli's equation.

Table C.2. Normal Doppler Ultrasound Intracardiac Velocities

Location	Children	Adults
Mitral flow (m/sec)	1.00 (.08–1.3)	0.90 (0.6–1.3)
Tricuspid flow (m/sec)	0.60 (0.5–0.8)	0.50 (0.3–0.7)
Pulmonary artery (m/sec)	0.90 (0.7–1.1)	0.75 (0.6–0.9)
Left ventricle (m/sec)	1.00 (0.7–1.2)	0.90 (0.7–1.1)
Aorta (m/sec)	1.50 (1.2–1.8)	1.35 (1.0–1.7)

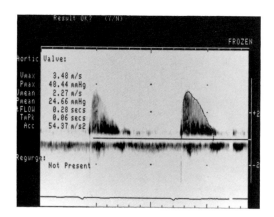

Figure C.4. An automatic tracing of the spectral display. Peak velocity, peak gradient, mean velocity, mean gradient, flow duration, time to peak, and acceleration are all displayed on the screen.

can be measured by tracing the spectral envelope (Fig. C.4). This system automatically calculates the peak pressure gradient (48.4 mm Hg).

CALCULATING THE PEAK PRESSURE GRADIENT IN AORTIC STENOSIS

Figure C.5 is an example of Doppler examination in a patient with aortic stenosis. The peak velocity is 3 m/sec, and the calculated peak pressure is 36 mm Hg.

CALCULATING THE SEVERITY OF AORTIC STENOSIS

A transvalvular gradient of more than 50 mm Hg represents significant aortic stenosis. However, a gradient of less than 50 mm Hg does not preclude significant stenosis. In the presence of severe left ventricular dysfunction, this lesser gradient can represent critical stenosis.

Recent investigations have attempted to develop quantitative Doppler methods for classifying aortic stenosis. This has resulted in several proposed formulas to calculate aortic valve area (AVA).

The first formula is:

$$AVA = \frac{SV}{(.09)(V_{max})(SEP)} \qquad \text{Eq. C.3}$$

where SV is the stroke volume and SEP is the systolic ejection period.

The second formula is:

$$A_1 \times V_1 = A_2 \times V_2 \qquad \text{Eq. C.4}$$

$$A_2 = \frac{A_1 \times V_1}{V_2}$$

A_1 and V_1 represent the cross-sectional area and the mean velocity at the nonstenotic portion in the left ventricular outflow tract, and A_2 and V_2 represent the cross-sectional area and the mean velocity at the aortic valve. An example of cal-

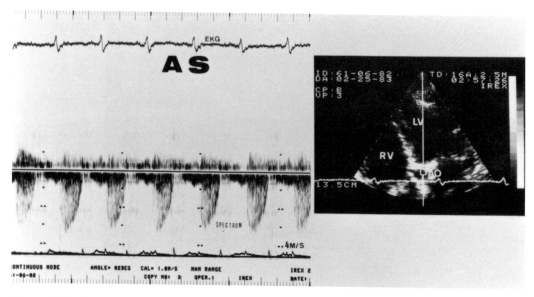

Figure C.5. A continuous wave Doppler beam is directed toward the left ventricular outflow tract. Using the audio signal, a 3 m/sec jet is recorded in this patient with aortic stenosis (*AS*). The pressure gradient is calculated by the formula, $P = 4V^2$. *AO* = aorta, *LV* = left ventricle, *RV* = right ventricle.

Figure C.6. Normal systolic flow from the descending aorta.

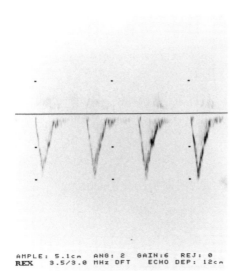

```
AMPLE:  5.1cm   ANG: 2   GAIN:6   REJ: 0
REX    3.5/3.0 MHz DFT     ECHO DEP: 12cm
```

culated AVA using this continuity equation appears in Figure C.11.

Another method used to evaluate severity involves the time it takes to reach peak velocity during systole as a reflection of severity of the lesion. The time to peak measurement provides additional qualitative information, since normal aortic peak velocity occurs in the first third of the systolic ejection period (SEP) (Fig. C.6). In patients with aortic stenosis, peak velocity usually occurs later in the SEP (Fig. C.7).

Figure C.8 shows two patients with the same peak velocity in systole (4.0 m/sec), with a peak pressure gradient of 64 mm Hg. However, the patient in Figure C.8, *upper recording*, has a longer time to peak, indicating a more severe lesion.

DOPPLER- VERSUS CARDIAC CATHETERIZATION-DERIVED GRADIENTS

Pressure gradients obtained at cardiac catheterization are measured by the peak-to-peak difference of the peak aortic pressure and the left ventricular pressure (Fig. C.9). The pressure gradient obtained by cardiac Doppler is the measurement of instantaneous pressure drop across the valve (Fig. C.10).

In moderate to severe aortic stenosis, differences are minimal between Doppler- and catheterization-derived gradients. This is because peak left ventricular (LV) pressure occurs later in systole. In patients with mild aortic stenosis or a combined lesion (such as aortic insufficiency) where detected velocity in the LV outflow tract may be increased, peak-to-peak and instantaneous gradients may show a significant difference. This can be minimized by calculating the mean pressure gradient or using a more complete Bernoulli equation.

The standard equation for Doppler determination of gradient is:

$$\text{Gradient} = 4\,(V_2^2 - V_1^2) \qquad \text{Eq. C.5}$$

where V_2 is the maximal transvalvular aortic gra-

Figure C.7. Flow velocities (*left* and *right*) are identical. However, the peak velocity indicated on the *left* occurs later in systole than that indicated on the *right*. This indicates a more severe lesion for the patient indicated on the *left*.

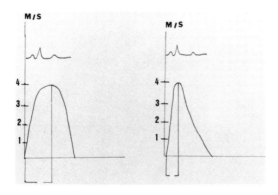

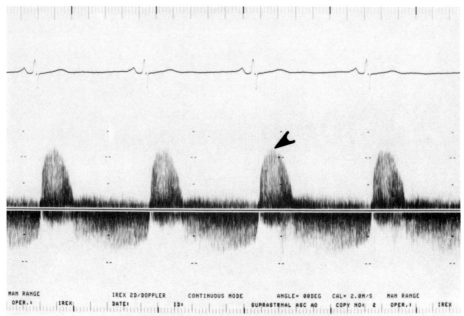

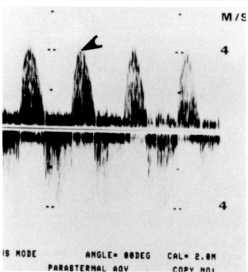

Figure C.8. *Upper recording*, Aortic flow, at a velocity of 4 m/sec, recorded from the suprasternal notch. Even though the peak gradient in both the *upper* and *lower recordings* is 64 mm Hg, the time to peak is shorter in the *lower recording*. This indicates the aortic stenosis is less severe as indicated in the *upper recording*. (Courtesy of Nancy Dalton, University of California at San Diego.)

CATH

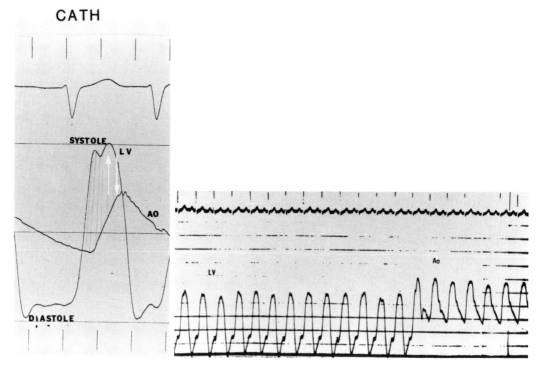

Figure C.9. Gradients determined by catheterization are measured as peak-to-peak gradients. *AO* = aorta, *LV* = left ventricle.

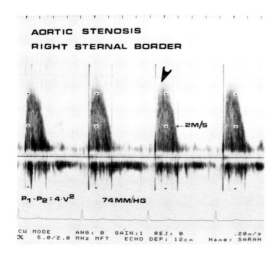

Figure C.10. Using the Doppler technique to calculate a pressure gradient across a valve, the clinician measures the instantaneous pressure drop across the orifice.

dient by continuous wave Doppler and V_1 is velocity in the LV outflow tract by pulsed wave Doppler.

Using this formula on the information in Figure C.11, V_2 is 3.5 m/sec and V_1 is 1.4 m/sec. The gradient is then given as:

$$\text{Gradient} = 4\,[(3.5)^2 - (1.4)^2]$$
$$= 4\,(12 - 1.96)$$
$$= 40.16 \text{ mm Hg}$$

CALCULATING THE MEAN PRESSURE GRADIENT

Several commercial systems automatically calculate mean velocity. The user simply traces the spectral envelope and the calculations are displayed on the screen (Fig. C.12).

The mean pressure gradient can be calculated manually. Several peak velocities must be taken along the spectral envelope. The pressure gradient is calculated at each point by using $P = 4V_m^2$. The mean pressure gradient is obtained by

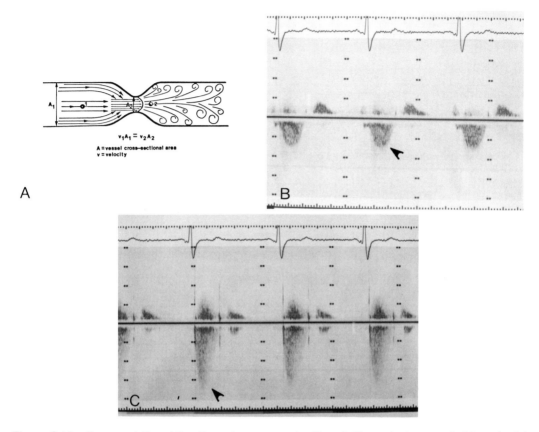

Figure C.11. Representation of flow through a narrowed orifice. *A*, Flow velocity recorded from the left ventricular outflow tract (V_1 = 1.4 m/sec). *B*, Flow velocity recorded using continuous wave Doppler (V_2 = 3.5 m/sec). The calculated gradient is 40.16 mm Hg. In this patient (A_1 = 2.2), the cross-sectional area is 3.8 cm². Using the formula $A_1V_1 = A_2V_2$, the calculated aortic valve area is 1.52 cm².

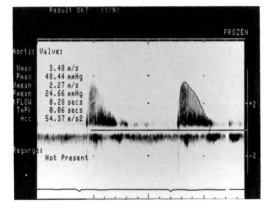

Figure C.12. Automatic calculation of the mean gradient. Each point along the tracing is calculated using $4V^2$. The mean of these calculations is reported.

summing the gradients and dividing by the number of points sampled.

Table C.3 calculates the mean pressure gradient in a patient with aortic stenosis (Fig. C.13).

Table C.3. Mean Pressure Gradient for Patient Shown in Figure C.13

V_m at Sampled Points (m/sec)	Pressure Gradient at Sample Points (mm Hg)[a]
1.2.0	16
2.3.0	36
3.4.0	64
4.4.2	70.56
5.3.0	36
6.2.0	16
Total	238.56

[a]Mean pressure gradient = 238.56/6 = 39.76 mm Hg.

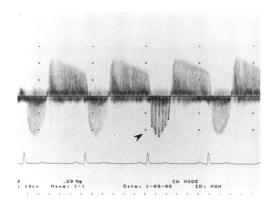

Figure C.13. An example of a patient with aortic stenosis and aortic regurgitation. The mean pressure gradient across the valve was calculated manually.

Figure C.14 is an example of a patient with mitral stenosis. The peak velocity is 2 m/sec, with an instantaneous pressure gradient of 16 mm Hg. The calculated mean pressure gradient is 1.2 mm Hg.

AORTIC INSUFFICIENCY

Doppler quantitation of aortic insufficiency is still under investigation. This procedure requires pulsed wave Doppler to map the flow, continuous wave Doppler to detect the peak velocity, and color Doppler to visualize flow.

Color Doppler is being used to provide a less qualitative assessment of the severity of aortic insufficiency. This technique uses the extension and width of the flow area in relationship to the left ventricle. Color Doppler imaging visualizes flow throughout the cardiac cycle and in several tomographic views.

Figure C.15 shows a patient with moderate aortic insufficiency determined by catheterization. The peak velocity of the aortic insufficiency jet is 4.0 m/sec.

A new method to quantify severity of aortic insufficiency involves calculating the regurgitant fraction using spectral Doppler. The regurgitant fraction (RF) is derived from the difference between the forward stroke volume at the aortic valve (ASV) and the pulmonic valve (PSV). The RF is calculated by the equation:

$$RF = \frac{ASV - PSV}{ASV} \qquad Eq.\ C.6$$

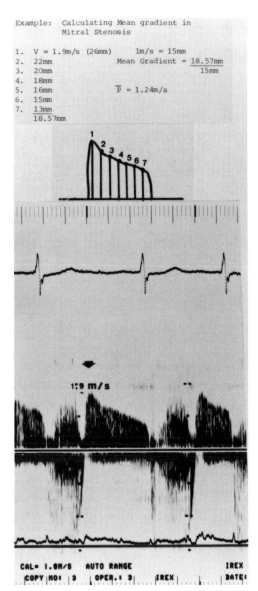

Figure C.14. An example of a patient with mitral stenosis and mitral regurgitation. Several points along the spectrum are measured, the pressure gradient is calculated, and a mean pressure gradient is computed.

STROKE VOLUME BY DOPPLER

Doppler calculation of stroke volume is derived from the flow velocity integral or the area under the Doppler spectral envelope. Flow velocity in-

Figure C.15. An example of a patient with moderate aortic insufficiency (*AI*). *A*, The spectral display demonstrates a 4 m/sec jet. *B*, The color flow Doppler shows the jet extending across the anterior leaflet of the mitral valve. *AS* = aortic stenosis. See this figure in Color Atlas.

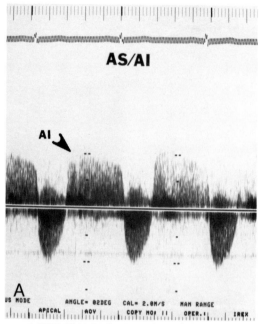

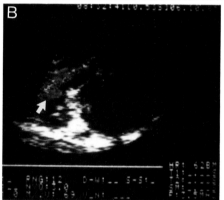

tegral is directly proportional to stroke volume and is expressed in units of distance (centimeters). Several commercially available systems can calculate the flow velocity integral, or it can be estimated by the equation:

Flow velocity integral (FVI)
$$= \frac{(PV) \times (ET)}{2} \quad \text{Eq. C.7}$$

where PV = peak velocity (cm/sec), ET = ejection time (seconds), and SV = (FVI) × (CSA) or

$$SV = \frac{(ET)(PV) \times CSA}{2}$$

where ET is ejection-time and CSA is cross-sectional area.

Figure C.16 shows flow in the ascending aorta, visualized from the suprasternal notch. The flow velocity integral is displayed automatically.

CALCULATING THE LEFT VENTRICULAR END-DIASTOLIC PRESSURE

In the presence of aortic insufficiency (AI), left ventricular end-diastolic pressure (LVEDP) is calculated by the formula:

LVEDP = ΔP (AI jet)
           − Diastolic cuff pressure   Eq. C.8

Figure C.17 shows a patient with aortic stenosis

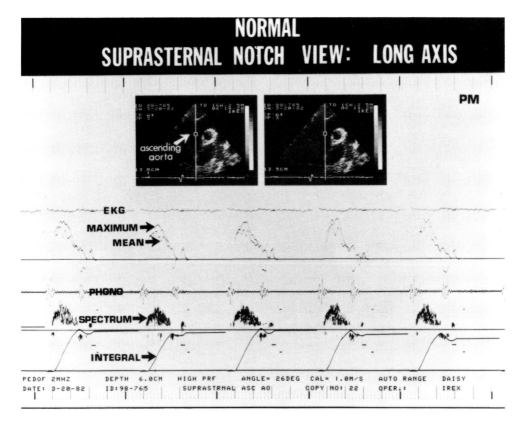

Figure C.16. A suprasternal notch view of the ascending aorta.

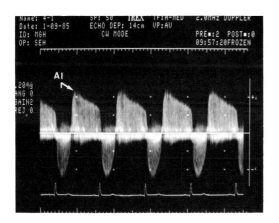

Figure C.17. An example of a patient with aortic stenosis (displayed *below* the baseline) and aortic insufficiency (*AI*) (*above* the baseline). The peak velocity is 5 m/sec for the aortic stenosis jet and 5 m/sec for the aortic insufficiency jet. The calculated left ventricular end-diastolic pressure is 10 mm Hg.

and aortic insufficiency. The peak velocity, recorded from the apex of the aortic insufficiency jet, is 5 m/sec. The patient's blood pressure is 140/90. Using $P = 4V_m^2$ and the blood pressure, left ventricular end-diastolic pressure can be calculated (Fig. C.16).

PULMONIC STENOSIS AND INSUFFICIENCY

Peak and mean pressure gradients are calculated just as in aortic stenosis. Pulmonic insufficiency can be mapped using pulsed wave Doppler and visualized by color flow imaging (Fig. C.18). Quantitative determination of pulmonary hypertension is still investigational. Color Doppler imaging has added another tool to determine the hemodynamic state of patients with pulmonary hypertension.

MITRAL STENOSIS

Figure C.19 shows the typical flow pattern of mitral stenosis, recorded from the cardiac apex.

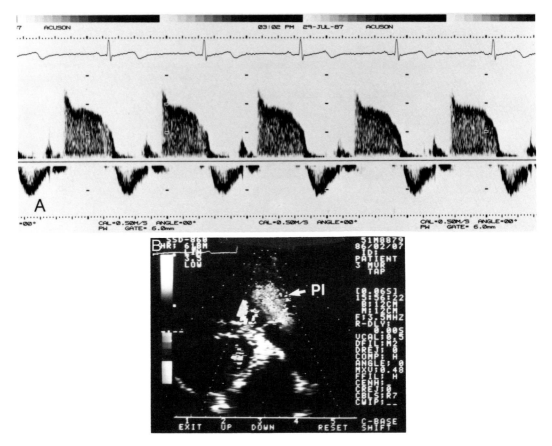

Figure C.18. Spectral display of a patient with pulmonary insufficiency, indicated by the broad spectrum *above* the baseline in diastole. *B,* Color flow Doppler display of the pulmonary insufficiency (*PI*) jet, showing variance in flow. See this figure in Color Atlas.

The recording was made in pulsed wave with a peak velocity of 2.0 m/sec. The initial velocity in diastole is higher than normal. This valvular obstruction is significant because velocity decreases slowly prior to atrial contraction.

Figure C.20 demonstrates the calculation of peak pressure gradient of the mitral valve in a patient with mitral stenosis. Peak pressure gradient can also be calculated in mitral stenosis by use of the Bernoulli equation (Fig. C.21).

Color flow imaging demonstrates a mitral stenosis jet in red (Fig. C.22). A continuous wave Doppler beam placed in the center of that jet records peak velocity (2.5 m/sec in this example).

Figure C.23 shows a view from the apex of a patient with mitral stenosis and mitral regurgitation. Table C.4 calculates the mean pressure gradient in this patient.

PRESSURE HALF-TIME FOR CALCULATING MITRAL VALVE AREA

Pressure gradients are affected by heart rate; i.e., the faster the heart rate, the higher the observed pressure drop. Doppler may show a day-to-day variation in pressure drop, especially in atrial fibrillation. Hatle et al. described a method where the time is measured from the initial pressure drop across an obstructed orifice to half that pressure. This is termed pressure half-time.

Pressure half-time can be obtained by dividing maximal velocity by 1.4 (the square root of two) and measuring the time from peak velocity to where this velocity decrease occurs. Pressure half-time correlates with mitral valve area and is independent of flow across the valve. In nonobstructive conditions, the half-time will be between

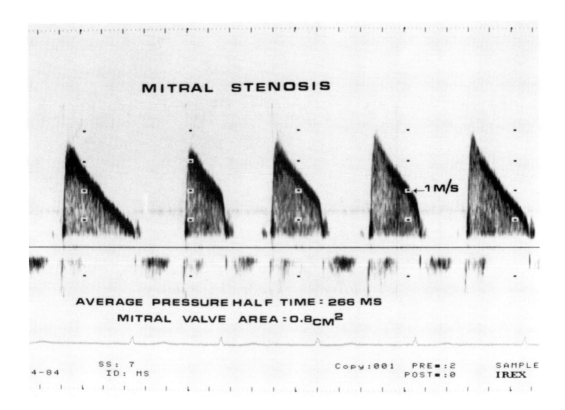

Figure C.19. An example of a patient with mitral stenosis and atrial fibrillation. The pressure half-time averaged over several beats is 266 msec, and the mitral valve area is 0.8 cm^2.

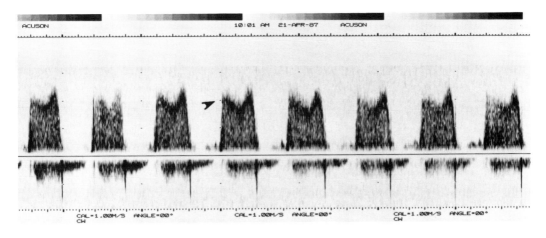

Figure C.20. Mitral stenosis and normal sinus rhythm.

Figure C.21. Mitral stenosis (*MS*) with a calculated pressure gradient of 19.4 mm Hg across the valve. (Courtesy of Nancy Dalton.)

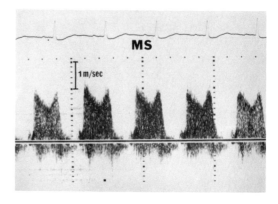

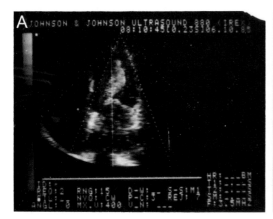

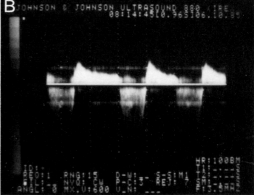

Figure C.22. A color flow Doppler display of a mitral stenotic jet (*A*) with a bright red flame-like appearance. The peak velocity (2.5 m/sec) is recorded by placing the continuous wave beam in the center of the jet. See this figure in Color Atlas.

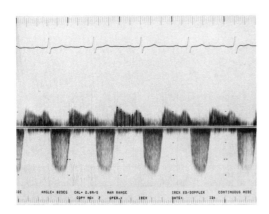

Figure C.23. Mitral stenosis jet recorded from the apex. (Courtesy of Nancy Dalton.)

20 and 60 msec. In the presence of an obstruction, the half-time is greater than 100 msec.

A good estimate of mitral valve area (in square centimeters) is given by the formula:

$$\text{Mitral valve area} = \frac{220}{P_{1/2}T} \qquad \text{Eq. C.9}$$

where 220 msec = 1 cm².

This same formula can be used for tricuspid valves and prosthetic valves. Differentiation between obstruction and regurgitation then depends upon the length of the pressure half-time.

Pressure Half-Time Calculation Method

There are six steps in the pressure half-time calculation method:

Table C.4. Mean Pressure Gradient for Patient Shown in Figure C.23

Peak Velocities (m/sec)	Calculated Peak Gradient (mm Hg)
1. $V_m = 2.5$	25
2. $V_m = 2.0$	16
3. $V_m = 1.9$	14
4. $V_m = 1.5$	9
5. $V_m = 1.6$	10
6. $V_n = 2.1$	17
7. $V_m = 2.0$	16
8. $V_m = 1.0$	4

TOTAL = 111/8 = 13.8 mm Hg

1. The peak velocity is the distance from the baseline to the initial peak of the spectrum.
2. Peak velocity divided by the square root of 2 (1.4) yields half the peak pressure difference ($V_{max}/1.4$).
3. A horizontal line is drawn at the point of the pressure half.
4. A line is drawn down the slope of the velocity curve, similar to the procedure of M-mode E-F slope determination (Figure C.24*D*).
5. The pressure half-time is the distance between the point of the initial peak velocity to the point where the lines drawn in Steps 3 and 4 intercept.
6. This distance is then measured against time markers.

Figure C.25 shows an automatically calculated pressure half-time using a commercially available ultrasound system. Figure C.26 is an example of manual calculation of pressure half-time in a patient with mitral stenosis and mitral regurgitation.

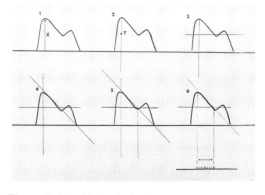

Figure C.24. Method of calculation for pressure half-time.

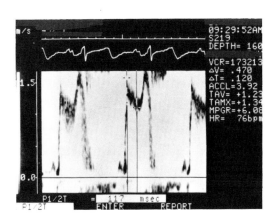

Figure C.25. Pressure half-time calculated automatically.

MITRAL REGURGITATION

There are no formulas to determine accurately by Doppler the regurgitant fraction from a mitral regurgitant jet. However, combined continuous wave, pulsed wave, and color flow imaging can assess severity of regurgitation. Relative changes can be determined by serial examination.

Although criteria differ among laboratories, a rating scheme has emerged for qualitatively assessing the severity of mitral regurgitation. The following are general criteria:

1+ Flow detected at the level of the mitral valve annulus
2+ Flow extending ~2 cm into the left atrium
3+ Flow extending >2 cm into the left atrium and lasting most of systole
4+ Flow extending back to the pulmonary veins and lasting throughout systole

Pulsed wave Doppler is used to map regurgitant flow back into the left atrium. Continuous wave Doppler records the peak velocity.

Figure C.27 shows a 5 m/sec jet mapped as far as 2 cm into the left atrium. Figure C.28 demonstrates a 3 m/sec mitral regurgitant jet mapped back to the pulmonary veins. The flow profiles are quite different: The first jet peaks earlier than the second. Using the above criteria, we would consider the lesion shown in Figure C.27 to be the more significant.

Figure C.29 is an example of trace mitral regurgitation, normally seen with prosthetic valves.

Color flow imaging allows visualization of a regurgitant jet. This additional Doppler modality

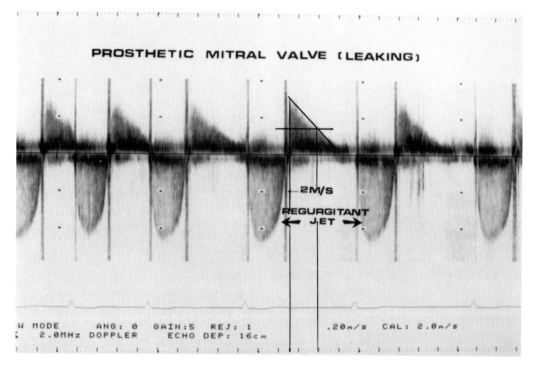

Figure C.26. A patient with a heterograft mitral prosthetic valve and mitral regurgitation. Peak velocity across the valve is 3.3 m/sec with a pressure gradient of 43.56 mm Hg.

allows investigation of the ratio of flow area to chamber size. Using the width and length of the jet, the severity of the lesion can be assessed. Color flow imaging is useful in mitral regurgitation (Figs. C.30 and C.31), aortic insufficiency (Fig. C.32), pulmonary insufficiency (Fig. C.33), and tricuspid regurgitation (Fig. C.34).

TRICUSPID STENOSIS

Mean and peak pressure gradients are calculated in the tricuspid valve by the same technique

used in the aortic and mitral valves. Also, the pressure half-time method employed to determine mitral valve area is being investigated for use on the tricuspid valve.

TRICUSPID REGURGITATION

The characteristic jet of tricuspid regurgitation is detected easily by Doppler. A high velocity regurgitant jet can indicate high pressure in the right ventricle and pulmonary artery. Doppler-calculated right ventricular systolic pressure

Figure C.27. A mitral regurgitant (*MR*) jet of 5 m/sec, peaking very early in systole.

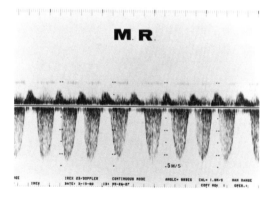

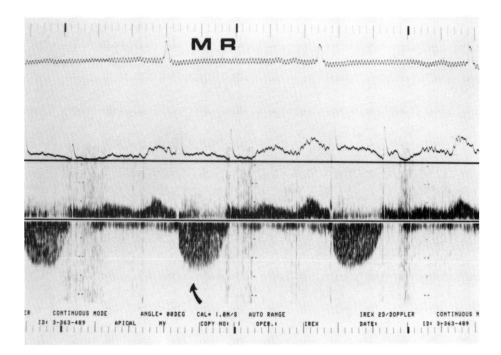

Figure C.28. A patient with a mitral regurgitant (*MR*) jet, also of 5 m/sec, peaking much later in systole. This indicates a more severe lesion than that seen in Figure C.27.

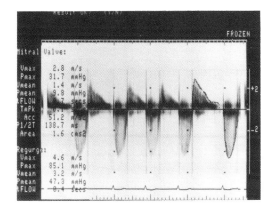

Figure C.29. A prosthetic mitral valve with a mitral regurgitant jet of 4 m/sec.

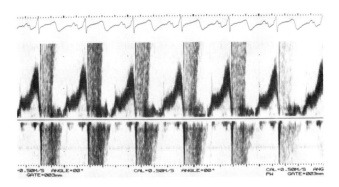

Figure C.30. An example of pulsed wave Doppler mapping a mitral regurgitant jet back into the left atrium. A typical disturbed flow pattern is seen in systole.

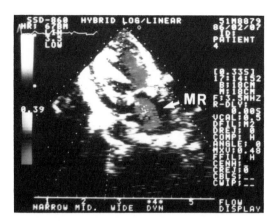

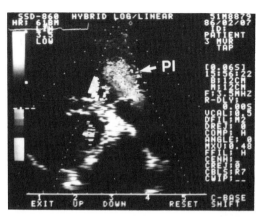

Figure C.31. The mosaic pattern seen in the left atrium is characteristic of mitral regurgitation (*MR*). See this figure in Color Atlas.

Figure C.33. An example of pulmonary insufficiency (*PI*). The color flow Doppler shows a wide jet in the right ventricular outflow tract. See this figure in Color Atlas.

(RVSP) has been found to correlate well with invasively derived systolic pressure. The Doppler formula is:

$$RVSP = \overline{RA} + 4V_m^2 \qquad \text{Eq. C.10}$$

$$P_1 - P_2 = 4V_m^2$$

where V_m = maximum velocity during systole in the right atrium (regurgitant jet), P_1 = peak right ventricular pressure, and P_2 = right atrial pressure (jugular venous pressure normally 5–6 mm Hg).

If the jugular venous pressure by physical examination is not available, the height of the ve-

nous pulse in the neck can be used to estimate right atrial systolic pressure. As a general rule, add 1 mm Hg for each centimeter above the clavicle.

Figure C.35 demonstrates a right atrial mean pressure of 5 mm Hg. The right systolic pressure calculated by Doppler is:

$$\text{Mean RA} = 5 \text{ mm Hg}$$
$$V = 3 \text{ m/sec}$$
$$P_1 - P_2 = 4V^2$$
$$RVSP = RA + 4V^2$$
$$= 5 + 4 \ (3)^3$$
$$RVSP = 39 \text{ mm Hg}$$

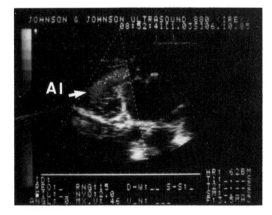

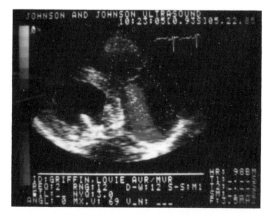

Figure C.32. An example of aortic insufficiency (*AI*). The jet can be seen extending across the anterior leaflet of the mitral valve in diastole. See this figure in Color Atlas.

Figure C.34. An example of tricuspid regurgitation. The color flow Doppler shows a jet extending all the way to the pulmonary veins. See this figure in Color Atlas.

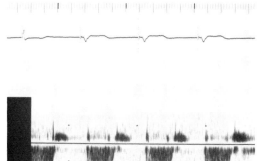

Figure C.35. A patient with tricuspid regurgitation secondary to mitral stenosis (Courtesy of Nancy Dalton).

Figure C.36 demonstrates a mean right atrial pressure of 7 mm Hg and a peak velocity of 3.5 m/sec in the right atrium. The RVSP calculation, demonstrated below, yields a value of 56 mm Hg.

Mean right atrial pressure = 7 mm Hg

$$V_m = 3.5 \text{ m/sec}$$
$$RVSP = \overline{RA} = 4V_m^2$$
$$RVSP = 7 + 4 (3.5)^2$$
$$RVSP = 56 \text{ mm Hg}$$

CALCULATING CARDIAC OUTPUT BY DOPPLER ECHOCARDIOGRAPHY

Cardiac output—or the product of stroke volume (SV) and heart rate (HR)—can be approximated by Doppler-derived stroke volume. The flow velocity integral, or the area under the Doppler spectral envelope, is multiplied by the cross-sectional area of the vessel to yield stroke volume. The problem is obtaining an accurate cross-sectional area (CSA), and much research attention has been focused on this question. The formula for Doppler derivation of cardiac output is:

$$SV = \text{Flow velocity integral} \qquad \text{Eq. C.11}$$
$$\times \text{ cross } = \text{ sectional area}$$

$$CSA = pi \times (D/2)^2 \qquad \text{Eq. C.12}$$

where pi(π) = 3.14 D = vessel diameter.

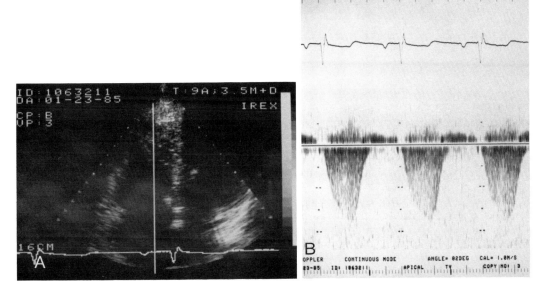

Figure C.36. Using the two-dimensional image to direct the continuous wave beam into the right atrium, a tricuspid regurgitant jet is revealed.

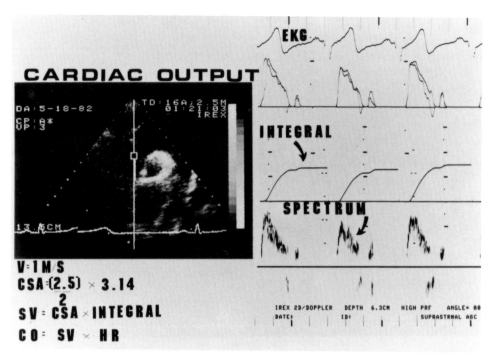

Figure C.37. Example of an automatic (flow velocity) integral.

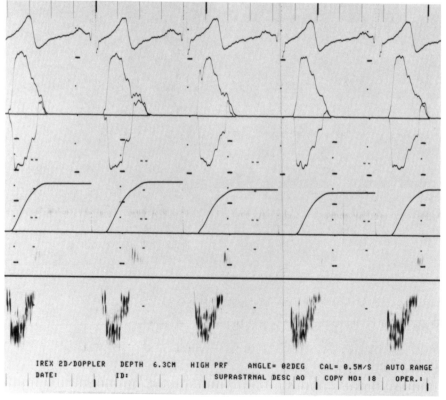

Figure C.38. Cardiac output can be calculated using the cross-sectional area of the vessel, the flow velocity integral (*area under curve*), and the heart rate.

Cardiac output = Stroke volume   Eq. C.13
× heart rate

The area under the spectral envelope is automatically calculated by some commercially available systems (Fig. C.37). The formula for calculating the integral manually is:

$$\text{Integral} = \frac{V_{max} \times \text{ET}}{2} \quad \text{Eq. C.14}$$

The diameter (D) should be derived from the area of the Doppler interrogation. Several areas can be used, the aortic, mitral, or pulmonic. You must take into account that the geometric flow area can be different than the effective flow area. Doppler information allows us to serially follow a patient and calculate the relative changes in cardiac output.

Figure C.38 shows how cardiac output can be calculated manually. The vessel diameter is 2.3 cm, heart rate is 70 beats/min, ET is 0.24 sec, and V is 0.9 m/sec.

$$\text{CSA} = \text{pi} \times (D/2)^2$$
$$\text{CSA} = 3.14 \times (2.3/2)^2$$
$$\text{CSA} = 3.14 \times 1.32$$
$$\text{CSA} = 4.15 \text{ cm}^2$$

$$\text{Integral} = V_m \times \text{ET}/2$$
$$= \frac{(0.90) \times (0.24)}{2}$$
$$= 0.108$$

Stroke volume = CSA × integral
= 4.15 × 0.108
= .4482 1/min

Cardiac output = SV × HR
CO = .4482 × 70
CO = 3.13 1/min

REFERENCES

Hatle L, Angelsen BAJ: *Doppler Ultrasound in Cardiology.* Philadelphia, Lea & Febiger, 1982.

Stam RB, Martin RP: Use of continuous wave Doppler for evaluation of stenotic aortic and mitral valves. *Am J Cardiol* 49:943, 1982.

Skjaerpe T, Hatle L: Diagnosis and assessment of tricuspid regurgitation with Doppler ultrasound. In Rijsterborgh H (ed): *Echocardiology: Developments in Cardiovascular Medicine.* The Netherlands, Martinus Nijhoff, Kluwer Academic, 1981.

Hatle L, Angelsen BAJ, Tromsdal A: Non-invasive assessment of atrioventricular pressure-time by Doppler ultrasound. *Circulation* 60:1097–1104, 1979.

Hatle L, Brubakk A, Tromsdal A, Angelsen B: Non-invasive assessment of pressure drop in mitral stenosis by Doppler ultrasound. *Br Heart J* 40:131–140, 1978.

COLOR ATLAS

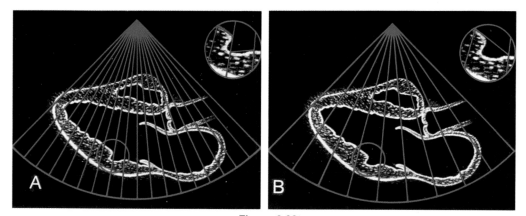

Figure 2.29.

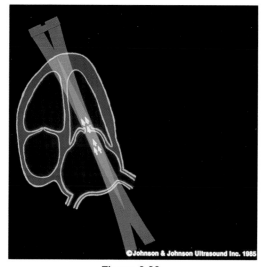

Figure 2.39.

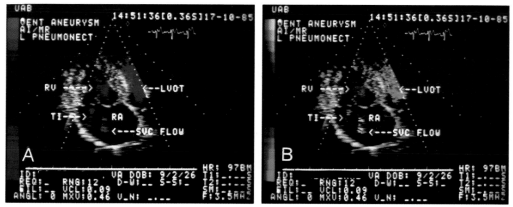

Figure 2.48.

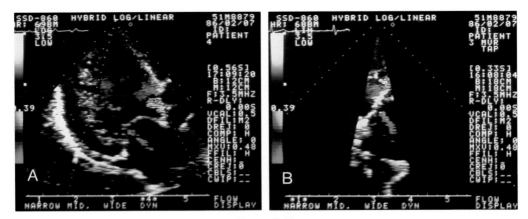

Figure 2.49.

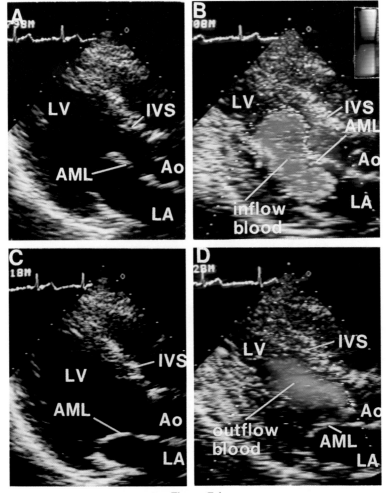

Figure 7.1.

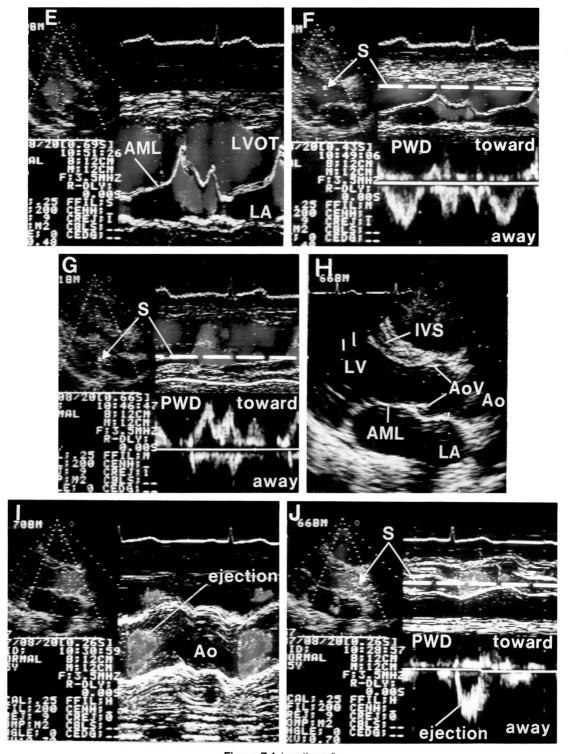

Figure 7.1 (*continued*).

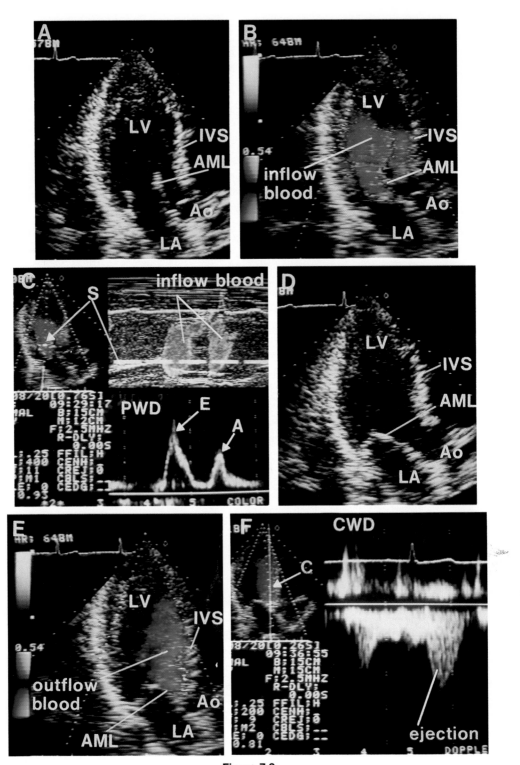

Figure 7.2.

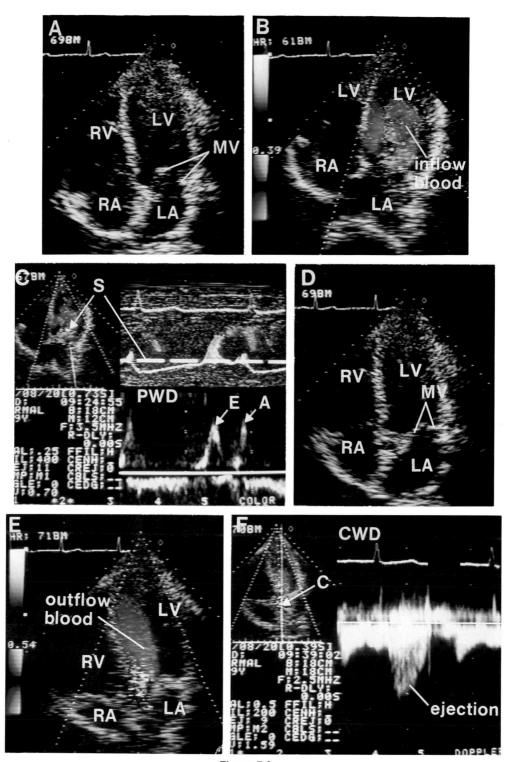

Figure 7.3.

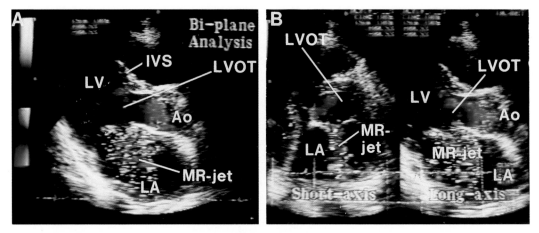

Figure 7.4.

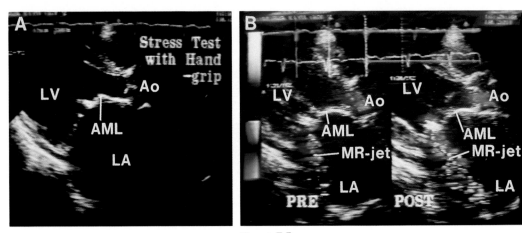

Figure 7.5.

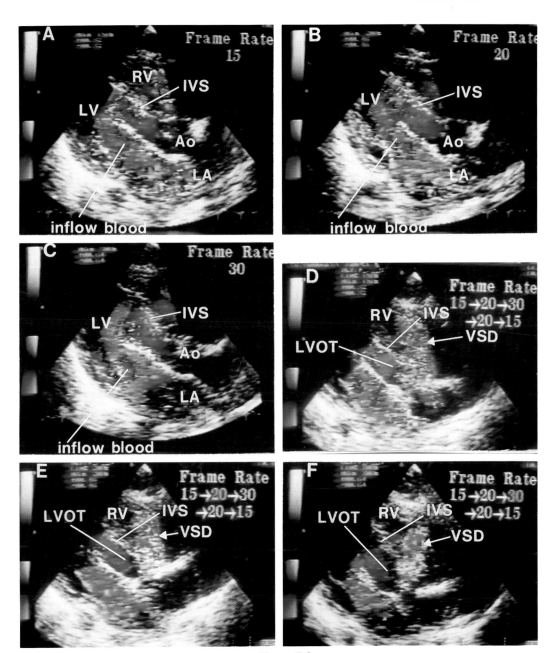

Figure 7.6.

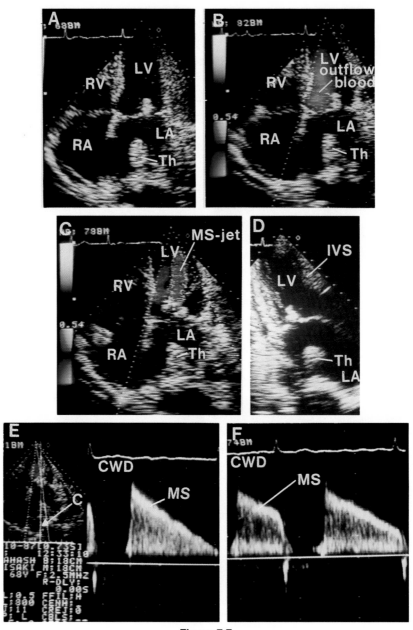

Figure 7.7.

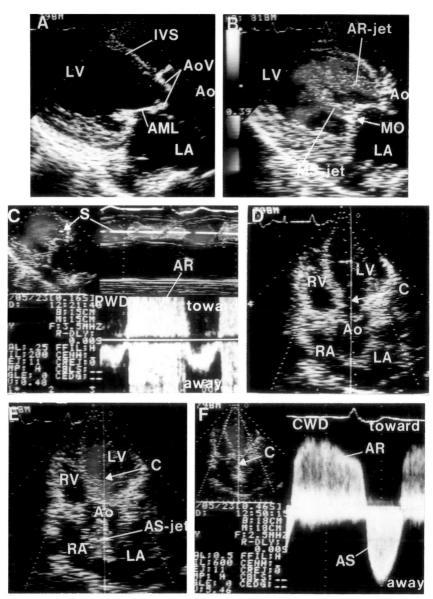

Figure 7.8.

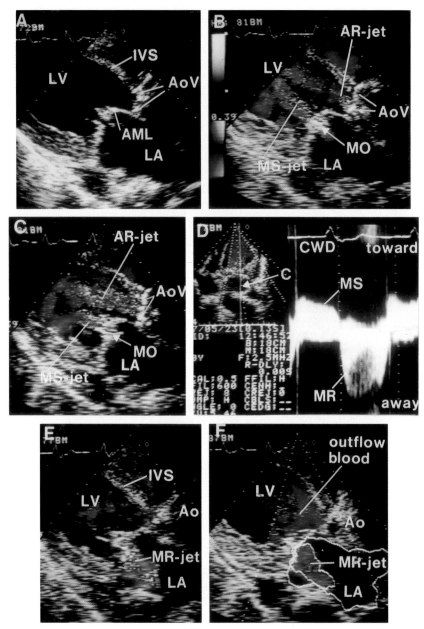

Figure 7.9.

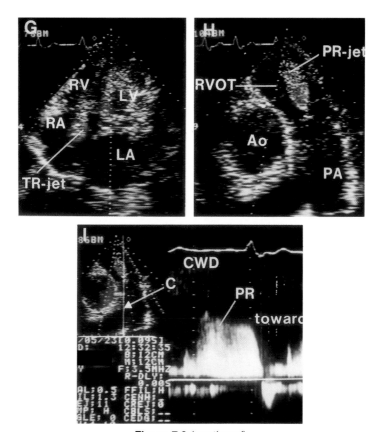

Figure 7.9 (*continued*).

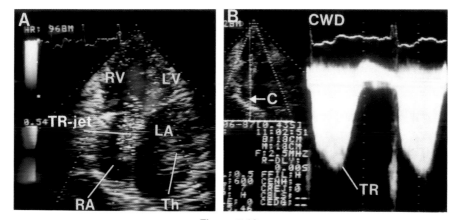

Figure 7.12.

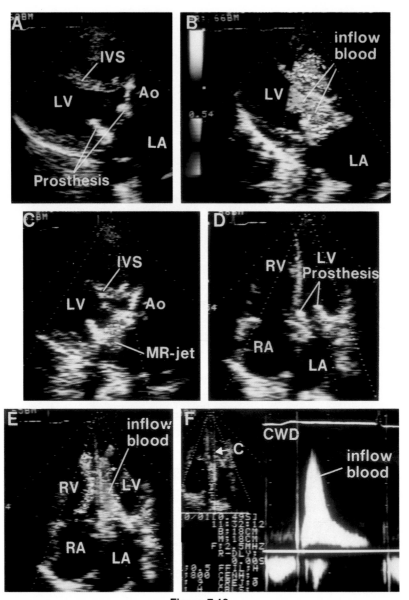

Figure 7.13.

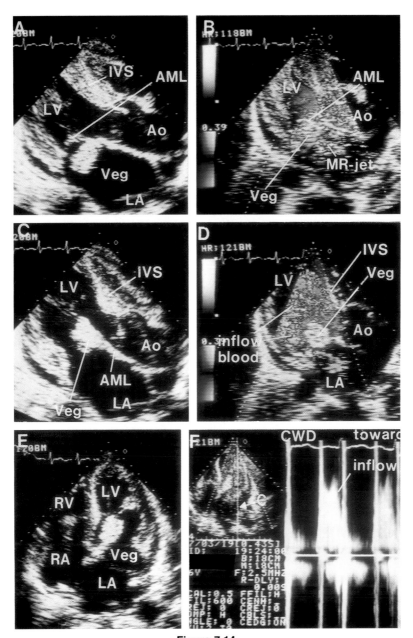

Figure 7.14.

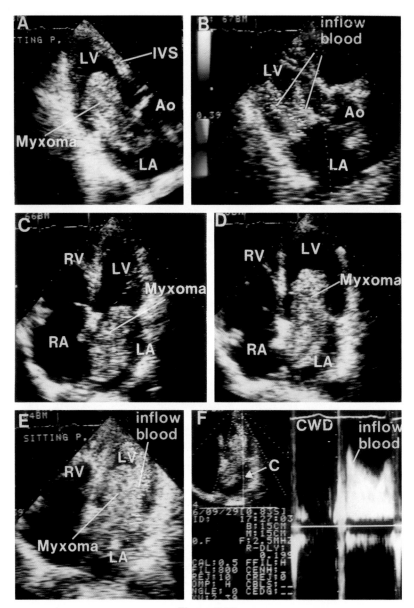

Figure 7.15.

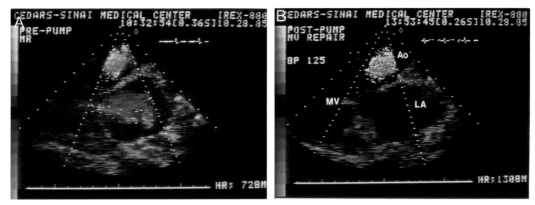

Figure 8.4.

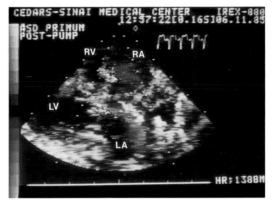

Figure 8.5.

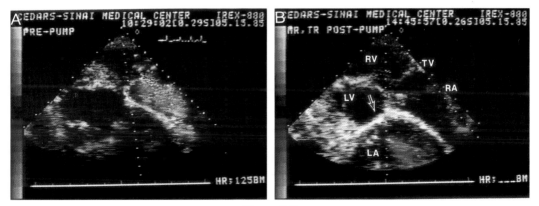

Figure 8.7.

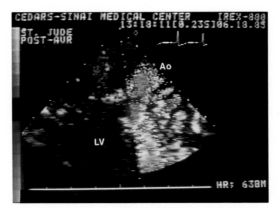

Figure 8.8.

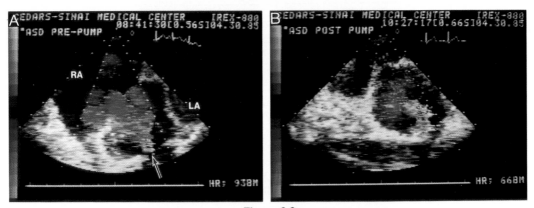

Figure 8.9.

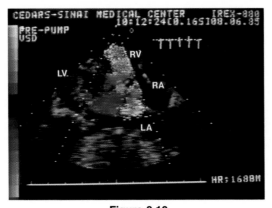

Figure 8.10.

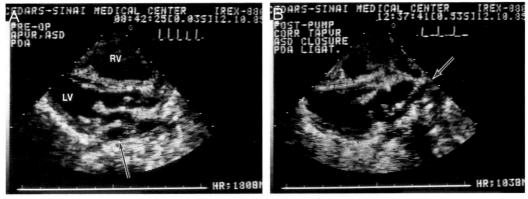

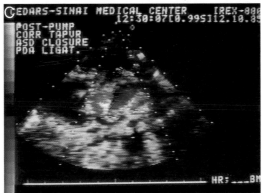

Figure 8.11.

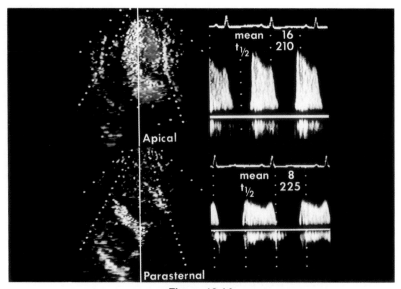

Figure 12.14.

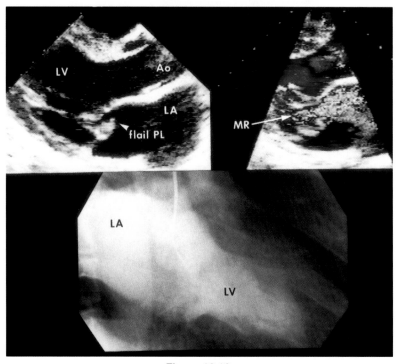

Figure 12.16.

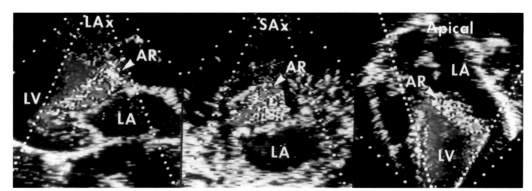

Figure 12.17.

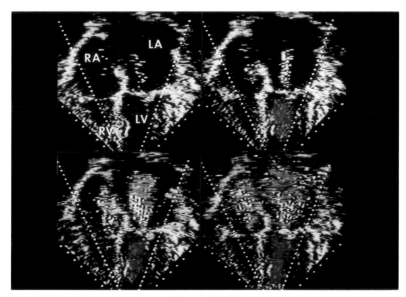

Figure 12.18.

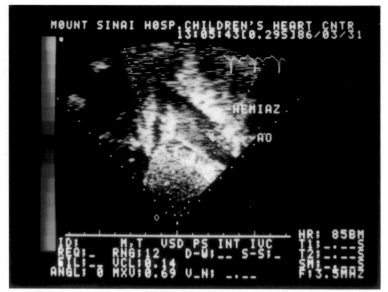

Figure 23.1*E.*

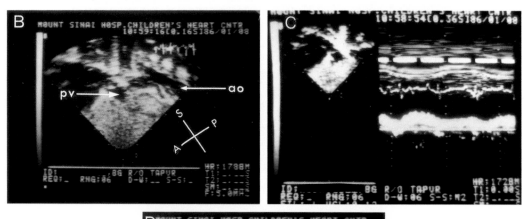

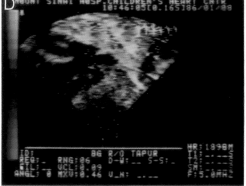

Figure 23.2, *B, C, D.*

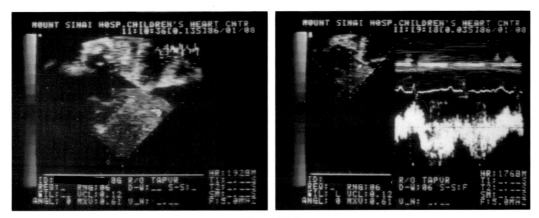

Figure 23.2.

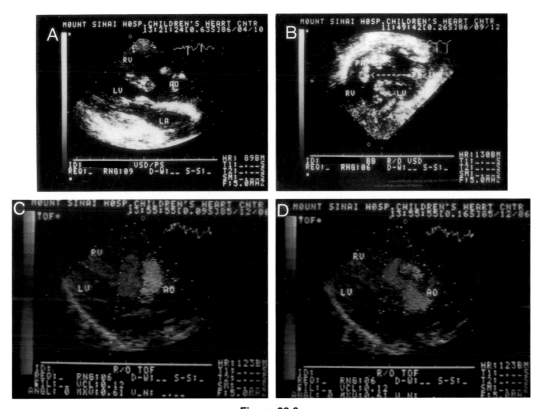

Figure 23.6.

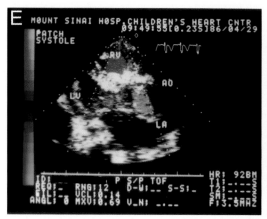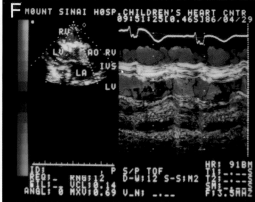

23.6, *E–F*

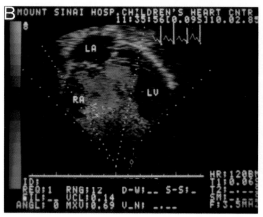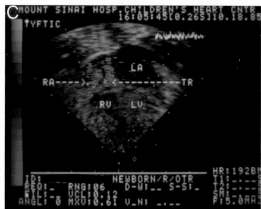

Figure 23.7.

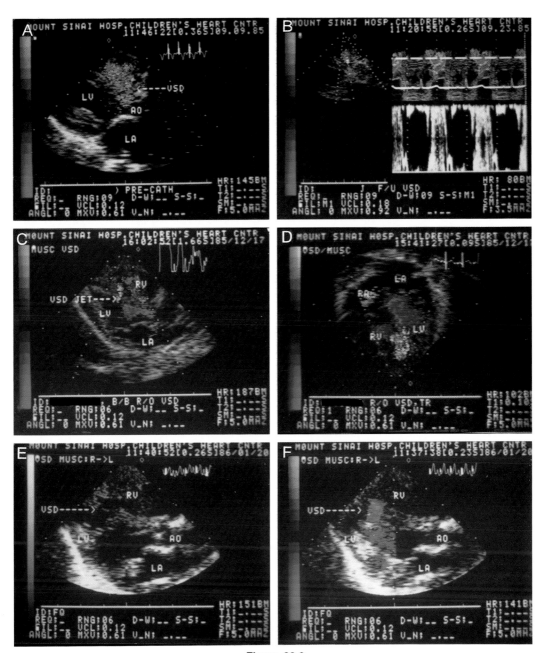

Figure 23.9.

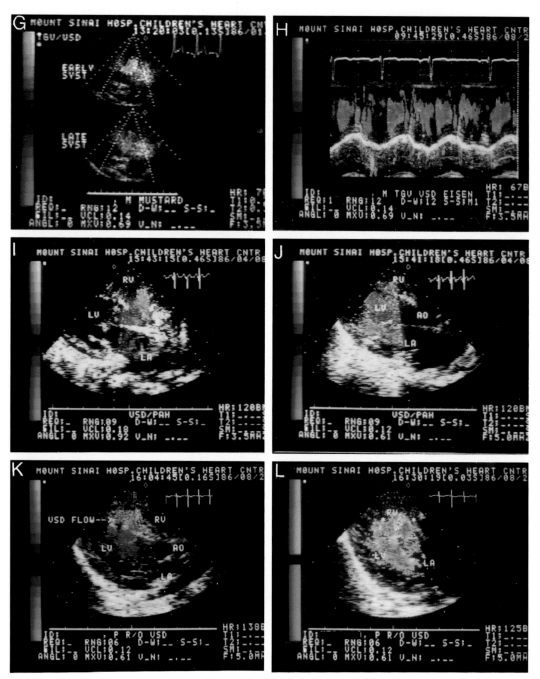

Figure 23.9 (continued).

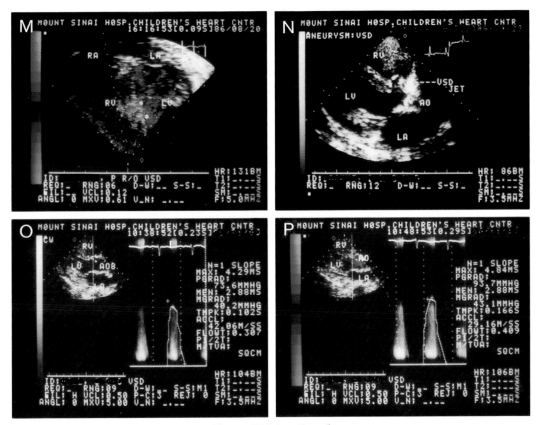

Figure 23.9 (*continued*).

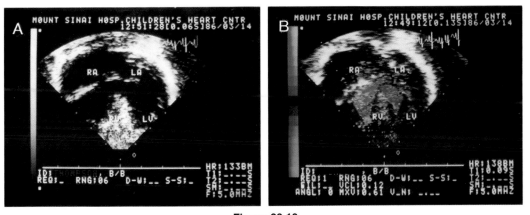

Figure 23.10.

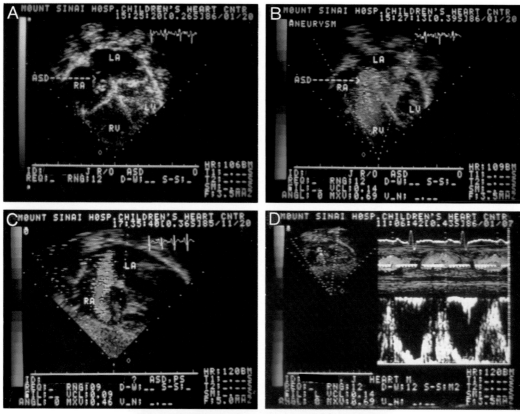

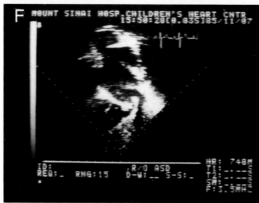

Figure 23.11, *A–D and F.*

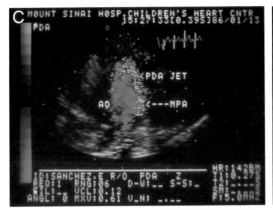

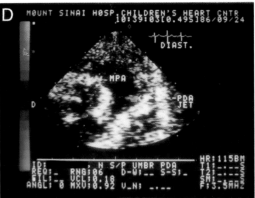

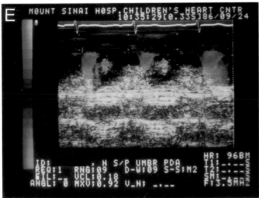

Figure 23.12, *C–E.*

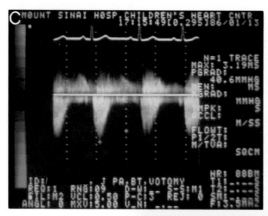

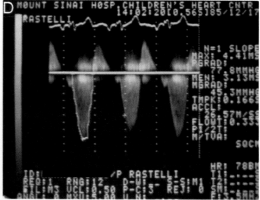

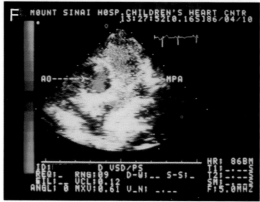

Figure 23.14, *C, D,* and *F.*

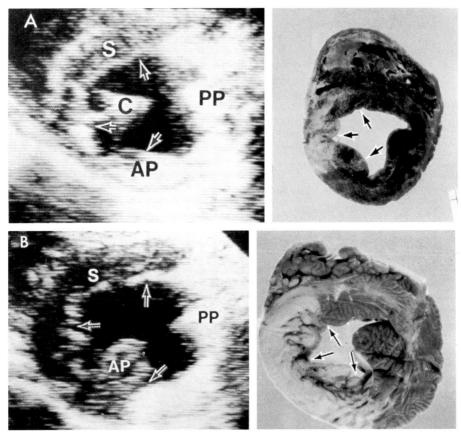

Figure 26.17.

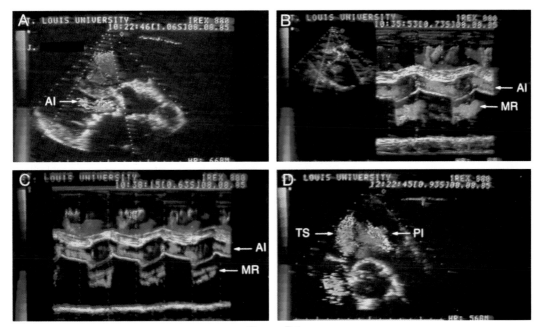

Figure B.1.

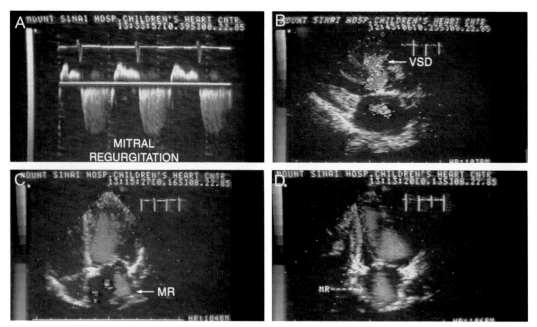

Figure B.2.

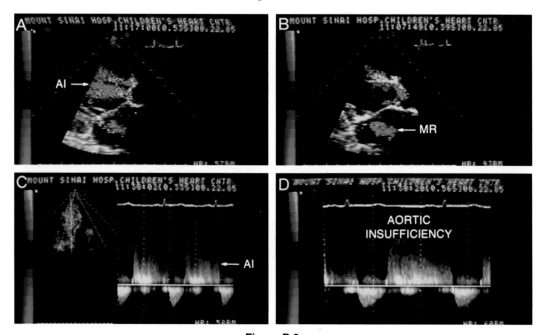

Figure B.3.

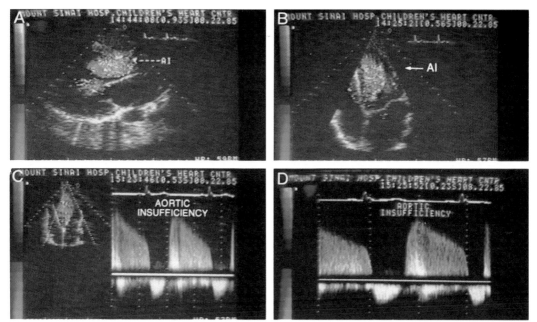

Figure B.4.

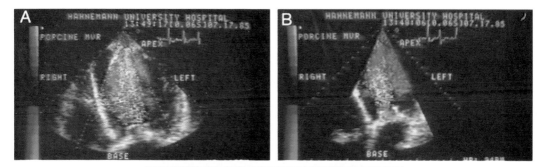

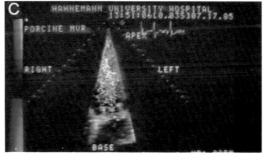

Figure B.5.

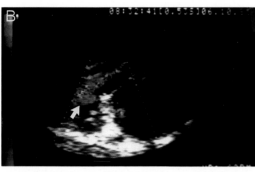

Figure C.15.

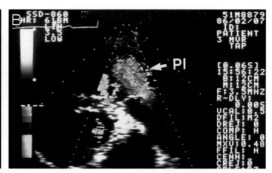

Figure C.18.

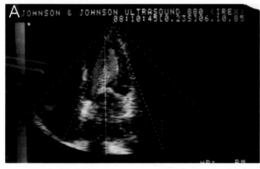

Figure C.22.

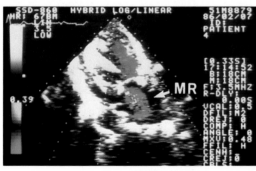

Figure C.31.

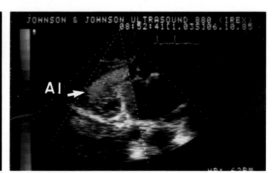

Figure C.32.

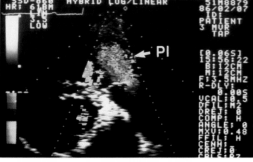

Figure C.33.

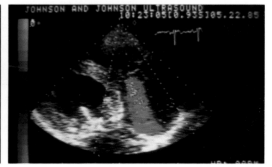

Figure C.34.

INDEX

Page numbers in *italics* denote figures.